Prepared for Eternity

A study of human embalming techniques in ancient Egypt using computerised tomography scans of mummies

Robert Loynes

Archaeopress Egyptology 9

Archaeopress Publishing Ltd
Gordon House
276 Banbury Road
Oxford OX2 7ED

www.archaeopress.com

ISBN 978 1 78491 110 2
ISBN 978 1 78491 111 9 (e-Pdf)

© Archaeopress and R Loynes 2015

Printed and bound in Great Britain by
Marston Book Services Ltd, Oxfordshire

All rights reserved. No part of this book may be reproduced, stored in retrieval system,
or transmitted, in any form or by any means, electronic, mechanical, photocopying or otherwise,
without the prior written permission of the copyright owners.

This book is available direct from Archaeopress or from our website www.archaeopress.com

Contents

List of Figures v

List of Tables xiii

Acknowledgements xvii

Terminology xix

Chronology xix

Chapter One: Introduction 1
    1.1 Mummification – The afterlife 1
        1.1.1 Religious beliefs and the afterlife 1
        1.1.2 Historical References to Mummification in Ancient Egypt 1
    1.2 Mummification – Types and Pathology 2
        1.2.1 Classification of mummies 2
        1.2.2 Experimental mummification 3
        1.2.3 Ancient Egyptian Knowledge of Anatomy 3
    1.3 The journey – From death to museum 4
        1.3.1 In Egypt 4
        1.3.2 In Continental Europe 4
        1.3.3 In Museums 4
    1.4 Research Disciplines in Mummy Studies 5
        1.4.1 Nineteenth and twentieth centuries 5
        1.4.2 Twenty first century 5
    1.5 Medical Imaging 5
        1.5.1 History and development 5
        1.5.2 Other Imaging Methods 6
        1.5.3 Current use of radiography in mummy studies 7
    1.6 Aims and Objectives 8
        1.6.1 Current Literature 8

Chapter Two: Methods 9
    2.1 Source of Materials 9
        2.1.1 Location of material 9
        2.1.2 Formats of Material 11
        2.1.3 Dicom readers 11
    2.2 Constraints 11
        2.2.1 Intellectual Property Considerations 11
        2.2.2 Technical Constraints 11
        2.2.3 Provenance 12
    2.3 Age at death 13
    2.4 Estimation of sex 13
    2.5 Palaeopathology 13
    2.6 Individual Reports 13
        2.6.1 Principle of Reports 13

Chapter Three: Results – General 25
    3.1 Comparison of Xrays, Older CT scans and Modern CT scans (digital format) 25
        3.1.1 X-ray of Exeter Mummy (Shepenmut – Cat. No. 11/3) 25
        3.1.2 Older Generation CT scans of Nesitanebetasheru and Djedma'atiuesankh in Sheffield Museum: 25
    3.2 Distribution of the mummies 30
    3.3 Analyses of various factors 32
        3.3.1 Topics to be considered 32

Chapter Four: Results – The Head 33
    4.1 Excerebration 33
        4.1.1 Trans-nasal route 34
            4.1.1.2 Ethmoid and sphenoid perforation 49

    4.1.1.3 Sphenoid only perforation.. 53
    4.1.1.4 Trans-nasal/orbital perforation.. 57
  4.1.2 Trans-foraminal route 58
  4.1.3 Trans-basal route.. 62
  4.1.4 Trans-orbital route 63
  4.1.5 No excerebration.. 64
 4.2 Treatment of the eyes 66
  4.2.1 Removal.. 66
  4.2.2 Desiccation 67
  4.2.3 Packing 69
  4.2.4 Eye Plates – 'False Eyes'... 73
 4.3 Treatment of the mouth 77
  4.3.1 Empty mouth 77
  4.3.2 Linen packing 77
  4.3.3 Linen plus resin 79
  4.3.4 Linen plus 'granular material' – possibly clay 80
  4.3.5 Granular material alone (possibly clay).. 81
  4.3.6 Resin alone 81
  4.3.7 A metal plate over the tongue (possibly gold) 82
 4.4 Treatment of the ears.. 83

Chapter Five: Results – The Trunk 84
 5.1 Introduction 84
 5.2 Grouping.. 84
  5.2.1 Abdominal incision... 84
  5.2.2 Perineal Approach... 150
  5.2.3 No evidence of incision or evisceration 156
  5.2.4 Evisceration. The extent of visceral clearance 172
    5.2.4.1 Thorax 172
    5.2.4.2 Abdomen 172
    5.2.4.3 Pelvic cavity... 172
    5.2.4.4 Evisceration of the thorax 172
    5.2.4.5 Evisceration of the abdomen.. 174
    5.2.4.6 Evisceration of the pelvic cavity.. 176
  5.2.5 The use of canopic packages 179
  5.2.6 Materials inserted into the body cavity after evisceration.. 180

Chapter Six: Results - Treatment of the skin, subcutaneous tissues and position of the arms 184
 6.1 The use of resin externally 184
 6.2 Subcutaneous packing 184
 6.3 Amulets... 185
 6.4 Position of the arms.. 185

Chapter Seven: Results related to Demographics and Palaeopathology 189
 7.1 Age at Death 189
  7.1.1 Results 189
 7.2 Sex 191
  7.2.1 Results 191
 7.3 Palaeopathology 192
  7.3.1 Results – Causes of death 193
  7.3.2 Results – Non-Fatal Pathologies... 196

Chapter Eight: Discussion of mummification techniques related to era, geographic location and age at death 197
 8.1 Introduction 197
 8.2 Patterns of mummification related to era 197
  8.2.1 Middle Kingdom... 199
  8.2.2 Dynasty 18.. 199
  8.2.3 Dynasty 19.. 200
  8.2.4 Dynasty 20.. 200
  8.2.5 Dynasty 21.. 200
  8.2.6 Dynasty 22.. 200
    8.2.6.1 Treatment of the Head and Neck 201

        8.2.6.2 Treatment of the Trunk 201
    8.2.7 Dynasty 25 201
        8.2.7.1 Treatment of the Head and Neck 202
        8.2.7.2 Treatment of the Trunk 203
    8.2.8 Mummies assigned to the 'Third Intermediate Period' (Dynasty 21-25) 203
        8.2.8.1 Treatment of the Head and Neck 203
        8.2.8.2 Treatment of the Trunk 203
    8.2.9 Dynasty 26 203
        8.2.9.1 Treatment of the Head and Neck 204
        8.2.9.2 Treatment of the Trunk 204
    8.2.10 Ptolemaic Period 204
        8.2.10.1 Treatment of the Head and Neck 204
        8.2.10.2 Treatment of the Trunk 205
    8.2.11 Roman Period 206
        8.2.11.1 Treatment of the Head and Neck 206
        8.2.11.2 Treatment of the Trunk 207
  8.3 Analysis of Specific Mummies 208
    8.3.1 Mummy XXV – TjesMoutPert 208
    8.3.2 Mummy LI – Khary 208
  8.4 Patterns of mummification related to location 209
    8.4.1 The Fayum and Hawara 211
    8.4.2 Gurob 211
    8.4.3 El-Hibe 211
    8.4.4 Assiut 212
    8.4.5 Akhmim 212
    8.4.6 Thebes 213
        8.4.6.1 Thebes in Dynasties 21-24 – the delta capitals 213
        8.4.6.2 Thebes in Dynasty 25 – Kushite rule 214
        8.4.6.3 Thebes in Dynasty 26 215
        8.4.6.4 Thebes in the Roman Period 216
    8.4.7 Deir El Bahari 216
  8.5 Techniques related to age at death 217

Chapter Nine: Discussion of specific mummification techniques 225
  9.1 Introduction 225
  9.2 Variations in the trans-nasal route of excerebration 225
  9.3 No excerebration 227
  9.4 More unusual routes used for excerebration 227
    9.4.1 Trans-basal route 227
    9.4.2 Trans-orbital route 228
  9.5 Treament of the eyes 228
  9.6 Use of the perineal route for evisceration 230
  9.7 Techniques used in the Roman Period 231
    9.7.1 Thoracic disruption 231
    9.7.2 Lack of an evisceration route 233
    9.7.3 Pelvic disruption 233
  9.8 Stiffeners within the wrappings and mummies. 234
    9.8.1 Stiffeners within the wrappings 234
    9.8.2 Stiffeners within the body 236
  9.9 The effect of foreign rule in various eras 237
    9.9.1 Introduction 237
    9.9.2 New Kingdom to Third Intermediate Period 237
    9.9.3 Dynasty 25 237
    9.9.4 The Late Period 238
    9.9.5 The Ptolemaic Period 238
    9.9.6 The Roman Period 238
  9.10 Practicalities from a surgeon's aspect 238

Chapter Ten: Conclusions 239
  10.1 Introduction 239
  10.2 The head 239

    10.3 The body 242
    10.4 Caveats 243
    10.5 The Future 244

Bibliography 245

Appendix I: Museums and other institutions contacted 248

List of Figures

Fig. 1.1 The Body Planes. 6
Fig. 2.1 External appearance of Graeco-Roman Mummy – BMAG...14
Fig. 2.2 3D reconstruction of skull showing the teeth in Graeco-Roman mummy 15
Fig. 2.3 Axial view of male genitalia in Graeco-Roman mummy..15
Fig. 2.4 Coronal view of skull - cribriform plate perforation 15
Fig. 2.5 Sagittal view of skull showing brain remnants in posterior fossa.....................................15
Fig. 2.6 Axial view of skull showing ocular remnants 15
Fig. 2.7 Coronal view of skull base showing foreign body...16
Fig. 2.8 Sagittal view of skull base showing foreign body. 16
Fig. 2.9 Coronal view of skull base showing multiple foreign bodies 16
Fig. 2.10 Axial view of skull base showing multiple foreign bodies 17
Fig. 2.11 Axial view of mid thoracic region - costo-vertebral dislocation 17
Fig. 2.12 Axial view of mid thoracic region - costo-vertebral dislocation 18
Fig. 2.13 Axial view of thorax showing asymmetry with anterior padding on left..........................18
Fig. 2.14 Coronal view of thorax showing chest asymmetry with anterior padding on left 19
Fig. 2.15 Axial view of thorax showing thoracic contents..19
Fig. 2.16 Axial view of abdomen - left flank incision...20
Fig. 2.17 Axial view of pelvis - sacro-iliac joint disruption 20
Fig. 2.18 Coronal view of pelvis - pubic symphysis disruption 21
Fig. 2.19 Coronal view of pelvis - bilateral hip dislocation..21
Fig. 2.20 Coronal view of pelvis - bilateral hip dislocation..21
Fig. 2.21 Axial view of pelvis - incision anterior to left hip 22
Fig. 2.22 Axial view of pelvis - incision anterior to right hip 22
Fig. 2.23 Axial view demonstrating detail of right wrist..22
Fig. 2.24 Coronal view illustrating detail of anterior wrappings 23
Fig. 2.25 Coronal view illustrating terracotta studs 23
Fig. 2.26 Murphy's skid 24
Fig. 2.27 Possible method of dislocation. Stage 1..24
Fig. 2.28 Possible method of dislocation. Stage 2..24
Fig. 3.1 Axial view of skull showing resin levels 26
Fig. 3.2 Axial view at level of mandible showing ear ring..26
Fig. 3.3 Axial view showing thoracic packing...26
Fig. 3.4 Axial view - symmetry of thoracic wall and exterior packing. 27
Fig. 3.5 Coronal view of thorax - possible canopic packages 27
Fig. 3.6 Axial view of pelvis - ischial tuberosity epiphyses...28
Fig. 3.7 Axial view of skull demonstrating perforation of the cribriform plate 28
Fig. 3.8 Axial view of skull showing brain material in posterior cranial cavity. 28
Fig. 3.9 Axial view of thorax showing the mediastinum. 29
Fig. 3.10 Axial view of the abdomen showing packing. 29
Fig. 3.11 Axial view of pelvis and contents. 29
Fig. 3.12 Axial view of thorax - radio-opaque objects anteriorly. 30
Fig. 4.1 Diagram of skull – the foramina in base of skull..33
Fig. 4.2 Diagram of inferior surface of the brain - the cranial nerves 33
Fig. 4.3 Sagittal view of skull - excerebration in Middle Kingdom Mummy XXVIII 34
Fig. 4.4 Coronal view of a 'false mummy'. 34
Fig. 4.5 Coronal view of skull illustrating cribriform plate perforation 35
Fig. 4.6 Sagittal view of skull - brain remnants in posterior fossa 35
Fig. 4.7 Axial view of skull illustrating limited damage to nasal structures..................................36
Fig. 4.8 Axial view of skull showing perforation of the cribriform plate 36
Fig. 4.9 Axial view of skull - brain material in posterior cranial cavity. 36
Fig. 4.10 Axial view of skull - retained meninges and empty cranial cavity. 37
Fig. 4.11 Sagittal view of skull - limited perforation of ethmoid and cribriform plate...................37
Fig. 4.12 Axial view of skull illustrating excerebration and loose linen packing.............................37
Fig. 4.13 Sagittal view of skull - excerebration and loose packing. 37
Fig. 4.14 Sagittal view of skull showing excerebration..38
Fig. 4.15 Sagittal view of skull - excerebration and packing..38
Fig. 4.16 Axial view of skull - perforation of cribriform plate..38
Fig. 4.17 3D reconstruction showing perforation of cribriform plate from the intra-cranial surface. 39
Fig. 4.18 Coronal view of skull - perforation of cribriform plate...39
Fig. 4.19 Sagittal view of skull - excerebration and packing..39
Fig. 4.20 Coronal view of skull - resin in maxillary sinuses. 39
Fig. 4.21 Sagittal view of skull - cribriform plate perforation..40
Fig. 4.22 Sagittal view of skull showing the large defect in the cribriform plate. 40
Fig. 4.23 Axial view of skull - perforation of cribriform plate and resin in the posterior cranial fossa. 40
Fig. 4.24 Sagittal view of skull - perforation of cribriform plate and resin in the posterior cranial fossa. 41
Fig. 4.25 Sagittal view of skull - cribriform plate perforation, packing and atlanto-occipital disruption. 41
Fig. 4.26 Sagittal views of skull showing bone and tooth within intra-cranial packing...................41

Fig. 4.27	Axial view of skull - debris in posterior cranial fossa.	42
Fig. 4.28	Axial view of skull - perforation of the cribriform plate.	42
Fig. 4.29	Axial view of skull - trans-nasal excerebration.	42
Fig. 4.30	Coronal view of skull - trans-nasal excerebration.	42
Fig. 4.31	Axial view of skull showing meningeal remnants.	43
Fig. 4.32	Sagittal view of skull demonstrating linen in nose and cranial cavity.	43
Fig. 4.33	Axial view of skull - excerebration via right nostril.	43
Fig. 4.34	Axial view of skull - resin with contained air.	43
Fig. 4.35	Axial view of skull - excerebration and packing.	44
Fig. 4.36	Sagittal view of skull demonstrating trans-nasal excerebration.	44
Fig. 4.37	Small coronal section of skull showing cribriform plate perforation.	44
Fig. 4.38	Axial view of skull showing cribriform plate perforation.	44
Fig. 4.39	Sagittal view of skull showing empty cranial cavity.	44
Fig. 4.40	Axial view of skull illustrating trans-nasal excerebration.	45
Fig. 4.41	Coronal view of skull - perforation of cribriform plate.	45
Fig. 4.42	Sagittal view of skull - cracked resin in posterior cranial fossa.	45
Fig. 4.43	Sagittal view of skull - perforation of ethmoid with intact sphenoid.	45
Fig. 4.44	Coronal view of skull showing limited perforation of cribriform plate.	46
Fig. 4.45	Sagittal view of skull - posterior ethmoid perforation and resin levels.	46
Fig. 4.46	Axial view of skull - meninges and resin levels.	46
Fig. 4.47	Sagittal view of skull - nasal tampons.	46
Fig. 4.48	Axial view of skull - nasal tampons and resin 'levels'.	46
Fig. 4.49	Sagittal view of skull showing excerebration route via ethmoid air sinuses.	47
Fig. 4.50	Sagittal view of skull - excerebration route and resin.	47
Fig. 4.51	Sagittal view of skull demonstrating cribriform plate perforation.	47
Fig. 4.52	Coronal view of skull showing cribriform plate perforation.	47
Fig. 4.53	Sagittal view of skull - fragment of cribriform plate in posterior cranial fossa.	48
Fig. 4.54	Coronal view of skull - ethmoid perforation.	48
Fig. 4.55	Sagittal view of skull - ethmoid perforation.	48
Fig. 4.56	Sagittal view of skull - meninges and brain tissue.	48
Fig. 4.57	Sagittal view of skull - cribriform perforation, resin and nasal tampon.	49
Fig. 4.58	Axial view of skull - ethmoid sinus and cribriform plate perforation.	49
Fig. 4.59	Axial view of skull - resin levels	49
Fig. 4.60	Sagittal view of skull - excerebration and resin	50
Fig. 4.61	Axial view of skull showing route of excerebration	50
Fig. 4.62	Sagittal view of skull - excerebration and resin	50
Fig. 4.63	Axial view of skull demonstrating resin	50
Fig. 4.64	Sagittal view of skull demonstrating two materials in resin packing	51
Fig. 4.65	Sagittal view of skull showing nasal tampon, ethmoid perforation and resin.	51
Fig. 4.66	Sagittal view of skull showing movement of the resin	51
Fig. 4.67	Coronal view of skull - ethmoid perforation	51
Fig. 4.68	Coronal view of skull - nasal tampon	51
Fig. 4.69	Axial view of skull - ethmoid perforation	52
Fig. 4.70	Sagittal view of skull - cribriform plate perforation	52
Fig. 4.71	Coronal view of skull - cribriform plate perforation	52
Fig. 4.72	Sagittal view of skull demonstrating the excerebration route	52
Fig. 4.73	Coronal view of skull demonstrating the excerebration route	53
Fig. 4.74	Coronal view of skull demonstrating the excerebration route	53
Fig. 4.75	Sagittal view of skull - excerebration route and resin.	53
Fig. 4.76	Axial view of skull - debris in posterior cranial fossa	54
Fig. 4.77	Axial view of skull - sphenoid perforation	54
Fig. 4.78	Sagittal view of skull - sphenoid perforation	54
Fig. 4.79	Axial view of skull - sphenoid perforation	55
Fig. 4.80	Sagittal view of skull - sphenoid perforation and linen packing	55
Fig. 4.81	Axial view of skull demonstrating linen packing	55
Fig. 4.82	Sagittal view of skull - foreign material in posterior cranial fossa	55
Fig. 4.83	Sagittal view of skull - route of cranial perforation	56
Fig. 4.84	Coronal view of skull - route of cranial perforation	56
Fig. 4.85	Sagittal view of skull showing the excerebration route	56
Fig. 4.86	Coronal view of skull - excerebration route in one plane	57
Fig. 4.87	Coronal view of skull - excerebration route in second parallel plane	57
Fig. 4.88	Coronal view of skull - excerebration route in third parallel plane	57
Fig. 4.89	Axial view of skull - excerebration route	57
Fig. 4.90	Sagittal view of skull - trans-nasal/orbital route of excerebration	58
Fig. 4.91	Coronal view of skull - trans-nasal/orbital route	58
Fig. 4.92	Axial view of skull - trans-nasal/orbital route	58
Fig. 4.93	Axial view of skull - granular material	58
Fig. 4.94	Axial view of skull - teeth in granular material	59
Fig. 4.95	Axial view of skull base - enlarged foramen magnum	59
Fig. 4.96	Axial view inferior to base of skull - anteriorly displaced atlas	59
Fig. 4.97	Sagittal view of skull demonstrating trans-foraminal route	60

Figure	Description	Page
Fig. 4.98	Axial view of skull showing cervical spine displacement	60
Fig. 4.99	Axial view close to skull base showing foramen magnum alignment	60
Fig. 4.100	Axial view close to skull base showing foramen magnum and atlas alignment	60
Fig. 4.101	Coronal view of skull demonstrating meninges	61
Fig. 4.102	Coronal view of cervical spine showing malalignment	61
Fig. 4.103	Sagittal view of skull showing a possible trans-foraminal route	61
Fig. 4.104	Sagittal view of skull in a mummy where the trans-basal route was used with an intact cribriform plate and a small amount of cerebral tissue in the posterior cranial fossa	62
Fig. 4.105	Coronal view of skull showing the trans-basal route with an intact cribriform plate	62
Fig. 4.106	Sagittal view of skull - trans-basal route	62
Fig. 4.107	Axial view of skull - trans-basal route	63
Fig. 4.108	Sagittal view of skull - foreign material in posterior fossa	63
Fig. 4.109	Sagittal view of skull - trans-orbital route	63
Fig. 4.110	Coronal view of skull showing distorted eyes in trans-orbital route	63
Fig. 4.111	Coronal view of skull - intact cribriform plate	64
Fig. 4.112	Sagittal view of skull - cerebral material in posterior cranial cavity	64
Fig. 4.113	Sagittal view of skull with intact cribriform plate and retained brain.	64
Fig. 4.114	Sagittal view of skull with intact cribriform plate and retained brain	64
Fig. 4.115	Sagittal view of skull with intact cribriform plate and retained brain	65
Fig. 4.116	Sagittal view of skull with intact cribriform plate and retained brain	65
Fig. 4.117	Sagittal view of skull with intact cribriform plate	65
Fig. 4.118	Sagittal view of skull with brain in posterior cranial fossa	65
Fig. 4.119	Sagittal view of skull with eye replaced by resin-soaked linen	66
Fig. 4.120	Axial view of skull - linen rolls in orbits and eye plates anteriorly	67
Fig. 4.121	Coronal view of skull with linen rolls in orbits	67
Fig. 4.122	Axial view of skull - desiccation of left eye and loss of right eye.	68
Fig. 4.123	Axial view of skull - remnants of the globes and muscles, but empty globes	68
Fig. 4.124	Axial view of skull with large remaining cavity in eyeball in Mummy XLV	68
Fig. 4.125	Axial view of skull. Small anterior compartment	69
Fig. 4.126	Sagittal view of orbit - linen packing within the globe of the eye	69
Fig. 4.127	Coronal view of skull - eyes tightly packed with linen	69
Fig. 4.128	Sagittal view of orbit demonstrating outer layer of the eye (sclera and cornea)	70
Fig. 4.129	External appearance of the damaged left eye	70
Fig. 4.130	Coronal view of skull - loosely packed eyes	71
Fig. 4.131	Sagittal view of orbit with small amount of packing through anterior wall of globe	71
Fig. 4.132	Coronal view of skull showing both packed eyes	71
Fig. 4.133	Sagittal view of skull - linen packing of right eye	71
Fig. 4.134	Sagittal view of skull - resin soaked linen packing of left eye	71
Fig. 4.135	Axial view of skull - eyes packed from anterior incisions	72
Fig. 4.136	Sagittal view of orbit - eyes packed from anterior incisions	72
Fig. 4.137	Axial view of skull - tight packing of linen into globes	72
Fig. 4.138	Coronal view of orbits showing tight packing of linen into globes	72
Fig. 4.139	Axial view of skull - packed eyes. More resin in the linen on the right than the left	73
Fig. 4.140	Axial view of skull showing packed eyes and eye plate over right eye	73
Fig. 4.141	Sagittal view of orbit - packed eye with eye plate	73
Fig. 4.142	3D reconstruction showing eye plates	74
Fig. 4.143	3D reconstruction showing eye plates	74
Fig. 4.144	Axial view of orbits showing detail of the embalming process of the eyes	75
Fig. 4.145	Sagittal view of orbits showing detail of the embalming process of the eyes	75
Fig. 4.146	Eye plates in 3D image	75
Fig. 4.147	Axial view of skull - eye plates – arrows	76
Fig. 4.148	Axial view of skull - eye plates and packed eyes	76
Fig. 4.149	Coronal view of skull demonstrating packed eyes	76
Fig. 4.150	3D reconstruction showing eye plates	76
Fig. 4.151	Sagittal view of orbits - embalming method for eyes	76
Fig. 4.152	Sagittal view of skull showing empty mouth with desiccated tongue	77
Fig. 4.153	Sagittal view of pharynx - loose linen packing within the mouth.	78
Fig. 4.154	Sagittal view of the skull - loose linen packing within the mouth.	78
Fig. 4.155	Sagittal view of skull - loose linen packing within the mouth.	78
Fig. 4.156	Sagittal view of skull - tight linen packing within the mouth in Mummy XXXI	78
Fig. 4.157	Coronal view of skull - tight linen packing within the mouth in Mummy XXXI. Also shown is the linen within the cheeks.	79
Fig. 4.158	Sagittal view of skull - tight linen packing in the mouth – Mummy XLV	79
Fig. 4.159	Sagittal view of skull showing the use of resin and linen in the mouth	80
Fig. 4.160	Axial view of skull demonstrating the use of both linen and 'granular' material	80
Fig. 4.161	Sagittal view of skull - use of both linen and 'granular' material	80
Fig. 4.162	Sagittal view of pharynx - packing in mouth and neck	81
Fig. 4.163	Sagittal view of pharynx – excess amorphous material in the mouth causing the teeth to be forced apart.	81
Fig. 4.164	Sagittal view of skull - resin in the mouth and packing in the neck	82
Fig. 4.165	Axial view at level of mandible - resin packing within the mouth.	82
Fig. 4.166	Coronal view of skull - metal plate over the tongue (possibly Gold)	82
Fig. 4.167	Sagittal view of skull - metal plate over the tongue (possibly Gold)	83

Fig. 4.168 3D reconstruction of metal plate lying over tongue..83
Fig. 5.1   Axial view of thorax showing costo-vertebral dislocation..85
Fig. 5.2   Axial view of thorax showing costo-vertebral dislocation..85
Fig. 5.3   Axial view of thorax - asymmetry with anterior padding on left..86
Fig. 5.4   Coronal view of thorax - asymmetry with anterior padding on left..86
Fig. 5.5   Axial view of thorax showing chest contents 87
Fig. 5.6   Axial view of lower abdomen - left flank incision 87
Fig. 5.7   Axial view of lower thorax - perforation in posterior wall..88
Fig. 5.8   Sagittal view of lower thorax - perforation in posterior wall..88
Fig. 5.9   Sagittal view of lower thorax – plug of material in perforation 88
Fig. 5.10   Coronal view of thorax showing remnants of pleura and mediastinum 88
Fig. 5.11   Axial view of lower abdomen - material hanging free from abdominal incision...89
Fig. 5.12   Sagittal view of abdomen - material in abdominal incision 89
Fig. 5.13   Axial view of thorax - fluid levels in 'resin'..89
Fig. 5.14   Coronal view of thorax - heart in mediastinum 90
Fig. 5.15   Axial view of thorax - heart in mediastinum 90
Fig. 5.16   Axial view of lower abdomen showing contents..90
Fig. 5.17   Axial view of thorax showing packing 91
Fig. 5.18   Axial view of thorax demonstrating asymmetrical chest wall and exterior packing...91
Fig. 5.19   Coronal view of thorax - probable canopic packages...92
Fig. 5.20   Axial view of thorax including the mediastinum..92
Fig. 5.21   Axial view of abdomen..92
Fig. 5.22   Axial view of pelvis showing contents..93
Fig. 5.23   Axial view of right shoulder - fractured acromion...93
Fig. 5.24   Axial view of right shoulder - scapular fractures 94
Fig. 5.25   Axial view of thorax showing viscera...94
Fig. 5.26   Axial view of pelvic organs 95
Fig. 5.27   Axial view of pelvis showing tubular structures and diastasis of symphysis pubis 95
Fig. 5.28   Sagittal view of trunk – compressed anterior thoracic wall 96
Fig. 5.29   Axial view of thorax - position of sternum 96
Fig. 5.30   Axial view of right lower thorax - organ containing vascular structures 97
Fig. 5.31   Axial view of lower thorax - tubular structures within resin 97
Fig. 5.32   Axial view of pelvis - constraining structures within pelvis 97
Fig. 5.33   Axial view of thorax - intra-thoracic viscera and 'loose' sternum 97
Fig. 5.34   Coronal view of trunk- remnants of diaphragm 98
Fig. 5.35   Sagittal view of abdomen showing intact abdominal wall 98
Fig. 5.36   Sagittal view of abdomen showing incision 98
Fig. 5.37   Sagittal view of thorax - mediastinum and diaphragm 99
Fig. 5.38   Sagittal view of trunk - canopic package 99
Fig. 5.39   Coronal view of trunk - canopic package 99
Fig. 5.40   Axial view of lower thorax - position of packages 100
Fig. 5.41   Axial view of lower thorax - position of packages - original image 100
Fig. 5.42   Coronal view of thorax – mediastinum 100
Fig. 5.43   3D reconstruction showing fractured left ribs 100
Fig. 5.44   Coronal view of abdomen - pack in abdominal incision 100
Fig. 5.45   Axial view inferior to pelvis - double structure of phallus 101
Fig. 5.46   More distal axial view inferior to pelvis – single structure of phallus 101
Fig. 5.47   Axial view of thorax...101
Fig. 5.48   Coronal view of torso..101
Fig. 5.49   Coronal view of upper thorax- rolls of material on the right 102
Fig. 5.50   Sagittal view of thorax - Sibson's fascia 102
Fig. 5.51   Axial view of thorax showing two layers of material...102
Fig. 5.52   Axial view of abdomen - extent of abdominal incision 102
Fig. 5.53   Sagittal view of pelvis showing structures 103
Fig. 5.54   Sagittal view of lower abdomen - fractured iliac crest 103
Fig. 5.55   Sagittal view showing thoracic structures 104
Fig. 5.56   Axial view lower thorax - mediastinum and posterior defect 104
Fig. 5.57   Coronal view thorax - great vessels, mediastinum and diaphragm..104
Fig. 5.58   Axial view of lower abdomen - abdominal incision...104
Fig. 5.59   Sagittal view of pelvis showing femoral head biopsy 105
Fig. 5.60   Coronal view of pelvis showing femoral head biopsy 105
Fig. 5.61 3D reconstruction - right fractured ribs – posterior view 106
Fig. 5.62   Sagittal view of trunk - returned viscera 106
Fig. 5.63   Coronal view of trunk - linen in abdominal incision 106
Fig. 5.64   Sagittal view of lower abdomen - visceral package...106
Fig. 5.65   Sagittal view of pelvis - perineal plug, resin and linen in abdomen 107
Fig. 5.66   Coronal view of trunk - canopic packages...107
Fig. 5.67   Coronal view of abdomen - solid organ – possibly liver...108
Fig. 5.68   Sagittal view of trunk - granular material and resin 108
Fig. 5.69   Coronal view of abdomen – left flank incision 108
Fig. 5.70   3D reconstruction showing disruption of rib cage – anterior aspect 109

Fig. 5.71	3D reconstruction showing disruption of rib cage – posterior aspect	109
Fig. 5.72	Coronal view of trunk - false breast in wrappings	109
Fig. 5.73	Coronal view of trunk - canopic packages	109
Fig. 5.74	Axial view of abdomen - left flank incision	110
Fig. 5.75	Sagittal view of pelvis - destroyed, featureless perineum	110
Fig. 5.76	Axial view of pelvis - disorganised sacro-iliac joints	111
Fig. 5.77	Coronal view of pelvis - dislocated symphysis pubis	111
Fig. 5.78	Axial view of pelvis - fractured inferior pubic ramus	111
Fig. 5.79	Axial view of pelvis - acetabular fractures	112
Fig. 5.80	Coronal view of thorax - empty apart from linen packs	112
Fig. 5.81	Coronal view of trunk - canopic packages in abdomen	112
Fig. 5.82	Sagittal view of lower abdomen - material in lower pelvis	112
Fig. 5.83	Axial view of thorax - mediastinum, heart and resin	113
Fig. 5.84	Axial view of lower thorax with returned viscera	113
Fig. 5.85	3D reconstruction of object possibly Wadjet eye	113
Fig. 5.86	Axial view lower abdomen – left flank incision and packing	113
Fig. 5.87	3D reconstruction at level of pelvis showing possible amulet	114
Fig. 5.88	3D reconstruction at level of pelvis showing possible amulet	114
Fig. 5.89	Coronal view of pelvis showing female shape of the pelvis	114
Fig. 5.90	Axial view of thorax showing contents	115
Fig. 5.91	3D reconstruction of heart scarab	115
Fig. 5.92	Axial view showing abdominal incision and amulet	115
Fig. 5.93	3D reconstruction of sistrum shaped amulet	115
Fig. 5.94	Coronal view of pelvis - canopic package	115
Fig. 5.95	Sagittal view of pelvis - perineum and false phallus	115
Fig. 5.96	3D reconstruction of false phallus and amulet	116
Fig. 5.97	Axial view of thorax and mediastinum	116
Fig. 5.98	Axial view of abdominal incision	116
Fig. 5.99	Axial view of thorax - mediastinum and resin	117
Fig. 5.100	Axial view of abdominal incision and canopic packages	117
Fig. 5.101	Axial view of pelvis – pubic symphysis	117
Fig. 5.102	Sagittal view of pelvis - left femoral head	117
Fig. 5.103	Sagittal view of pelvis - right femoral head	117
Fig. 5.104	Coronal view of pelvis - external genitalia and left femoral head	117
Fig. 5.105	Axial view of thorax - dislocated costo-vertebral joints	118
Fig. 5.106	Axial view of thorax - intact costo-vertebral joints	118
Fig. 5.107	3D reconstruction of compressed rib cage	119
Fig. 5.108	3D reconstruction of compressed rib cage	119
Fig. 5.109	Axial view of compressed thorax	119
Fig. 5.110	Axial view of lower abdomen showing folds in abdominal wall	119
Fig. 5.111	Axial view of pelvis - dislocated sacro-iliac joints (SIJ)	119
Fig. 5.112	Axial view of pelvis - dislocated symphysis pubis	120
Fig. 5.113	Sagittal view of pelvis - perineal structures	120
Fig. 5.114	Axial view of thorax - anterior thoracic wall damage	120
Fig. 5.115	Coronal view of trunk showing position of carpus	121
Fig. 5.116	Sagittal view of trunk showing position of carpus	121
Fig. 5.117	Axial view of lower thorax - canopic packages	122
Fig. 5.118	Sagittal view of trunk showing posterior penetration of resin	122
Fig. 5.119	Axial view of lower abdomen showing left flank incision	122
Fig. 5.120	Axial view of lower abdomen showing damage to anterior abdominal wall	122
Fig. 5.121	Coronal view of thorax – position of left 2nd rib	123
Fig. 5.122	Sagittal view of thorax – left 6th rib fracture	123
Fig. 5.123	Sagittal view of thorax – fractured right ribs	123
Fig. 5.124	Coronal view of trunk – contents of torso	123
Fig. 5.125	Axial view of lower abdomen – left flank incision	123
Fig. 5.126	Coronal view of pelvis – fractured right iliac bone	124
Fig. 5.127	Sagittal view of perineum	124
Fig. 5.128	Coronal view of trunk – fragments of ribs and sternum	124
Fig. 5.129	Axial view of thorax - rib fragments and resin casts	125
Fig. 5.130	Coronal view of thorax – vertebrae and resin casts	125
Fig. 5.131	Coronal view of thorax – indentations in the resin cast	125
Fig. 5.132	Axial view lower abdomen - shape of linen from abdominal incision	126
Fig. 5.133	Axial view of pelvis – dislocated SIJs	126
Fig. 5.134	Coronal view of pelvis - dislocated symphysis pubis	126
Fig. 5.135	Coronal view of pelvis and lower abdomen - canopic packages	126
Fig. 5.136	Coronal view of thorax – left 1st rib lying free	127
Fig. 5.137	Coronal view of sternum lying free within the thorax	127
Fig. 5.138	Axial view showing material within the thorax	127
Fig. 5.139	Coronal view of superior mediastinum	127
Fig. 5.140	Axial view of superior mediasinum	127
Fig. 5.141	Axial view of abdominal incision	128

Figure	Description	Page
Fig. 5.142	Sagittal view of trunk showing compressed abdomen	128
Fig. 5.143	Axial view of pelvis - subluxed right SIJ	128
Fig. 5.144	Axial view of thorax -remnants of viscera	129
Fig. 5.145	Coronal view of thorax showing diaphragms	129
Fig. 5.146	Axial view showing abdominal incision	130
Fig. 5.147	Coronal view of abdominal incision	130
Fig. 5.148	Coronal view showing material within abdomen	130
Fig. 5.149	Axial view showing material within abdomen	131
Fig. 5.150	Axial view of lower abdomen - viscera	131
Fig. 5.151	Sagittal view showing an organ within pelvis - possibly uterus	131
Fig. 5.152	Coronal view of trunk - fractured right ribs	132
Fig. 5.153	Coronal view of trunk - canopic packages	132
Fig. 5.154	Sagittal view of thorax - facetted objects – probably gallstones	132
Fig. 5.155	Coronal view of thorax - facetted objects – probably gallstones	132
Fig. 5.156	Axial view showing abdominal incision and incision plate	132
Fig. 5.157	Axial view of abdomen demonstrating material on posterior wall	133
Fig. 5.158	Axial view of pelvis - left hip joint articular cartilage	133
Fig. 5.159	Sagittal view showing pelvic contents and plate over perineum	133
Fig. 5.160	Axial view showing abdominal incision and contents	134
Fig. 5.161	Axial view of pelvis - acetabular fractures	134
Fig. 5.162	Axial view of pelvis - fractured inferior pubic rami	134
Fig. 5.163	Axial view of thorax - mediastinum and canopic packages	135
Fig. 5.164	Axial view showing abdominal incision	135
Fig. 5.165	Axial view of pelvis - disrupted left SIJ	135
Fig. 5.166	Axial view of pelvis - disrupted pubic symphysis	135
Fig. 5.167	Axial view inferior to pelvis - cross section of phallus	135
Fig. 5.168	Axial view of thorax - mediastinum	136
Fig. 5.169	Axial view of thorax - mediastinum and great vessels	136
Fig. 5.170	Axial view of thorax demonstrating diaphragm	136
Fig. 5.171	Axial view of lower thorax - probable canopic packages	136
Fig. 5.172	Coronal view of thorax - canopic packages and 'cuboid' structure	136
Fig. 5.173	Axial view of lower thorax - biopsy site in right rib posteriorly	137
Fig. 5.174	Sagittal view of pelvis - linen pack in perineum	137
Fig. 5.175	Coronal view of pelvis showing hip joints	137
Fig. 5.176	Coronal view of thorax - comparison of 1st ribs	137
Fig. 5.177	Sagittal view of thorax - posterior position of sternum	137
Fig. 5.178	Axial view of thorax - tissues and material on posterior wall	138
Fig. 5.179	Axial view - viscera and material in abdomen	138
Fig. 5.180	Coronal view of pelvis - disruption of symphysis pubis	138
Fig. 5.181	Coronal view of thorax - outline of right lung and dilated heart	139
Fig. 5.182	Sagittal view of thorax - defect in diaphragm	139
Fig. 5.183	Axial view showing viscera within the abdominal cavity	139
Fig. 5.184	Axial view of lower abdomen - lower abdominal wall defect (incision)	140
Fig. 5.185	Axial view of lower abdomen - lower abdominal wall defect (incision)	140
Fig. 5.186	Axial view of lower abdomen - lower abdominal wall defect (incision)	140
Fig. 5.187	3D reconstruction - lower abdominal wall defects	141
Fig. 5.188	Sagittal view of pelvis - perineal structures	141
Fig. 5.189	Axial view showing thoracic shape and packing	141
Fig. 5.190	Axial view of lower abdomen showing incision	141
Fig. 5.191	Axial view of thorax - mediastinum and lungs	142
Fig. 5.192	Coronal view of trunk - remnants of diaphragm	143
Fig. 5.193	Axial view of thorax demonstrating shape of rib cage	143
Fig. 5.194	Axial view showing abdominal wall incision	143
Fig. 5.195	Axial view - viscera on posterior pelvic wall	143
Fig. 5.196	Axial view of thorax - mediastinum	144
Fig. 5.197	Axial view of lower thorax - canopic packages	144
Fig. 5.198	Coronal view of trunk - canopic packages in abdomen	145
Fig. 5.199	Axial view of abdomen - metal plate covering incision	145
Fig. 5.200	3D reconstruction of incision plate	145
Fig. 5.201	Sagittal view of pelvis - canopic package at brim of pelvis	145
Fig. 5.202	Sagittal view of pelvis - perineal structures and material in pelvis	145
Fig. 5.203	Axial view showing loose packing in thorax	146
Fig. 5.204	Axial view of thorax - resin over anterior surface of vertebrae	146
Fig. 5.205	Coronal view of trunk - fragmented resin	147
Fig. 5.206	Axial view showing abdominal incision	147
Fig. 5.207	Coronal view of abdomen - canopic packages	147
Fig. 5.208	Sagittal view of pelvis - fragments of resin in pelvis	147
Fig. 5.209	Sagittal and coronal views of pelvis - perineal floor	147
Fig. 5.210	Axial view of thorax demonstrating shape and contents	148
Fig. 5.211	Axial view showing abdominal incision	148
Fig. 5.212	Coronal view of abdomen - canopic packages	148

Fig. 5.213	Coronal view of pelvis - canopic package within the pelvis	148
Fig. 5.214	Sagittal view of pelvis - coccyx and pelvic floor	149
Fig. 5.215	Sagittal view of pelvis - symphysis pubis and false phallus	149
Fig. 5.216	3D reconstruction demonstrating false phallus	149
Fig. 5.217	Oblique axial view of pelvis - false phallus	149
Fig. 5.218	Oblique sagittal view of pelvis - false phallus	150
Fig. 5.219	Axial view of upper thorax - costo-vertebral dislocation and rib fracture	150
Fig. 5.220	Coronal view of trunk - mediastinal structures and Ibis	151
Fig. 5.221	Axial view showing structures in thorax	151
Fig. 5.222	Coronal view - granular material within pelvis	151
Fig. 5.223	Axial view of abdomen - Ibis	151
Fig. 5.224	Sagittal view of abdomen - Ibis	151
Fig. 5.225	Axial view of pelvis - acetabular fractures	151
Fig. 5.226	Axial view of upper thorax - great vessels	152
Fig. 5.227	Axial view of thorax - heart and right lung	152
Fig. 5.228	Axial view of lower thorax - remains of diaphragm	152
Fig. 5.229	Axial view of lower abdomen - tissues in paraspinal gutters	152
Fig. 5.230	Axial view of pelvis - healed fracture of right pubic ramus	152
Fig. 5.231	Axial view of pelvis - pack in upper perineum	153
Fig. 5.232	Axial view of pelvis - pack in lower perineum	153
Fig. 5.233	Axial view of thorax - imbricated ribs	153
Fig. 5.234	Sagittal view of trunk - antero-posteriorly compressed thorax	154
Fig. 5.235	Coronal view of trunk - asymmetry of thorax	154
Fig. 5.236	Axial view of thorax - tissue on posterior wall	154
Fig. 5.237	Axial view of pelvis - sacro-iliac joint (SIJ) disruption	155
Fig. 5.238	Axial view of pelvis - dislocation of symphysis pubis	155
Fig. 5.239	Axial view of pelvis - superior pubic ramus fracture	155
Fig. 5.240	Axial view of pelvis - inferior pubic ramus fracture	155
Fig. 5.241	Axial view of pelvis - ischial fracture	156
Fig. 5.242	Sagittal view of pelvis - perineal pad	156
Fig. 5.243	Axial view of thorax - viscera in thoracic cavity	157
Fig. 5.244	Sagittal view of thorax - depressed and distorted sternum	157
Fig. 5.245	Sagittal view of abdomen - extruded lumbar vertebrae	157
Fig. 5.246	Axial view of pelvis - bladder and rectum	157
Fig. 5.247	Axial view - thoracic wall compression and thoracic visceral contents	158
Fig. 5.248	Coronal view of abdomen - atlas within abdominal wrappings	158
Fig. 5.249	Coronal view of trunk - spinal curvature - scoliosis	159
Fig. 5.250	Coronal view of trunk - disrupted ribs	159
Fig. 5.251	Axial view of thorax - viscera in thoracic cavity	159
Fig. 5.252	Axial view of pelvis - metal plate over genitalia	160
Fig. 5.253	Coronal view of trunk - metal plate over genitalia	160
Fig. 5.254	Axial view of thorax - costo-vertebral joints	160
Fig. 5.255	Axial view of thorax - viscera overlying thoracic vertebral body	161
Fig. 5.256	Axial view of abdomen - viscera in abdomen	161
Fig. 5.257	Sagittal view of trunk - compression of abdominal wall against the spine	161
Fig. 5.258	Sagittal view showing viscera within pelvic cavity	161
Fig. 5.259	Coronal view showing intra-thoracic structures	162
Fig. 5.260	Axial view of abdomen - compression of abdomen and contained structures	162
Fig. 5.261	Coronal view of trunk - liver and calcified node	163
Fig. 5.262	Coronal view of pelvis - hip joints	163
Fig. 5.263	Sagittal view showing pelvic viscera	163
Fig. 5.264	Axial view demonstrating intra-thoracic contents	164
Fig. 4.265	Sagittal view showing intra-thoracic contents	164
Fig. 5.266	Axial view of lower abdomen - viscera on posterior abdominal wall	164
Fig. 5.267	Axial view of pelvis - slight disruption of the bony pelvis	165
Fig. 5.268	Coronal view of hip joints	165
Fig. 5.269	Sagittal view of pelvic contents	165
Fig. 5.270	Axial view of thorax - slight asymmetry of thoracic wall	166
Fig. 5.271	Axial view of thorax - mediastinum	166
Fig. 5.272	Axial view showing abdominal compression and viscera	166
Fig. 5.273	Axial view of sacro-iliac joints	166
Fig. 5.274	Sagittal view of thorax showing compression	167
Fig. 5.275	Coronal view of disrupted ribs and spine	167
Fig. 5.276	Axial view of compressed thorax and contents	167
Fig. 5.277	Axial view of compressed abdomen and contained viscera	168
Fig. 5.278	Axial and sagittal views of pack in rectum	168
Fig. 5.279	Axial view showing asymmetry of rib cage	169
Fig. 5.280	Axial view of thorax - costo-vertebral joints	169
Fig. 5.281	Axial view of thorax - mediastinum – great vessels	169
Fig. 5.282	Sagittal view of thorax - mediastinum - heart	170
Fig. 5.283	Coronal view of thorax - mediastinum - heart	170

Fig. 5.284	Coronal view of trunk and axial view of thorax - diaphragm and liver	170
Fig. 5.285	Axial view of pelvis - disrupted SIJ	170
Fig. 5.286	Coronal view of pelvis - disrupted symphysis pubis and fractured acetabulum	170
Fig. 5.287	Coronal view of congruous hip joints	171
Fig. 5.288	Axial view of thorax - sternum lying against vertebral bodies	171
Fig. 5.289	Axial view of thorax - viscera lying over vertebral bodies	171
Fig. 5.290	Axial view of thorax - costo-vertebral dislocation	171
Fig. 5.291	Axial view of thorax - crowded ribs	172
Fig. 5.292	The anatomy of the thorax and mediastinum	173
Fig. 5.293	Coronal view of trunk - liver and canopic packages	175
Fig. 5.294	Axial view of lower abdomen - residual visceral tissue	175
Fig. 5.295	Axial view of abdomen - residual visceral tissue	176
Fig. 5.296	Coronal view of trunk - viscera returned after desiccation	176
Fig. 5.297	Coronal view of trunk - returned viscera and a canopic package	176
Fig. 5.298	Axial view of abdomen - canopic packages and retained viscera	177
Fig. 5.299	Coronal view of trunk - loose viscera and canopic package	177
Fig. 5.300	Sagittal view of trunk - canopic packages in a mummy with only a perineal approach	179
Fig. 5.301	Coronal view of trunk - canopic package – True or False?	179
Fig. 5.302	Coronal view of trunk - canopic package – True or False?	180
Fig. 5.303	Axial view of abdomen - an example of total filling of the body cavity with 'material' ('clay/mud')	181
Fig. 5.304	Axial view of abdomen - an example of a large amount of filling material	181
Fig. 5.305	Axial view of thorax - an example of a small amount of 'material' ('Resin')	182
Fig. 6.1	Axial view of cervical region - subcutaneous packing	184
Fig. 6.2	Sagittal view of cervical region - granular packing (Mummy XXXIII)	184
Fig. 6.3	Sagittal view of cervical region - linen packing (Mummy VIII)	185
Fig. 6.4	3D reconstruction showing arms flexed and across chest	185
Fig. 6.5	Arms extended and lateral to the thighs	185
Fig. 6.6	Arms extended and over upper thighs/hips	186
Fig. 7.1	Sagittal view of trunk - collapse of the first lumbar vertebra	194
Fig. 7.2	Sagittal view of abdomen - fourth lumbar vertebra pathology	194
Fig. 7.3	Coronal view of fourth lumbar vertebra pathology	194
Fig. 7.4	Sagittal view of fourth lumbar vertebra pathology	194
Fig. 7.5	Sagittal view of thoraco-lumbar junction - collapsed vertebrae	195
Fig. 7.6	3D reconstruction of facial fractures	195
Fig. 7.7	3D reconstruction of fractured right occiput	195
Fig. 7.8	3D reconstruction of fractured left angle of mandible and left humeral neck	195
Fig. 7.9	Sagittal view of infected cervical spine.	196
Fig. 8.1	Axial view of rope and reeds at one end of the mat 'coffin'	199
Fig. 8.2	The nasal profile of Mummy LI – Khary compared with Ramesses II	209
Fig. 8.3	Location of places of origin of mummies	209
Fig. 9.1	Sagittal view of skull - line drawn in the mid line from upper front teeth to posterior edge of hard palate	228
Fig. 9.2	Sagittal view of skull - parallel line to that in Fig. 9.1, shown on CT 'slice' showing trans-basal perforation	228
Fig. 9.3	Sagittal view of skull - mouth packing	228
Fig. 9.4	Sagittal view of the perineum with arrow showing the very straight linen 'membrane'.	231
Fig. 9.5	Coronal view of the perineum showing the linen wrappings.	231
Fig. 9.6	The costo-vertebral joints seen on a CT scan (axial) of the mid-thorax	232
Fig. 9.7	Axial view of thorax - double board used for support	234
Fig. 9.8	Coronal view of trunk - dowels in re-used wooden planks	234
Fig. 9.9	Axial view of knees - single board used for support	235
Fig. 9.10	Coronal and axial views showing two pericules used in Mummy LII	235
Fig. 9.11	Axial view of pelvis - cross-section of 'reeds' anterior to the abdomen	235
Fig. 9.12	Sagittal view of 'reeds' anterior to the abdomen	236
Fig. 9.13	Sagittal view of stick anterior to and supporting cervical spine	236
Fig. 9.14	Axial view of stick anterior to and supporting cervical spine	236
Fig. 9.15	Coronal view of metal rod through skull into thoracic spine	236
Fig. 9.16	Axial view of point of trepanation in skull, used for rod insertion	237
Fig. 9.17	Sagittal view of cervical region - metal rod and point of separation of the head from the torso	237

List of Tables

Table 2.1 Current locations, origins and era of mummies	10
Table 2.2 Grouping of current locations	10
Table 3.1a Distribution in time	31
Table 3.1b Distribution in time	31
Table 3.2 Distribution in time	32
Table 3.3 Distribution by location	32
Table 4.1 Mummies with ethmoid perforation only	35
Table 4.2 Mummies with ethmoid and sphenoid perforation	49
Table 4.3 Treatment of eyes by removal	66
Table 4.4 Treatment of eyes by desiccation only	67
Table 4.5 Treatment of eyes by desiccation and enhancement by use of plates/linen	67
Table 4.6 Eyes opened and packed – some with the use of eye plates ('false eyes')	69
Table 4.7 Mummies with empty mouths	77
Table 4.8 Mouth packing with linen only	77
Table 4.9 Granular material in the mouth	81
Table 4.10 Treatment of the mouth - resin only	81
Table 5.1 Mummies with an abdominal incision	84
Table 5.2 Mummies with no incision and no evisceration	156
Table 5.3 Evidence of the presence of part of the diaphragm	173
Table 5.4 Thoracic evisceration complete, with the addition of packing	173
Table 5.5 Presence of lung and other tissues and packing material	173
Table 5.6 Retention of the heart, great vessels and lungs	174
Table 5.7 Mummies with an abdominal incision and some evidence of evisceration	175
Table 5.8 Mummies with retained viscera despite some evisceration	175
Table 5.9 Viscera returned to the body cavity after initial removal	176
Table 5.10 Pelvic contents after evisceration	178
Table 5.11 Presence of canopic packages	179
Table 5.12 Mummies with foreign material inserted into the body cavity	180
Table 5.13 Foreign materials in the body cavity	182
Table 5.14 Material used in packing the body cavity	183
Table 5.15 Distribution of amounts of material	183
Table 6.1 Mummies where resin is used to 'anoint' the skin	184
Table 6.2 The use of subcutaneous packing	184
Table 6.3 Position of arms	187
Table 6.4 Hand posture in mummies with flexed arms	188
Table 7.1 Age at Death	190
Table 7.2 Age distribution	190
Table 7.3 Age distribution of this cohort	190
Table 7.4 Age at death distribution of US males 2002	190
Table 7.5 Age at death model for the Roman Period	191
Table 7.6 Sex distribution in cohort analysed	192
Table 7.7 Causes of death in 2011 in UK – Men – Primary soft tissue cancers in grey	192
Table 7.8 Causes of death in 2011 in UK – Men	192
Table 7.9 Causes of death in 2011 in UK –Women – Primary soft tissue cancers in grey	193
Table 7.10 Causes of death in 2011 in UK – Women	193
Table 7.11 Distribution of observed probable causes of death	196
Table 7.12 Non-Fatal pathologies	196
Table 8.1 Distribution of mummies by era	198
Table 8.2 Numbers in each era	199
Table 8.3 Numbers in each era	199
Table 8.4 Mummies from Dynasty 22	200
Table 8.5 Mummification techniques used in the head	200
Table 8.6 Mummification techniques used in the trunk	201
Table 8.7 Mummies from Dynasty 25	201
Table 8.8 Mummification techniques used in the head	202
Table 8.9 Mummification techniques used in the trunk	202
Table 8.10 Mummies from the Third Intermediate Period	202
Table 8.11 Mummification techniques used in the head in Third Intermediate Period	202
Table 8.12 Mummification techniques used in the trunk in Third Intermediate Period	203
Table 8.13 Mummies from Dynasty 26	203
Table 8.14 Mummification techniques used in the head in Dynasty 26	204
Table 8.15 Mummification techniques used in the trunk in Dynasty 26	204
Table 8.16 Contents of mediastinum	205
Table 8.17 Mummies from the Ptolemaic Period	205
Table 8.18 Mummification techniques used in the head in the Ptolemaic period	205
Table 8.19 Mummification techniques used in the trunk in the Ptolemaic Period	205
Table 8.20 Contents of mediastinum	206

Table 8.21	Mummies from the Roman Period	206
Table 8.22	Mummies from the Roman Period grouped by location of origin	206
Table 8.23	Mummification techniques used in the head in the Roman Period	207
Table 8.24	Mummification techniques used in the trunk in the Roman Period	207
Table 8.25	Mummies arranged by location of origin	211
Table 8.26	Mummies from Fayum and Hawara	211
Table 8.27	Mummies from Akhmim	212
Table 8.28	Mummies from Thebes	212
Table 8.29	Theban mummies from Dynasty 20 to 24	213
Table 8.30	Mummification techniques used in the head in Dynasty 20 to 24	213
Table 8.31	Mummification techniques used in the trunk in Dynasty 20 to 24	214
Table 8.32	Theban mummies from Dynasty 25	214
Table 8.33	Mummification techniques used in the head in Dynasty 25	214
Table 8.34	Mummification techniques used in the trunk in Dynasty 25	214
Table 8.35	Mummification techniques used in the head of Mummy XVII	215
Table 8.36	Mummification techniques used in the trunk of Mummy XVII	215
Table 8.37	Theban mummies from Dynasty 26	215
Table 8.38	Mummification techniques used in the head in Theban Dynasty 26	215
Table 8.39	Mummification techniques used in the trunk in Theban Dynasty 26	216
Table 8.40	Theban mummies from the Roman Period	216
Table 8.41	Mummification techniques used in the head in Roman Period Thebes	216
Table 8.42	Mummification techniques used in the trunk in Roman Period Thebes	216
Table 8.43	Mummification techniques used in the head	217
Table 8.44	Mummification techniques used in the trunk	217
Table 8.45	Mummies sorted by age at death	218
Table 8.46	Children in order of age	218
Table 8.47	Children in order of era	219
Table 8.48	Treatment of the head in children in order of age	219
Table 8.49	Treatment of the head in children grouped by era	219
Table 8.50	Treatment of the trunk in children in order of age	220
Table 8.51	Treatment of the trunk in children grouped by era	220
Table 8.52	Mummies within the Young Adult group	221
Table 8.53	Mummies within the Middle Age group	221
Table 8.54	Mummies within the Elderly group	221
Table 8.55	Treatment of the head in Young Adults	222
Table 8.56	Treatment of the head in Middle Age	222
Table 8.57	Treatment of the head in the Elderly	222
Table 8.58	Treatment of the trunk in Young Adults	223
Table 8.59	Treatment of the trunk in Middle Age	223
Table 8.60	Treatment of the trunk in the Elderly	223
Table 9.1	Mummies with ethmoid sinus perforation only grouped by era	225
Table 9.2	Mummies with ethmoid sinus perforation only grouped by location	226
Table 9.3	Mummies with ethmoid and sphenoid sinus perforation by era	226
Table 9.4	Mummies with ethmoid and sphenoid sinus perforation by location	226
Table 9.5	Mummies with exclusively sphenoid perforation	226
Table 9.6	Mummies with a trans-nasal orbital route for excerebration	226
Table 9.7	Effect of excerebration route on efficiency of excerebration	227
Table 9.8	Mummies with no excerebration	227
Table 9.9	Distribution of treatment of the eyes	229
Table 9.10	All mummies with desiccated eyes	229
Table 9.11	Mummies with eye desiccation alone by era	229
Table 9.12	Mummies with packed globes – in order of era	229
Table 9.13	Mummies in which the eyes were removed	230
Table 9.14	Mummies with use of the perineal route for evisceration	230
Table 9.15	Mummies from the Roman Period and their locations	231
Table 9.16	Roman mummies with damage to the chest wall and its detail	232
Table 9.17	Mummies of the Roman Period without chest compression	232
Table 9.18	Chest injury in Non-Roman mummies	233
Table 9.19	Pelvic injury with compression of the chest and abdomen	233
Table 9.20	Sex, age and location of mummies with chest and abdominal compression	234
Table 9.21	Stiffeners in mummies	234
Table 10.1	Structure perforated during Trans-nasal Excerebration	239
Table 10.2	Structure perforated during Trans-nasal Excerebration	240
Table 10.3	Vertical 'strike' c.f. Horizontal 'strike'	240
Table 10.4	Vertical 'strike' c.f. Horizontal 'strike'	240
Table 10.5	Change in percentage of vertical c.f. horizontal 'strike'	240
Table 10.6	Frequency of Eye Plate usage	241
Table 10.7	Revised frequency of Eye Plate usage	241
Table 10.8	Evisceration routes	242
Table 10.9	Evisceration routes	242
Table 10.10	Evisceration routes as percentages of each cohort	243

Table 10.11	Evisceration routes as percentages of each era.	243
Table 10.12	Evisceration routes as percentages of each era.	243
Table 10.13	Incidence of chest compression.	244
Table 10.14	Incidence of chest compression.	244

Acknowledgements

My first expression of gratitude has to be to my wife Peta for all her help and her unwavering support, encouragement, patience and tolerance.

I would also like to express gratitude to my supervisor, Prof. Rosalie David. She has provided direction, advice and support throughout the whole project.

My thanks are due to Dr. Joyce Tyldesley who helped to supervise and guide my efforts during the early part of this research.

My thanks are also due to Prof. Andrew Chamberlain who took over supervision for the final half of the project. His help and guidance are much appreciated.

My advisors Mrs. Angela Thomas and Dr. Nick Ashton have both been very supportive and helpful throughout the project.

My gratitude also goes to Prof. Frank Ruhli and his staff who made the collection of mummy CT scans held in the IEM, Zurich freely available to me and encouraged my efforts in this field of endeavour.

Dr. Cristina Martina and her colleagues at the Ospedale Mollinette must not be forgotten for their help during my stay in Turin.

My thanks go to Prof. Judy Adams whose advice and whose help in arranging sessions at the Royal Manchester Children's Hospital were invaluable.

Without the help and cooperation of curators in Manchester, Liverpool, London and Birmingham museums none of this would have been possible. They are Dr. Campbell Price, Dr. Ashley Cooke, Dr. John Taylor and Dr. Phil Watson. Thanks also go to the conservators, Sam Sportun, Tracey Seddon and Deborah Cane for their help.

Thanks go to radiographers from Royal Manchester Children's Hospital (Superintendent Suzie Crimmins and the staff of the CT department), the Royal Liverpool and Broadgreen University Hospital (Superintendent Julie Houghton and the staff of the CT department) and Stafford Hospital (Superintendent Brenda Sharwin and the staff of the CT department). Without their cooperation and willingness to work out of hours many of the CT scans would never have materialized.

Thanks are due for the permissions to reproduce copyright images from Manchester and the British Museum.

Finally I would like to thank the staff of Archaeopress Publishing Ltd. and, in particular, Rajka Makjanic for the tireless effort to convert my original manuscript into a presentable form for publication.

Terminology

The anatomical terminology used throughout this document is taken from Gray's Anatomy Ed 32 (Johnston, Davies and Davies, 1958).

The medical terminology used can be found in any standard medical dictionary.

Chronology

Period	Dynasty	Date
Early Dynastic	I - II	3000 – 2686 BC
Old Kingdom	III - VIII	2686 - 2160 BC
First Intermediate	IX - XI	2160 – 2055 BC
Middle Kingdom	XI - XIV	2055 – 1650 BC
Second Intermediate	XV - XVII	1650 – 1550 BC
New Kingdom	XVIII - XX	1550 – 1069 BC
Third Intermediate	XXI - XXV	1069 – 664 BC
Late Period	XXVI - XXXI	664 – 332 BC
Ptolemaic		332 – 30 BC
Roman		30 BC – AD 395

(AFTER SHAW [ED.], 2000: 480 -482).

Chapter One

Introduction

1.1 Mummification – The afterlife

1.1.1 Religious beliefs and the afterlife

It is generally accepted that the ancient Egyptians held a strong belief in life after death and that this 'afterlife' could be eternal assuming that the correct conditions were met (Ikram, Dodson, 1998: 18). It was also accepted that what is currently called the 'soul' or 'spirit' was comprised of various aspects, including the *ba* (the personality of the deceased), the *ka* (the life force) and the *Akh* (representing the immortality of the deceased), (Tyldesley, 2010: 114). Whilst the *ka* had to remain close to the body to receive sustenance, the *ba* and *akh* could leave the body to return later. (David, 2002: 116). It was, therefore, necessary to preserve the body after death so that it would survive for all eternity. Ideally the body would be 'perfectly' preserved and completely whole and intact.

The body would be transformed, after mummification/embalming, into a living entity by the utterance of spells. Today the most recognized of these spells is probably 'the Opening of the Mouth Ceremony'. This ceremony, contained in spells 21-23, was designed to activate the mouth, eyes and ears of the deceased, preparing them for the afterlife and contained such phrases as 'My mouth is opened, my mouth is split open by Shu with that iron harpoon of his with which he split open the mouths of the gods' – shown in the papyrus of Nebqed- N3068, found in the Louvre Museum (Taylor, 2010: 88).

Whilst it is clear that the compromises necessary to achieve preservation of the body would, inevitably, render the body less than 'whole', it was (presumably) believed that the spells would adequately compensate for this and, once more, create a 'whole, intact' body that would be useful in the afterlife.

1.1.2 Historical References to Mummification in Ancient Egypt

Contemporary records of embalming/mummification have not been found and mummification is rarely depicted in any specific or informative detail: see, for example, the scenes on the Late Period coffin of Djed-Bastiuf-Ankh (Hildesheim Museum) which show the body being purified by water, the body heaped with natron, the mummy with its canopic jars, and the god Anubis working with the mummy. Occasional, brief references to mummification may be found in Egyptian texts, but there is nothing that helps our understanding of the process. Some references from the classical authors briefly mention mummification but in scant detail. For example Strabo: Geographica XVII.1.1-10. 795 (Jones, 1917: 795) states '…and then one comes to the suburb Necropolis, in which are many gardens and groves and halting-places fitted up for the embalming of corpses'. Pliny the Elder in Historia Naturalis (Bostock, Riley, 1855: Book 11, 70) states '…this is the notion entertained by the Egyptians, whose custom it is to embalm the bodies of the dead, and so preserve them'. Porphyry of Tyre is slightly more detailed – as follows: '… the Egyptians, when they buried those that were of noble birth, privately took away the belly and placed it in a chest, and together with other things which they performed for the sake of the dead body, they elevated the chest towards the sun, whom they invoked as a witness; an oration for the deceased being at the same time made by one of those to whose care the funeral was committed.' (Taylor, 1823: 110-138). Plutarch's description is slightly less detailed: 'the Egyptians, who cut open the dead body and expose it to the sun, and then cast certain parts of it into the river, and perform their offices on the rest of the body, feeling that this part has now at last been made clean.' (Plutarch, 1928: 16.1). Finally, Cicero adds the detail that 'condiunt Aegyptii mortuos et eos servant domi' – 'the Egyptians embalm their dead and keep them in their houses' (Cicero, XLV.108).

The earliest useful records are therefore those provided by the Classical authors Herodotus and Diodorus Siculus. For example Herodotus, in his *Histories* (Book 2: 86), describes some methods of mummification as recounted to him by priests during his visit to Egypt in the fourth century BC during the occupation by the Persians in the Late Period. He describes three methods of mummification including what is generally known as the 'classical' method. This will be described in detail (as much as was given by Herodotus at that time!) below. However, Diodorus Siculus (*Diodorus Siculus: Book 1, 69*) was less than complimentary about Herodotus' description and the validity of his reports and adds some of his own observations.

To reiterate, the 'classical' description of mummification as described by Herodotus is as follows (*The Histories* 2: 86):

> The most perfect process is as follows: as much as possible of the brain is extracted through the nostrils with an iron hook and what the hook cannot reach is rinsed out with drugs; next the flank is laid open with a flint knife and the whole contents of the abdomen removed; the cavity is then thoroughly cleansed and washed out, first with palm wine and again with an infusion of pounded spices. After that it is filled with pure bruised myrrh, cassia and every other aromatic substance with the exception of frankincense, and sewn up again, after which the body is placed in natron, covered entirely over, for seventy days - never longer.

When this period, which must not be exceeded, is over, the body is washed and wrapped from head to foot in linen cut into strips and smeared on the underside with gum, which is commonly used by the Egyptians instead of glue. In this condition the body is given back to the family, who have a wooden case made shaped like the human figure, into which it is put.

When, for reasons of expense, the second quality is called for, the treatment is different: no incision is made and the intestines are not removed, but oil of cedar is injected with a syringe into the body through the anus which is afterwards stopped up to prevent the liquid from escaping. The body is then cured in natron for the prescribed number of days, on the last of which the oil is drained off. The effect of it is so powerful that as it leaves the body it brings with it the viscera in a liquid state, and as the flesh has been dissolved by the natron, nothing of the body is left but the skin and bones. After this treatment, it is returned to the family without further attention.

The third method, used for embalming the bodies of the poor, is simply to wash out the intestines, and keep the body for seventy days in natron.

Diodorus Siculus' contribution was prefaced by the words:

'Now as for the stories invented by Herodotus and certain writers on Egyptian affairs, who deliberately preferred to the truth the telling of marvellous tales and the invention of myths for the delectation of their readers'.

However he gives the following information, which does add to Herodotus' description.

First, he who is called the scribe, laying the body down, marks on the left flank where it is to be cut. Then he who is called the cutter takes an Ethiopian stone, and cuts the flesh as the law prescribes, and forthwith escapes running, those who are present pursuing and throwing stones and cursing, as though turning the defilement [of his act] on to his head. For whosoever inflicts violence upon, or wounds, or in any way injures a body of his own kind, they hold worthy of hatred. The embalmers, on the other hand, they esteem worthy of every honor and respect, associating with the priests and being admitted to the temples without hindrance as holy men. When they have assembled for the treatment of the body that has been cut, one of them inserts his hand through the wound in the corpse into the breast and takes out everything excepting the kidneys and the heart. Another man cleanses each of the entrails, sweetening them with palm-wine and with incense. Finally, having washed the whole body, they first diligently treat it with cedar oil and other things for over thirty days, and then with myrrh and cinnamon and [spices], which not only have the power to preserve it for a long time, but also impart a fragrant smell. Having treated it, they restore it to the relatives with every member of the body preserved so perfectly that even the eyelashes and eyebrows remain, the whole appearance of the body being unchangeable, and the cast of the features recognizable.

The translation of Herodotus' original document given above is that of Selincourt (Selincourt 1954: 115). It is recognized that there are many translations of this document but the difference in the detail of the description of mummification is only minor (although there are wider differences in other parts of the texts).

Several embalmers' caches have been found which give details of the materials used and the cost thereof. One such find in Saqqara describes dates ascribed to the use of the materials (Janak and Landgrafova, 2011: 30-45). However, reference to the communication from Eaton-Krauss indicates that many other caches have been discovered in a variety of types of location and have been described with differing levels of detail (Eaton-Krauss M., 2008: 288-293).

A group of papyri known as 'the Embalmers Archives' from the Ptolemaic Period, currently in the Ashmolean Museum, Oxford only describes the organisation of the embalmers' profession and deals with ownership of land and tombs by the embalmers (Clarysse, Depauw, 1973: 125-128). These papyri do not contain any insight into the processes of mummification.

1.2 Mummification – Types and Pathology

1.2.1 Classification of mummies

It would be appropriate to discuss the origin of the word 'mummy' at this point. The word is derived from the Persian-Urdu *'mum'* (Aufderheide, 2003: 1) meaning wax. A substance from the Middle East, bitumen, was also referred to as 'mumiya' – probably because of its similarity to wax. In the Middle Ages, it was noted for its medicinal properties. Initial observations of Egyptian 'mummies' erroneously attributed their dark external appearance to the result of the use of bitumen (rather than resin) to cover them. The name was then adopted to describe the preserved bodies of ancient Egyptians and, subsequently, to describe any preserved body.

Mummies can be classified into two broad groups, namely naturally occurring (spontaneous) and artificial (anthropogenic) (Aufderheide, 2010: 41). The result of mummification is to resist decay of the tissues. This may be a delay of a short time of, for example, months or as long as several millennia (as in the case of Egyptian mummies).

The processes of decay or putrefaction are the result of enzyme and bacterial action. Enzymes are released by the breakdown of cells following cell death and by bacteria that occur naturally in the body, for example in the gut. The result is a chemical breakdown of the proteins, fats and carbohydrates into smaller molecules that are either water soluble or gaseous. As a result the soft tissues are destroyed. The effects of external influences such as insects and their larvae can then sometimes be added to the equation.

Natural mummification can occur when the ambient conditions are suitable. These conditions include desiccation by drying, thermal effects (extremes of high or low temperatures) and chemical effects (e.g. bog bodies).

Of particular interest is the fate of the brain within an intact skull. Initially the brain becomes somewhat softened by autolysis, sinking to the most dependent part of the cranial cavity (posterior cranial cavity if the body is supine). It then shrinks and becomes harder. The effects of bacterial action are absent if the skull is not opened, leaving the gross anatomy of the brain visible (the gyri are usually clearly seen).

Artificial (anthropogenic) mummification has been practiced in many geographical locations. In Egypt, the process essentially consisted of excerebration, evisceration, desiccation and subsequent 'treatment' with various chemicals such as resin. Whilst these 'phases' of mummification/embalming conform to the 'classical' description, variations from this theme will be explored in this project. To précis the process, it consists of

(i) Physical/surgical treatment.

This includes in some cases, but not all, the removal of the brain (excerebration) and removal of the thoracic, abdominal and pelvic viscera (evisceration) – again not in all cases.

(ii) Chemical Treatment.

This includes treatment in natron (solid or possibly in solution) for a period of time (probably forty days) and the application of 'resin' or other unguents to the surface and internal cavities of the body – in some cases, but not all.

(iii) Bandaging/wrapping.

This was accompanied by the reciting of spells (Budge, 1899: 185).

1.2.2 Experimental mummification

In an attempt to clarify and confirm the assumed processes of mummification, some scientists have undertaken experiments on tissues. The most useful of these have been the mummification of whole human corpses. Unfortunately, the laws governing the treatment of human bodies (for example in the UK, The Human Tissue Acts 1961 and 2004) make such experimental work extremely rare. A recent experiment by Buckley was reported on British television (Channel 4, 24 October, 2011) and, subsequently, in the press but has not, as yet, been reported in the scientific literature. Brier and Wade performed a complete embalming experiment in 1994 (Brier, Wade, 1997: 89-100 and Brier, Wade, 1999: 89-97). Embalming instruments were fashioned to reproduce those presumed to have been used in ancient Egypt. They performed excerebration and evisceration followed by desiccation in natron for 35 days. The resulting 'mummy' was described as having the 'excellent visual appearance of a mummy'. It was then wrapped in linen and placed in a 'tomb' for eighteen weeks after which it received its final wrappings. It was noted that the major joints of the arms and legs were flexible after initial desiccation (but not the small joints of the fingers or toes) but had become rigid after the eighteen weeks in the 'tomb'.

Experimental mummification using animals (Garner in David, 1979: 19-24) and occasionally human parts (Panzer et al., 2013: 1527-1535) has been performed. The latter example from Zurich combines the experimental mummification process (all be it with a single limb rather than a whole body) with sequential CT imaging to follow the progress of the anatomical changes.

Other experiments have been performed on the skull to investigate the process of trans-nasal excerebration. In the often-quoted experiment (Leek, 1969: 112-116) Leek used replica instruments to perforate the cribriform plate and macerate the brain tissue with a hooked rod. Although he did not, in fact, remove the brain successfully, Brier did so and concluded that maceration was the key to removal rather than irrigation. However, his successful brain removal required both the use of irrigation and swabbing out the cranial cavity with linen strips.

Further useful experiments and analyses have been performed on the resin used for the final stages of mummification such as the 'anointing' of the body surface and its use with the bandages. One such analysis by Buckley and Evershed (Buckley, Evershed, 2001: 837-841) showed that coniferous resins were used but in combination with beeswax. The percentage of beeswax increased from 38% in a Dynasty 26 mummy to 87% in a Ptolemaic mummy. The ability of the compounds to 'dry' (polymerize) and seal was noted, as were the antibacterial properties.

1.2.3 Ancient Egyptian Knowledge of Anatomy

The question as to why the Egyptians chose certain methods to preserve the body is open to discussion. Early burials in Egypt were in shallow pit graves with the body in direct contact with the hot desert sand (Raven and Taconis, 2005:37). The result of this was natural desiccation of the body and, hence, its preservation. As the graves were shallow, 'rediscovery' of them and their contents may have been frequent. It has been suggested that such 'rediscovery' may have been the result of the activities of either (or both) animals or grave robbers (Tyldesley, 2010:114). With the increasing sophistication of the population, those who could afford it probably wished to be buried in more luxurious surroundings such as stone lined tombs (Tyldesley, 2010: 115). Unfortunately, with the removal of the direct contact with hot desiccating sand, the bodies (like any other unpreserved body tissue, e.g. meat) started to putrefy. It was, therefore, necessary to develop a methodology/technology to overcome this problem. This would appear to have been the driver for the development of mummification.

It would be well known from experience with animal carcasses intended for food that one of the potent sources of the putrefaction process was the viscera. Therefore, removal of the viscera (evisceration) became one of the important processes in mummification.

There have been, commonly, three sources of anatomical knowledge available throughout history. One is the dissection of human bodies, another is knowledge gained through the treatment of war wounds and finally observations of the structure of animals and extrapolation to humans. The systematic dissection of bodies is usually fundamentally influenced by religious belief and the strength of belief in the 'sanctity' of the body. Given the importance of the survival of the body for the benefit of the *Ka* and its continuing need for food and drink and the deceased's future in the afterlife, it is difficult to believe that dissection of the human body would have been sanctioned in Pharaonic Egypt (Snape, 2011: 21) unless dissection of executed criminals was permitted. This leaves one other possibility (but nothing more) that war and its injuries were a major source of anatomical knowledge along with knowledge gained from the dismemberment (butchery) of animals.

Following evisceration and excerebration, the next step in preserving the body was desiccation. In the absence of the hot sand, the preferred method developed was the use of natron. Natron is a mixture of sodium carbonate, sodium bicarbonate, sodium sulphate and sodium chloride (David, 1979:19). The commonly accepted method was to cover the body in natron for 40 days. The body was subsequently anointed with various unguents and, on occasions, made to look more lifelike by subcutaneous 'packing'. In certain eras the desiccated viscera were returned to the body cavity either loose or in packages or placed in sets of canopic jars. The body was then wrapped/ bandaged.

1.3 The journey – From death to museum

It can be seen from the following sections that damage to the mummy is an ever-present threat to its pristine integrity. It is important that such influences are borne in mind at all stages when interpreting the medical image appearance of the mummies studied.

A further threat to the integrity of provenance is that caused by the false pairing of mummies with coffins other than the original, a practice that was sometimes performed in both Egypt and collections in Europe.

1.3.1 In Egypt

The hope of ancient Egyptians was that they would enjoy eternal life following death on earth. To this end a variable (and probably increasing number) of them opted for mummification and burial in a tomb. Whilst assuming that the mummification process would be performed properly to ensure eternal life, no subsequent disturbance of the body would have been welcomed. In particular, the desecration of the burial by tomb robbers was feared. However, the utterance of the name of the deceased would be taken as 'bringing them to life' so would be regarded positively.

Despite this there are many recorded instances of tomb and grave robbery in Pharaonic Egypt. A good example of this practice from antiquity is found in the record of the trial of tomb robbers that took place in the reign of Ramesses IX, mentioned in the Amherst, Abbott, Mayer and BM Papyri (Peet, 1915a: 173-177; Peet, 1915b: 204-206; Peet T, 1925a: 37-55; Peet, 1925b: 162-164; Capart et al., 1936: 169-193).

In subsequent centuries, the trade in Egyptian antiquities encouraged the continued pilfering of tombs along with the inevitable damage to the contents including the mummies themselves. It is doubtful that the robbers would have any concept of care of the artifacts.

Those mummies that were not damaged were then often transported to other countries including the UK and Continental Europe. This would represent another part of the 'journey' when damage could be sustained.

1.3.2 In Continental Europe

Once acquired for collectors or collections in continental Europe (and the UK) the mummies were curated by a wide variety of methods. This resulted in some being well kept and preserved and others deteriorating to the point where they were destroyed as being of no value. In the 19th century they were often traded as art objects (Raven, Taconis, 2005: 19) and the accurate preservation of the mummies was of secondary importance, as long as the external appearance was 'valuable'.

1.3.3 In Museums

Once in museums or well curated private collections the mummies were, largely, reasonably cared for including the use of controlled environments and secure storage facilities. An increasing desire developed to perform scientific studies on the mummies. There were several accepted scientific methods used to explore mummies, but initially they usually involved destructive techniques such as dissection and removing samples for chemical, histological and other analyses.

It was only with the advent of medical imaging and its use on mummies that alternative, non-invasive methods of investigation came to be used. The fact that the mummies have to be transported from museum display or storage to a medical facility adds further risk of damage (although nowadays this risk is significantly reduced by very careful specialist handling).

1.4 Research Disciplines in Mummy Studies

1.4.1 Nineteenth and twentieth centuries

During these centuries the initial method of scientific research was in the form of dissection. Clearly, whilst this produced information and tissue samples, it was totally destructive. However, it was a significant improvement on the practice of 'unrolling', previously performed – largely for the purposes of entertainment rather than true science (Raven, Taconis, 2005: 41).

With the progress of the twentieth century other disciplines were introduced. These were largely from the field of medical science and included chemical analysis, histology and bacteriology as well as the use of X-rays. As the twentieth century advanced, other disciplines were added, such as immunology, DNA analysis, radiocarbon dating, endoscopy and CT scanning.

With the exception of CT scanning, all these methodologies still required invasive procedures into the mummy, however slight.

1.4.2 Twenty first century

During the thirteen years of the twenty first century, there has been a continuous refinement of the above disciplines but no completely new ones. Such advances include the ability to analyse ever-smaller samples of material to determine the content and pattern of ancient DNA for purposes of either genealogical analysis or to detect the presence of certain infecting agents such as TB.

1.5 Medical Imaging

1.5.1 History and development

Only since the discovery of X-rays by Wilhelm Konrad Roentgen in 1895 have non-invasive methods of examination been available (Firkin / Whitworth, 1989: 454).

Whilst 'conventional' X-rays were employed with increasing frequency during the first half of the 20th century, as time has passed and the sophistication of and definition provided by X-rays have improved, they have become a routine tool for non invasive investigation in both the medical and Egyptological arenas.

Over the past 50 years or so the quality of the images has improved immeasurably. Therefore the detail provided has allowed a much more sophisticated analysis of the contained information. However, it was the advent of computed axial tomography (CAT) scanning, developed by pioneers such as Hounsfield that allowed a quantum leap forward in the amount of information available in the images. A CAT scan of the brain was first performed at the Atkinson Morley Hospital in 1971 reported to a meeting of the British Institute of Radiology in the following year and was published in the BJR in 1973 (Housfield, 1973: 1016-1022). The first Whole Body Scanner was built in 1975. Because the cost of CAT Scanners was initially very high, the availability of such machines was only relatively slowly adopted throughout the UK. However, they can now be found in virtually all District General Hospitals. More recently machines have been introduced into a few national museums, although not all CT machines (the acronym CAT scanner gradually became shortened by common usage to CT scanner during the nineteen-nineties) are of medical diagnostic type.

The basic principles of the technology of X-rays and CAT/CT scans are relatively easy to understand. The X-ray is simply a shadowgram taken in one direction. Indeed, one of the earlier names for an X-ray is a Skiagram as demonstrated in the title of one of the early influential works in Radiology, 'Roentgenology. The Borderlands of the Normal and Early Pathological in the Skiagram' (Kohler, 1931). Clearly X-rays produce a two-dimensional image of a three-dimensional object and to be able to diagnose most abnormalities it is necessary to take a second X-ray in another plane. Because the film is taken in one direction the image outlines of superimposed structures can be confusing. This can lead to some features being obscured and therefore being missed, even though further views are taken in one or more different directions or planes.

In an attempt to overcome this problem, a technique called tomography was developed in the 1930s by Alessandro Vallebona (Vallebona, 1930) and refined by Ziedses des Plantes whereby the X-ray image was of structures in one plane and at a single distance through the body (or a predetermined plane section of the body while blurring the images of other planes), similar to imaging a single 'slice' of the body. This was effected by swinging the X-ray tube back and forth whilst moving the film in the opposite direction. The fulcrum point determined the level of the plane imaged. This left the structures in that plane in focus, but structures in other planes blurred. (Sutton, 1969) The distance between the image planes varied from time to time in history, but was in the region of 1 cm. in the 1960s.

The next major leap forward was the development of the CAT scanner, Computerised Axial Tomography. In this technique, the X-ray tube is rotated around the body and many images/measurements are taken from thousands of angles. Instead of photographic film being used to acquire the image, sensors are used for this purpose. The body was then moved a distance and a further set of images created. This was repeated many times and a composite picture constructed by computer. The distance between 'slices' was in the region of 2 or 3 mms in the 1990s but nowadays more modern machines are able to take image 'slices' of 0.6 mms. In fact, the more modern machines produce Spiral Tomograms. That is to say, the body continues to move whilst the X-ray tube rotates around it. With these modern machines the computer software is such that the images are not only much more detailed, but 3D images can be reconstructed from the data. Furthermore, with the conventional computer reconstructions it is possible to produce images that represent 'slices' of the body in three planes, that is axial (transverse), sagittal and coronal planes. The axial plane is transverse across the body, whilst the sagittal plane runs 'back to front', i.e. forehead to back of skull. Finally the coronal plane runs across the body 'left to right'(See Fig.1.1). Although the software can reconstruct other planes (at infinitely variable angles from those described), these are usually used to correct for rotation of the body or to 'follow' a particular structure through its course, and have to be used with caution.

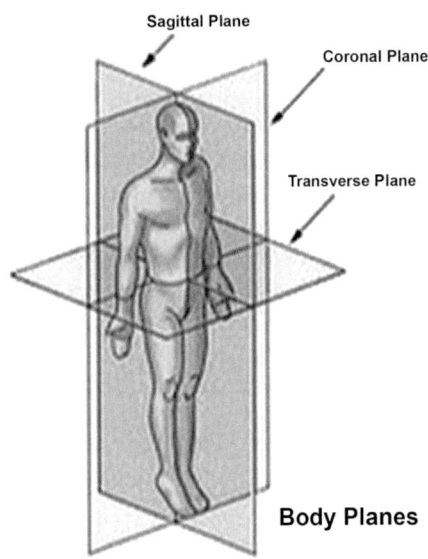

FIG. 1.1 THE BODY PLANES.
(IN PUBLIC DOMAIN)

By analysing all the available information it is possible to detect abnormalities of the structure of the human anatomy.

The evolution of X-ray technology has resulted in the significant progress of medical knowledge. For example, prior to its use, pain in the hip was often regarded as being the result of tuberculosis or a variant of tuberculosis. The use of X-rays allowed people like Perthes to differentiate a form of childhood hip disease, Osteochondritis Deformans Juvenilis, from tuberculosis (Perthes, 1910: 111). The cause is a form of avascularity of the femoral head growth centre and has an entirely different course and end result from that of TB. Many more examples of new diagnoses discovered with the use of X-rays are available in the orthopaedic and radiological literature.

With the advent of CT scanning it has been possible to locate, measure and diagnose lesions far more accurately, so assisting not only in diagnosis but also in treatment.

More recent advances in CT technology have been largely within the field of diagnostic and image manipulation software programmes. The majority of the information regarding these diagnostic programmes is found within the manufacturers' literature, the details of the programmes themselves being regarded as 'commercially sensitive' and not open to description in the scientific literature. However, it is fair to say that there are several versions of the image manipulation software (called Dicom readers) currently available.

1.5.2 Other Imaging Methods

Other methods of medical imaging deserve mention and discussion with regard to their relevance to the study of mummies.

MRI or Magnetic Resonance Imaging produces excellent images of the soft tissues. Unfortunately, it depends on the presence of hydrogen atoms in water (normally present to the extent of approximately 65% of the human body). Clearly, water is the one thing that has been deliberately removed as thoroughly as possible from a mummy. Therefore this modality of imaging was thought unlikely to be productive. This has been reported to be the case by Cockburn, Cockburn and Reyman (1998:364) and Ruhli et al (2004:218-227). However, Karlik et al, found that 'by using a strategy that was optimized for tissues with very short water relaxation times' it was possible to generate useful images of a desiccated brain (Karlik, Bartha, Kennedy and Chhem, 2007: 105-110). It should be noted, however, that the brain was not in situ within the skull and it was not discussed how difficult this technique would be with a brain (or other soft tissue organs) when contained within a body cavity.

Ultrasound Imaging is frequently used in medical practice today, but depends on the reflection of sound waves to produce images (Cobbold, 2007: 422-423). The ultrasound waves are reflected back by 'hyper-echoic' structures such as bone or, for example, gallstones, thus producing a bright or white acoustic image. Unfortunately this reflection also produces a dark acoustic 'shadow' behind it. Fluid filled spaces (such as cysts) are hypo-echoic or anechoic and do not reflect the ultrasound signal, thus resulting in a low signal image (black) with an apparently enhanced, lighter, signal behind. It is reported by Ruhli et al (v.s.) that this technique fails to produce acceptable images in mummified bodies.

Positron Emission Tomography (PET scanning) (Adam and Dixon [Eds], 2008: 135-146) is useful in assessing physiology and metabolism and therefore appropriate in living bodies but of no use in the dead.

Terahertz imaging has also been investigated with regard to its use in mummy studies. Unfortunately its value is limited to the surface and near surface appearance as the definition of deeper structures is not good (Ohrstrom et al., 2010: 497-500).

One final influence on imaging which has appeared within the last decade is the development of PACS, Picture Archiving and Communication System. PACS enables images such as x-rays and scans to be stored electronically and viewed on screens (so replacing analogue images with digital ones), creating a near filmless process and improved diagnostic methods (PACS 2011). The software enables the images to be manipulated. For example, they can be magnified and the contrast and brightness altered. Viewing window sizes can be reduced to allow comparison of two or more images at the same time. It is possible to create 3D type images with shadows that can give a very lifelike, solid representation of the part that can also be rotated. Furthermore, it is possible to rapidly scroll through a series of images, so gaining an enhanced appreciation of the anatomy of the part. The transport of images is also made simpler in that it is no longer necessary to send hard copy films from one location to another. Transport of images is now on CD ROMs with significant amounts of image material in one disc or on portable external hard drives (up to 2Tb). Alternatively, image data can be sent over the Internet. With this sort of data transfer the issue of data security arises. Although this may not be an issue in Egyptology, it is a serious concern when dealing with patients and 'patient confidentiality'.

It should be noted, however, that although images shown as 3D reconstructions are very impressive (some years ago the reconstructions looked rather 'pixelated' as if constructed with miniature Lego bricks, whereas they are now smooth and lifelike), they only demonstrate the outer 'solid' appearance rather than the internal structure of a part which might otherwise have been seen in a planar view (sagittal, axial or coronal). They do, nevertheless, have their place, for example in examining the teeth and assessing periodontal disease. More recently, image manipulation development has allowed a technique called 'virtual fly through' which reconstructs '3D' images of the internal cavities of the body.

1.5.3 Current use of radiography in mummy studies

The abnormalities to be found in mummies include those resulting from pre-mortem disease or trauma, those resulting from the embalming/mummification process and those that have resulted from the subsequent handling, transport and treatment of the subject. Changes resulting from disease should be easily recognisable and will be well described in radiology textbooks. Trauma should be recognisable as matching the known patterns of injury as described in orthopaedic textbooks and literature in general. If these two groups of changes are eliminated then the other changes seen can be attributable to either mummification or the subsequent 'treatment' of the mummies. Changes due to damage relating to handling and transport will be influenced by the integrity of the mummy. For example, if a mummy is fully wrapped and otherwise undisturbed, then transport damage is likely to be generalised and not localised, whereas localised change is more likely to be the result of locally induced damage such as would occur during mummification (unless there is clear evidence of damage to an area of overlying bandaging or cartonnage which would indicate localised handling damage). However, the susceptibility to such damage would inevitably be influenced by the durability and strength of the body – an attribute which is related and in proportion to the excellence or otherwise of the mummification process. Unfortunately, the picture can be complicated by previous invasive archaeological/biomedical examination such as endoscopy or tissue sampling. However, these procedures would be expected to have been recorded and therefore it should be possible to unravel the evidence.

Given that the process of mummification will almost certainly have involved extraction of the viscera (+/- the brain), examination of body images can be restricted to the structure of the head, neck, body wall of the trunk and the limbs. There may also be evidence of objects within the cavities of the skull, trunk and wrappings. These may be of a variety of origins, for example, returned mummified viscera or packing with or without amulets etc. With regard to the tissues of the body wall and limbs, these will inevitably be distorted from the normal expected anatomy by the process of desiccation during mummification. The amount of distortion will be proportional to the volume of water normally found within those tissues. Hence the distortion of bone will be undetectable, whilst that of fat and muscle will be significant.

Positional abnormalities in the body during life can be due to muscle activity (e.g. torticollis), to soft tissue contractures (e.g. a long standing claw hand following a stroke) or to abnormal bone shape (e.g. following fracture mal-union). However, interpretation of abnormal posture in mummies must be undertaken with care. For example, there are instances of reported scoliosis in museum exhibits where there is only lateral curvature of the spine. In fact, in life, scoliosis consists of both curvature and rotation of the spine. Pahor and Cole reported a case of supposed torticollis where the torticollis was supposed to be secondary to infection following a wound (Pahor and Cole, 1995:273-276). This is clearly unlikely as such a deformity is due to muscle spasm and this would have ceased upon death.

Analysis of combinations of abnormalities/injuries can help in the detection of those that could have occurred during life and those that are unlikely to be pre-mortem. An example will be given later where there is a combination of disruption of the pelvic ring (complete dislocation of a sacro-iliac joint with disruption of the pubic symphysis) with dislocation of both hip joints. This is almost impossible as the result of trauma (and a combination of injury never seen by the author in forty years of clinical orthopaedic practice). Both the bony pelvis and the hip joint are very stable, strong structures because of the intrinsic shape of the constituent bones and the strength of the ligaments. Because of this, the force necessary to cause the initial injury to one of these structures (pelvic ring or hip joint) can only result in further displacement of the resulting separated parts (if there is any residual energy) rather than being transferred to the other structure (the path of least resistance).

The timing of fractures in relation to the time of death requires knowledge of the fracture healing process. The following comments apply to most bones with the exception of the skull and spine. After a bone has been fractured bleeding occurs. This causes swelling which may be observed in the proximity of the fracture. Evidence of swelling may remain after desiccation. Within a short time (varying from about a week in children to two weeks in adults) calcium will be laid down within the haematoma. This will be seen in Xray images. The calcium in the callus renders it more prominent on Xray as time progresses. Eventually the fracture is healed by callus that then undergoes remodeling resulting in the final appearance of the healed fracture. From this description it can be seen that any visible callus indicates that the fracture occurred at least one or two weeks prior to death. The absence of callus indicates that the fracture occurred within a week or two prior to death or after death. Although the presence of swelling may help to differentiate the timing, its absence does not.

The integrity of the skeleton as a whole within a mummy will depend upon the ligaments. In turn the integrity of the ligaments will be influenced by the excellence or otherwise of the original mummification process and by subsequent handling. Alternatively, the ligaments may have been damaged pre-mortem by disease or trauma or post-mortem during the mummification process.

1.6 Aims and Objectives

Although much has been written concerning mummy studies and, in particular, the use of modern medical imaging techniques in those studies, the current literature concentrates on confirming (or otherwise) pre-existing concepts regarding the techniques used. These consist of historical descriptions from Herodotus and Diordorus. The detailed analysis of CT image files (Dicom data files) by a trained medical professional presents the opportunity for a fresh approach. This gives the chance to change the parameters of the data.

Whilst excerebration has previously been classified as either trans-nasal or trans-foraminal (or excerebration absent), this research will also assess the direction of the trans-nasal approach with particular reference to the structures perforated / damaged during the process.

The treatment of the eyes during embalming has not been studied to any great extent in the past and will be analysed in this document.

Evisceration has received attention in the past, but a detailed analysis of organ removal, treatment and return in various forms will be performed.

The use of embalming 'unguents' such as resin will be identified and patterns of usage (if any) will be noted.

Having acquired the necessary data, it will be evaluated to identify any patterns of technique related to era and location. An initial aim to assess the relationship of mummification technique to status was not pursued because of the fragmentary descriptions of status in the provenance data available.

Any new techniques observed will be described and techniques that appear to be related to specific locations and/or eras will be identified.

Previously accepted techniques will be critically assessed where the evidence justifies this.

1.6.1 Current Literature

Although other studies have sought to analyse the presence, absence or variation from 'classical' techniques in mummification they have been based, largely, on meta-analyses of previous observers (Wade et al, 2011: 248-269 and Wade, Nelson, 2013: 1-28). The method in the current study is the personal observation and analysis of CT images to form independent opinion rather than rely upon the observations and interpretations of others.

Previous reports of the CT examination of mummies have frequently concentrated on the analysis of one, two or three mummies rather than an extensive series. These are often published in the medical journals and four examples of such publications are given, although many more exist (Ruhli, Chhem, Boni, 2004:218-227), (Chhem, 2006: 803-804) , (Gupta et al, 2008: 705-713) , (Cavka et al, 2012: 2151-2157).

Chapter Two

Methods

2.1 Source of Materials

2.1.1 Location of material

In the first instance, museums in the UK were located using a combination of personal knowledge, web searches for 'museums in the UK' and reference to the Museums and Galleries Year Book. An initial approach was made by email to ascertain whether the institution had any Egyptian mummies. This resulted in an 'uptake', i.e. response, in about 50% of cases. Of these responses only a few museums were found to possess Egyptian human mummies. The question was then posed as to whether these mummies had been subjected to medical imaging.

An initial decision was made to investigate all responses, including those where only plain X-ray films were available. This resulted in an early visit to the Royal Albert Memorial Museum and Art Gallery, Exeter. As a result, a report was compiled on those films and the data provided. This was compared with CT data collected from mummies in the Birmingham Museum and Art Gallery. The result of this comparison will be discussed below.

As a result of the paucity of responses from the UK (with the exception of the British Museum [BM], Birmingham, Liverpool and Manchester) a decision was made to widen the field of enquiry to include Europe and the USA. Whilst positive responses were initially received from a couple of locations in the USA, the agreement to provide data was, eventually, not forthcoming. Therefore, no material from the USA is included in this study.

Appendix 1 shows a list of the museums contacted.

Positive responses were received from the Centre of Evolutionary Medicine (IEM), the University of Zurich and from the Egyptian Museum in Turin.

Table 2.1 (on pages 9-10) shows the distribution of mummies included in this study with their current locations, historical era and original locations. Table 2.2 shows the grouping of the current locations.

NUMBER	MUSEUM	MUMMY NAME	ORIGIN	PERIOD
I	Birmingham	Graeco-Roman	Unknown	Roman
II	Birmingham	Namenkhetamun	Thebes	D26
III	Birmingham	Padimut	Thebes	D20-21
IV	Exeter	Shepenmut	Thebes	D22
V	Sheffield	Nesitanebetasheru	Thebes	D25
VI	Sheffield	Djedma'atiuesankh	Thebes	D26
VII	Ipswich	Tahathor	Thebes	D25
VIII	Liverpool	Padiamun - 53.72a	Thebes	D22
IX	Liverpool	Padiamunnebnesuttauwy	Thebes	D25
X	Liverpool	Nesmin	Akhmim	Ptolemaic
XI	Liverpool	Padiamun - M14003	Thebes	D26
XII	Manchester	MM1768	Faiyum	Roman
XIII	Manchester	MM1767	Faiyum	Roman
XIV	Manchester	MM1777 - Asru	Thebes	D26
XV	Liverpool	13.10.11.25	Hawara	Roman
XVI	Liverpool	M13997a	Thebes	Roman
XVII	Liverpool	Ankhesenaset – M 14000	Thebes	3IP
XVIII	Liverpool	M14048	Thebes	Roman
XIX	Zurich	Altdorf Child	Unknown	Roman
XX	Zurich	TaDjIsis - K1205	Thebes	D26
XXI	Zurich	Lausanne - 490	Unknown	3IP
XXII	Zurich	Bern - 00/2	Unknown	Unknown
XXIII	Zurich	Yverdon - Nes-Shou - MY/3775	Akhmim	Ptolemaic
XXIV	Zurich	Basel - BSAE.1030	El-Hibe	Roman
XXV	Zurich	Geneva - TjesMoutPert - D0242	Thebes	D22-25
XXVI	Zurich	Geneva - Infant	Unknown	Unknown

NUMBER	MUSEUM	MUMMY NAME	ORIGIN	PERIOD
XXVII	Manchester	Demetria - MM11630	Hawara	Roman
XXVIII	Manchester	Sheri-Ankh – MM13783	Akhmim	Ptolemaic
XXIX	BM	Hor - EA6659	Thebes	D22
XXX	BM	Ankh-Unen-Nefer - EA6681	Thebes	D25
XXXI	BM	Padiamunet - EA6682	Thebes	D25
XXXII	BM	EA20744	Deir El Bahari	D22
XXXIII	BM	EA22939	Thebes	D22
XXXIV	BM	EA25258	Thebes	D22
XXXV	BM	EA29577	Thebes/Faiyum	D22
XXXVI	Zurich	Bern - AE9	Akhmim	Ptolemaic
XXXVII	Zurich	Lenzburg - Sherit-Min	Akhmim	Ptolemaic
XXXVIII	Zurich	St. Gallen - Shepenese	Thebes	D26
XXXIX	Zurich	St. Gallen - C3530	Thebes	D21
XL	Zurich	Lausanne - 492	Unknown	3IP
XLI	Zurich	Lenzburg - K10351	Unknown	Roman
XLII	Turin	Taaset - Suppl.9480	Faiyum	Ptolemaic
XLIII	Turin	(Tebtynis) - Suppl.19691	Faiyum	Ptolemaic ??
XLIV	Turin	Provv.610	Unknown	Ptolemaic ??
XLV	Manchester	MM1766	Hawara	Roman
XLVI	Manchester	MM10881	Thebes	D26
XLVII	Manchester	MM1769	Hawara	Roman
XLVIII	Manchester	MM3496	Gurob	D18
IL	Manchester	MM5053.a - Perenbast	Thebes	D22
L	Perth	23/1936	Akhmim/Thebes	D26
LI	Manchester	MM9354a - Khary	Unknown	D19/ Ptolemaic?
LII	Manchester	MM9319 - child	?Hawara	Roman
LIII	Manchester	MM1976.51a	Thebes	D25
LIV	Manchester	Salford 2	Unknown	3IP
LV	Manchester	MM13011	Unknown	Ptolemaic
LVI	Manchester	MM2109	Hawara	Roman
LVII	Manchester	MM1775 - Artemidorus	Hawara	Roman
LVIII	Manchester	MM13784	Unknown	Middle Kingdom
LIX	BM	EA 22108 Child	Hawara	Roman
LX	BM	EA 6704	Thebes	Roman

TABLE 2.1 CURRENT LOCATIONS, ORIGINS AND ERA OF MUMMIES

M/C	Zur.	L'pool	BM	B'ham	Tur	Shffld	Exet	Perth	Ipsw	TOT
18	14	8	9	3	3	2	1	1	1	60

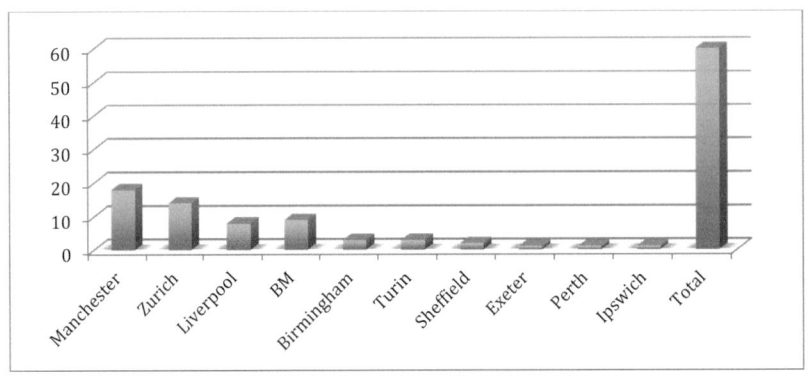

TABLE 2.2 GROUPING OF CURRENT LOCATIONS

2.1.2 Formats of Material

The format of the X-rays from Exeter is, clearly, hard copy X-ray film analysed using a light box.

The CT scans from Sheffield were in analogue form. That is they were displayed as 'thumbnails' on X-ray film (20 thumbnails to each film) and, again, analysed on a light box.

All other mummy data was provided in digital form. However, the CT scanning machines used to acquire data varied from location to location.

The Manchester mummies were scanned on a Siemens Somatom Definition AS+ machine.

The Zurich mummy collection was, in fact, taken from nine different museums in Switzerland and the CT scans were performed on at least six different types of machine, including models of Siemens, Toshiba and Philips manufacture.

The mummies from Liverpool were scanned using a Siemens Somatom Definition Flash machine.

Those from the British Museum were scanned using a GE Lightspeed Pro 32 machine and a Siemens Somatom Definition Flash machine.

The mummies from Birmingham were scanned on a Toshiba Aquilion 64 machine.

Turin mummies were scanned at the Ospedale Molinette, Turin on 5/5/12 on a GE Lightspeed Pro 16.

The mummy from the Ipswich Museum was scanned on a Siemens Definition AS scanner.

The Sheffield mummies were scanned on a Siemens Somatom CR machine.

The slice thicknesses used varied from 3.0 mms to 0.6 mms.

2.1.3 Dicom readers

In all cases of digital format image, there was a requirement to have a Dicom Reader available. On some occasions, (for example in the case of the Birmingham mummies) the Dicom Reader used was that provided by the hospital PACS supplier. In the case of Birmingham the PACS was a GE PACS and the Reader was GE Centricity, whilst the mummy from Ipswich had the data supplied via a Kodak Reader.

Clearly, with a number of potentially different formats to deal with, it was necessary to find a Dicom Reader that could accommodate the different formats. The result was that Osirix was chosen for its flexibility and overall versatility of performance. This required the use of an Apple computer as Osirix only works on such a machine.

The Osirix 64-bit programme was chosen part way through the study as being superior in performance to the 32-bit version. This superiority is seen particularly when processing 3D image reconstructions, especially when using the clipping tool, these being functions requiring significant processing power.

2.2 Constraints

2.2.1 Intellectual Property Considerations

Until recently, Intellectual Property rights were rarely considered and CT scans on mummies from museums were performed largely as a result of the 'goodwill' of hospital staff. On many occasions no fee was paid for the service and staff were happy to do the work free and gratis. However, with the increasing concerns of people to 'protect' their interests, the subject of IP rights has to be considered. In some cases, in this study, permission was given to the author to copy the full CT scan data so that analysis could be performed without time constraints (and the possibility of re-examination of the 'raw' data was always possible). However in the case of the Zurich collection, the full data set was made available, but only on site in Zurich – necessitating two visits to the University of Zurich, where full facilities were made available.

In the case of Turin, access to the Dicom files was only permitted on the hospital computers (within a busy department and outside normal working hours when accompanied by a member of staff). Furthermore, image copying was restricted to one image per mummy. For a variety of reasons access to the files was only made available on one occasion – so restricting the number of analyses to three. Further access is currently under discussion, but unlikely to occur within the next twelve months.

2.2.2 Technical Constraints

The CT scans used in this study were acquired over a period of twenty years. This resulted in there being a considerable difference in the quality of images between those acquired in 1992 and those acquired in 2013. This is reflected in the amount of detail available in each case and in the clarity of image.

Further issues were encountered as the result of the radiographic parameters used on various occasions. For example, the slice thickness chosen was not always the thinnest and the file contents were variable, in that on some occasions a file would be of the CT 'run' of the head and neck only, followed by the thorax and so on. On one occasion, this resulted in very small collections of slices making reconstructions (particularly 3D reconstructions) very difficult to the point where they were meaningless.

Images were made available, in the case of Manchester, Liverpool, the British Museum and Zurich (IEM) in the format of either direct access to the files on External Hard Drive or by direct access to the server holding the files.

In other cases, for example some from Turin (for one of the three mummies), that from Ipswich and those from Birmingham, the Dicom files were on CD ROM. The time to download from a CD is considerably longer than from an External Hard Drive – on one occasion forty-five minutes from a CD ROM as opposed to a maximum of five minutes from an External Hard Drive.

Whilst the software within Osirix allowed easy manipulation in three planes and in 3D (and other more sophisticated modes), other Dicom Readers were less flexible and more constrained.

'Single observer errors' may have been reduced by engaging two or more observers. However, the use of other observers would have conflicted with the ethos of author originality in Ph.D. research and engaging observers with the necessary experience could have proved difficult.

2.2.3 Provenance

The provenance of a mummy is taken from the museum records. On some occasions this is incomplete and on others it is open to discussion and question. However, in the absence of any more robust information about a mummy, the records are taken on face value. The museum records are a combination of notes made by curators at the time of donation of the artifact (including correspondence and diary notes from the donors) and subsequent notes made when further information about the mummy became available. There are a few occasions when the mummy has been studied further and any resulting publications are mentioned in the Provenance list immediately below. There are occasions on which the entire provenance is not available and this is reflected most often in the absence of the identity and status of the individual. This has resulted in relating the styles/methods of embalming to status to be possible in only a few cases. Overall provenance is a weak point relating to several mummies but, apart from those mummies donated to museums by the archeologists who discovered them (a minority of mummies in museums except for royal mummies), it is the only source of data available to any and all researchers. The further study of mummies and revision of provenance as and when it happens has been embodied within this volume.

Provenance

I – III – Birmingham

Location and date from museum records. Pers. Comm. Curator, Dr. Phil Watson.

IV – Exeter

Location from museum records. Pers. Comm. Curator, Jenny Durrant. Date from Aidan Dodson - *Catalogue of Egyptian Coffins in Provincial Collections of the United Kingdom*, I: *the South West*. (Dodson, 2014: 8-15).

V and VI (J93.1283, J93.1284) - Sheffield

Location and date from museum records. Pers. Comm. Curator, Helen Harman

VII Tahathor (COLEM 1871.3.7) – Ipswich

Location from diary of George H Errington purchaser and donor (museum records).

Date D25 - from museum records and paper Bennett J., 1967: The symbolism of a mummy case. *Journal of Egyptian Archeology.* 53 P 165-166.

VIII Padiamun (53.72a) – Liverpool

Dated by Taylor J to 8th. Century BC and from Thebes from coffins.

IX Padiamunnebnesuttauwy (M14050) – Liverpool

Location and date from museum records. Pers. Comm. Curator, Dr. Ashley Cooke.

X Nesmin (56.22.79a) – Liverpool

Location and date from museum records. Pers. Comm. Curator, Dr. Ashley Cooke.

XI Padiamun (M14003) – Liverpool

Location and date from museum records. Pers. Comm. Curator, Dr. Ashley Cooke.

XV Unnamed (13.10.11.25) – Liverpool

Date and location from Flinders Petrie who presented the mummy to the museum. Flinders Petrie W M., 1911: Roman Portraits and Memphis (IV). *British School of archeology in Egypt and Egyptian Research Account Seventeenth Year. 1911.* P 1-2 and 14-15.

XVI Unnamed (M13997a) – Liverpool

Location and date from museum records. Pers. Comm. Curator, Dr. Ashley Cooke.

XVII Ankhesenaset (M14000) – Liverpool

Location and date from museum records. Pers. Comm. Curator, Dr. Ashley Cooke.

XVIII Unnamed (M14048) – Liverpool

Location and date from museum records. Pers. Comm. Curator, Dr. Ashley Cooke.

XII, XIII, XIV, XXVII, XXVIII, XLV – IL, LI – LVIII – Manchester

Location and date from museum records. Pers. Comm. Curator, Dr. Campbell Price.

XXIX – XXXV + LIX and LX – British Museum

Dates and locations from museum records. Pers. Comm. Curator, Dr. J Taylor.

XLII, XLIII, XLIV – Egyptian Museum, Turin

Dates and locations from museum records. Pers. Comm. Dr. Matilde Borla, Director of Archeology. Egyptian Museum, Turin. Also data within *'Catalogo Generale dei Musei di Antichita e degli Oggetti d'arte'. 1881. Vol. I. – Piedmonte.* Rome.

L – Perth

Location and dates from. Dr. Campbell Price, Manchester Museum (vs) – Pers. Comm. Also from Museum records in Perth. Pers. Comm. History Officer, Mark Hall, Perth Museum and Art Gallery.

XIX – XXVI, XXXVI – XLI – IEM, Zurich

Dates and locations from IEM records except those shown below as K and S taken from Kuffer and Siegmann (Kuffer, Siegmann, 2007 – pages shown below).

XIX – XXVI and XL - IEM

XXXVI – K and S P152-156

XXXVII – K and S P138-146

XXXVIII – K and S P110-121

XXXIX – K and S P93-99

XLI – K and S P189. Carbon 14 dating to 3BC – 128AD.

2.3 Age at death

The age at death was estimated, in adults, by dental wear and pathology such as loss of teeth and periodontal pathology. It is recognized that this method has limited accuracy. This was combined with skeletal degenerative changes such as osteophyte formation. Loss of joint space was regarded as of no value in view of the probable effects of desiccation. This resulted in the characterization of adult age as being young adult, middle aged or elderly.

In children the age was estimated by a combination of dental eruption and ossific centre appearance and fusion. Data for this was taken from Gray's Anatomy (Johnston, Davies and Davies, 1958: 226-449 and 1371). Occasional cross-references were made to Greulich and Pyle (Greulich and Pyle, 1959). Other methods of age assessment were considered but regarded as unnecessary as a 'forensic' accuracy was not required and the whole method could be criticized in that the estimates are made with reference to modern European or USA children. This resulted in an age for children being given as a range of years probable. If a conflict occurred between the two methods an assessment was made as to the more likely occurrence of the pathology to explain the outlier estimation. For example if there was a dental age of, say, eleven and a bone age of seventeen or more, then the options to explain this phenomenon were either a delay in dental eruption or advanced skeletal age due to a pituitary tumour. In the absence of a pituitary tumour (with expansion of the pituitary fossa) then delayed dental eruption was regarded as the more likely explanation. Discussion with Paediatric Radiologists (Dr. H. Foster and Dr. C. Johnson, Pers. Comm. 2013) confirmed this decision.

It is accepted that both methods of age estimation are vague and of limited accuracy.

2.4 Estimation of sex

Although the sex of the individual was sometimes given in the information on a coffin or other document, this was not taken as a certain fact. Therefore the estimation of the sex of an individual was always attempted. The most obvious marker was the presence of external genitalia. This provided more certainty in the male than the female as the detail of the perineum was sometimes obscured by desiccation. In the case of females, the presence of breasts was rarely seen conclusively or convincingly. However more indirect methods of sex estimation were also used. These included the presence of bold muscle origin and insertion bone markings and the presence of prominent brow ridges and the glabella in males. The shape of the pelvic inlet, the sub-pubic angle and the shape of the sciatic notch were also used as markers.

2.5 Palaeopathology

During the analysis of each mummy, any pathology was noted. However, it was not the intent of this study to record all pathologies. The fact that the cause of death is so frequently not shown is a reflection of the fact that the majority of deaths are reflected in the soft tissues (which are, by definition, distorted by desiccation). Deaths due to infection and cancers without bone metastases will not be shown with any degree of reliability. However, pathologies such as skeletal degenerative disease, fractures and deformities were noted. If possible, the relationship to the time of death was also noted.

2.6 Individual Reports

2.6.1 Principle of Reports

As each CT scan data set became available it was analysed in three planes (axial, sagittal and coronal) and in 3D reconstruction. Whilst the three planes provided the most useful information, 3D reconstruction did allow better evaluation of the dental state and the anatomy of the ribs than planar views. It was also possible to cut away superficial structures such as bandages to allow better visualization of the underlying features.

A unique number was assigned to each report for ease of reference.

Each report was designed to be of maximum value to the museum possessing the mummy and to this end more information was gathered than strictly necessary for this study.

A copy of an unfilled report is given below.

No. - Name Museum - Catalogue Number
General Introduction and description
General
Sex, age, state, other damage, dental status
Regional Review
Head
Cavity, perforation, eyes, mouth, etc.
Neck
Thorax
Abdomen
Pelvis and Hips
Spine

Limbs

Preparation of mummy

Wrapping

Embalming

Cause of death

Conclusion

An example of a completed report is given below.

I The Graeco-Roman Mummy – Birmingham Museum (Cat. No. 1894A15)

This mummy is identified as Graeco-Roman by the style of the wrappings. Little is known about it other than the fact that Mr. Albert Phillips, a local businessman, donated it to Birmingham Museum and Art Gallery in 1894. Unfortunately, there is no associated anthropoid coffin or label to give a more definitive identity. This, unfortunately, means that not only do we not have a name, but we also do not have a precise location of origin. However, on the positive side, the mummy wrappings are intact and there has been no attempt at unwrapping or other interference. The only damage is thermal damage to the front of the legs and this is superficial (see Fig. 2.1).

As nothing was known about the contents of the mummy wrappings, a CT scan was arranged at Stafford Hospital. This took place on 12/12/08 using a Toshiba Aquilion 64 (multi slice scanner). The quantum detectors deliver 64 simultaneously acquired 0.5mm thin slices facilitating isotropic data sets. The software also allows 3D reconstructions to be performed.

General

The body is that of a young adult male. There has been a certain amount of damage to the body, but whether this is pre-mortem or the result of the embalming processes will be discussed later. However, the overall state of the skeleton is extremely good with normal continuity in all places except those mentioned below.

The skull contains 31 teeth (lower right 8 not erupted) – all in good condition. There is no evidence of periodontal pathology, caries or wear (there are well rounded cusps).

This indicates that, whilst the body is that of a mature adult (there is no evidence of open epiphyseal plates), the age is probably not above 30 years – and, maybe younger (see Fig. 2.2).

With regard to the sex of the individual, this is evident from the image of the soft tissues of the genitalia. There is no doubt that this is a male body. (See Fig. 2.3).

Regional Review

Head

A variety of features are found in the head. The first is that there is perforation of the cribriform plate, indicating removal of the brain tissue via the transnasal route. However, it is only the cribriform plate that is perforated

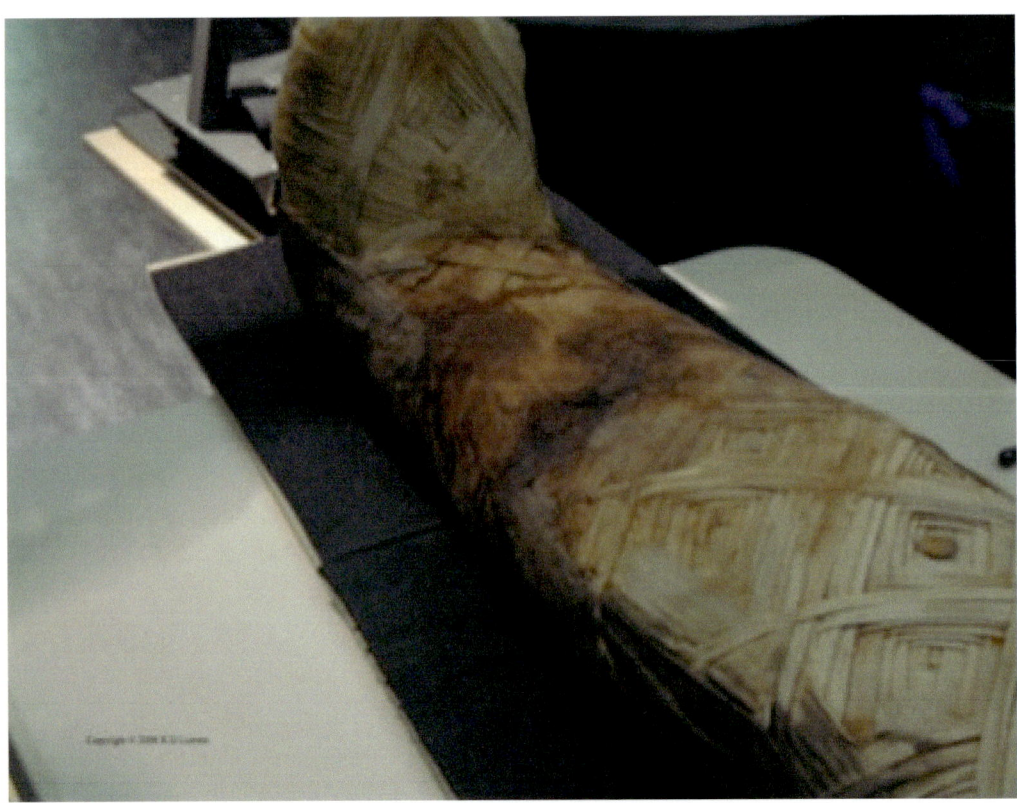

FIG. 2.1 EXTERNAL APPEARANCE OF GRAECO-ROMAN MUMMY – BMAG

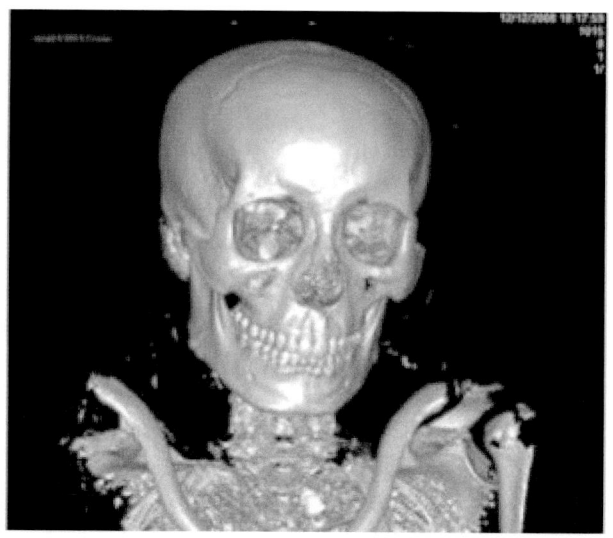

FIG. 2.2 3D RECONSTRUCTION OF SKULL SHOWING THE TEETH IN GRAECO-ROMAN MUMMY

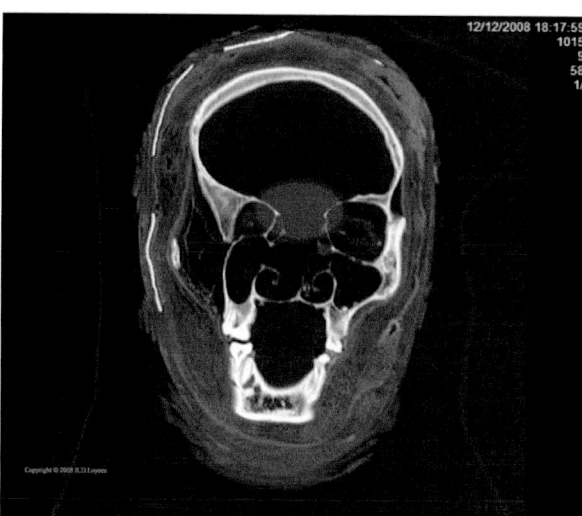

FIG. 2.4 CORONAL VIEW OF SKULL - CRIBRIFORM PLATE PERFORATION

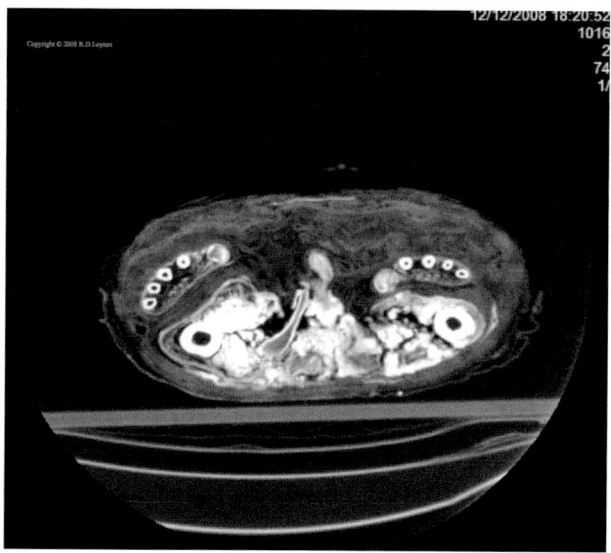

FIG. 2.3 AXIAL VIEW OF MALE GENITALIA IN GRAECO-ROMAN MUMMY

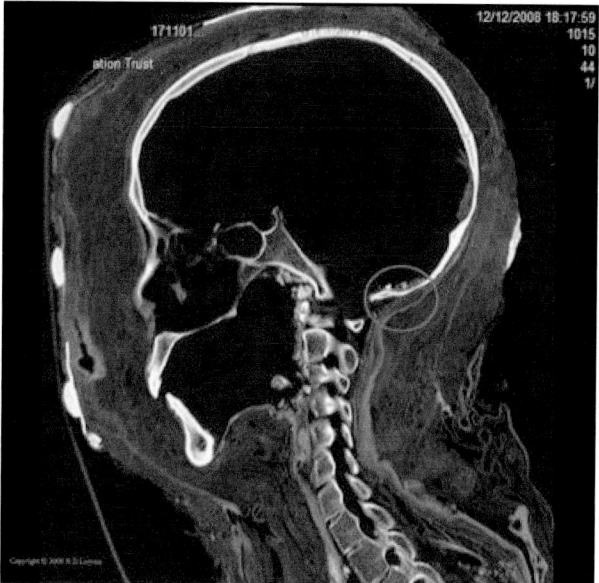

FIG. 2.5 SAGITTAL VIEW OF SKULL SHOWING BRAIN REMNANTS IN POSTERIOR FOSSA

and not the more posterior sphenoid air sinuses indicating that the perforation was made by a more or less vertical strike via the nose. It also indicates that the area of bone removed is in the region of 2.0x1.0cms limiting the access to the cranial cavity by any instrument subsequently used. (See Fig. 2.4)

Furthermore, there is only minimal evidence of any brain tissue. This indicates that the brain removal has been very thorough, perhaps indicating washing out of the cranial cavity with some sort of lytic or caustic material. (See Fig. 2.5).

Examination of the orbits allows visualisation of the remains of the globes of the eyes. These appear to be intact, with evidence of not only the globes but also the optic nerves and muscles. There is even a suggestion of the presence of lenses. There are, however, no 'eye plates' or false eyes in front of the eyes. (See Fig. 2.6).

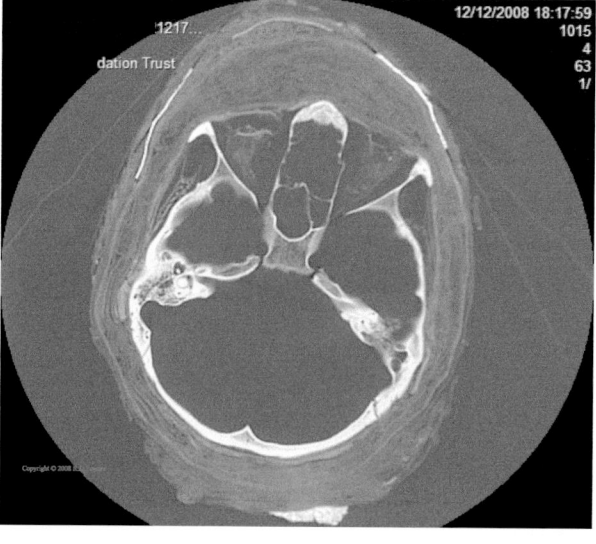

FIG. 2.6 AXIAL VIEW OF SKULL SHOWING OCULAR REMNANTS

Neck

The cervical spine is unremarkable in that there is, unsurprisingly, no evidence of degenerative change or of any injury. For the record there is only minimal tissue within the spinal canal.

The subject of interest in the neck lies at the base of the skull. In this location, close to the right jugular foramen, there are multiple radio-dense objects. These may lie either in the wall of the posterior naso-pharynx or just outside it. The largest of these was found on X-ray, in the past and was interpreted as being a possible arrowhead and was queried as the possible cause of death (Pahor and Cole, 1995: 273-276).

However, with the benefit of more modern imaging, it is possible to see that the object does not really fit the shape of an arrowhead. It is very dense and may be of metal, although this has yet to be proven conclusively. Further analysis in the form of estimating the Hounsfield Unit value of the object/s may help in identifying these objects. (See Fig. 2.7 – 2.10).

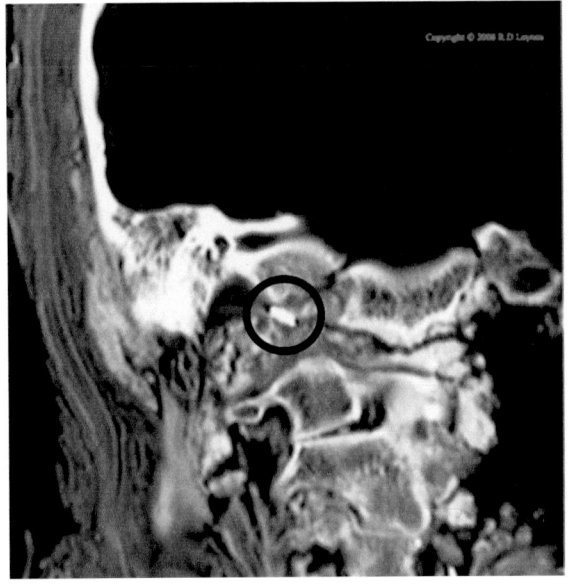

FIG. 2.7 CORONAL VIEW OF SKULL BASE SHOWING FOREIGN BODY.

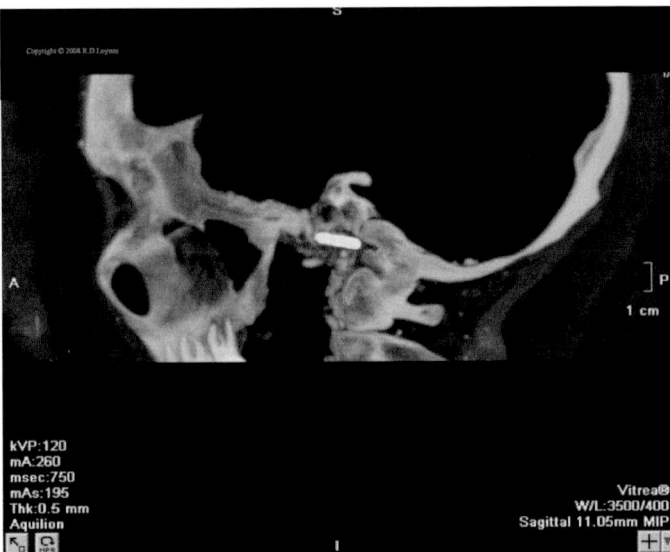

FIG. 2.8 SAGITTAL VIEW OF SKULL BASE SHOWING FOREIGN BODY.

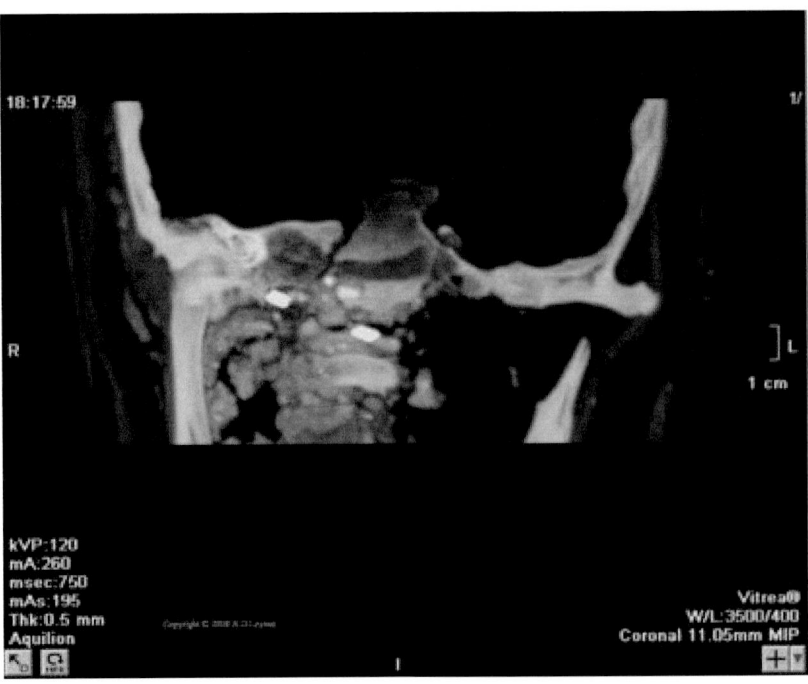

FIG. 2.9 CORONAL VIEW OF SKULL BASE SHOWING MULTIPLE FOREIGN BODIES

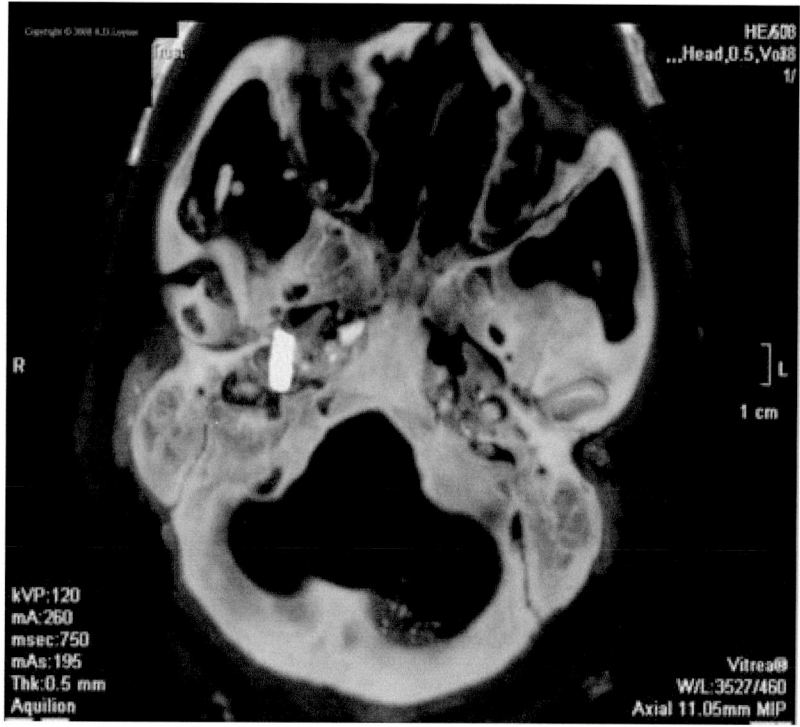

FIG. 2.10 AXIAL VIEW OF SKULL BASE SHOWING MULTIPLE FOREIGN BODIES

The size of the largest object is in the region of 1.0x0.5x0.3cms and, on this more sophisticated investigation, there are found to be at least 3 other objects that are smaller.

Being so deeply embedded at the base of the skull begs the question as to how they got there! Were they introduced during the process of embalming or were they introduced before death? The likelihood of these being part of some sort of weapon is very small. There is no evidence of any bony damage locally. Therefore, there is a high likelihood of the introduction being via the pharynx at the time of mummification. It is not known why this happened.

Thorax

There is some subluxation of both shoulder joints. The tight bandaging towards the end of the mummification process could well have caused this. There is no evidence of incisions around the shoulders (as will be described

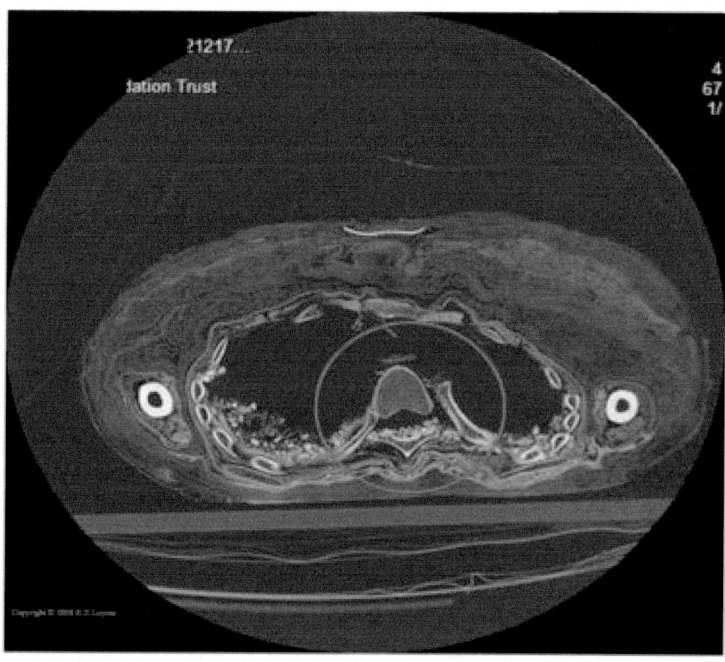

FIG. 2.11 AXIAL VIEW OF MID THORACIC REGION - COSTO-VERTEBRAL DISLOCATION

later in relation to the hips). The thoracic cage and cavity both show interesting features. The thoracic cage comprising of the ribs, spine, sternum and costo-vertebral junctions, shows significant asymmetry. This is the result of posterior dislocation of the left 6th to 10th ribs inclusive and subluxation of the left 4th and 5th ribs. There is also dislocation of the right 8th, 9th and 10th ribs, all at the costo-vertebral joints. Finally there are dislocations of the left 2nd, 3rd and 4th costo-chondral junctions. (See Fig. 2.11 and 2.12).

There is, however, no evidence of <u>bony</u> damage associated with these dislocations/subluxations. It takes a significant force to cause dislocations of the costo-vertebral joints and it would be very unlikely to happen, as the result of trauma, in the absence of bony damage. It seems more likely, therefore, that the damage to the costo-vertebral joints took place after death, i.e. during the mummification process. This could be achieved by dissecting the costo-vertebral joints from the inside of the thoracic cavity, accessed from the incision in the abdomen. However, the necessary 'surgery' to divide

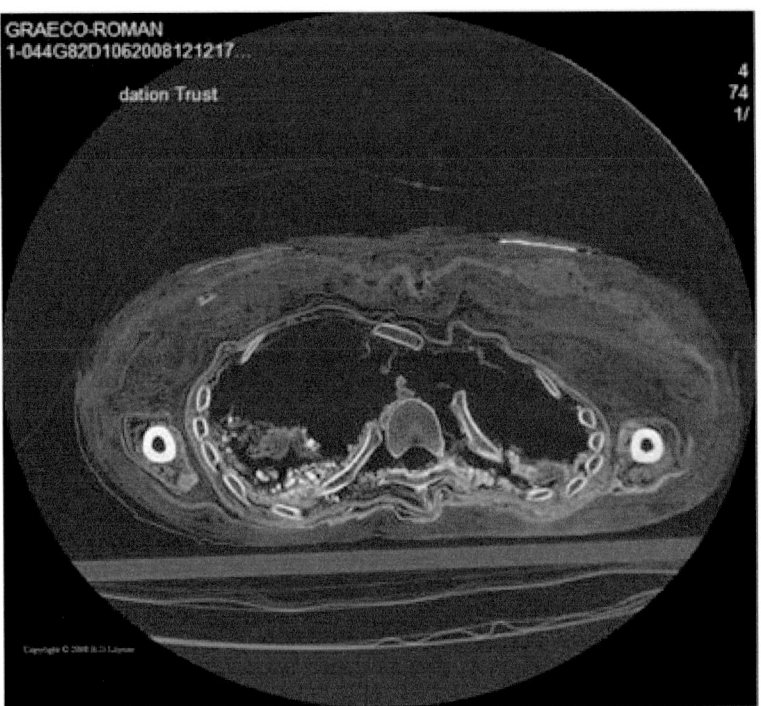

FIG. 2.12 AXIAL VIEW OF MID THORACIC REGION - COSTO-VERTEBRAL DISLOCATION

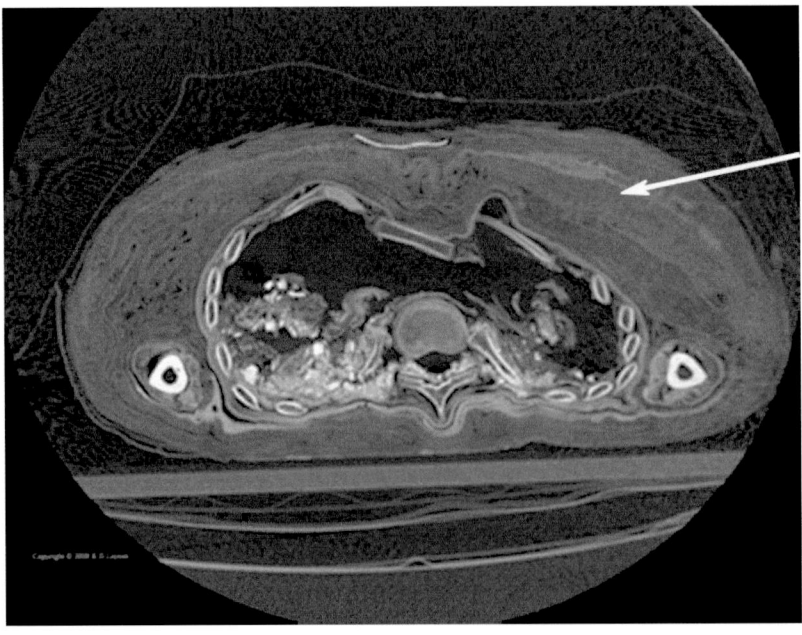

FIG. 2.13 AXIAL VIEW OF THORAX SHOWING ASYMMETRY WITH ANTERIOR PADDING ON LEFT

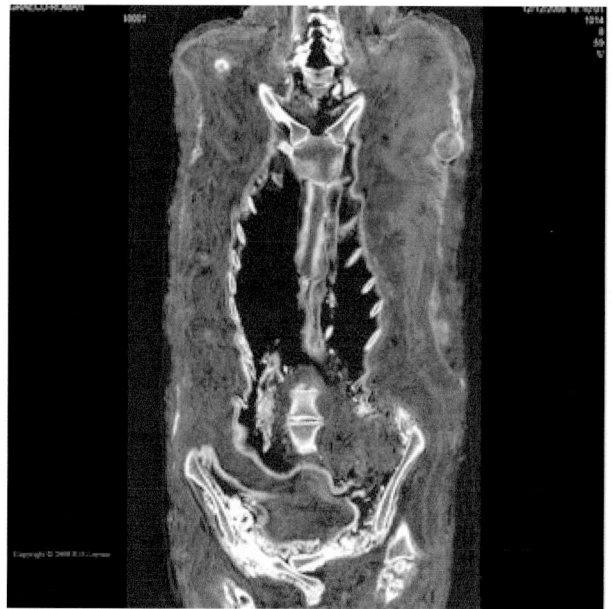

FIG. 2.14 CORONAL VIEW OF THORAX SHOWING CHEST ASYMMETRY WITH ANTERIOR PADDING ON LEFT

Why this was performed remains a matter of conjecture, but it is noticeable that the afore-mentioned dislocations are accompanied by an attempt at compression of the left rib cage, making the thorax somewhat smaller. Unfortunately, this has resulted in asymmetry that has been corrected in the final form of the mummy by padding out the resultant defect! (See Figs. 2.13 and 2.14).

The thoracic cavity itself is loosely 'filled' with a mixture of granular material and body tissues – probably bowel (certainly the appearance is tubular). The granular material is of varying density with both high and low radio-dense constituents. The cavity contains only a modest amount of material with more on the right than the left side. There is no evidence of layers of material or of fluid levels, such as might be associated with the use of resin. (See Fig. 2.15).

There is no evidence of the diaphragm remaining and presumably it was removed during the evisceration process, allowing easier access. There is little convincing evidence of the presence of the heart.

the costo-transverse ligaments (following disruption of the costo-vertebral joints) to allow this degree of movement of the ribs, would be extremely difficult to perform blind with access only through the abdomen! To re-enforce the concept of a trans-abdominal/thoracic approach it is noted that there is no convincing evidence of an incision through the skin of the posterior wall of the thorax. There is a continuous extension of the granular material from the thoracic cavity to the para-vertebral and sub-scapular spaces on the left side (opposite the dislocated ribs) and to a lesser extent on the right side.

Abdomen

The anterior abdominal wall contains an incision in the left side. This runs from the upper abdomen laterally to the lower abdomen in the region of the Symphysis Pubis in or near the mid line. The incision has not been closed and there is evidence of the material used for wrapping crossing from the outside to the inside of the abdomen through this incision. (See Fig. 2.16).

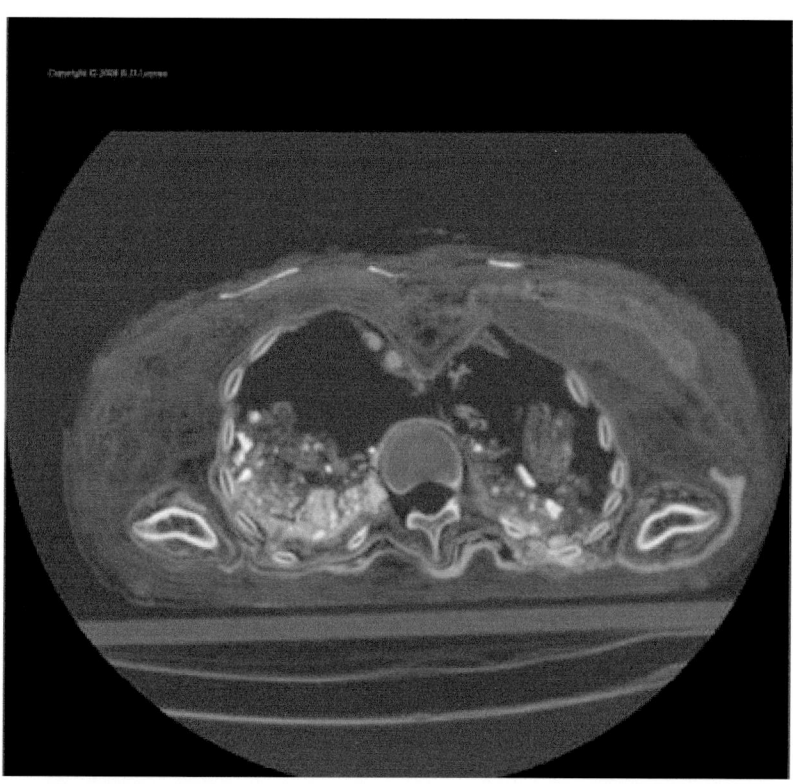

FIG. 2.15 AXIAL VIEW OF THORAX SHOWING THORACIC CONTENTS

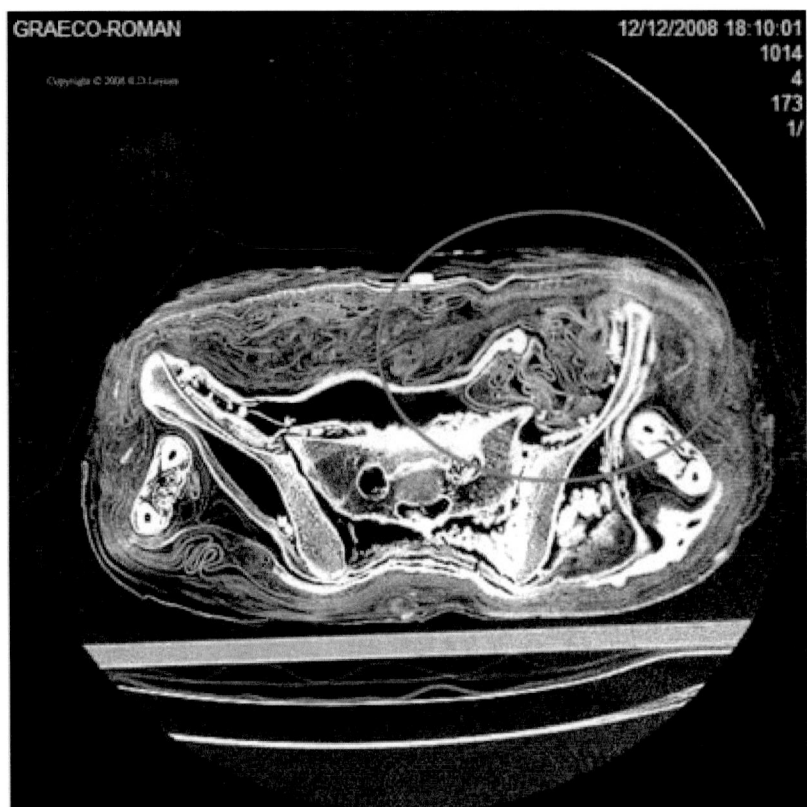

FIG. 2.16 AXIAL VIEW OF ABDOMEN - LEFT FLANK INCISION

The abdominal cavity contains a mixture of granular, radio-dense material similar to that seen in the thorax (presumably 'mummification material' - packing) and material that appears tubular and is therefore likely to be human tissue such as bowel. As in the thorax, the abdomen is loosely packed. There is also a significant amount of material (possibly linen) within the thoracic/ abdominal cavity that is in continuity with that passing through the abdominal embalming incision. Finally, there is the presence, in the trunk cavity, of two packages that might

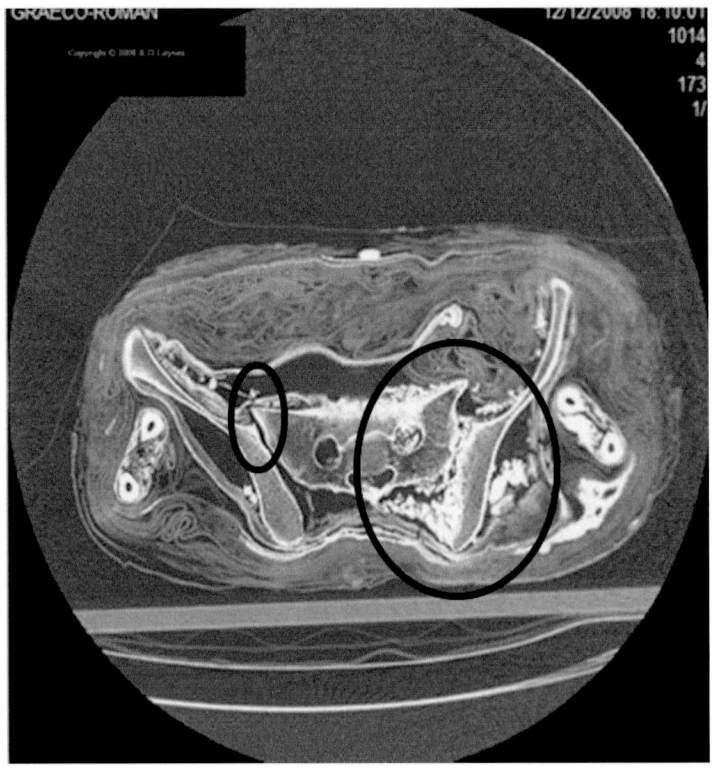

FIG. 2.17 AXIAL VIEW OF PELVIS - SACRO-ILIAC JOINT DISRUPTION

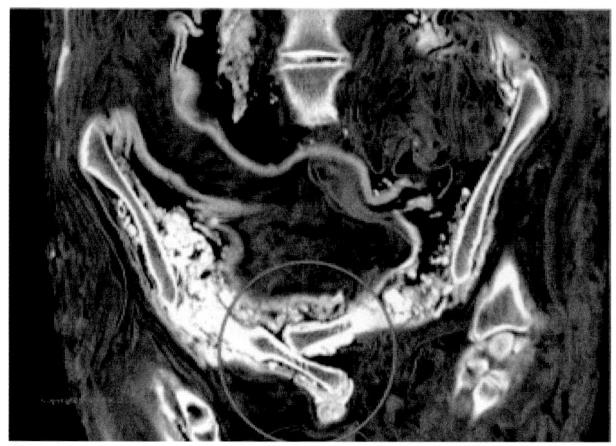

FIG. 2.18 CORONAL VIEW OF PELVIS - PUBIC SYMPHYSIS DISRUPTION

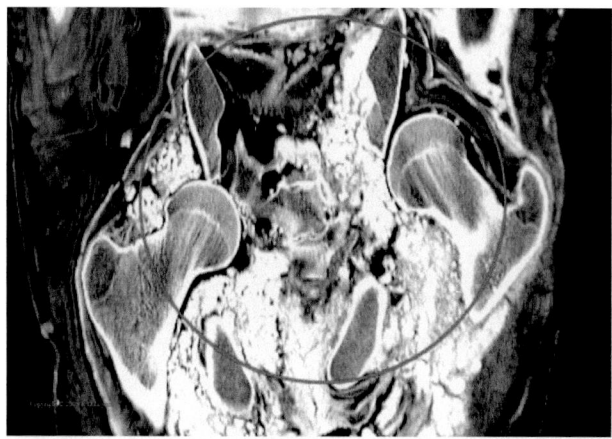

FIG. 2.19 CORONAL VIEW OF PELVIS - BILATERAL HIP DISLOCATION

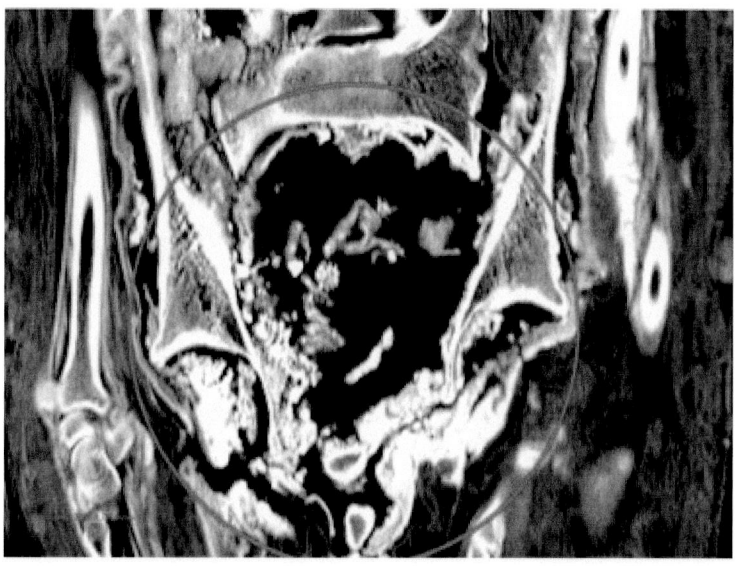

FIG. 2.20 CORONAL VIEW OF PELVIS - BILATERAL HIP DISLOCATION

represent canopic packages (although there are usually four of these, it can be conjectured that the other two may have disintegrated and not be readily visible as entities).

Pelvis and Hips

There is evidence of significant damage to both the left sacro-iliac joint (SIJ) and to both hips. The right SIJ is also abnormal but not to the same extent as on the left side and these latter appearances may be the result of either slight movement after wrapping or traumatic subluxation before or after death (See Fig. 2.17).

The left SIJ is completely disrupted and there is evidence of radio-dense 'mummification' material within the gap, indicating that the damage occurred prior to the final packing of the body cavity. Whilst the right SIJ is abnormal, the displacement is mild and there is no evidence of 'foreign' material within the joint.

The pubic symphysis is also completely disrupted, with overlapping of the pubic rami. (See Fig. 2.18).

However, in conjunction with these major pelvic disruptions, there is bilateral dislocation of the hips with postero-superior displacement. Despite these very severe disruptions of both the pelvic ring and the hip joints, there is no evidence of a fracture in the vicinity! Under these circumstances, it is considered highly unlikely that this extensive damage to the skeleton is all traumatic, i.e. accidental, in origin (see Fig. 2.19 and 2.20).

As can be seen from Fig. 2.20, there is granular material in both hip joints, lying within the acetabular cavities. This, again, would indicate that the disruption of these joints occurred prior to wrapping of the body.

Further, there is evidence of incisions anterior to both hip joints (see Fig. 2.21 and 2.22).

The implications of all this evidence will be discussed later.

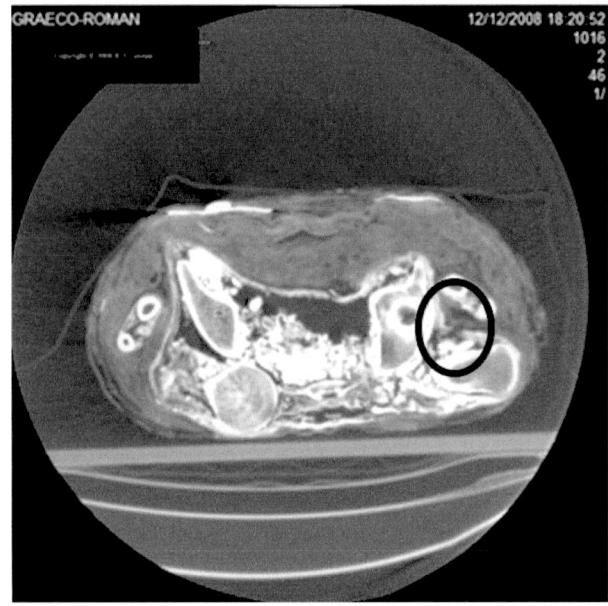
FIG. 2.21 AXIAL VIEW OF PELVIS - INCISION ANTERIOR TO LEFT HIP

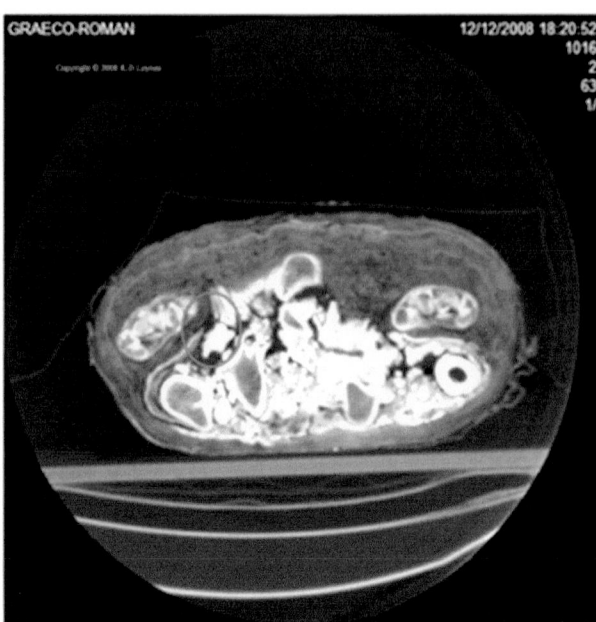
FIG. 2.22 AXIAL VIEW OF PELVIS - INCISION ANTERIOR TO RIGHT HIP

Spine

Examination of the spine shows no evidence of degenerative change. This accords well with the previously stated opinion that this mummy is that of a young man. However, it must also be added that there is no evidence of traumatic abnormality in the spine but material is seen within the spinal canal – presumably the remains of the spinal cord.

Limbs

The upper and lower limbs are well visualised and show no evidence of pathology. The level of general detail that is available is demonstrated by the clear visualisation of the flexor tendons and bony details at the wrist. The arms lie beside the body with the hands over the front of the hips (see Fig. 2.23).

Preparation of the Mummy

Wrapping

The wrappings of the body are well visualised but do not show any unexpected characteristics. There do not appear to be any objects such as amulets or jewellery within the bandages. Evidence of striation within the material used is present. There is a diagonal distribution of bandaging across the shoulders akin to stoles used in some mummies.

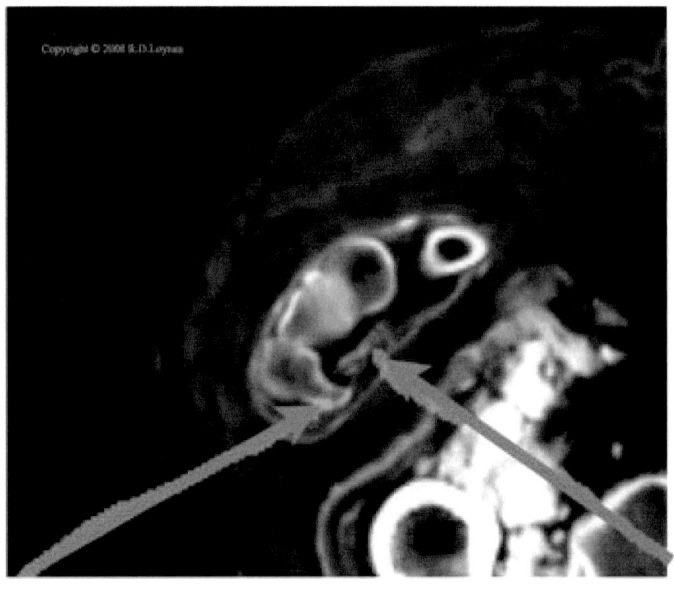
FIG. 2.23 AXIAL VIEW DEMONSTRATING DETAIL OF RIGHT WRIST

METHODS

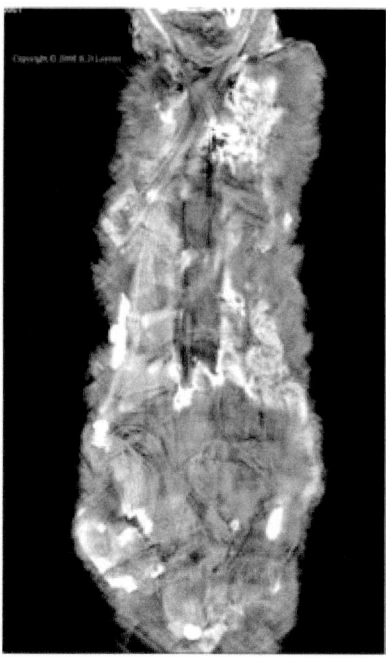

FIG. 2.24 CORONAL VIEW ILLUSTRATING DETAIL OF ANTERIOR WRAPPINGS

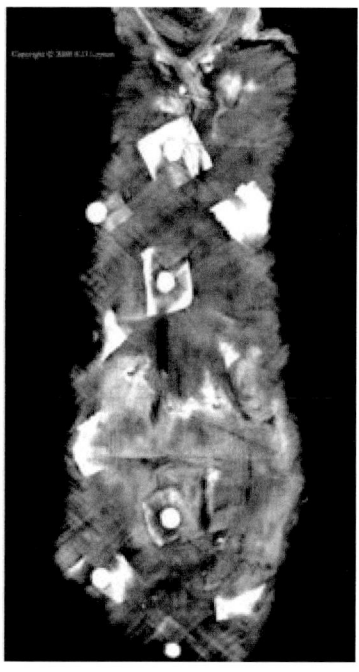

FIG. 2.25 CORONAL VIEW ILLUSTRATING TERRACOTTA STUDS

(Taylor, 2004:33) (See Fig. 2.24). The arms are individually wrapped prior to being bandaged with the trunk. The legs are, likewise, wrapped separately before being bound together.

The position of the arms is noted to be at the sides, with the hands overlying the front of the hips, but with the forearms lying behind the pelvis. Finally, there are gilded terracotta studs attached to metal sheets within the superficial bandages (see Fig. 2.25).

Embalming

The excerebration process seems to have been performed in the accepted conventional way, with removal of the brain through the nose (via the cribriform plate). This was carried out through a limited opening, although this did not prevent virtually complete removal of the tissue.

The internal organs have been removed through an incision in the left flank and appear to have been returned to the body cavity via the same route, presumably after desiccation. The body cavity has then been packed in a peremptory fashion with further material of unknown origin but of a radio-dense and granular nature. It may or may not be possible to identify this material by reference to Hounsfield Units in the future and further investigation along these lines is recommended.

The curious feature of this mummy is the apparently deliberate dismemberment of parts of the skeleton. In the first place, the left rib cage has been deformed by dislocation of several ribs posteriorly. It is difficult to find any reference in the medical literature to such an 'injury' being caused by trauma. Furthermore it would (in the experience of the author) require a very significant force to cause such a type of damage and it is difficult to imagine such a force not also causing fractures to the adjacent ribs and / or spine.

However, to cause a posterior dislocation at the costo-vertebral joints would require division of the soft tissues (capsule and ligaments) of the costo-vertebral joints themselves and, quite probably, the costo-transverse ligaments. This, in turn, would require a detailed knowledge of the anatomy of the part and a significant dexterity to carry out such 'surgery' blind (i.e. by palpation) from an incision in the abdomen. It is open to conjecture as to whether this was an experiment in an attempt to make the rib cage smaller for some reason (possibly commercial) but that it failed because access to the right side was too difficult to allow performance of the same procedure to any great and useful extent. This would explain the abandonment of the procedure and the subsequent packing out of the chest externally to make the finished mummy symmetrical.

In the case of the pelvis and hip joint mutilation, there is a unique combination of abnormalities. It is recognised that, as the result of trauma, there is a possibility of bilateral hip dislocation or of disruption of the pelvic ring in two places, but both of these unusual combinations occurring at the same time is unheard of and mechanically inexplicable. The reason for this is that once either the hip joint restraining structures or the pelvic joint ligaments have been 'overcome', it is not possible for the forces to continue acting in a manner to cause such damage to the other structure/s. This fact, combined with the presence of 'mummification' material at these sites, would indicate that these 'injuries' probably occurred at the time of embalming. This possibility is further supported by the presence of incisions over the anterior aspect of both hips. However, even after the incision is made, it requires a sophisticated knowledge of anatomy and special instruments to effect the dislocation of the hips. The anterior capsule of the hip joint, which is itself 2 or 3 mms thick, would have to be incised and an instrument inserted to perform the dislocation as illustrated in Figs. 2.26 – 2.28. The instrument used in this illustration is a Murphy's skid, which is used to the present day during surgery to dislocate joints such as the hip and shoulder.

Cause of Death

There is no obvious certain cause of death demonstrated within these findings. Although, if either the damage to the hip joints, or more likely the damage to the pelvic ring were to have occurred pre-mortem, the level of violence required could well have caused major internal haemorrhage. In the days before blood transfusion this alone could have caused death.

Conclusion

This mummy is that of a young male adult who has no evidence of ill health. There is evidence of extensive skeletal damage. It is likely that the process of mummification would have caused most of this. There is the presence of metallic (almost certainly) objects in the neck at the base of the skull (probably within or just outside the wall of the naso-pharynx). There is little evidence that these represent the remains of a weapon as previously surmised, but how they got there is at present a mystery. It is possible that they were introduced at the time of mummification. One is left, therefore, with the remaining possibility that death was secondary to a major pelvic injury – such as is seen in a crushing/ very severe twisting injury of the pelvis.

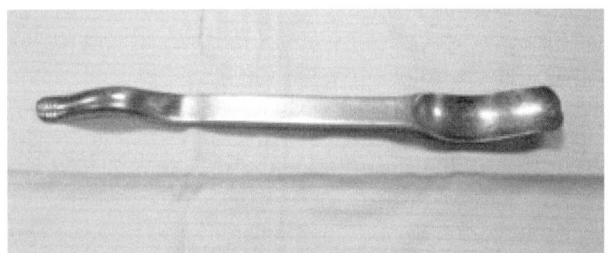

FIG. 2.26 MURPHY'S SKID

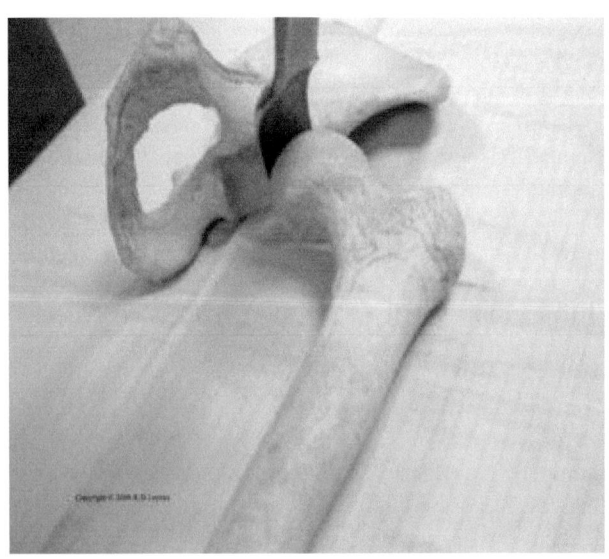

FIG. 2.27 POSSIBLE METHOD OF DISLOCATION. STAGE 1

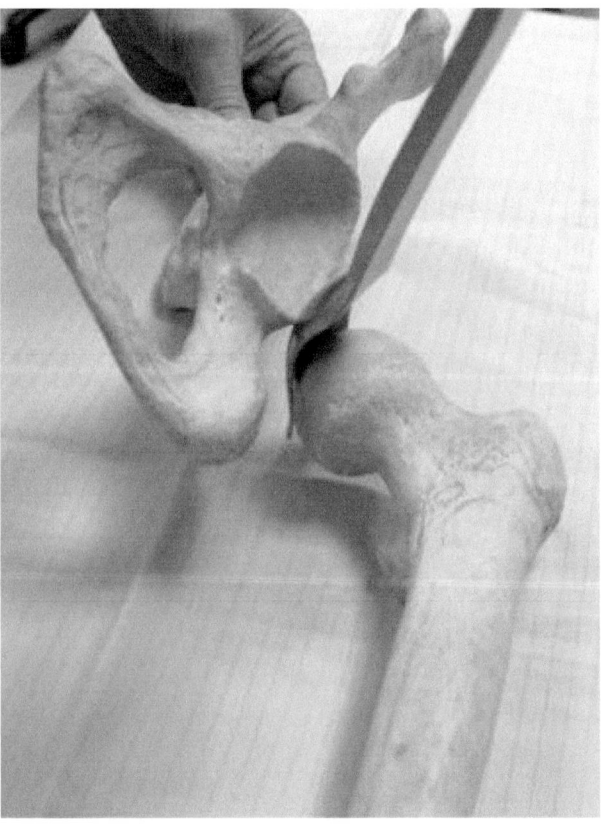

FIG. 2.28 POSSIBLE METHOD OF DISLOCATION. STAGE 2

Chapter Three

Results – General

A total of sixty individual reports have been prepared. However, of these one is of X-rays of a mummy in Exeter and will be used in the next section to illustrate the constraints of this method of investigation when compared with the data afforded by modern CT scans.

Of the remaining fifty nine scans, two were available only in analogue form and, therefore, analysis was restricted to viewing 'thumbnail' images of axial views without the opportunity to 'reconstruct' images in other planes or in 3D.

Fifty-seven CT image data sets are in digital format.

3.1 Comparison of Xrays, Older CT scans and Modern CT scans (digital format)

3.1.1 X-ray of Exeter Mummy (Shepenmut – Cat. No. 11/3)

The information on this mummy from the plain X-rays is so sparse that the following report contains only a small amount of information – but all that was available.

IV Shepenmut – Exeter Mummy (Museum Catalogue No:11/3)

This mummy lies within a cartonnage case that has previously been opened to allow examination and investigation. The cartonnage was then resealed and the mummy is not, currently, available for examination. Museum records show that it is the body of Shepenmut, a priestess in the temple of Amun Re at Thebes in or around 800 BC. That is during the Third Intermediate Period - probably Dynasty 22. The mummy was donated by a Mr. West of Exeter in 1897. In the early 1960s the mummy was X-rayed and subsequently underwent examination by the curator, Mr. Adams. This examination in 1965/66 included an 'operation' to remove part of the spine. This was performed because a likely diagnosis of ochronosis was made radiologically. The spine, once removed, was send to a Professor Dent in London for analysis. Unfortunately, there is no record of the results of this investigation – if it ever took place! Mr. Adams described the whole procedure in 1990 (Adams, 1990: 9-19).

General

Unfortunately, the only images are X-rays and their quality is barely average. Whilst the skull is seen, it is not possible to determine whether or not the cribriform plate was perforated. It is also impossible to determine the state of the teeth other than the fact that they are present. The long bone epiphyses are fused indicating that this is an adult. The pelvis shows a wide sub-pubic angle and a round pelvic brim, indicating that it is that of a female. There are canopic packages within the body cavity. The hands are seen overlying the hip area.

Unfortunately, there is little more that can be extracted from the X-rays other than the presence of mild arthritic change. The mummy itself was returned to the cartonnage case, which was then sealed so preventing further direct examination.

As can be seen the information on mummification technique is virtually absent with no evidence relating to excerebration or evisceration methods. The only information of value is that there are two canopic packages within the torso.

3.1.2 Older Generation CT scans of Nesitanebetasheru and Djedma'atiuesankh in Sheffield Museum

Both reports follow to illustrate the level of information available in analogue Dicom files.

V Nesitanebetasheru – Sheffield Museum (Cat. No. J93.1283)

This mummy consists of a wrapped body sealed inside a cartonnage case and placed within a wooden anthropomorphic coffin. The museum records indicate that the body is that of a middle aged female from Dynasty 25 and from Thebes. The mummy was acquired in 1858 by a Mr. Bateman and incorporated into his collection. It was, subsequently, bought for the Sheffield Museum collection.

The mummy was CT scanned on 7/7/92 and the resulting images are available as thumbnails on X-ray film. It was also X-rayed on 29/6/92. The CT scan was performed on a Siemens Somatom CR machine.

General

The body is that of an adult female as shown by the pelvic shape. The epiphyses are closed.

Regional Review

Head

Excerebration has been carried out via the trans-nasal route. There is no evidence of residual brain material in the cranial cavity. However, there are 'levels' of radio-opaque material in the posterior part of the cavity – almost certainly due to the introduction of resin. The double level indicates preservation of the falx cerebri or falx cerebella. There is also evidence of the meninges having been retained (see Fig. 3.1).

Fig. 3.1 also shows perforation of the cribriform plate, but with retention of some of the structures of the nasal cavity and ethmoid and sphenoid air sinuses.

Whilst the images are not absolutely clear, there is good evidence of the treatment of the eyes. They appear to have been opened, packed with linen and covered at the front with eye plates (see Fig. 3.1). The teeth are fully erupted with a full set of 32 teeth present. The quality of the images precludes an assessment of their wear. The oral cavity contains linen packing along with some granular material at the back of the naso-pharynx and the oro-pharynx. On the right side of the head, level with the bottom of the chin there is a metallic object that could well be a displaced ear ring (see Fig. 3.2). There is also a metallic object lying in front of the bridge of the nose, within the wrappings. Its nature is unknown.

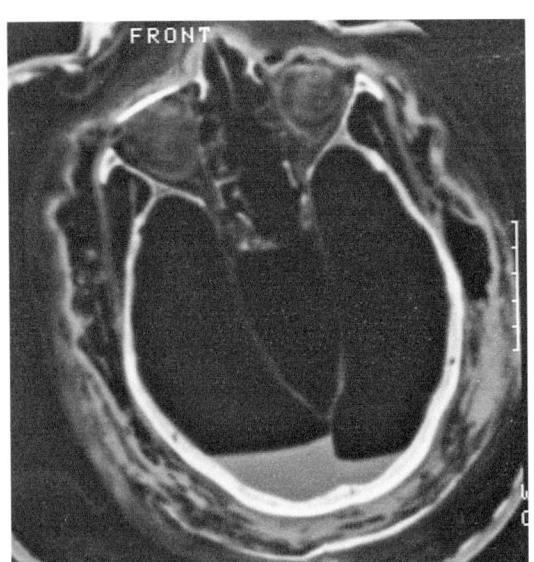

FIG. 3.1 Axial view of skull showing resin levels

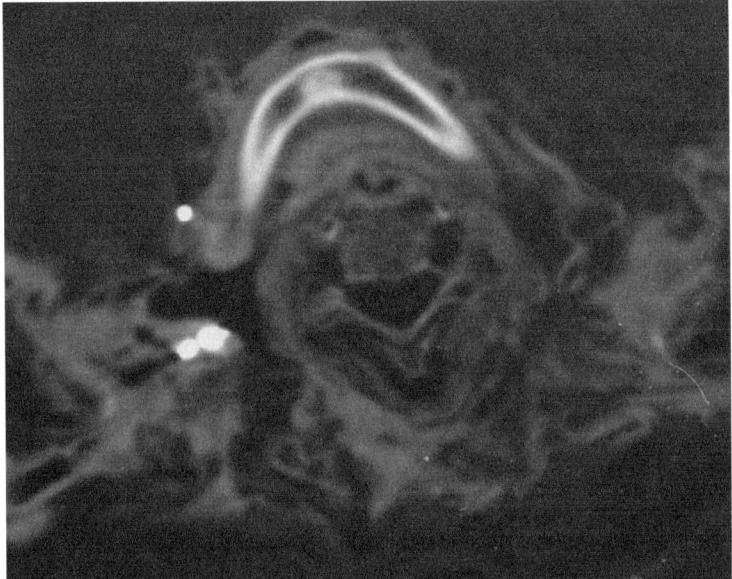

FIG. 3.2 Axial view at level of mandible showing ear ring

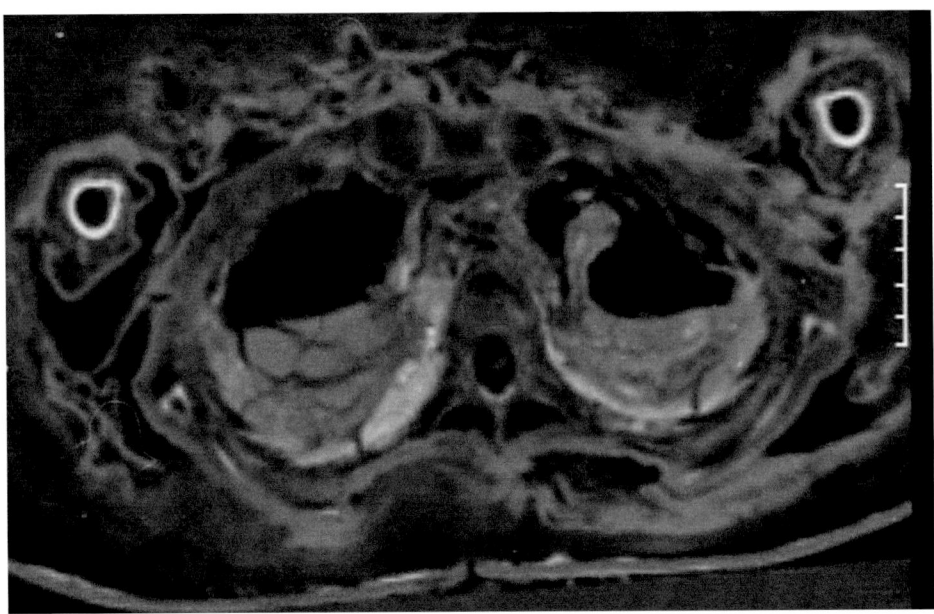

FIG. 3.3 Axial view showing thoracic packing

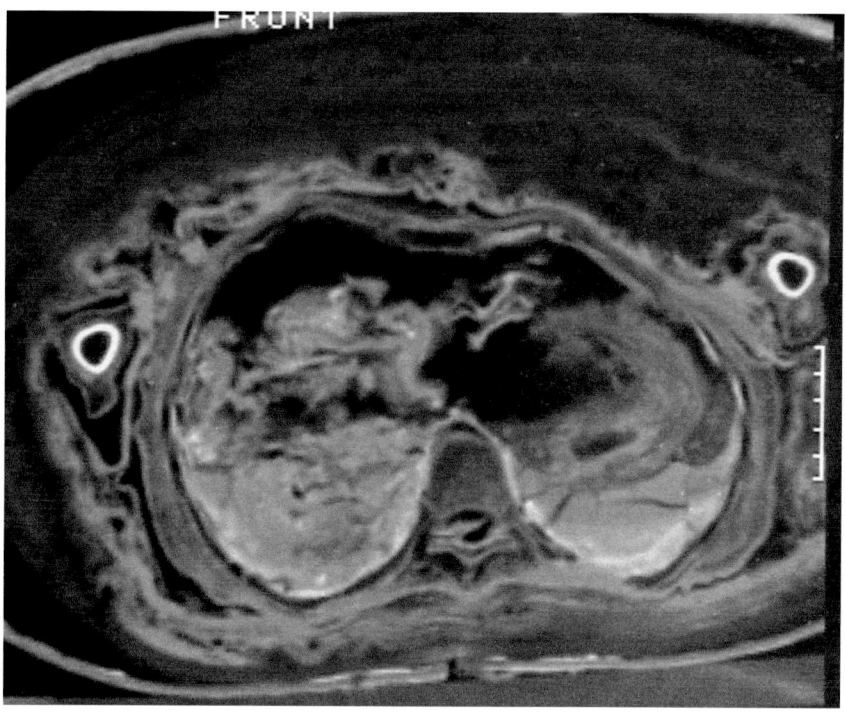

FIG. 3.4 AXIAL VIEW - ASYMMETRY OF THORACIC WALL AND EXTERIOR PACKING.

Neck

The available axial images do not show any unusual features in the neck. The state of the facet (apophyseal or zygapophyseal) joints is impossible to determine. There is evidence of material within the spinal canal, probably meninges.

Thorax

The thoracic cavity is asymmetrical in its upper part with a layer of granular material lying at the back with a fluid level. However, this material has cracked in several places. The asymmetry has resulted in asymmetrical bandaging, with different styles of packing outside the chest wall on each side. There is no evidence of abnormality of the costo-vertebral joints (see Fig. 3.3. and 3.4) or retention of the mediastinal structures.

The viscera have been returned to the body cavity in a somewhat somewhat random fashion but there is a suggestion of packages seen in one image (see Fig. 3.5).

Abdomen

There is only one axial image of the abdomen. This does not confirm an abdominal incision (nor refute one). The forearms are seen lying on the anterior abdominal wall.

Pelvis and Hips

The images are not clear enough to determine the state of the hip joints with regard to arthritis, but the joints appear to be congruous.

Spine

This is not shown in sufficient detail to draw any conclusions.

Limbs

The arms appear to be normal, in the limited views available. The knee joints are shown in X-rays. There is no evidence of arthritis in the available views.

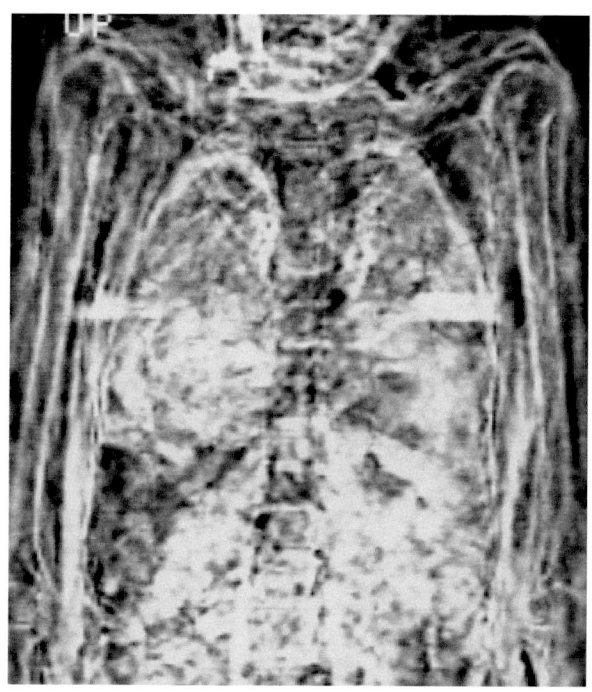

FIG. 3.5 CORONAL VIEW OF THORAX - POSSIBLE CANOPIC PACKAGES

Preparation of the mummy

Embalming

Excerebration has been performed and material, almost certainly resin, introduced into the cranial cavity. The eyes have been packed with linen and plates inserted in front of the globes. Granular material and linen strips have been introduced into the mouth.

Although there is no direct evidence of an abdominal incision, there is granular material in the body cavity, implying that there is an incision somewhere (the perineum is not clearly visualized). The viscera have been returned to the body cavity.

Wrapping appears to be intact but there is asymmetry of the interior packing beneath the outer bandages in the chest area.

VI Djedma'atiuesankh – Sheffield Museum (Cat. No. J93.1284)

This mummy consists of a wrapped body inside a wooden anthropomorphic coffin. The museum records indicate that the body is that of a teenage female from the Dynasty 26 and from Thebes. The mummy was acquired in 1854 by a Mr. Bateman and incorporated into his collection. It was, subsequently, bought for the Sheffield Museum collection.

The mummy was CT scanned on 16/3/92 and the resulting images are available as thumbnails on X-ray film. It was also X-rayed in March 1992. The CT scan was performed on a Siemens Somatom CR machine.

General

The body is that of a child. There are 12 teeth in each jaw, indicating an age of approximately 12 to 13 years (Johnson / Davies / Davies. 1958 : 1371). The only epiphyses clearly shown in the CT scans are those of the ischial tuberosities, but others are visible in the lower limbs in the X-rays. In these X-rays, the tibial epiphyses are shown clearly and are not fused. The tibial tuberosity epiphyses are not shown convincingly, but the views available do not exclude their presence. The elbows are not shown sufficiently clearly in the CT scans to allow assessment of the epiphyses to indicate the age of the child. The presence of the ischial tuberosity epiphyses indicates an age of 13 to 16 years (Scheuer and Black, 2000: 365) (see Fig. 3.6).

There is inadequate imaging of the pelvis or skull to allow an indication of the sex of the individual.

Regional Review

Head

There is evidence of perforation of the cribriform plate and removal of most of the brain with some residual brain tissue in the back of the cranial cavity (see Figs. 3.7 and 3.8).

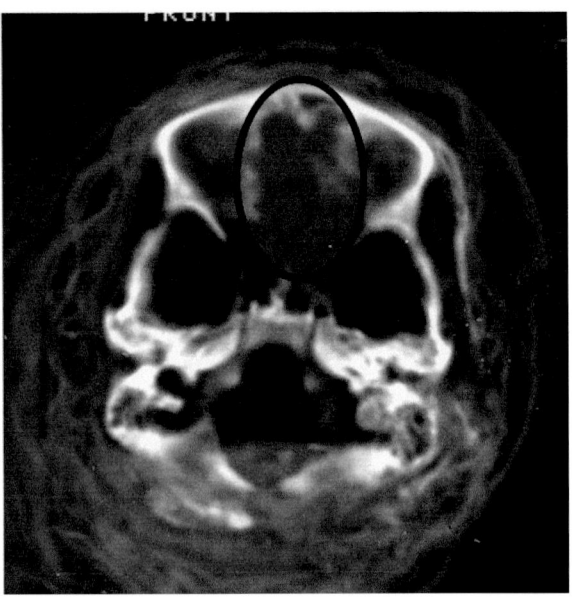

FIG. 3.7 AXIAL VIEW OF SKULL DEMONSTRATING PERFORATION OF THE CRIBRIFORM PLATE

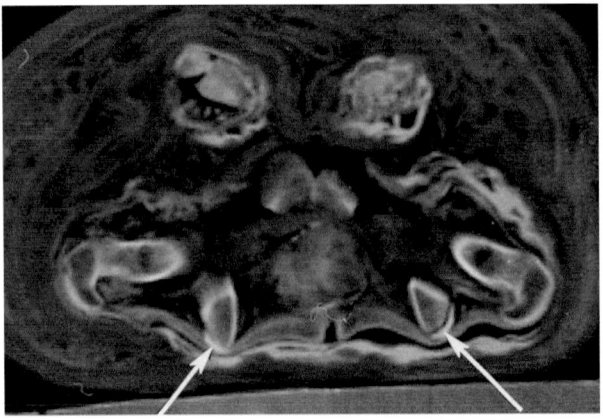

FIG. 3.6 AXIAL VIEW OF PELVIS - ISCHIAL TUBEROSITY EPIPHYSES.

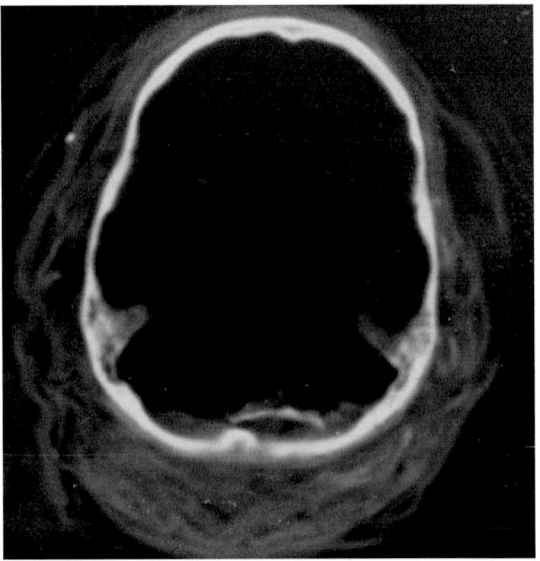

FIG. 3.8 AXIAL VIEW OF SKULL SHOWING BRAIN MATERIAL IN POSTERIOR CRANIAL CAVITY.

The eyes have been retained. They are only shown on one image, which is slightly blurred. It is not possible to be certain, but the eyes appear to have been packed. There are no eye plates. The CT scans demonstrate opaque material in the posterior aspect of the maxillary sinuses.

Neck

Not clearly visualised.

Thorax

The thorax is symmetrical and the wall intact. The midline structures are preserved throughout the thoracic cavity, indicating that the mediastinum has been retained (probably including the heart). The two thoracic cavities are filled completely with amorphous material containing cracks (see Fig. 3.9).

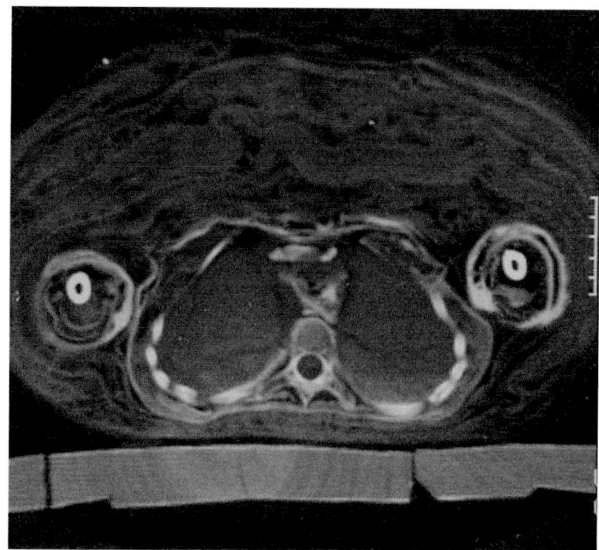

FIG. 3.9 AXIAL VIEW OF THORAX SHOWING THE MEDIASTINUM.

Abdomen

There is an incision in the left flank that has not been closed. The abdominal cavity is filled with the same amorphous material as in the thorax. The anterior abdominal wall is flattened. Linen material is seen crossing through the incision into the abdominal cavity. The viscera have not been returned to the thoracic or abdominal cavity (see Figs. 3.9 and 3.10).

Pelvis and Hips

There is no evidence of pelvic damage, the sacro-iliac joints and symphysis pubis being intact. The hips are also congruous. The upper femoral epiphysis is seen on the right side. Within the pelvic cavity, there are two types of filling. What this represents is uncertain. The demonstrated extent is only 6 cms but the pelvis is not fully shown. The material other than the amorphous matter is regular and round in cross section. It may be a package of viscera or a packed rectum (see Fig.3.11).

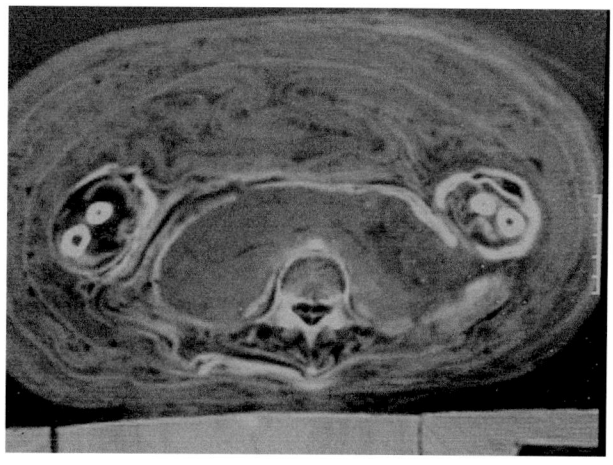

FIG. 3.10 AXIAL VIEW OF THE ABDOMEN SHOWING PACKING.

Spine

The spine is unremarkable. Some images do show material within the spinal canal, which is, presumably, spinal cord and meningeal remnants.

Limbs

The upper and lower limbs are normal.

Preparation of mummy

Wrapping

The limbs are initially wrapped separately and then enclosed in the outer bandaging which is regular and bulky enough to double the size of the body. There are radio-opaque objects on the front of the mummy just under the outer layers of bandages (see Fig. 3.12).

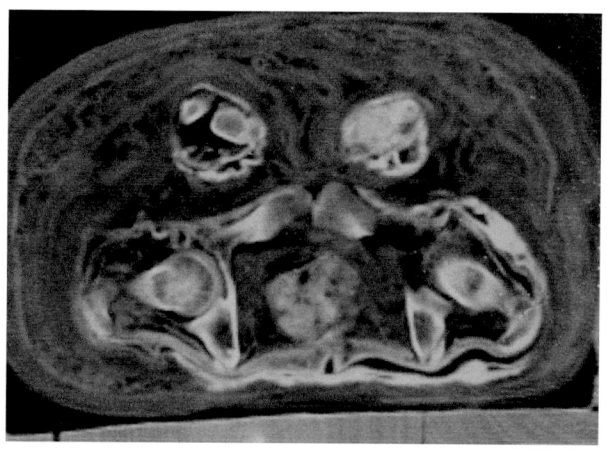

FIG. 3.11 AXIAL VIEW OF PELVIS AND CONTENTS.

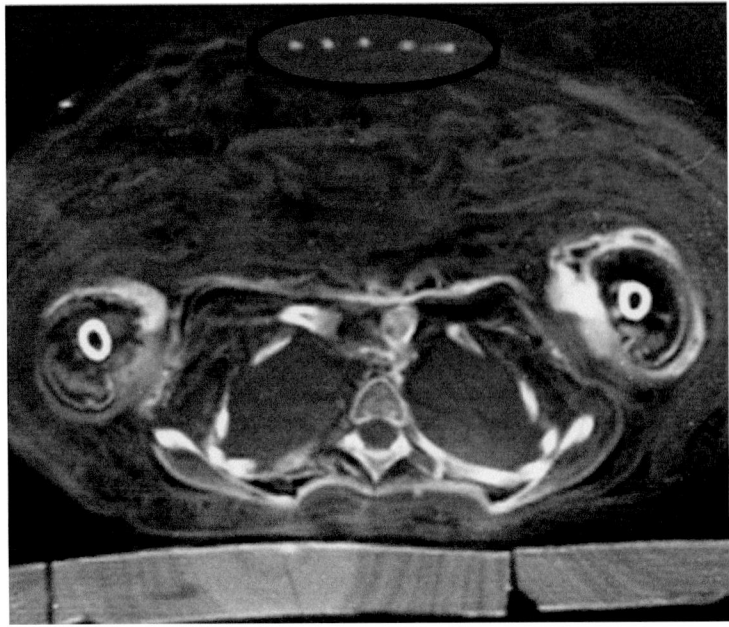

Fig. 3.12 Axial view of thorax - radio-opaque objects anteriorly.

Embalming

Excerebration has been performed, but no foreign material introduced into the cranial cavity afterwards. The eyes have almost certainly been incised and packed with material. No eye plates have been used. The viscera have been removed, but almost certainly not returned to the body cavity with the possible exception of the pelvic area. The mediastinum has been retained – probably including the heart. There is no evidence of damage to the body. The arms are lying on the front of the abdomen and hips.

Cause of Death

Unknown.

Conclusions

This is the body of a teenager. The museum records indicate that it is that of a girl (presumably from the coffin text). The 'classical' methods of mummification have been used. The points of note are the retention of the mediastinum, the complete filling of the body cavity with amorphous material, the stuffing of the eyes and the fact that the mummy is not unwrapped or damaged in any way.

As can be seen, the amount of information available is far superior to that in the X-rays of the preceding case, but there is still a considerable constraint resulting from the inability to manipulate the images in any way and from the wide spacing of the 'slices' (unspecified in the museum records, but approximately one centimetre).

It is clear that, although the information gleaned from analogue CT scan images gives a reasonable amount of information, there is a limit to its flexibility and completeness. Although gross assessment of excerebration and evisceration methods can be achieved, the finer details (to be demonstrated below) are not available. For example although it would be possible to assess the absence or presence of cribriform plate perforation, it would not be possible to determine if this had been exclusively via the ethmoid sinuses or had also involved part of the sphenoid sinuses.

The remaining mummies in the series have been CT scanned using more modern machines and, more importantly, the Dicom image data is in digital file format. As a result the information can be manipulated and can yield far more subtle data detail.

3.2 Distribution of the mummies

Although not all the desired information is available, an analysis of the distribution of the mummies in time and location is a useful background to assessing other features. Tables 3.1, 3.2 and 3.3 illustrate these points. Table 3.1 and 3.2 account for fifty-eight of the mummies, the remaining two being from un-known era. It will be noticed that Manchester mummy – MM9354a – Khary appears in two columns. This is because the provenance regarding era is currently in dispute.

Middle K.	New K.	3IP
MM13784	M3496	B'ham - Padimut
	MM9354a - Khary	Exeter - Shepenmut
		Sheffield - Nesitanebetasheru
		Ipswich - Tahathor
		L'pool - Padiamun - 53.72a
		L'pool - Padiamunnebnesuttauwy
		L'pool - Ankhesenaset
		Lausanne - 490
		Geneva - TjesMoutPert - D0242
		Hor - EA6659
		Pef-Tjau-Emawy-Khonsu- EA6681
		Padiamunet - EA6682
		EA20744
		EA22939
		EA25258
		EA29577
		St. Gallen - C3530
		Lausanne - 492
		MM5053.a - Perenbast
		MM1976.51a
		Salford 2
<u>1</u>	<u>2</u>	<u>21</u>

TABLE 3.1A DISTRIBUTION IN TIME

Late P.	Ptolemaic	Roman
Djedma'atiuesankh	Nesmin	B'ham - Graeco-Roman
Padiamun - M14003	Yverdon - Nes-Shou - MY/3775	M1768
M/C - Asru	Bern - AE9	M1767
TaDjIsis - K1205	Lenzburg - Sherit-Min	L'pool - 13.10.11.25
St. Gallen - Shepenese	Taaset - Suppl.9480	L'pool - M13997a
M10881	(Tebtynis) - Suppl.19691	L'pool- M14048
Perth - 23/1936	Provv.610	Altdorf Child
Namenkhetamun	**M9354a - Khary**	Basel - BSAE.1030
	MM13011	Demetria - 11630
	M/C – Ta-Sheri-Ankh – MM13783	Lenzburg - K10351
		M1766
		M1769
		M9319 - child
		MM2109
		MM1775 - Artemidorus
		EA 22108 Child
		EA 6704
<u>8</u>	<u>10</u>	<u>17</u>

TABLE 3.1B DISTRIBUTION IN TIME

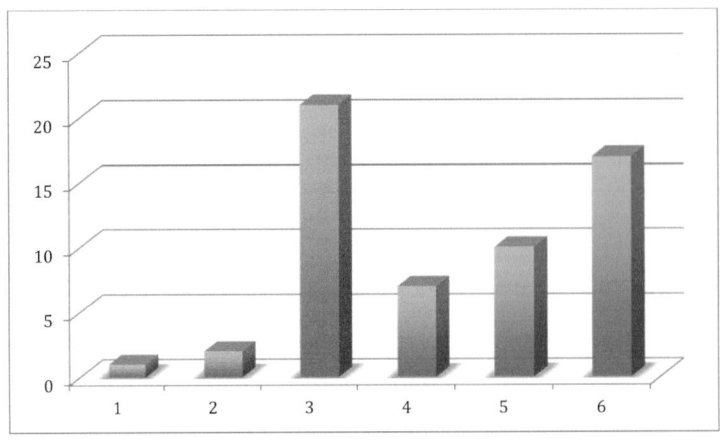

1= Middle Kingdom 2=New Kingdom 3=3rd. IP 4=Late Period
5=Ptolemaic 6=Roman
Table 3.2 Distribution in time

Complete List of locations

LOC	Th	Haw	Fay	Akh	Ass	El H	Gur	DeB	Un-k
3 IP	15		1					1	4
Late	7			1					
Ptol			1	5	1				3
Roman	2	8	2			1			4
Tot	24	8	4	6	1	1			

LOC=Location Th=Thebes Haw=Hawara Fay=Fayum Akh=Akhmim Ass=Assiutt El H=El Hibe Gur=Gurob
DeB=Deir el Bahari Un-k=Unknown
Table 3.3 Distribution by location

For completeness, the mummy from the Middle Kingdom is from an un-known location and the mummies from the New Kingdom are from Gurob and an un-known location. The two mummies without provenance of era also had no provenance of location. These figures include the double counting of the Manchester mummy – M9354a – Khary who may be from either the New Kingdom or the Ptolemaic Period.

3.3 Analyses of various factors

3.3.1 Topics to be considered

The advantage of a personal review of the complete CT data is that it is possible to expand the criteria of each factor as opposed to having to accept other authors' interpretations of the data, such as is the case in a metadata review. An example of the latter is the work of Wade et al (Wade, Nelson, Garvin, 2011: 248-269 and Wade, Nelson, 2013: 1-28).

The topics to be covered are:

Excerebration
Treatment of the eyes
Treatment of the mouth
Evisceration
Treatment of the perineum
Use of canopic packages and foreign material
The use of sub-cutaneous packing materials

Topics related to the head such as excerebration and the treatment of the eyes will be covered in chapter four. Subsequent chapters will cover the results related to the trunk and other areas.

Chapter Four

Results – The Head

4.1 Excerebration

The classical description of mummification / embalming as given by Herodotus (Herodotus, *The Histories* 2: 86.) mentions removal of the brain through the nose.

Before discussing this approach and other alternatives, it is appropriate to discuss the topic of brain removal in general. Whilst accepting that removal of the viscera is a necessary step in reducing the chances (or at least the progress) of putrefaction, the motive for removal of the brain is a little more obscure.

The brain is enclosed in a virtually sealed cavity, the cranial cavity. The only breaches in the wall of this cavity are the foramen magnum and the exits for the twelve pairs of cranial nerves. These 'exits' consist of the perforations in the cribriform plate, the optic canals, the superior orbital fissures and the various foramina in the base of the skull. Fig. 4.1 shows a diagram of the basal foramina and Fig. 4.2 shows some of the cranial nerves on the base of the brain in diagrammatic form (from Cull, 1989: 177, 181). In Fig. 4.1 the grey circles indicate the cribriform plate (A) and the foramen magnum (B). These have, until now been regarded as the sites of entry for excerebration. In effect, the skull is a closed box and would not permit the ingress of microorganisms. Under normal circumstances, there are no microorganisms existing within the cranial cavity.

The immediate question to be answered is 'why remove the brain'. If left in situ, there is little chance of it putrefying. Even if it did, the resulting smell of putrefaction would not be emitted, as there are no naturally patent openings in the skull. As mentioned above, the Ancient Egyptians did not harbor the notion that the brain was of any functional importance, the heart being the seat of the 'soul' – or its equivalent - in their eyes.

There is the possibility (but no proof) that experience with war wounds involving the cranium could have influenced their thinking. The example of the Pharaoh Seqenenre's mummy with its severe wounds to the skull and face indicates that this sort of injury occurred in the Second Intermediate Period (Dynasty 17) (Shaw, 2000: 211). That maces (and presumably other weapons used for striking the head) existed in Pre-Dynastic times is implied by the ceremonial mace head known as the Scorpion mace -head (Shaw, 2000: 65). Whatever the motive for the act, it is assumed that excerebration has been performed from an early stage in Egyptian history.

The earliest mummy in this study is from the Middle Kingdom and does have evidence of excerebration. This is the mummy from Manchester Museum (MM 13784), examined by CT scan on 26/9/13. The images revealed that excerebration has been performed, but there are intact ethmoid and sphenoid sinuses and cribriform plate. (See Fig. 4.3 - arrow 1). There is a moderately large amount of material in the posterior cranial fossa. This consists of two types of substance (Fig.4.3 - arrows 2 and 3) of which one may well be brain tissue (arrow 3). However, the presence of a fluid level as shown by arrow 2 in Fig. 4.3 does indicate the presence of a 'foreign' substance that was once liquid. The absence of the cervical spine (as shown in Fig. 4.3 – grey oval) prevents definite confirmation of a trans-foraminal excerebration, but it certainly cannot be excluded. Indeed, the very fact that the cervical spine has been disturbed may point to the possibility that the trans-foraminal route was used for excerebration.

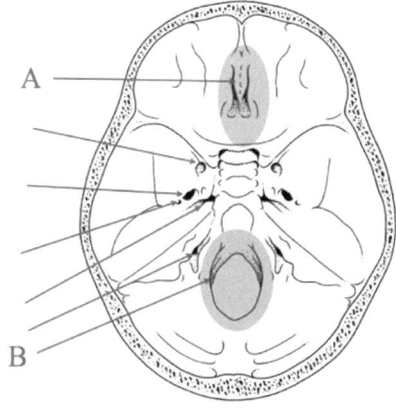

FIG. 4.1 DIAGRAM OF SKULL – THE FORAMINA IN BASE OF SKULL (AFTER IEM IMAGE)

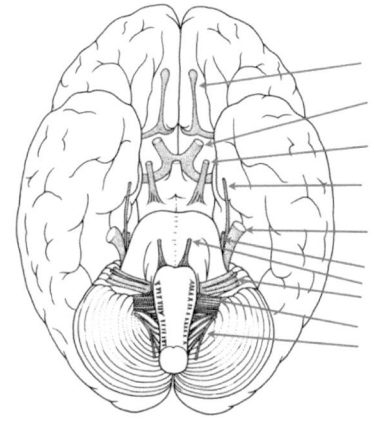

FIG. 4.2 DIAGRAM OF INFERIOR SURFACE OF THE BRAIN - THE CRANIAL NERVES (AFTER IEM IMAGE)

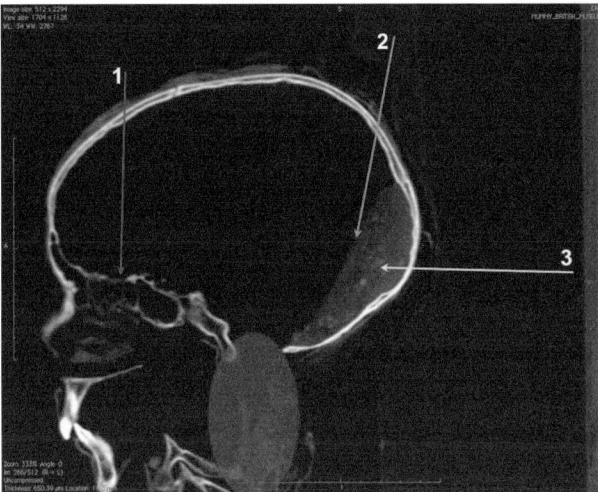

Fig. 4.3 Sagittal view of skull - excerebration in Middle Kingdom Mummy XXVIII

It has been recognized for some time that excerebration was not always performed (Wade, Nelson and Garvin, 2011: 251). The trans-foraminal route has also been recognized for some time. However, the attribution of this route has sometimes been by inference rather than actual proof of anatomical disturbance in the area (Wade, Nelson and Garvin, 2011: 250). If this route is considered from a surgical point of view, it will be realized that significant disturbance – actual disarticulation - of the atlanto-occipital area is necessary to expose the foramen magnum from below the skull. In the absence of such disturbance it would be difficult to imagine how excerebration could be achieved. The approach has to be either from posteriorly (the most likely) or anteriorly. A posterior approach requires division of all the posterior and lateral muscles of the neck below the skull. The incision would have to include structures anterior to the atlas (first cervical vertebra) to allow the skull to be rotated to allow proper access to the foramen magnum. An anterior approach would require access either through the mouth or behind the mandible and then upwards to the base of the skull. Such an approach has yet to be demonstrated in Ancient Egyptian mummies.

Excerebration will now be considered under the following headings.

- Trans-nasal route
- Trans-foraminal route
- Trans-basal
- Trans-orbital route
- No excerebration

4.1.1 Trans-nasal route

Of the fifty-nine mummies studied by CT scan one is of a 'false mummy' and forty-two of the remainder were found to have had trans-nasal excerebration. The sixtieth mummy was only examined by X-ray and the skull not visualised well enough to identify the presence or absence of the cribriform plate and, hence, determine the route used for excerebration.

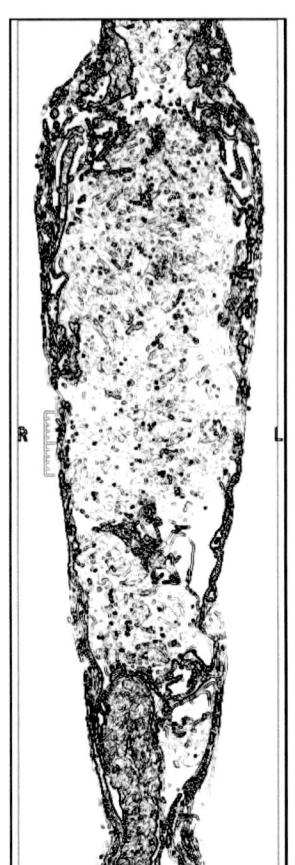

Fig. 4.4 Coronal view of a 'false mummy'. (After IEM image)

For the sake of completeness the 'false mummy' will be briefly described. It is Mummy XXI. The mummy is from Lausanne Museum (Accession No.490) and the CT scans were viewed in Zurich. Whilst the museum records show this to be the mummy of a female from the Third Intermediate Period, the CT scans reveal a completely empty set of bandages (See Fig.4.4). Further research revealed that the mummy had, in the past, been opened from the back and the body extracted so that it could be displayed along side the bandaging. The body itself had, subsequently, been lost. This is an excellent example of one of the hazards of what has been described above as ' The journey – From death to museum'.

The forty-two examples of the trans-nasal route were not all uniform. Although the commencement of the skull perforation was via the nasal passages, the direction taken and, therefore, the end point – and actual point of entry into the skull – varied. In the majority (that is in thirty examples) the perforation was of the ethmoid sinuses and the cribriform plate alone. These are recorded below.

4.1.1.1 Ethmoid perforation

The mummies involved are listed with their historical timeline and their place of origin, if known (see Table 4.1).

Extracts of the relevant reports follow.

NUMBER	ERA	LOCATION
I	Roman	Unknown
III	Dyn. 20-21	Thebes
VI	Dyn. 26	Thebes
XI	Dyn. 26	Thebes
XVII	3 IP	Thebes
XVIII	Roman	Thebes
XIX	Roman	Unknown
XXIII	Ptolemaic	Akhmim
XXV	Dyn. 22-25	Thebes
XXVI	Unknown	Unknown
XXVII	Roman	Hawara
XXVIII	Dyn. 21	Akhmim
XXIX	Dyn. 22	Thebes
XXX	Dyn. 25	Thebes
XXXI	Dyn. 25	Thebes
XXXIII	Dyn. 22	Thebes
XXXVI	Ptolemaic	Akhmim
XXXVII	Ptolemaic	Akhmim
XXXVIII	Dyn. 26	Thebes
XLI	Roman	Unknown
XLIII	Ptolemaic	Fayum
XLV	Roman	Hawara
L	Dyn. 26	Akhmim/Thebes
LI	Dyn. 19 / Ptolemaic	Unknown
LIII	Dyn. 25	Thebes
LIV	3 IP	Unknown
LVI	Roman	Hawara
LVII	Roman	Hawara
LX	Roman	Thebes

TABLE 4.1 MUMMIES WITH ETHMOID PERFORATION ONLY.

I The Graeco-Roman Mummy – Birmingham Museum (Cat. No. 1894A15)

Head

A variety of features are found in the head. The first is that there is perforation of the cribriform plate, indicating

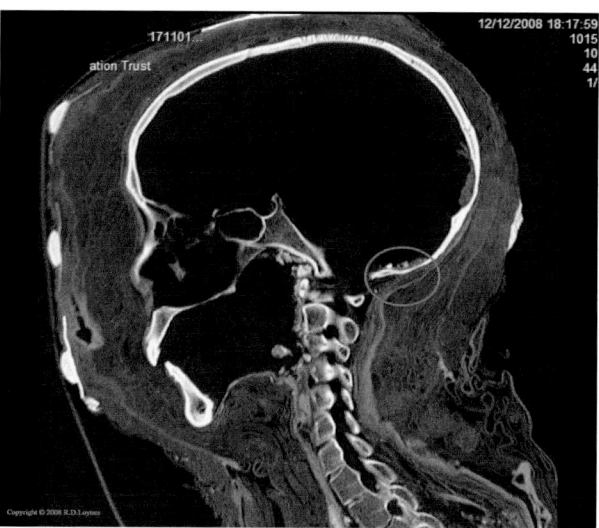

FIG. 4.6 SAGITTAL VIEW OF SKULL - BRAIN REMNANTS IN POSTERIOR FOSSA

removal of the brain tissue via the trans-nasal route. However, it is only the cribriform plate that is perforated and not the more posterior sphenoidal air sinuses. This indicates that the perforation was made by a more or less vertical strike up the nose. It also indicates that the area of bone removed is in the region of 2.0x1.0cms. This would, therefore, limit the access to the cranial cavity by any instrument subsequently used (See Fig. 4.5).

Furthermore, there is only minimal evidence of any brain tissue. This indicates that the brain removal has been very thorough, perhaps indicating washing out of the cranial cavity with some sort of lytic or caustic material (see Fig. 4.6).

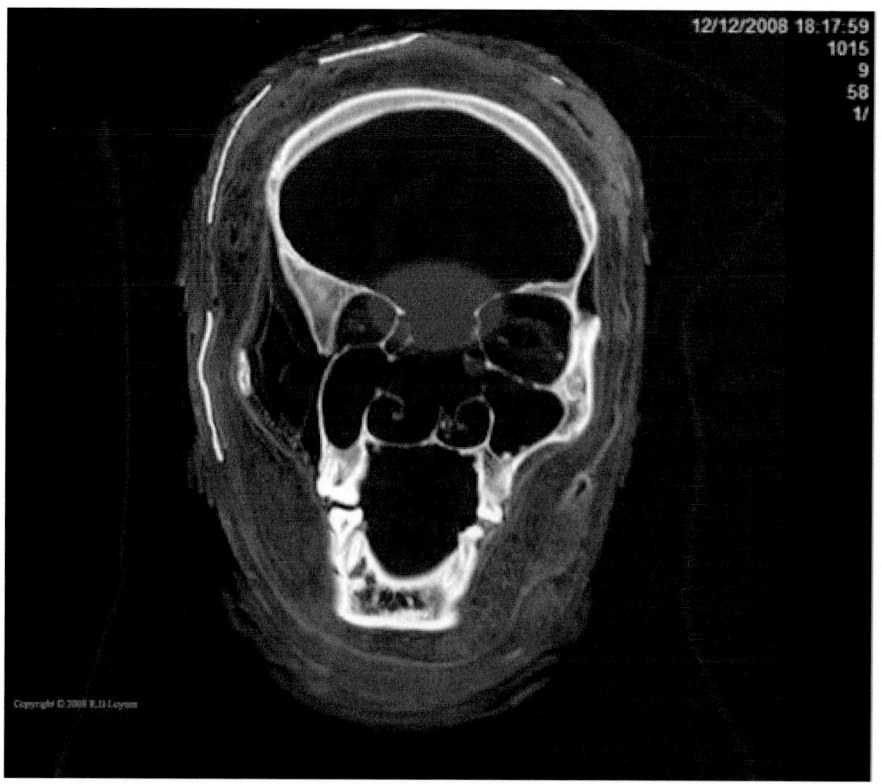

FIG. 4.5 CORONAL VIEW OF SKULL ILLUSTRATING CRIBRIFORM PLATE PERFORATION

III Padimut (BMAG – Cat. No. 1991W1)

Head

There is perforation of the cribriform plate, but no damage to the sphenoid air sinuses indicating limited damage and, therefore, access. Furthermore, there is minimal damage to the internal structures of the nose pointing to a very limited access to the skull cavity (See Fig. 4.7).

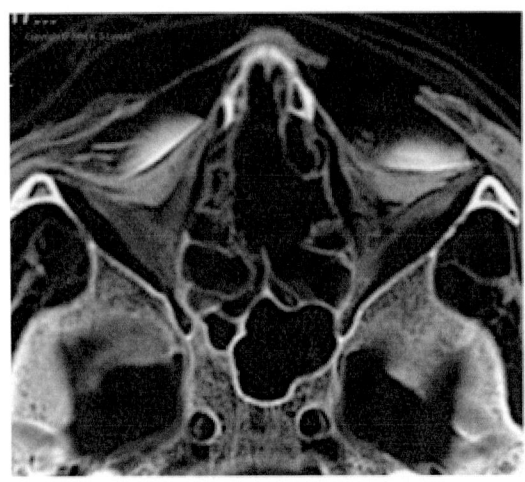

FIG. 4.7 AXIAL VIEW OF SKULL ILLUSTRATING LIMITED DAMAGE TO NASAL STRUCTURES

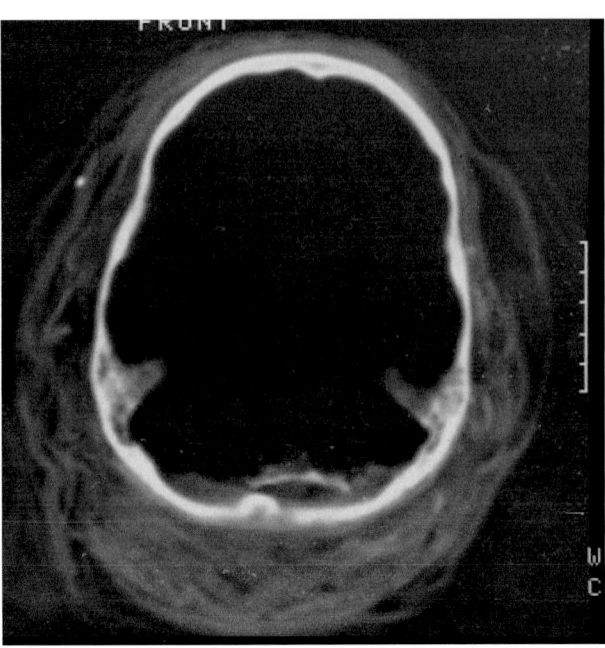

FIG. 4.9 AXIAL VIEW OF SKULL - BRAIN MATERIAL IN POSTERIOR CRANIAL CAVITY.

Despite this, the brain has been completely removed and there are no remnants of tissue within the skull. As mentioned elsewhere, the size and position of the perforation would indicate a vertical 'strike' upwards via the nose and subsequent use of a suitably caustic 'washout' to thoroughly remove the brain tissue.

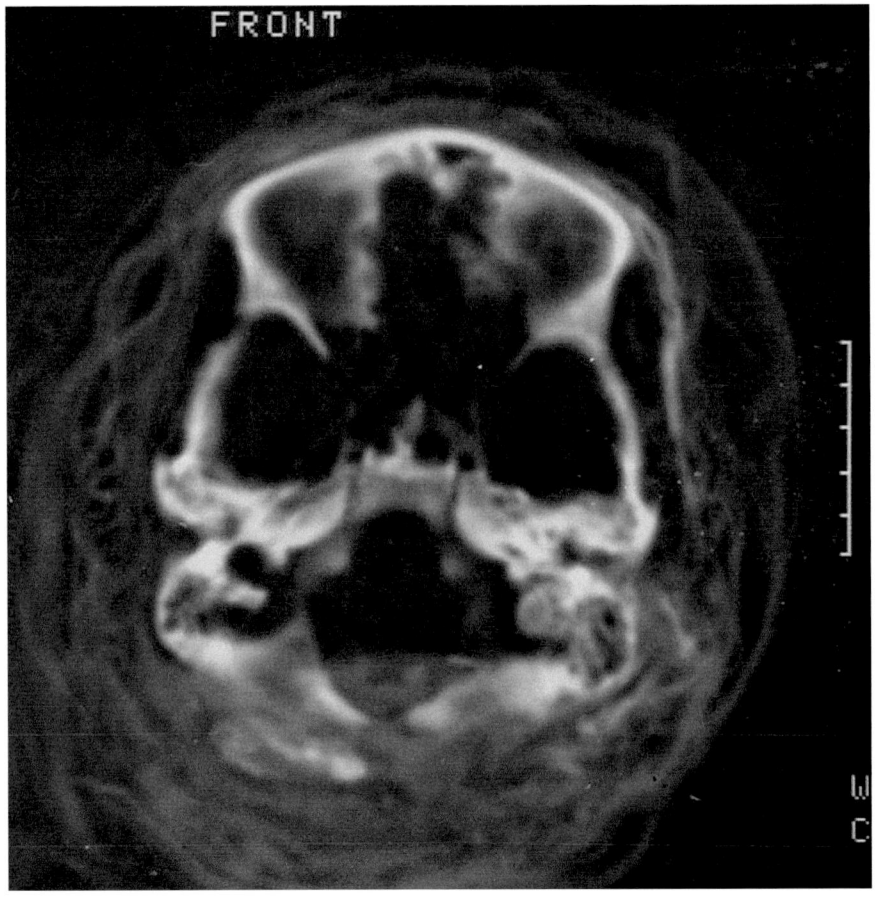

FIG. 4.8 AXIAL VIEW OF SKULL SHOWING PERFORATION OF THE CRIBRIFORM PLATE

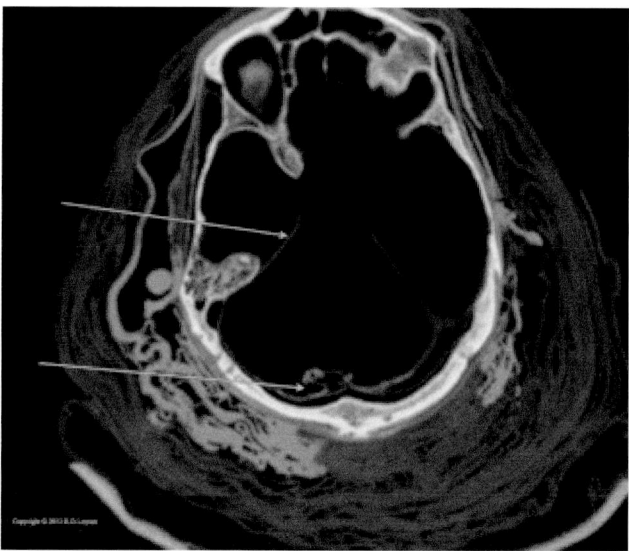

FIG. 4.10 AXIAL VIEW OF SKULL - RETAINED MENINGES AND EMPTY CRANIAL CAVITY.

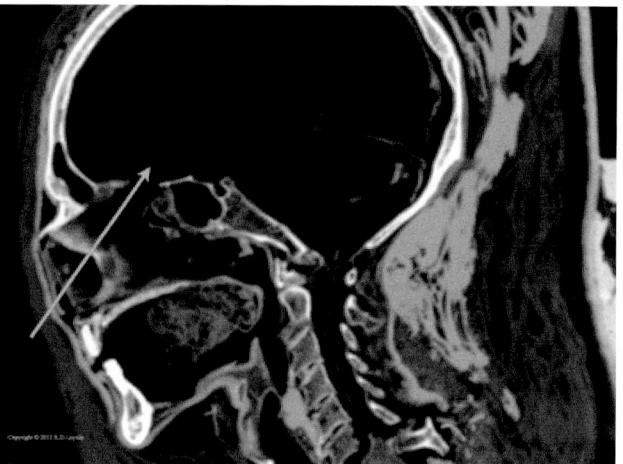

FIG. 4.11 SAGITTAL VIEW OF SKULL - LIMITED PERFORATION OF ETHMOID AND CRIBRIFORM PLATE.

VI Djedma'atiuesankh – Sheffield Museum (Cat. No. J93.1284)

Head

There is evidence of perforation of the cribriform plate and removal of most of the brain but with some residual brain tissue in the back of the cranial cavity (See Figs. 4.8 and 4.9).

XI. Padiamun – National Museums Liverpool (Accession No. M14003)

Head

There has been thorough excerebration via the trans-nasal route. The meninges have been retained and there is no material introduced into the cranial cavity (See Fig. 4.10 - arrows indicate the meninges).

Fig. 4.11 shows the small perforation in the cribriform plate and ethmoid sinuses. Arrow.

XVII. Ankhesenaset – National Museums Liverpool (Accession No. M14000)

Head

Trans-nasal excerebration (Black circles in Figs 4.12 and 4.13) has been performed thoroughly and the cranial cavity packed very loosely with linen (Arrows 1 in Figs. 4.12 and 4.13). A separate linen pack has been inserted into the nose (See Fig. 4.13 - arrow 2).

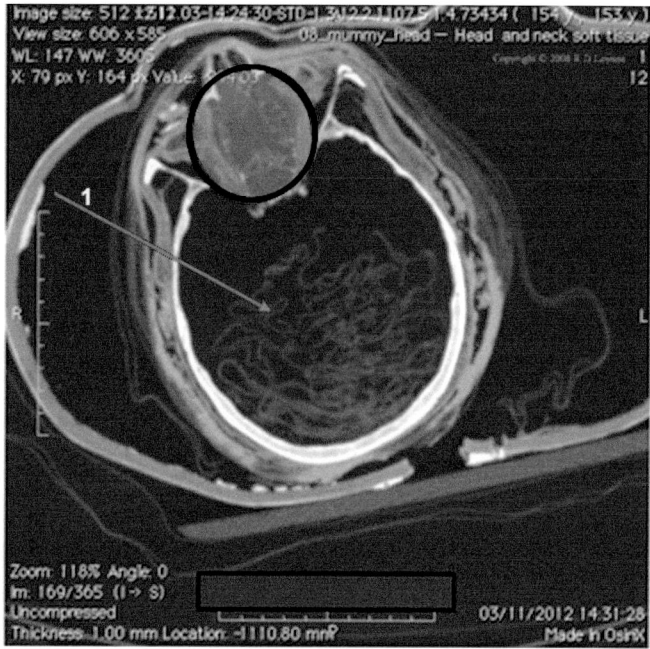

FIG. 4.12 AXIAL VIEW OF SKULL ILLUSTRATING EXCEREBRATION AND LOOSE LINEN PACKING.

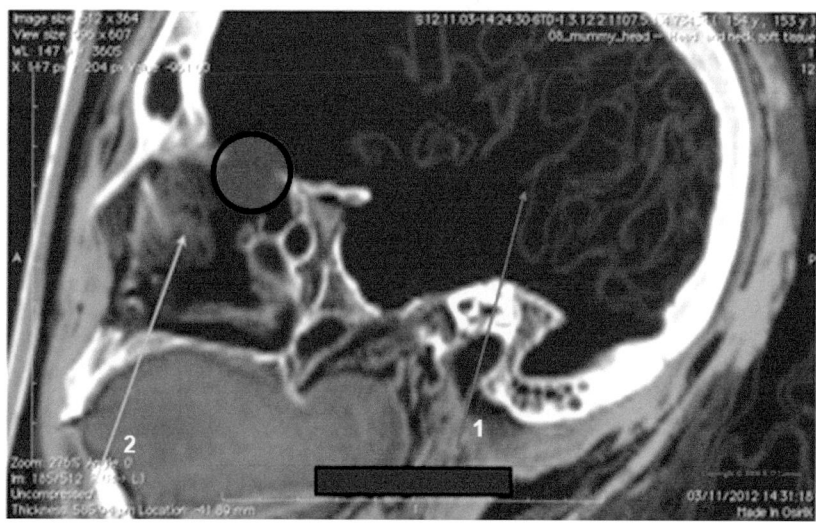

FIG. 4.13 SAGITTAL VIEW OF SKULL - EXCEREBRATION AND LOOSE PACKING.

XVIII. Unnamed – National Museums Liverpool – (Accession No. M14048)

Head

Excerebration via the trans-nasal route has been complete with the subsequent introduction of a small amount of resin (See Figs. 4.14 and 4.15).

In Fig. 4.15 arrow 1 indicates the resin and the arrow 2 indicates the Crista Galli that has been fractured off during perforation of the cribriform plate. The perforation is shown in Figs. 4.16 and 4.17.

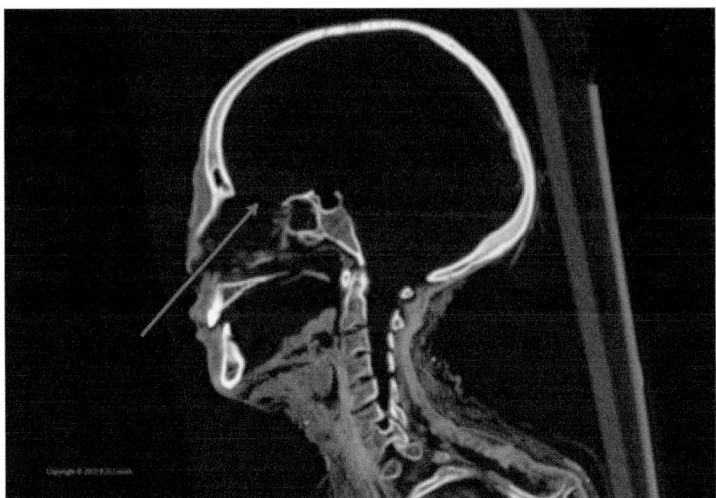

FIG. 4.14 SAGITTAL VIEW OF SKULL SHOWING EXCEREBRATION

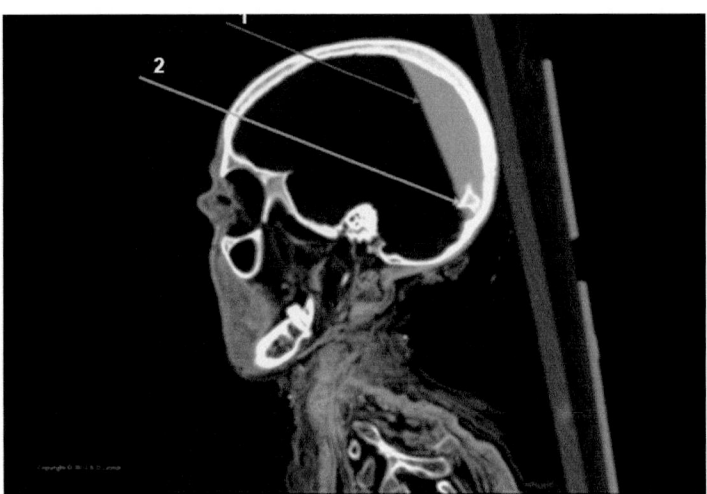

FIG. 4.15 SAGITTAL VIEW OF SKULL - EXCEREBRATION AND PACKING.

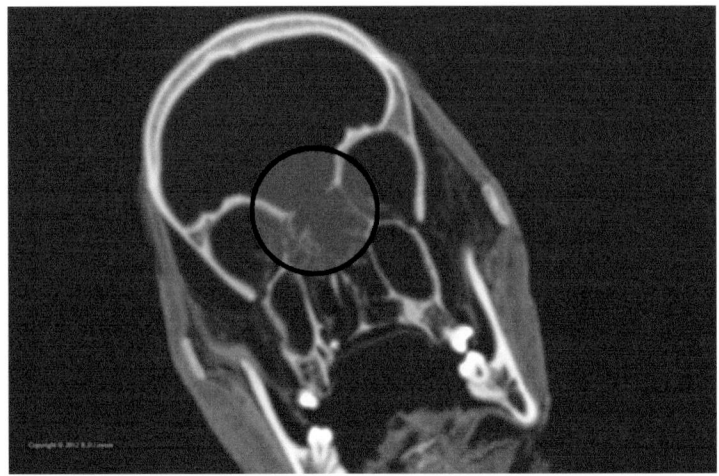

FIG. 4.16 AXIAL VIEW OF SKULL - PERFORATION OF CRIBRIFORM PLATE.

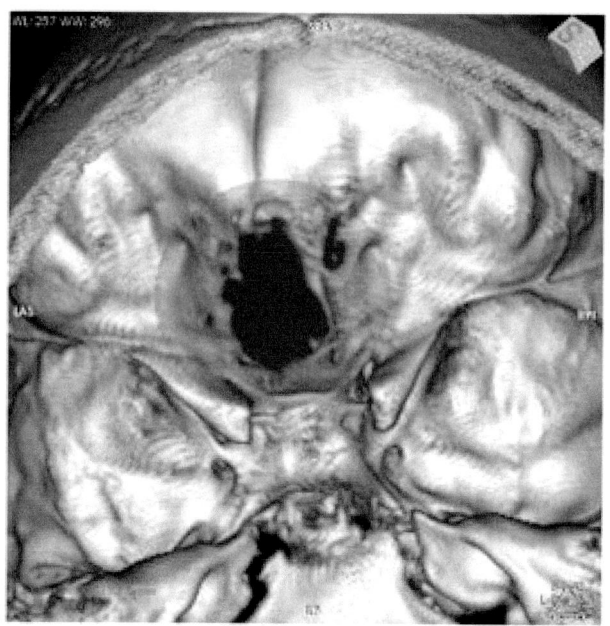

FIG. 4.17 3D RECONSTRUCTION SHOWING PERFORATION OF CRIBRIFORM PLATE FROM THE INTRA-CRANIAL SURFACE.

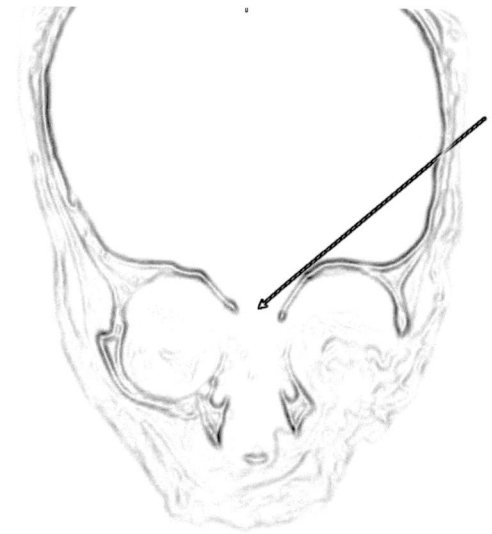

FIG. 4.18 CORONAL VIEW OF SKULL - PERFORATION OF CRIBRIFORM PLATE. (AFTER IEM IMAGE)

XIX. Unnamed (Child) – Altdorf Museum

Head

There has been excerebration via the trans-nasal route leaving an empty cranial cavity. (See Fig. 4.18. Arrow).

XXIII. Nes-Shou – Yverdon Museum (Accession No.MY/3775)

Head

There has been complete excerebration that may have been performed via the cribriform plate but, if so, the damage to the cribriform plate and the ethmoid sinuses has been limited (Fig. 4.19 - arrow 1). There is a thin sliver of tissue remaining in the floor of the anterior fossa (Fig. 4.19 - arrow 3). A plaque of resin over the front of the nose and upper lip (Fig. 4.19 - arrow 2) extends into the nostril. Resin has been poured into the cranial cavity after excerebration, and has separated into three layers prior to setting (Fig. 4.19 - white arrows). The inferior/posterior layer contains some granular material (Fig. 4.19 - wider of the white arrows). The maxillary and sphenoid sinuses contain resin (See Fig. 4.20).

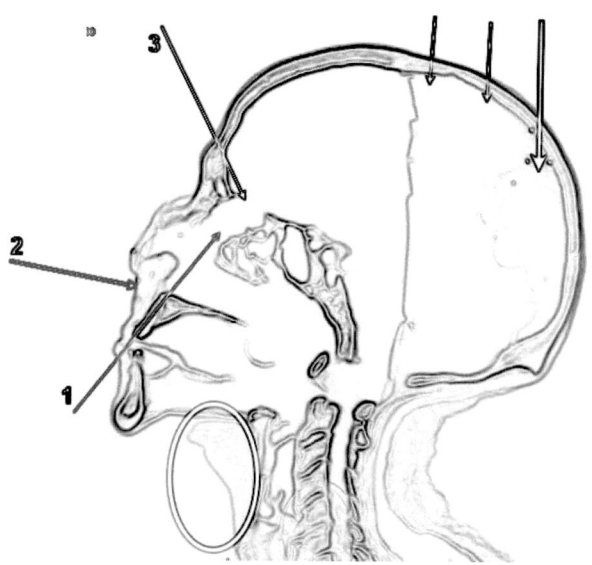

FIG. 4.19 SAGITTAL VIEW OF SKULL - EXCEREBRATION AND PACKING (AFTER IEM IMAGE)

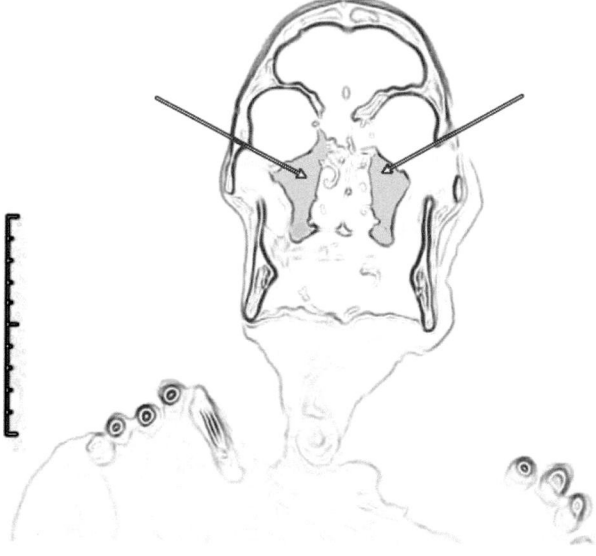

FIG. 4.20 CORONAL VIEW OF SKULL - RESIN IN MAXILLARY SINUSES. (AFTER IEM IMAGE)

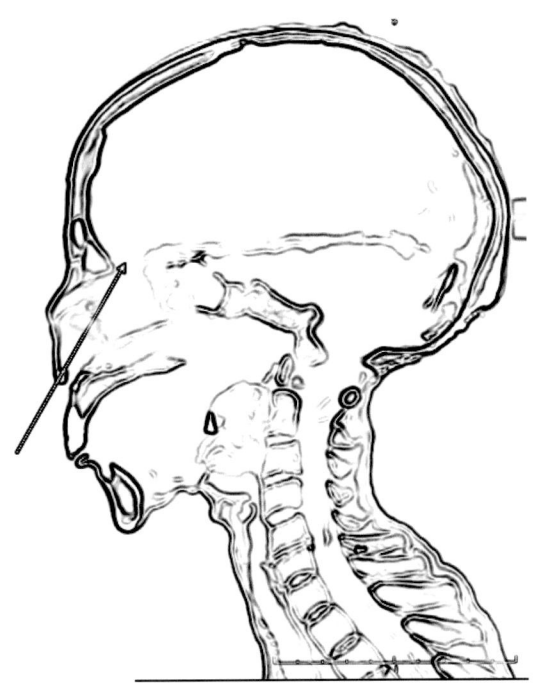

Fig. 4.21 Sagittal view of skull - cribriform plate perforation. (After IEM image)

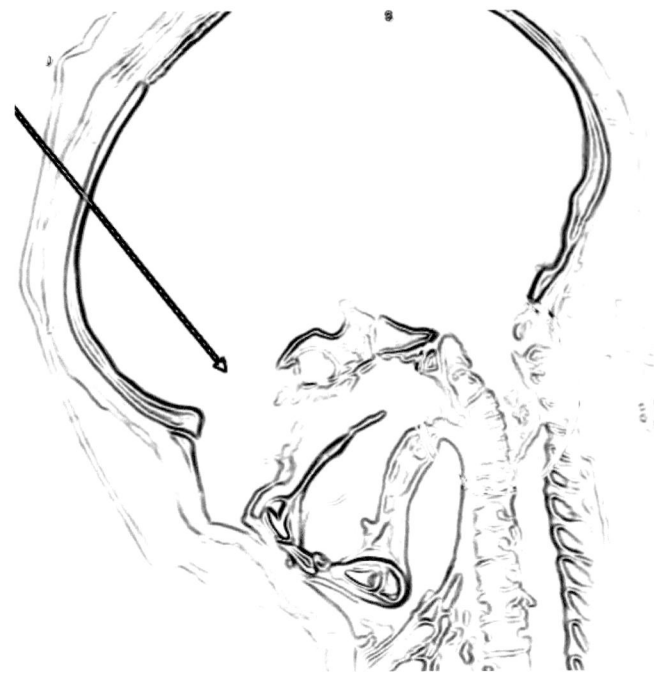

Fig. 4.22 Sagittal view of skull showing the large defect in the cribriform plate. (After IEM image)

XXV. TjesMoutPert – Geneva Museum (Cat. No.D0242)

Head

The cribriform plate has been perforated, excerebration performed and some resin, which has cracked, introduced into the posterior fossa (See Fig. 4.21).

XXVI. Unnamed – Geneva Museum (Cat. No. Infant)

Head

The cranial cavity is completely empty. Excerebration is via a trans-nasal approach with perforation of the cribriform plate (See Fig. 4.22).

XXVII. Demetria – Manchester Museum (Cat. No.MM11630)

Head

Complete excerebration has been performed via the trans-nasal route and a small amount of resin, which has cracked, inserted (See Fig. 4.23 - arrow 1 = Eyes on cartonnage; arrow 2 = perforation of cribriform plate; arrow 3 = resin; arrows 4 = desiccated eyes).

XXVIII. Ta-Shere-Ankh - Manchester Museum - (Cat. No. MM13783)

Head

Excerebration is via the trans-nasal route, with wide removal of the cribriform plate (See Fig. 4.24 - arrow 1). Resin has been inserted and is in two layers (Fig. 4.24 - arrows 2 and 3). Some of the meninges remain (See Fig.4.24 arrow 4).

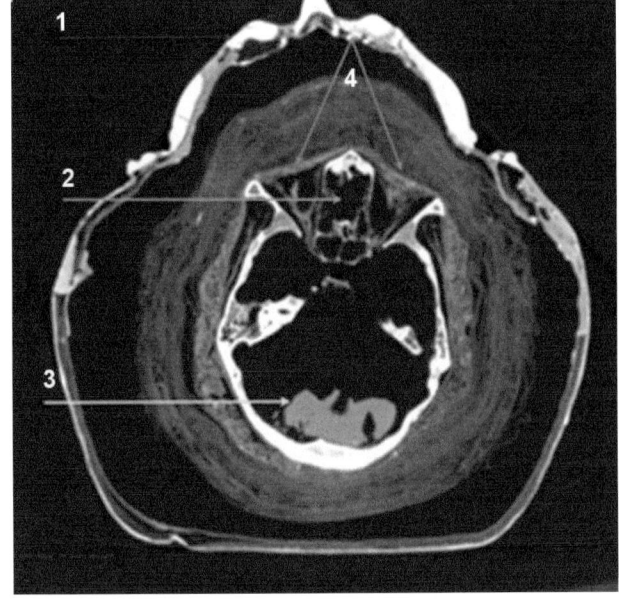

Fig. 4.23 Axial view of skull - perforation of cribriform plate and resin in the posterior cranial fossa.

XXIX. Hor - British Museum - (Accession No. EA 6659)

Head

Excerebration is via the trans-nasal route with perforation of the cribriform plate. (Fig. 4.25 - arrow 1), there is also displacement of the Atlas (first cervical vertebra) forwards (4 = margins of foramen magnum. 3 = peripheral margins of atlas). This is an abnormality usually seen in cases of trans-foraminal excerebration. In this case, there is no evidence of linen or other packing in the foramen magnum.

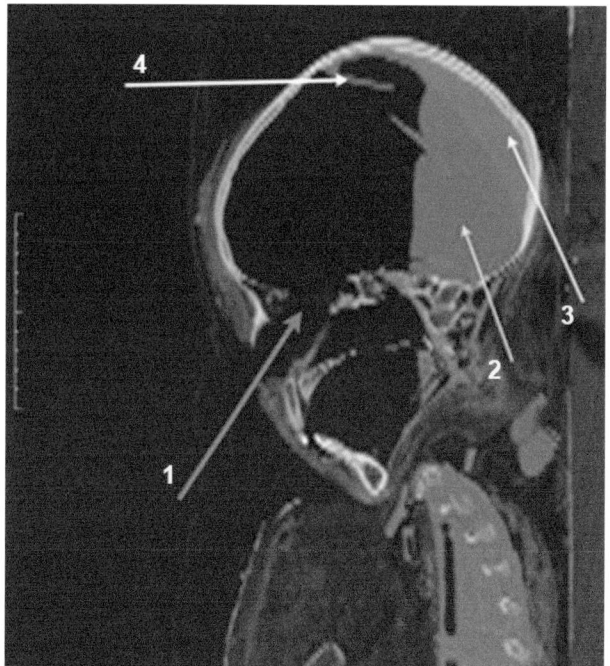

FIG. 4.24 SAGITTAL VIEW OF SKULL - PERFORATION OF CRIBRIFORM PLATE AND RESIN IN THE POSTERIOR CRANIAL FOSSA.

This indicates that the anterior movement of the atlas almost certainly occurred after bandaging. Excerebration has been thorough and a granular substance subsequently introduced into the cranial cavity (arrow 2 in Fig. 4.25). Within this granular substance (which may be clay) there are some objects. These consist of a tooth (Fig. 4.26- black circle) and some fragments of bone, one of which is seen in Fig. 4.26 (white circle).

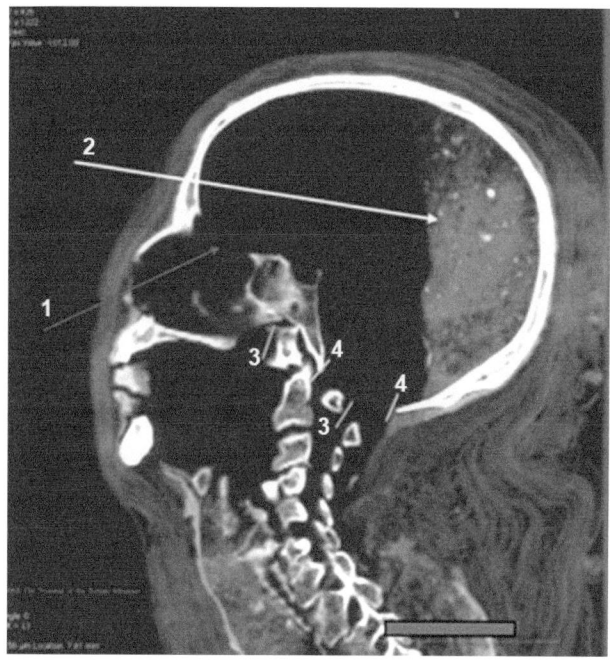

FIG. 4.25 SAGITTAL VIEW OF SKULL - CRIBRIFORM PLATE PERFORATION, PACKING AND ATLANTO-OCCIPITAL DISRUPTION. COURTESY OF THE TRUSTEES OF THE BRITISH MUSEUM

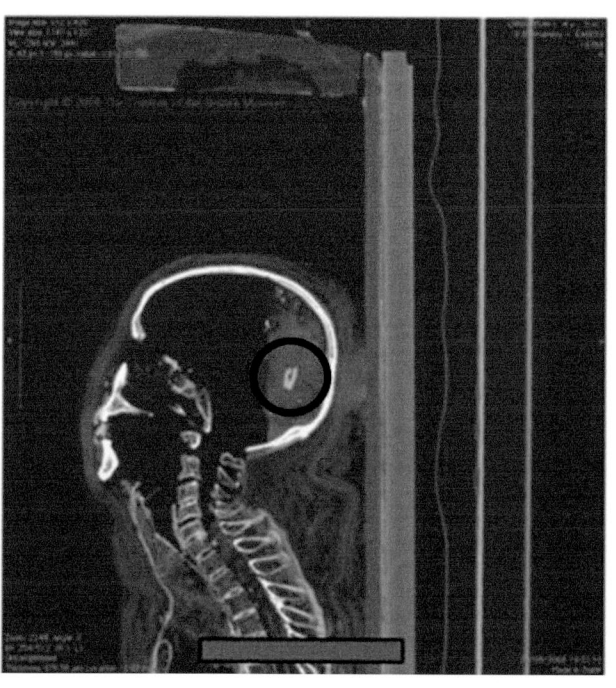
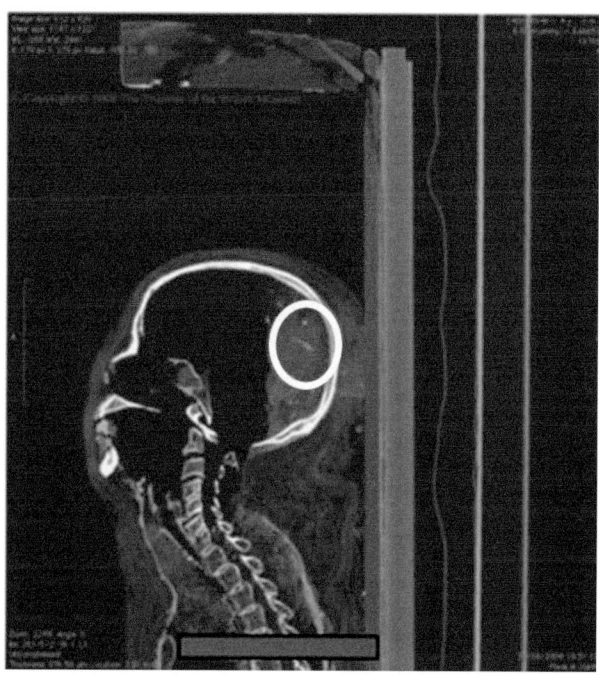

FIG. 4.26 SAGITTAL VIEWS OF SKULL SHOWING BONE AND TOOTH WITHIN INTRA-CRANIAL PACKING. COURTESY OF THE TRUSTEES OF THE BRITISH MUSEUM

XXX. Pef-Tjau-Emawy-Khonsu - British Museum - (Accession No. EA 6681)

Head

Excerebration has been performed thoroughly via the trans-nasal route, with perforation of the cribriform plate (See Figs. 4.27 and 4.28 - circle) and a small amount of debris remaining in the posterior fossa.

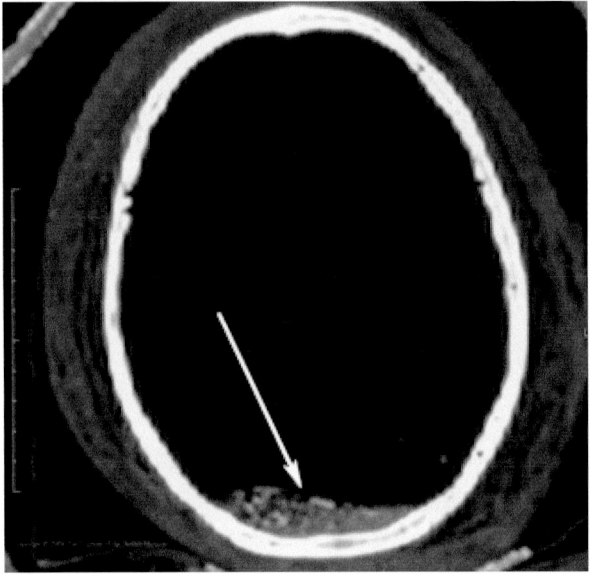

FIG. 4.27 AXIAL VIEW OF SKULL - DEBRIS IN POSTERIOR CRANIAL FOSSA.

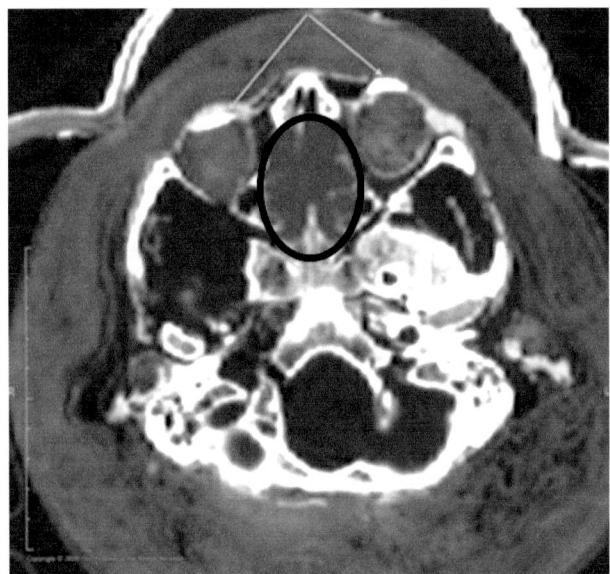

FIG. 4.28 AXIAL VIEW OF SKULL - PERFORATION OF THE CRIBRIFORM PLATE.

XXXI. Padiamun - British Museum - (Accession No.EA6682)

Head

Excerebration has been performed via the trans-nasal route (See Figs. 4.29 and 4.30), with complete removal of brain tissue, and a little meningeal tissue left in the cranial cavity (See Fig. 4.31 - arrow 1).

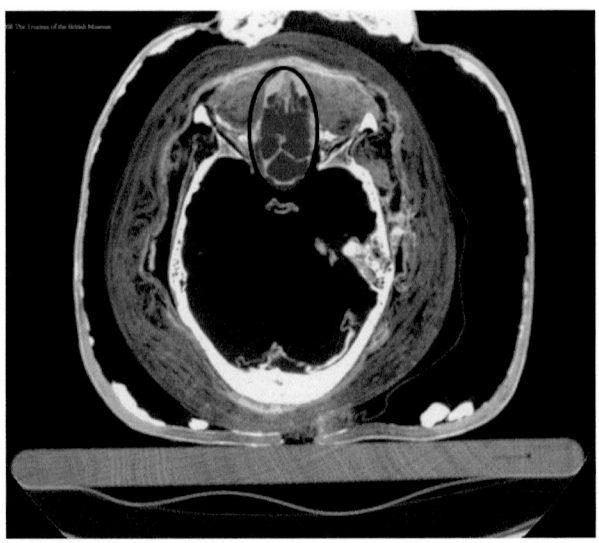

FIG. 4.29 AXIAL VIEW OF SKULL - TRANS-NASAL EXCEREBRATION.

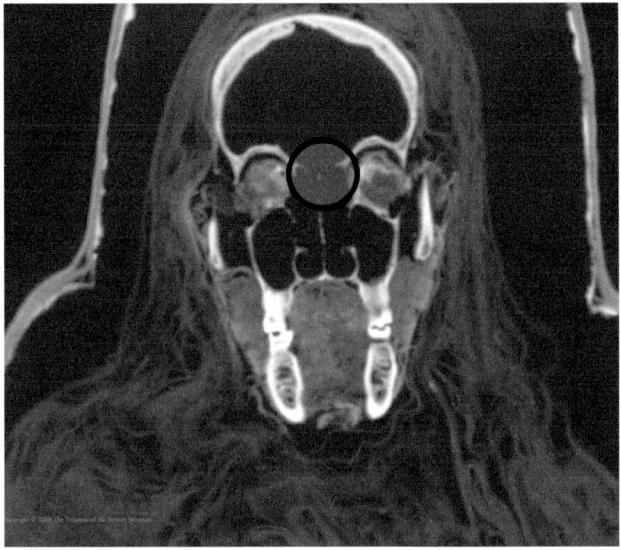

FIG. 4.30 CORONAL VIEW OF SKULL - TRANS-NASAL EXCEREBRATION.

XXXIII. Tjenmutengebtiu - British Museum - (Accession No. EA 22939)

Head

Excerebration is via the nose, the ethmoid sinuses and the cribriform plate. Brain removal has been thorough and the cranial cavity then lightly packed with linen introduced through the nose (See Fig. 4.32 - arrow 1).

XXXVI. Unnamed. - Bern (AE 9)

Head

Thorough excerebration is via the trans-nasal route (right nostril) (See Fig. 4.33) with the subsequent introduction of resin, which has set with a large number of air bubbles within it (See Fig. 4.34 - arrow 1).

Some remnants of the meninges are also seen (See Fig. 4.34 - arrows 2).

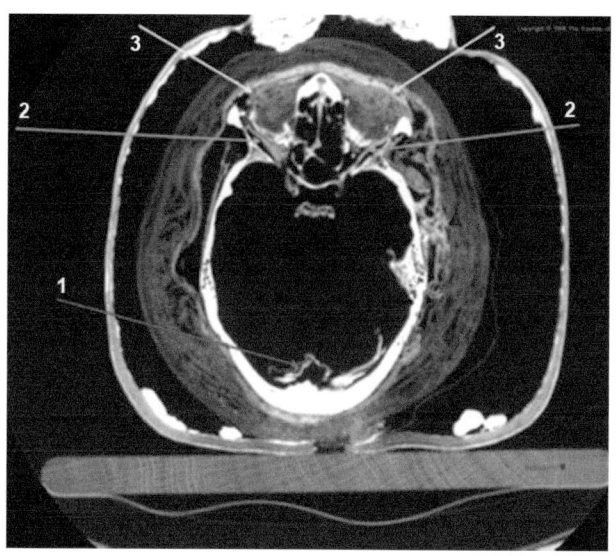

FIG. 4.31 Axial view of skull showing meningeal remnants.

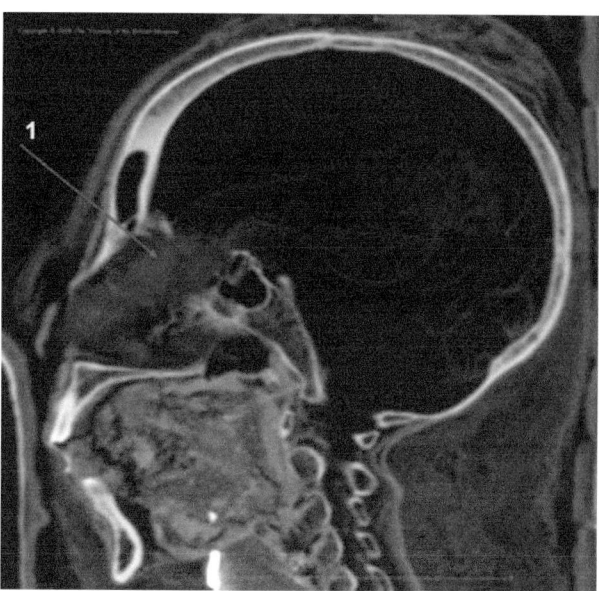

FIG. 4.32 Sagittal view of skull demonstrating linen in nose and cranial cavity.
Courtesy of the Trustees of the British Museum

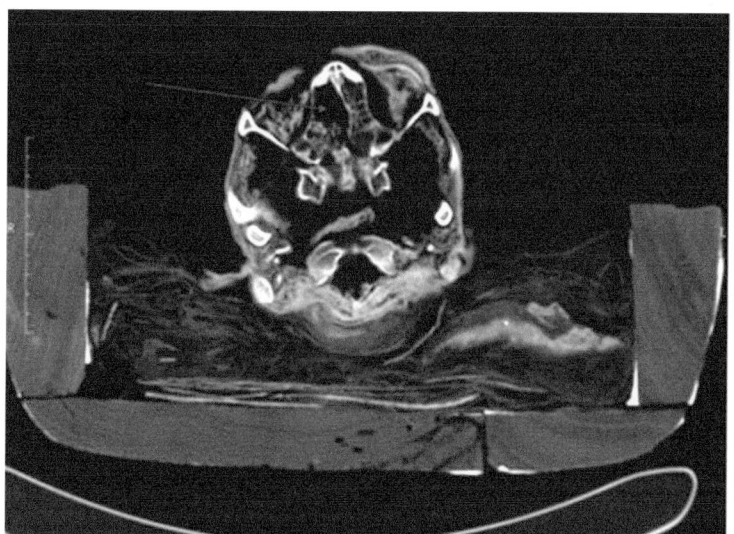

FIG. 4.33 Axial view of skull - excerebration via right nostril.

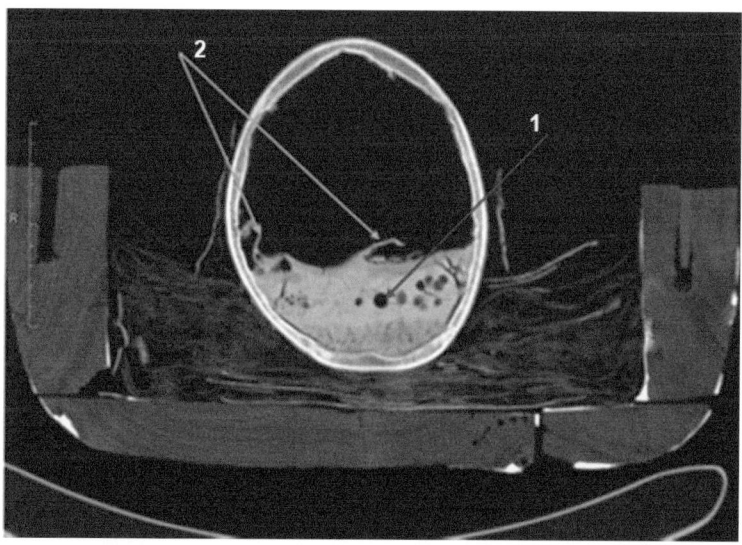

FIG. 4.34 Axial view of skull - resin with contained air.

XXXVII. Sherit-Min - Lenzburg (K10352)

Head

Excerebration has been via the trans-nasal route with complete removal of the brain and resin introduced in significant quantities (See Fig. 4.35 - arrow 1 = cribriform plate perforation; arrow 2 = resin layer)

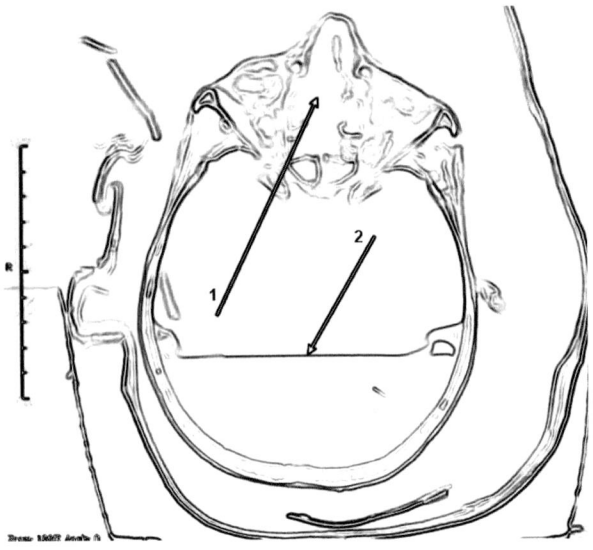

FIG. 4.35 AXIAL VIEW OF SKULL - EXCEREBRATION AND PACKING. (AFTER IEM IMAGE)

XXXVIII. Shepenese - St. Gallen (no Number)

Head

Excerebration has been thorough and performed via the trans-nasal route. No foreign material has been introduced into the cranial cavity (See Fig. 4.36).

XLI. Unnamed child - Lenzburg (Cat. No.K-10351)

Head

Complete excerebration has been performed via the trans-nasal route. No substance has been inserted subsequently (See Figs. 4.37, 4.38 and 4.39).

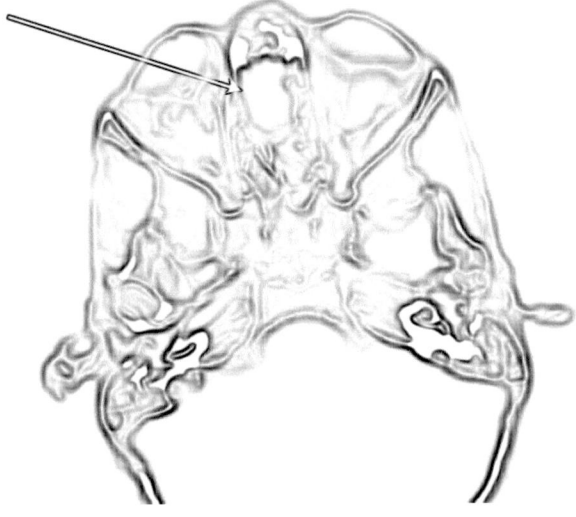

FIG. 4.38 AXIAL VIEW OF SKULL SHOWING CRIBRIFORM PLATE PERFORATION (AFTER IEM IMAGE)

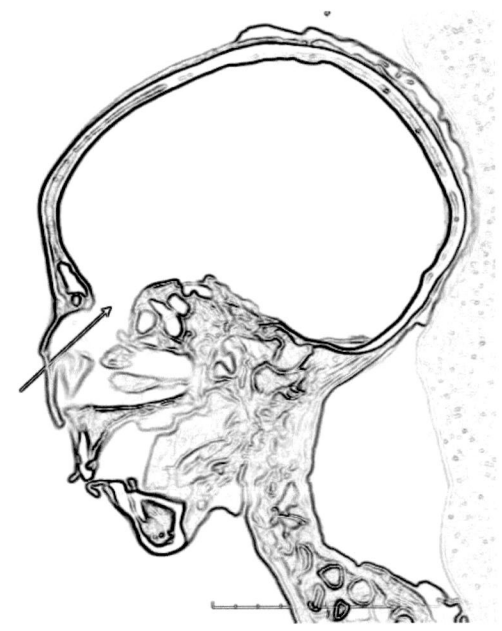

FIG. 4.36 SAGITTAL VIEW OF SKULL DEMONSTRATING TRANS-NASAL EXCEREBRATION (AFTER IEM IMAGE)

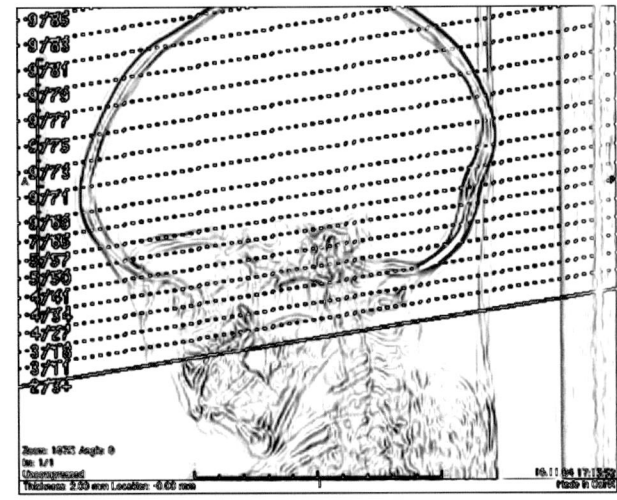

FIG. 4.39 SAGITTAL VIEW OF SKULL SHOWING EMPTY CRANIAL CAVITY (AFTER IEM IMAGE)

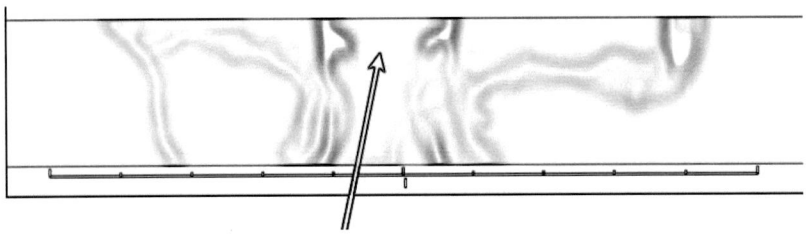

FIG. 4.37 SMALL CORONAL SECTION OF SKULL SHOWING CRIBRIFORM PLATE PERFORATION. (AFTER IEM IMAGE)

XLIII. Unnamed fromTebtynis - Turin (Cat. No. Suppl.19691)

Head

There is complete excerebration via the trans-nasal route (See Fig. 4.40). This Figure also shows some debris within the posterior aspect of the cranial cavity.

XLV. Unnamed - Manchester Museum (Cat. No.MM1766)

Head

Excerebration has been via the trans-nasal route, with complete perforation of the cribriform plate (See Fig. 4.41). The approach appears to have been predominantly via the left nostril.

Excerebration has been complete, with some resin introduced that has pooled and solidified in the occipital region of the cranial cavity and then cracked (See Fig. 4.42- arrow 1).

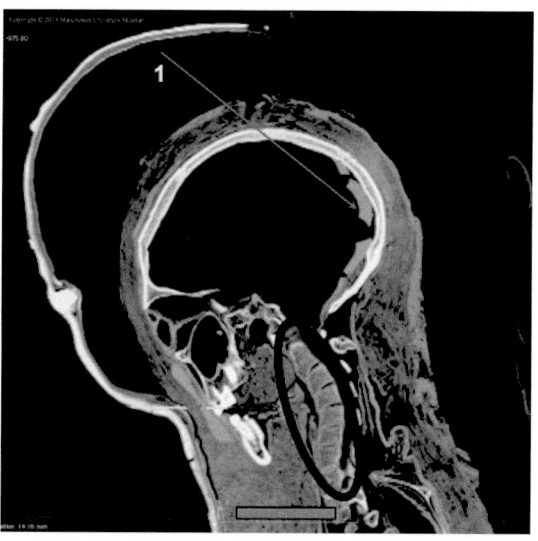

FIG. 4.42 SAGITTAL VIEW OF SKULL - CRACKED RESIN IN POSTERIOR CRANIAL FOSSA.

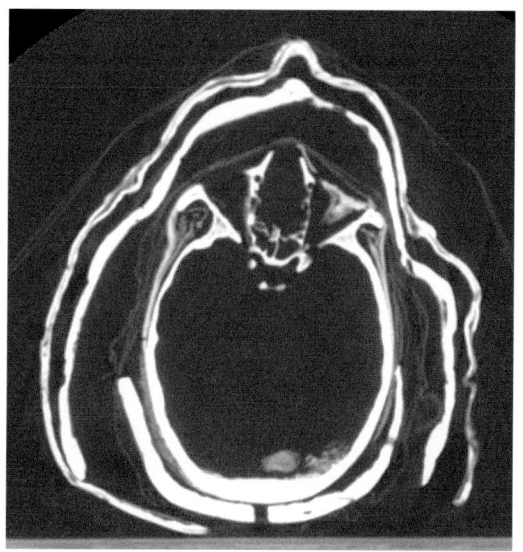

FIG. 4.40 AXIAL VIEW OF SKULL ILLUSTRATING TRANS-NASAL EXCEREBRATION.

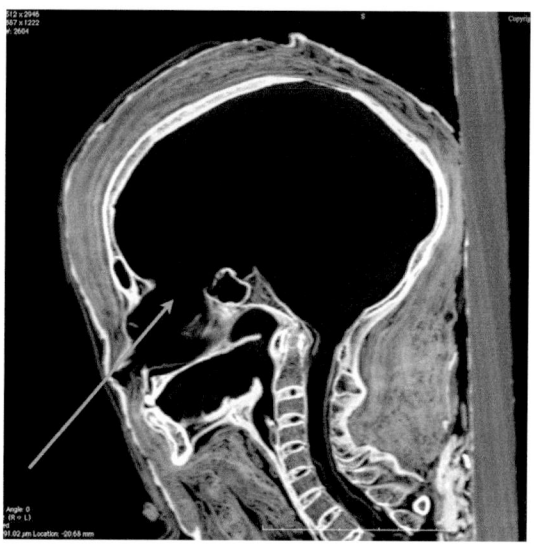

FIG. 4.43 SAGITTAL VIEW OF SKULL - PERFORATION OF ETHMOID WITH INTACT SPHENOID.

L. Ta-Kr-Hb - Perth Museum and Art Gallery (Cat. No. 23/1936)

Head

Complete excerebration has been performed via the trans-nasal route, through the ethmoid sinuses. The sphenoid sinus remains intact (See Fig. 4.43).

LI. Khary - Manchester Museum (Accession No. MM9354a)

Head

Excerebration with complete removal of the brain has been performed through a relatively small perforation of the cribriform plate via the posterior ethmoid air cells (See Figs. 4.44 and 4.45). These figures also show the subsequent introduction of resin into the cranial cavity.

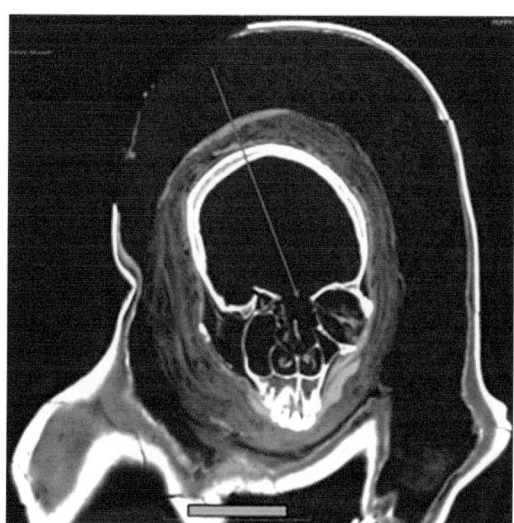

FIG. 4.41 CORONAL VIEW OF SKULL - PERFORATION OF CRIBRIFORM PLATE.

As the meninges have remained intact, the resin has been allowed to solidify in at least two levels, a third level appearing in the cervical spinal canal (See Figs 4.45 - arrows 2 and 4.46).

Fig. 4.46 also shows that the meninges from the clivus have been detached from the bone and reflected posteriorly to form a false cavity that has retained the resin. Subsequent to excerebration and the introduction of resin, the nasal cavity has been closed with two tampons of linen (See Figs 4.47 and 4.48 - circles).

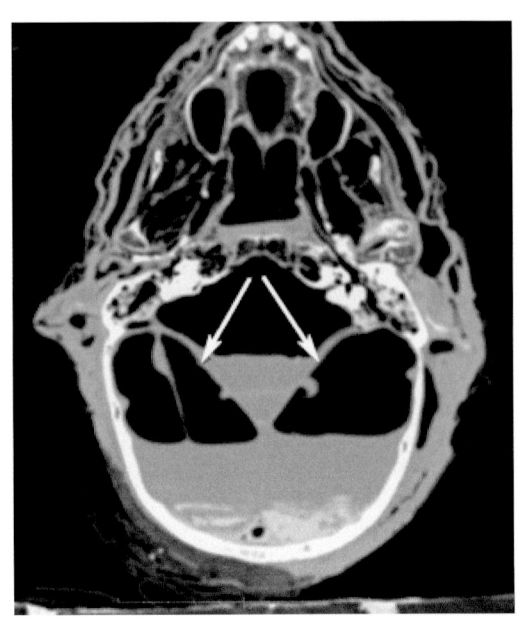

FIG. 4.46 AXIAL VIEW OF SKULL - MENINGES AND RESIN LEVELS.

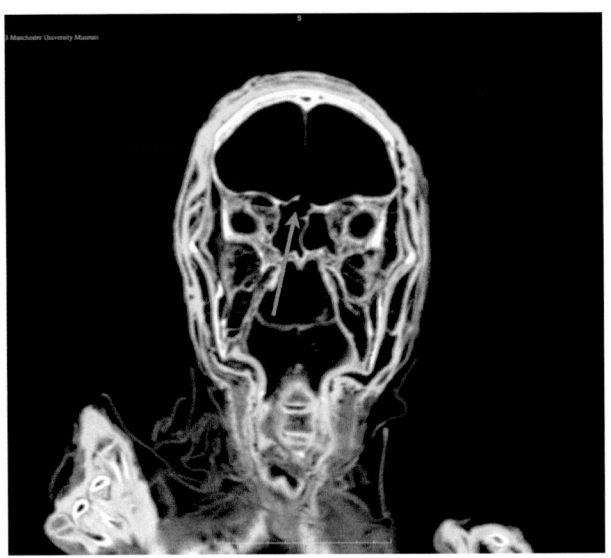

FIG. 4.44 CORONAL VIEW OF SKULL SHOWING LIMITED PERFORATION OF CRIBRIFORM PLATE.

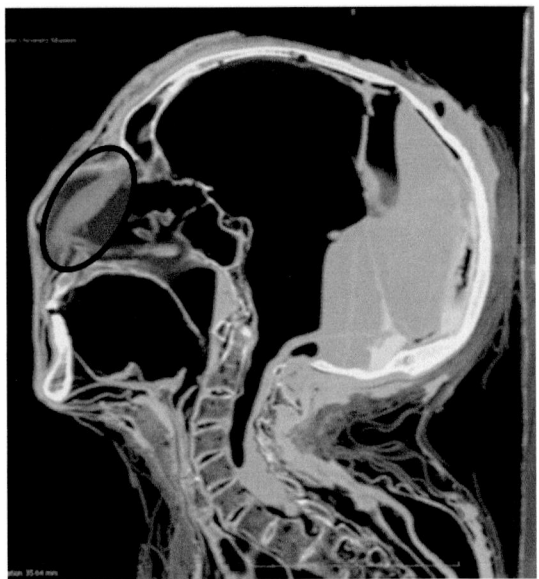

FIG. 4.47 SAGITTAL VIEW OF SKULL - NASAL TAMPONS.

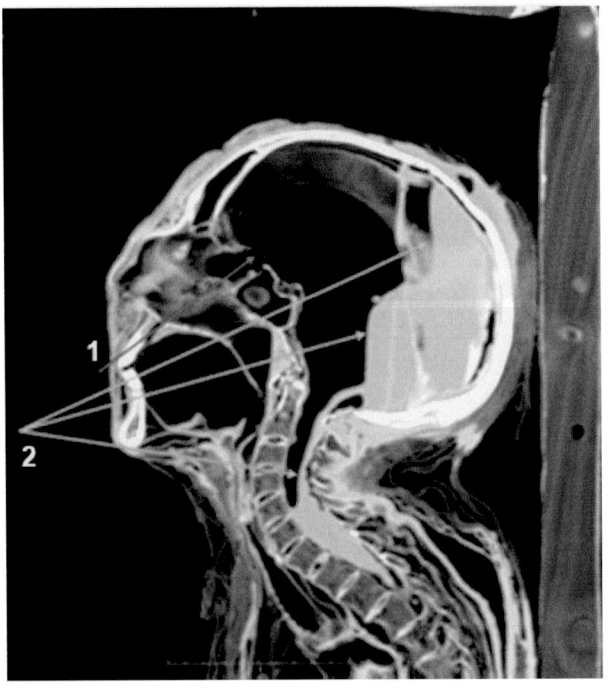

FIG. 4.45 SAGITTAL VIEW OF SKULL - POSTERIOR ETHMOID PERFORATION AND RESIN LEVELS.

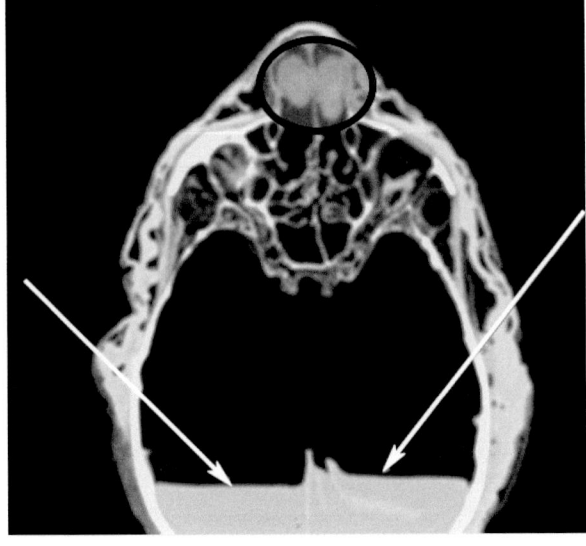

FIG. 4.48 AXIAL VIEW OF SKULL - NASAL TAMPONS AND RESIN 'LEVELS'.

LIII. Unnamed - Manchester Museum (Accession No. MM1976.51.a)

Head

Excerebration has been performed with complete removal of the brain tissue and the introduction of some substance that has 'set' and, subsequently, fractured into many pieces (the substance has at least two different radio densities) (See Fig. 4.49). As can be seen from this figure a trans-nasal route has been used with perforation of the cribriform plate via the ethmoid sinuses.

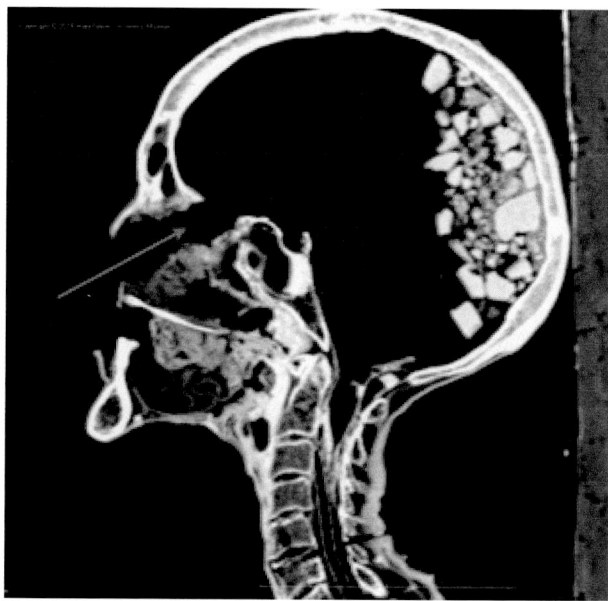

FIG. 4.49 SAGITTAL VIEW OF SKULL SHOWING EXCEREBRATION ROUTE VIA ETHMOID AIR SINUSES.

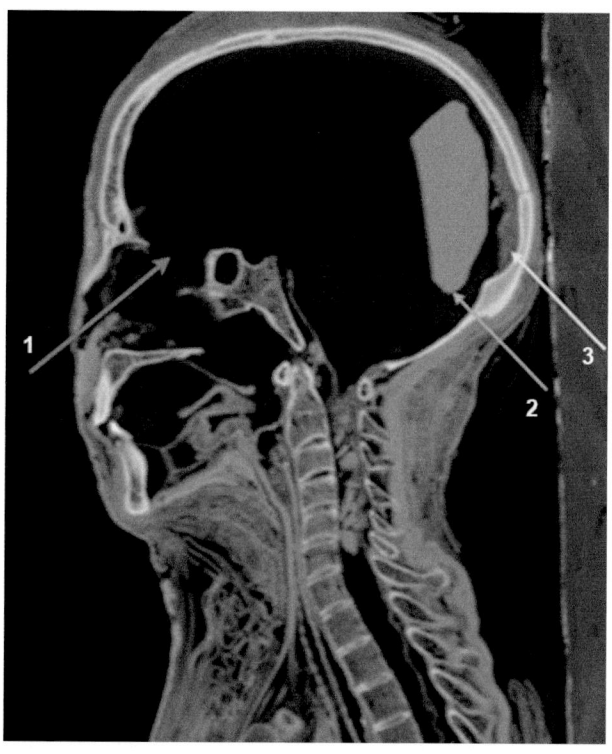

FIG. 4.50 SAGITTAL VIEW OF SKULL - EXCEREBRATION ROUTE AND RESIN.

LIV. Unnamed - Manchester Museum (Accession. No. Salford2)

Head

Trans-nasal excerebration has been via the ethmoid and cribriform plate with the brain almost completely removed and resin inserted. Remnants of this and other material (possibly brain tissue) are seen in the posterior cranial fossa (See Fig. 4.50 - where the arrow 1 shows the route for excerebration, the arrow 2 shows the resin and the arrow 3 shows the other material possibly brain tissue).

LVI. Unnamed child - Manchester Museum (Accession. No. MM 2109)

Head

Complete excerebration has been via the ethmoid sinus and cribriform plate (See Figs. 4.51 and 4.52). The plate of bone fractured from the cribriform plate is seen in the posterior fossa (See Fig. 4.53 - black circle). No material has been introduced following excerebration.

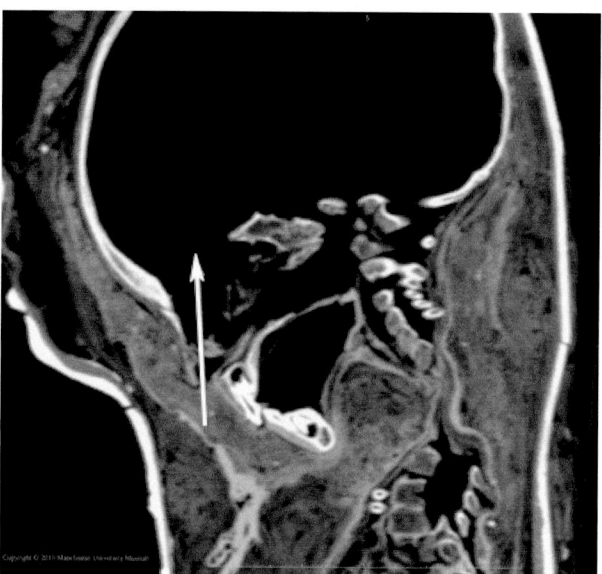

FIG. 4.51 SAGITTAL VIEW OF SKULL DEMONSTRATING CRIBRIFORM PLATE PERFORATION.

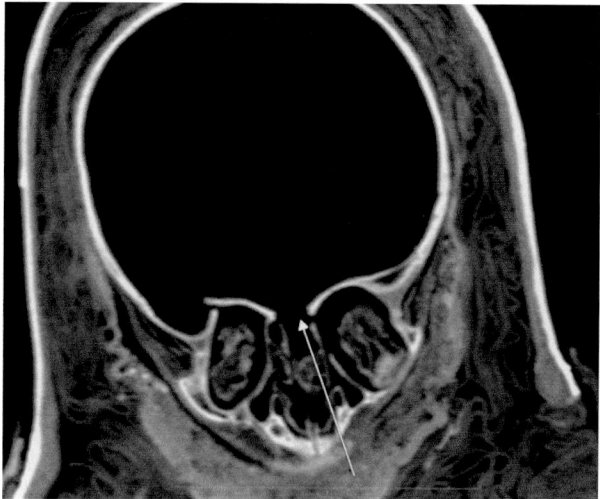

FIG. 4.52 CORONAL VIEW OF SKULL SHOWING CRIBRIFORM PLATE PERFORATION.

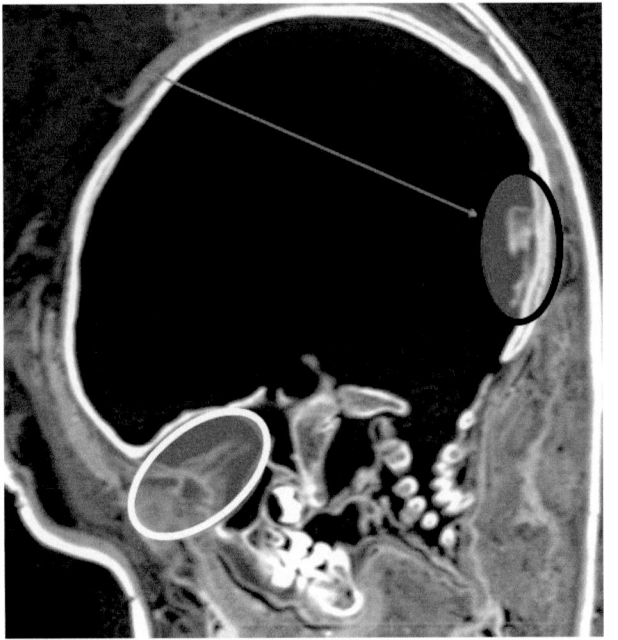

FIG. 4.53 SAGITTAL VIEW OF SKULL - FRAGMENT OF CRIBRIFORM PLATE IN POSTERIOR CRANIAL FOSSA.

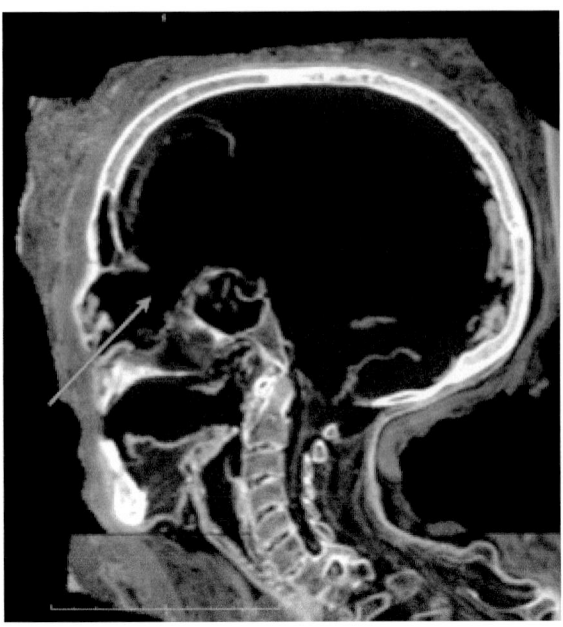

FIG. 4.55 SAGITTAL VIEW OF SKULL - ETHMOID PERFORATION.

LVII. Artemidorus - Manchester Museum (Cat. No. MM 1775)

Head

Excerebration has been performed via the ethmoid sinus and the cribriform plate. The sphenoid sinus has been spared (See Figs. 4.54 and 4.55).

Fig. 4.56 shows a small amount of residual brain tissue in the posterior fossa (arrow 2). There is, also, some remaining meningeal tissue. arrows 3.

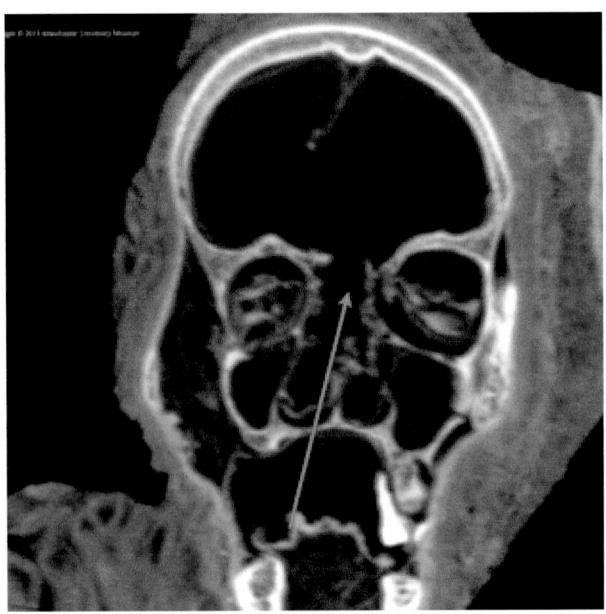

FIG. 4.54 CORONAL VIEW OF SKULL - ETHMOID PERFORATION.

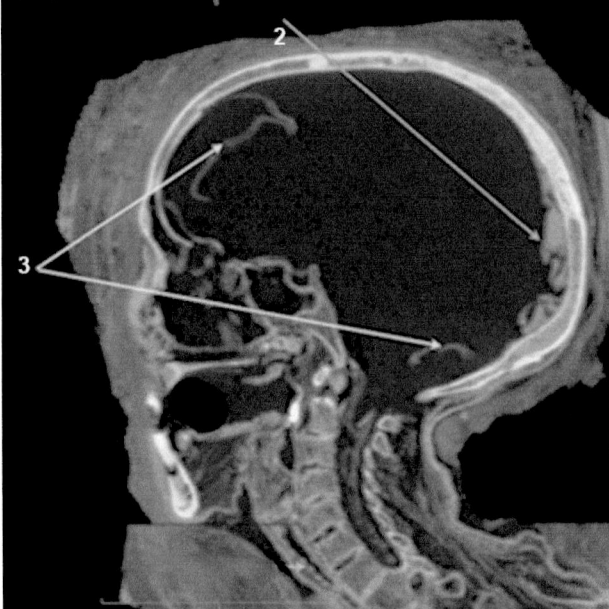

FIG. 4.56 SAGITTAL VIEW OF SKULL - MENINGES AND BRAIN TISSUE.

LX. Unnamed - British Museum (Cat. No. EA 6704)

Head

Excerebration has been performed via the ethmoid sinuses and the cribriform plate (See Figs. 4.57 and 4.58 - arrow 1) with a small amount of material - probably resin - in the posterior cranial fossa (See Fig. 4.57- arrow 3). A linen tampon has been inserted into the nose subsequently (See Fig. 4.57 - arrow 2).

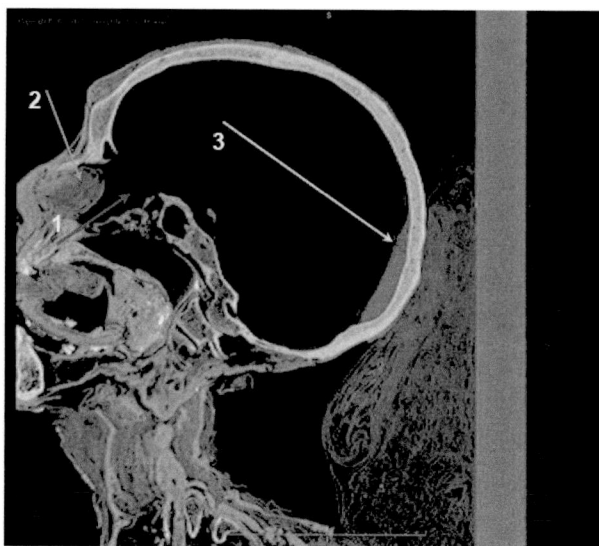

FIG. 4.57 SAGITTAL VIEW OF SKULL - CRIBRIFORM PERFORATION, RESIN AND NASAL TAMPON.
COURTESY OF THE TRUSTEES OF THE BRITISH MUSEUM

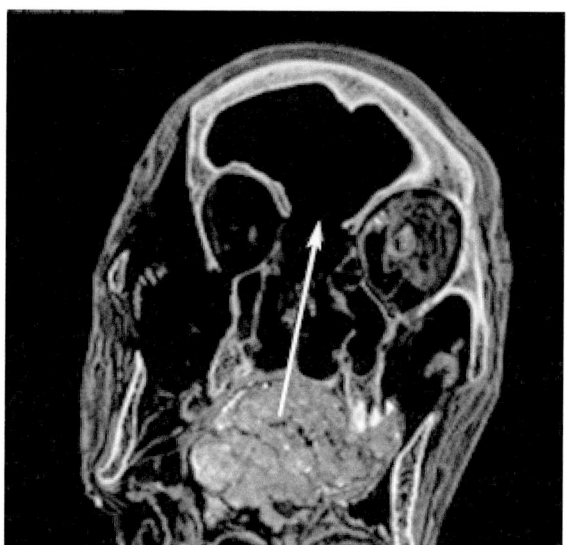

FIG. 4.58 AXIAL VIEW OF SKULL - ETHMOID SINUS AND CRIBRIFORM PLATE PERFORATION.
COURTESY OF THE TRUSTEES OF THE BRITISH MUSEUM

4.1.1.2 Ethmoid and sphenoid perforation

There are ten examples of more extensive perforation of the cribriform plate that is perforation of both the ethmoid and sphenoid sinuses. These will be set out below (Table 4.2) for comparison with Table 4.1 (P35).

NUMBER	ERA	LOCATION
V	Dyn. 25	Thebes
VIII	Dyn. 22	Thebes
X	Ptolemaic	Akhmim
XVI	Roman	Thebes
XXII	Unknown	Unknown
XXXIV	Dyn. 22	Thebes
XXXV	Dyn. 22	Thebes/Fayum
XL	3IP	Unknown
XLII	Ptolemaic	Fayum
XLIV	Ptolemaic	Unknown

TABLE 4.2 MUMMIES WITH ETHMOID AND SPHENOID PERFORATION

V Nesitanebetasheru - Sheffield Museum (Cat. No. J93.1283)

Head

Excerebration has been carried out via the trans-nasal route with no evidence of residual brain material in the cranial cavity. There are, however, 'levels' of radio-opaque material in the posterior part of the cavity – almost certainly due to the introduction of resin. The double level indicates preservation of the falx cerebri or falx cerebella. There is also evidence of the meninges having been retained (See Fig. 4.59).

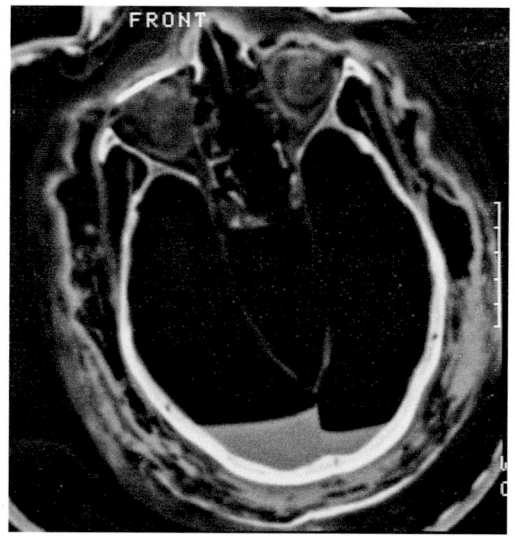

FIG. 4.59 AXIAL VIEW OF SKULL - RESIN LEVELS

Fig. 4.59 also shows perforation of the cribriform plate, but with retention of some of the structures of the nasal cavity.

VIII Padiamun - National Museums Liverpool (Accession No. 53.72a)

Head

There is an almost completely empty cranial cavity with a small amount of material in the posterior fossa, seen in Fig. 4.60, arrow 1. This figure also illustrates the absence of the cribriform plate, arrow 2 that would indicate a trans-nasal excerebration.

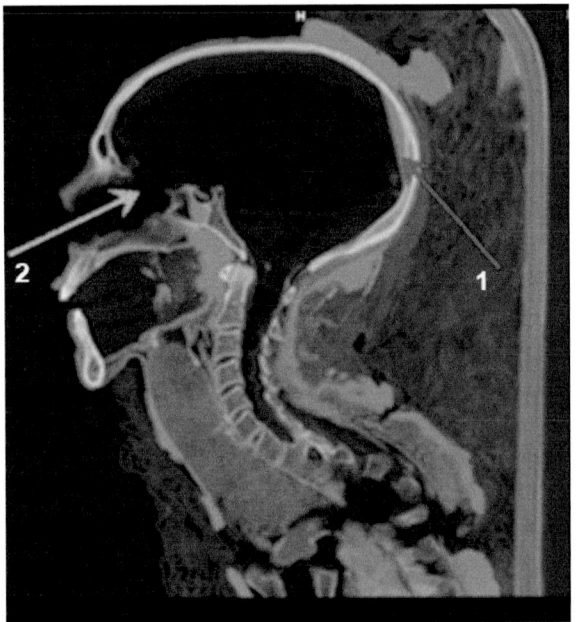

FIG. 4.60 SAGITTAL VIEW OF SKULL - EXCEREBRATION AND RESIN

X. Nesmin- National Museums Liverpool (Accession No. 56.22.79a)

Head

There is perforation of the cribriform plate on the right, with destruction of the ethmoid air sinuses and perforation of the anterior wall of the sphenoid sinuses. The brain has been completely removed (see Fig. 4.61 and Fig. 4.62 arrow 3). The sphenoid sinuses have resin in them (see Fig. 4.62 arrow 1).

The skull has a significant amount of resin in it with a fluid level corresponding to the posterior margin of the foramen magnum (See Fig. 4.62 - arrow 2). The resin has three distinct levels of material and there is a swirl of material running through the middle layer, suggesting that the posterior/lower layer has been poured later and 'subsided' through the middle layer or that the 'mixture' contains materials which become solid at different rates (See Fig. 4.63 arrow and Fig. 4.64 circle).

An alternative interpretation is that this represents a remnant of meninges.

Introduction of the resin has, presumably, been through the nose as there is evidence of resin in the pharynx, maxillary sinuses and sphenoid sinuses as well as in the posterior fossa of the cranium.

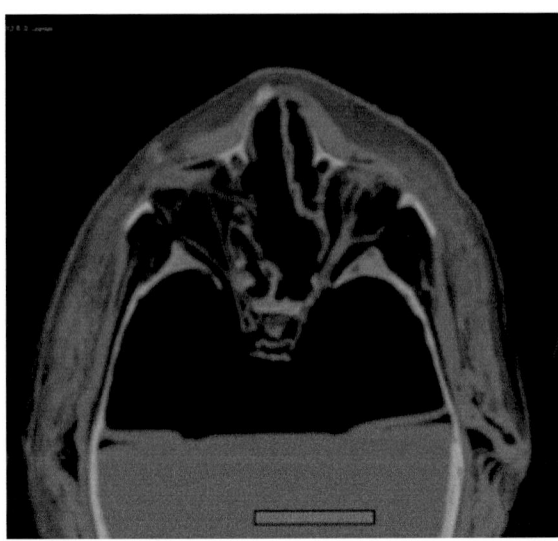

FIG. 4.61 AXIAL VIEW OF SKULL SHOWING ROUTE OF EXCEREBRATION

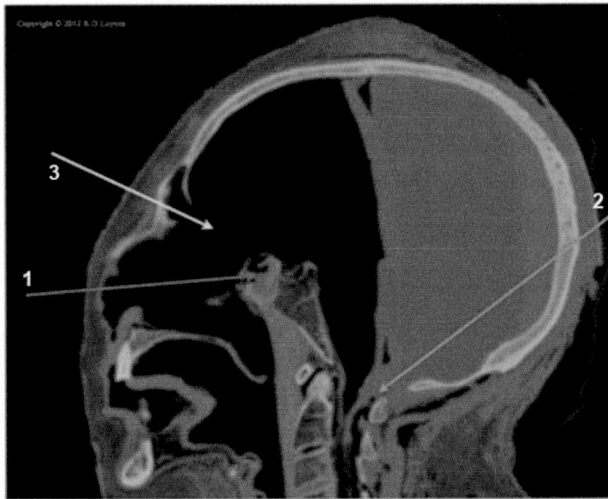

FIG. 4.62 SAGITTAL VIEW OF SKULL - EXCEREBRATION AND RESIN

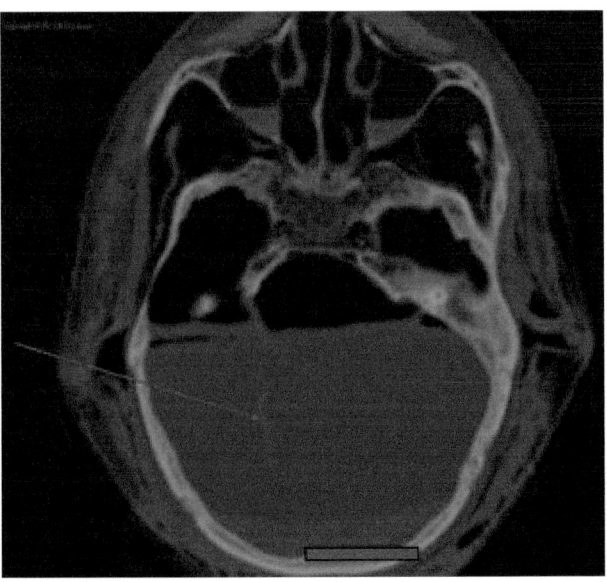

FIG. 4.63 AXIAL VIEW OF SKULL DEMONSTRATING RESIN

RESULTS – THE HEAD

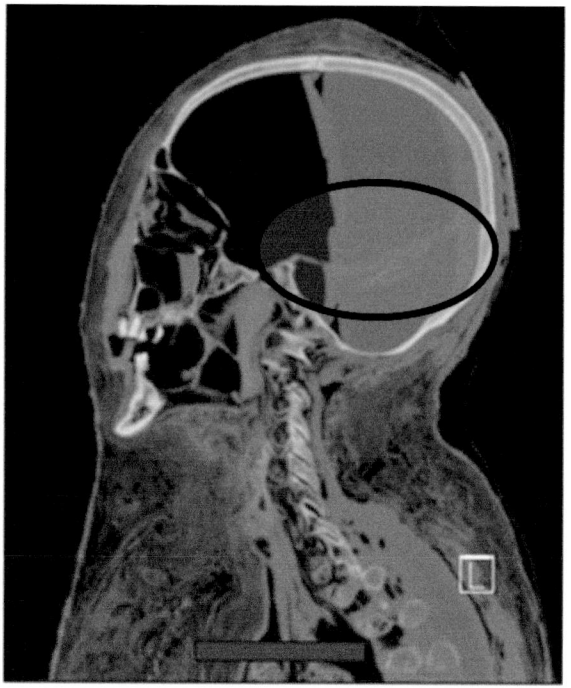

FIG. 4.64 SAGITTAL VIEW OF SKULL DEMONSTRATING TWO MATERIALS IN RESIN PACKING

Perforation of the ethmoid is also demonstrated in Fig. 4.67 and the nasal tampon in Fig. 4.68. In Figs. 4.65 and 4.66 the 'layering' of the resin can be seen, indicating the possibility of two different components of the resin.

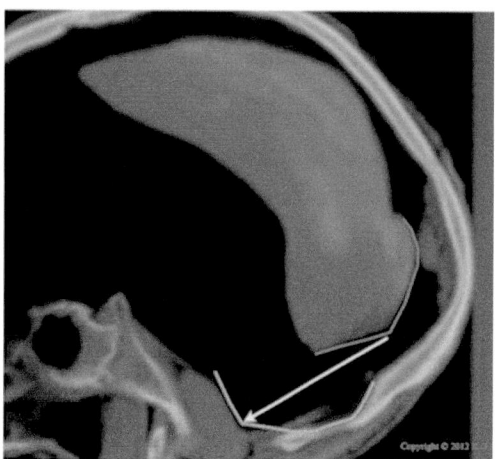

FIG. 4.66 SAGITTAL VIEW OF SKULL SHOWING MOVEMENT OF THE RESIN

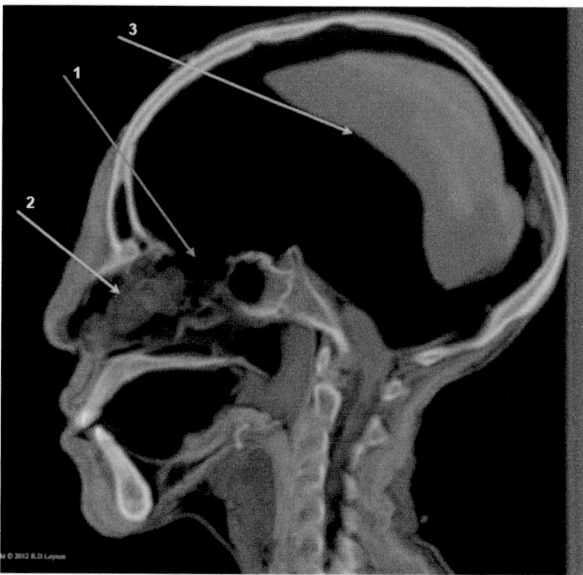

FIG. 4.65 SAGITTAL VIEW OF SKULL SHOWING NASAL TAMPON, ETHMOID PERFORATION AND RESIN

XVI. Unnamed - National Museums Liverpool (accession No. M13997a)

Head

Excerebration has been performed via the trans-nasal route, with perforation of the ethmoid and damage to the anterior wall of the sphenoid sinus (See Fig. 4.65 - arrow 1 to perforation of the ethmoid : arrow 2 to a pack ('tampon') in the nose and arrow 3 to solidified resin in the cranial cavity). Resin has been introduced into the cranial cavity after complete removal of the brain tissue. From the appearance of the 'fluid level' in the resin, it would appear that this has become detached from the back of the skull and has moved since its introduction (See Fig. 4.66).

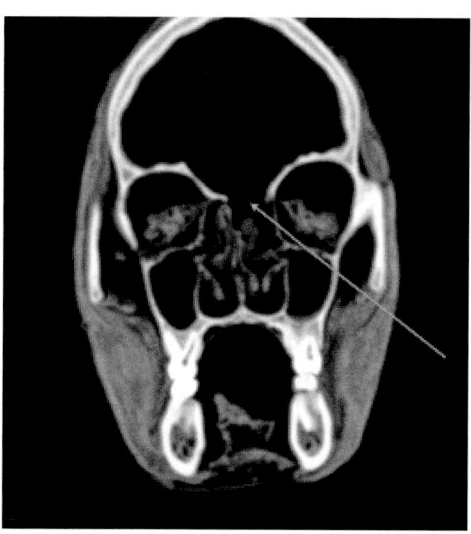

FIG. 4.67 CORONAL VIEW OF SKULL - ETHMOID PERFORATION

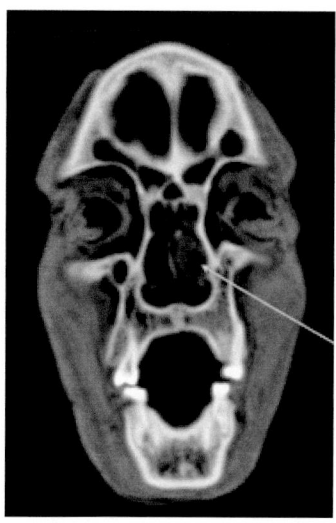

FIG. 4.68 CORONAL VIEW OF SKULL - NASAL TAMPON

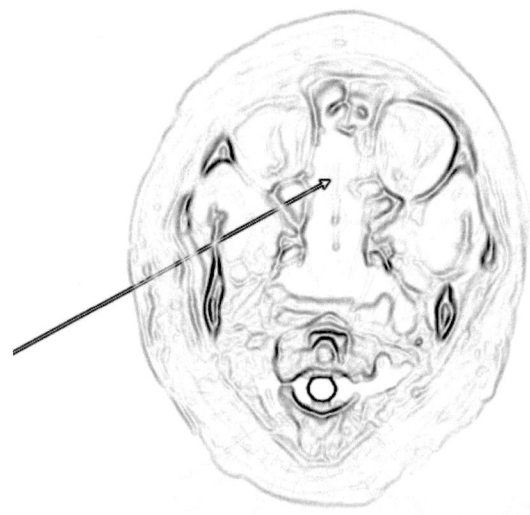

Fig. 4.69 Axial view of skull - ethmoid perforation (After IEM image)

XXII. Unnamed - Bern Museum - Cat. No. 00/2

Head

Excerebration has been performed via the cribriform plate, with complete removal of the brain (See Fig. 4.69 - arrow).

XXXIV. Unnamed - British Museum - (Accession No. EA 25258)

Head

There has been thorough trans-nasal excerebration via both ethmoid and sphenoid sinuses leaving no evidence of any brain tissue within the cranial cavity (See Figs. 4.70 and 4.71. - arrows).

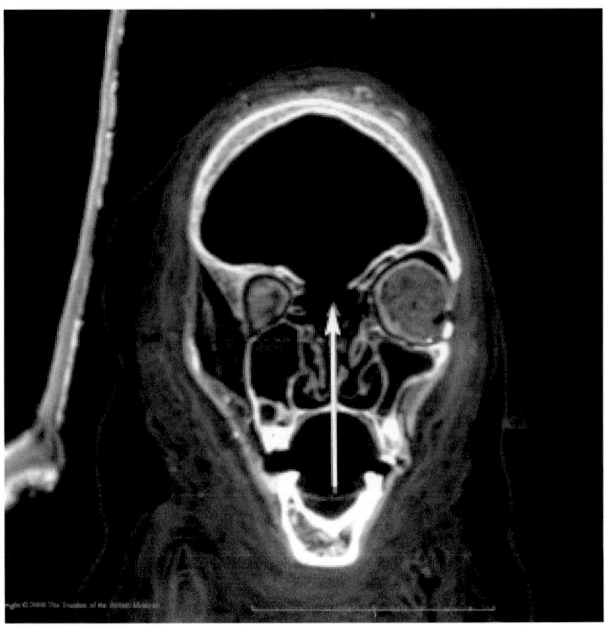

Fig. 4.71 Coronal view of skull - cribriform plate perforation.
Courtesy of the Trustees of the British Museum

XXXV. Djedameniufankh - British Museum - (Accession No. EA 29577)

Head

Although the head has clearly been disarticulated, and shows no evidence of soft tissues, excerebration has been performed via the trans-nasal route with perforation of the ethmoid and sphenoid air sinuses (See Figs. 4.72 and 4.73).

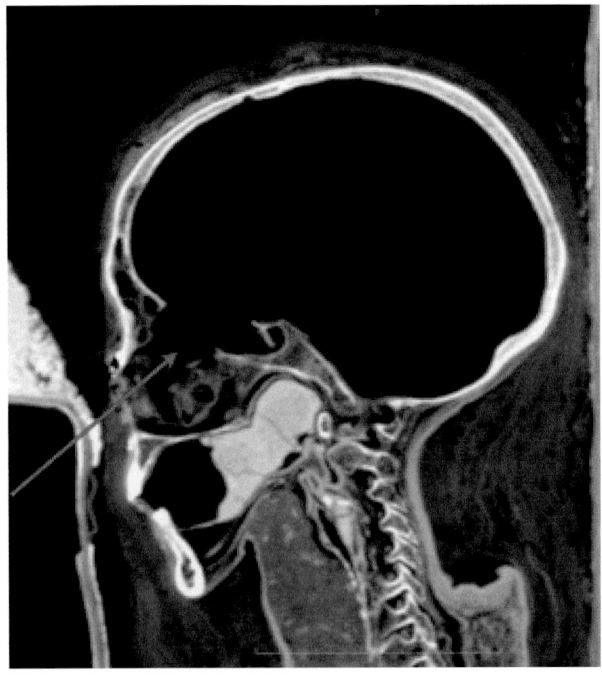

Fig. 4.70 Sagittal view of skull - cribriform plate perforation.
Courtesy of the Trustees of the British Museum

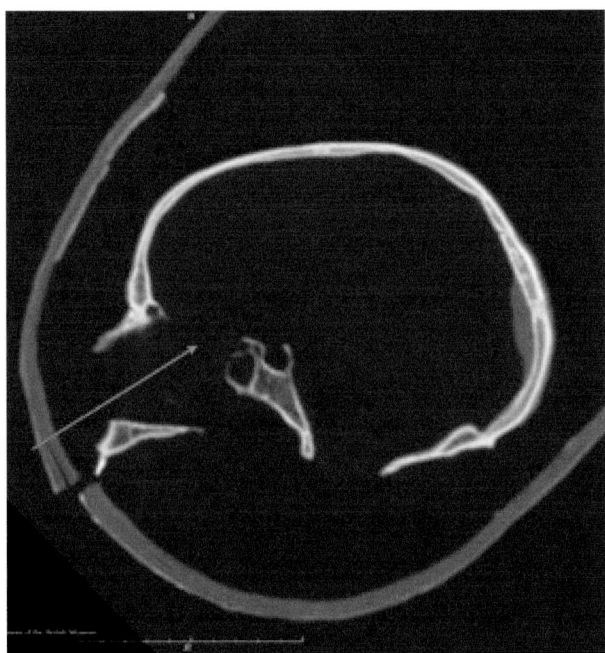

Fig. 4.72 Sagittal view of skull demonstrating the excerebration route.
Courtesy of the Trustees of the British Museum

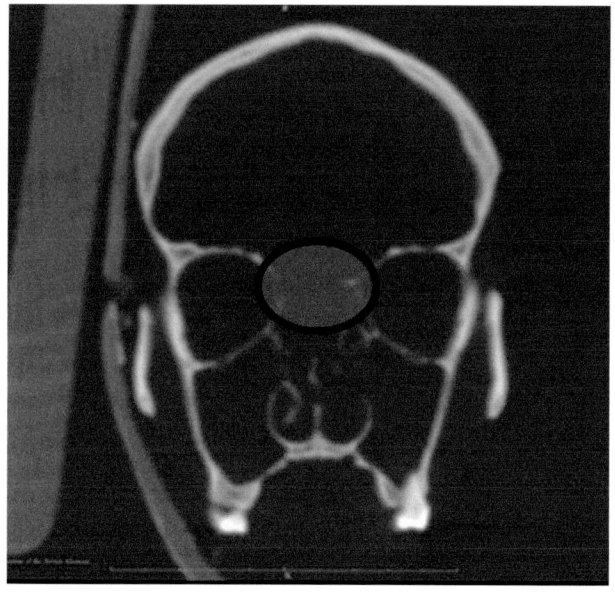

FIG. 4.73 CORONAL VIEW OF SKULL DEMONSTRATING THE EXCEREBRATION ROUTE.
COURTESY OF THE TRUSTEES OF THE BRITISH MUSEUM

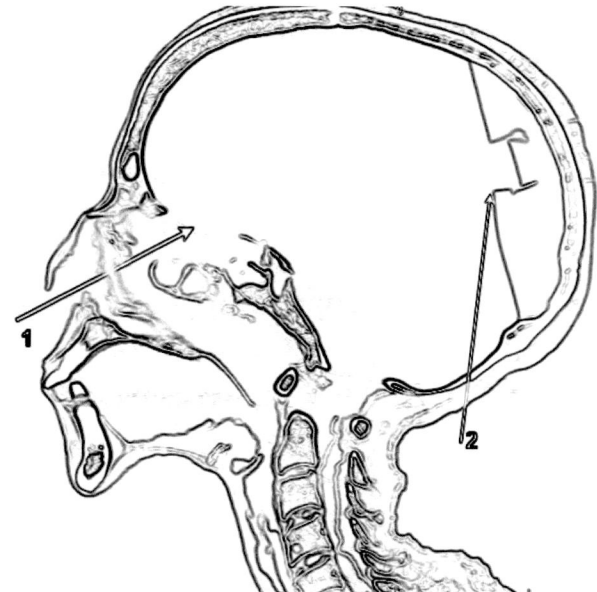

FIG. 4.75 SAGITTAL VIEW OF SKULL - EXCEREBRATION ROUTE AND RESIN (AFTER IEM IMAGE)

XL. Unnamed - Lausanne (Cat. No.492)

Head

Complete excerebration has been performed via a more horizontal route than is usually seen with perforation of the ethmoid and sphenoid sinuses (See Fig. 4.74; arrow and Fig. 4.75) followed by the introduction of resin into the cranial cavity. This has set and cracked (See Fig. 4.75; arrow 2).

XLII. Ta-aset - Turin (Cat. No. Suppl. 9480)

Head

The cranial cavity exhibits deep vascular markings and remnants of the meninges. Complete excerebration has been performed via the trans-nasal route. There is a small amount of radio-dense material in the back of the cranial cavity and the nose packed with two nasal tampons.

XLIV. Unnamed -Turin (Cat. No. Prov. 610)

Head

Complete trans-nasal excerebration has been performed with a very small amount of debris remaining in the posterior part of the cranial cavity, but no resin or other substance.

4.1.1.3 Sphenoid only perforation

There are three examples of perforation of the sphenoid sinus only without any intrusion into the ethmoid sinuses. In these cases, the exit point is either through or below the pituitary fossa.

The examples are given below.

XLVI. Ta-ath - Manchester Museum (Cat. No. MM10881)

Head

Thorough trans-nasal excerebration has been performed with a little debris and resin in the back of the skull (See Fig. 4.76). Although the trans-nasal route has been used it has been via the sphenoid rather than the ethmoid sinuses, thus leaving the cribriform plate intact (See Figs. 4.77 and 4.78).

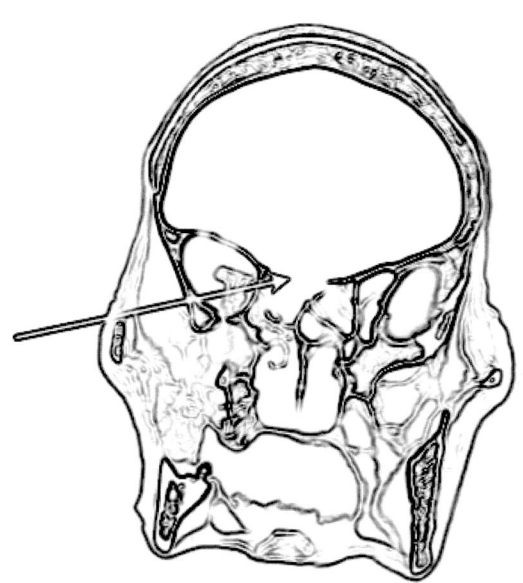

FIG. 4.74 CORONAL VIEW OF SKULL DEMONSTRATING THE EXCEREBRATION ROUTE (AFTER IEM IMAGE)

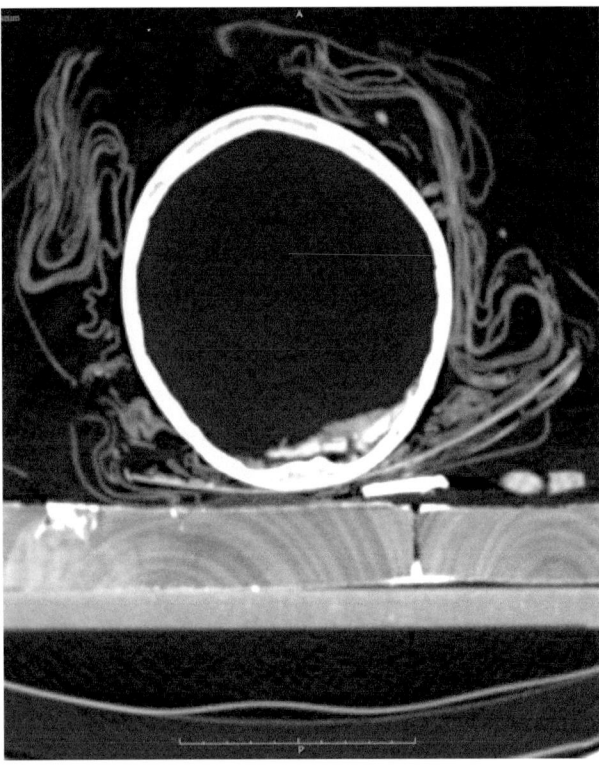

FIG. 4.76 AXIAL VIEW OF SKULL - DEBRIS IN POSTERIOR CRANIAL FOSSA

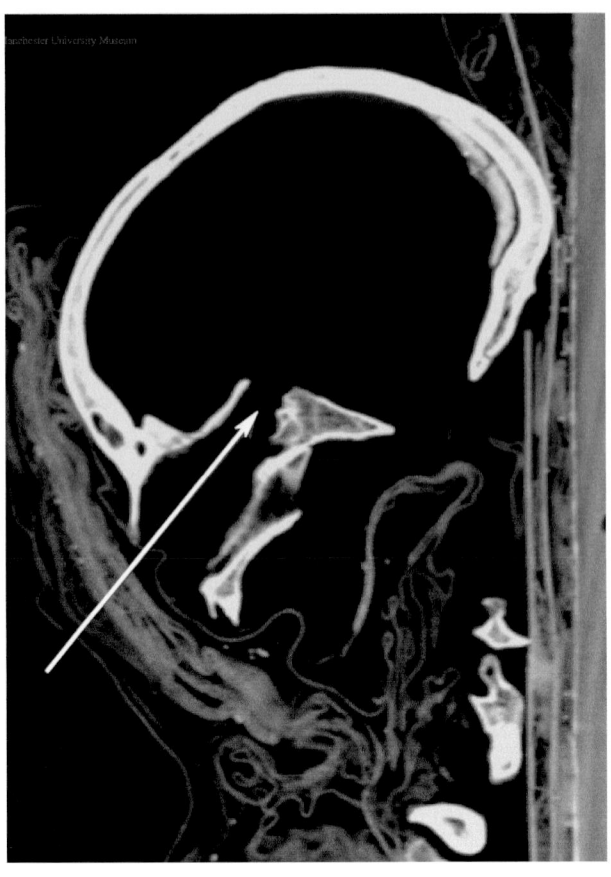

FIG. 4.78 SAGITTAL VIEW OF SKULL - SPHENOID PERFORATION

IL. Perenbast - Manchester University Museum (Accession No. MM5053.a)

Head

Excerebration has been performed thoroughly via the nose. The route is more horizontal than usual, resulting in perforation of the sphenoid sinus rather than the ethmoid sinus (See Fig. 4.79, which also shows remnants of the meninges, the brain having been completely removed). Fig. 4.80 shows the same features in the sagittal view. In this case, with the much more horizontal approach, the cribriform plate has not been perforated. Linen has been inserted into the cranial cavity - mostly on the right (See Fig. 4.81 – black circle).

LIX. Unnamed - British Museum (Cat. No.EA 22108)

Head

Excerebration has definitely been performed, there being a little residual foreign material in the posterior cranial fossa (See Fig. 4.82 - arrow). No perforation of the cribriform plate or disturbance of the atlanto-occipital region is seen but there is a ragged horizontal perforation through the base of the skull (See Figs. 4.83 and 4.84) which progresses through the sphenoid sinus on the right and on, posteriorly, into the cranial cavity inferior to the pituitary fossa. This is the most likely route for entry into the cranial cavity.

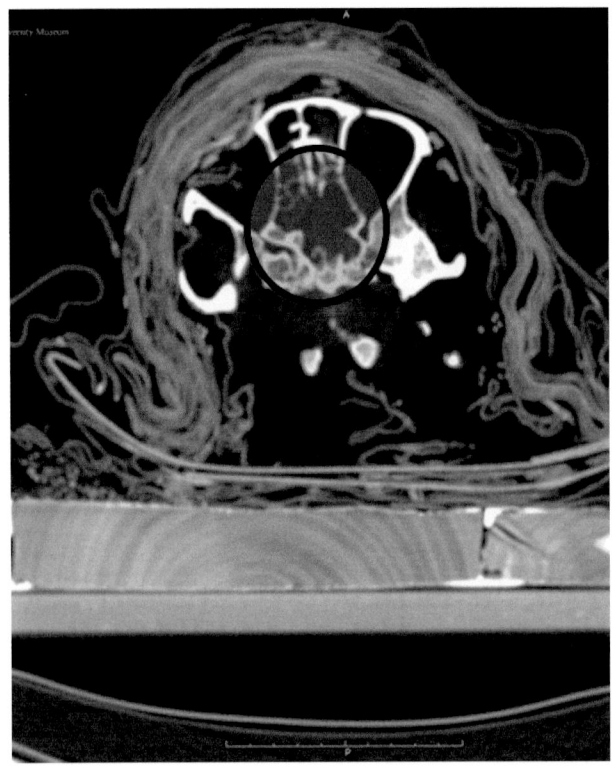

FIG. 4.77 AXIAL VIEW OF SKULL - SPHENOID PERFORATION

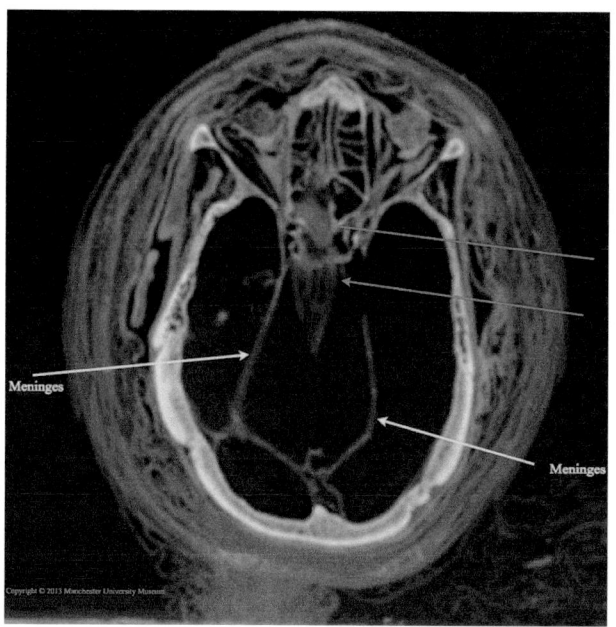

FIG. 4.79 AXIAL VIEW OF SKULL - SPHENOID PERFORATION

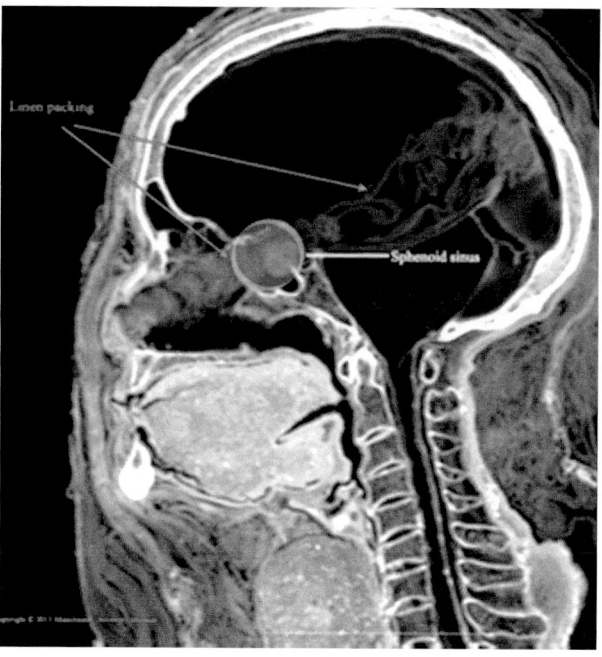

FIG. 4.80 SAGITTAL VIEW OF SKULL - SPHENOID PERFORATION AND LINEN PACKING

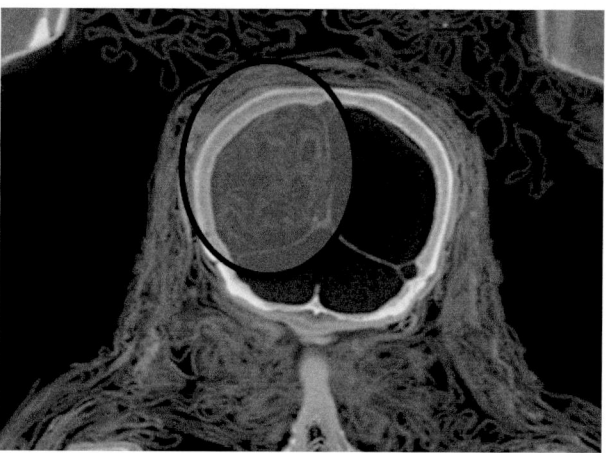

FIG. 4.81 AXIAL VIEW OF SKULL DEMONSTRATING LINEN PACKING

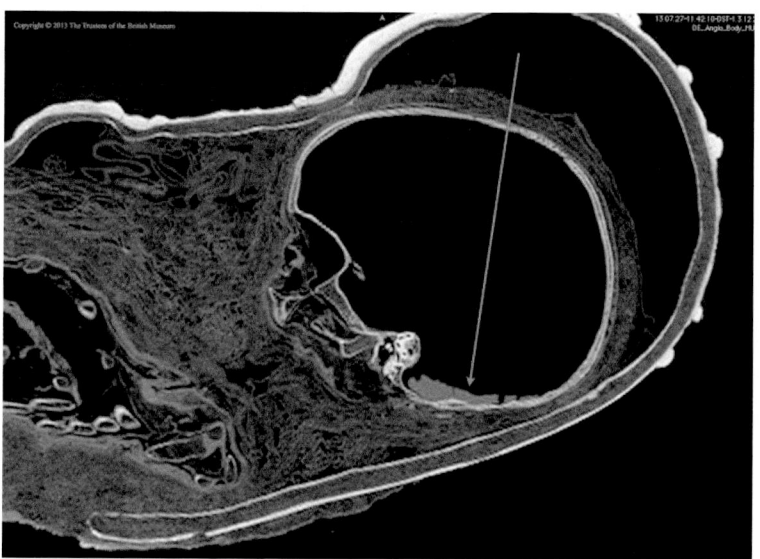

FIG. 4.82 SAGITTAL VIEW OF SKULL - FOREIGN MATERIAL IN POSTERIOR CRANIAL FOSSA.
COURTESY OF THE TRUSTEES OF THE BRITISH MUSEUM

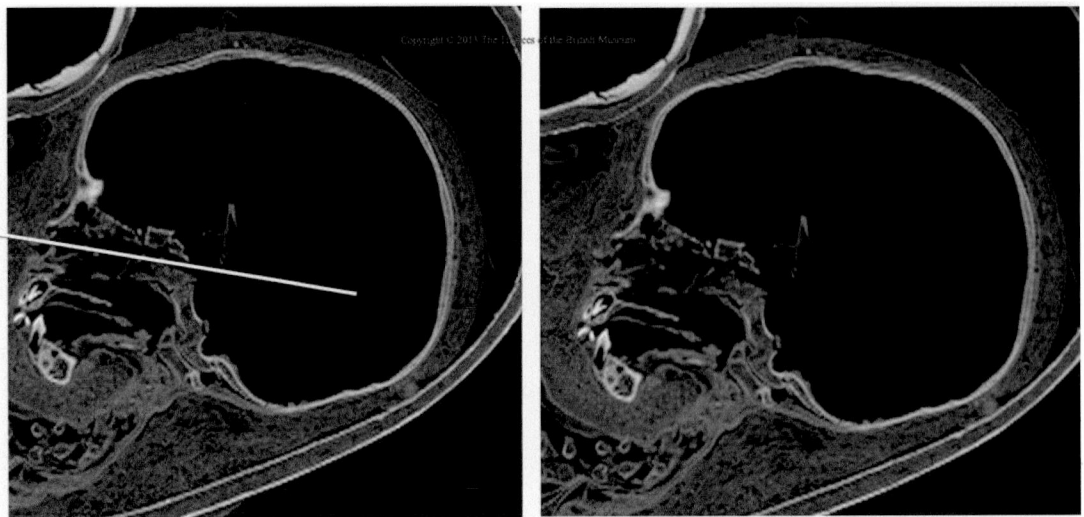

Fig. 4.83 Sagittal view of skull - route of cranial perforation
Courtesy of the Trustees of the British Museum

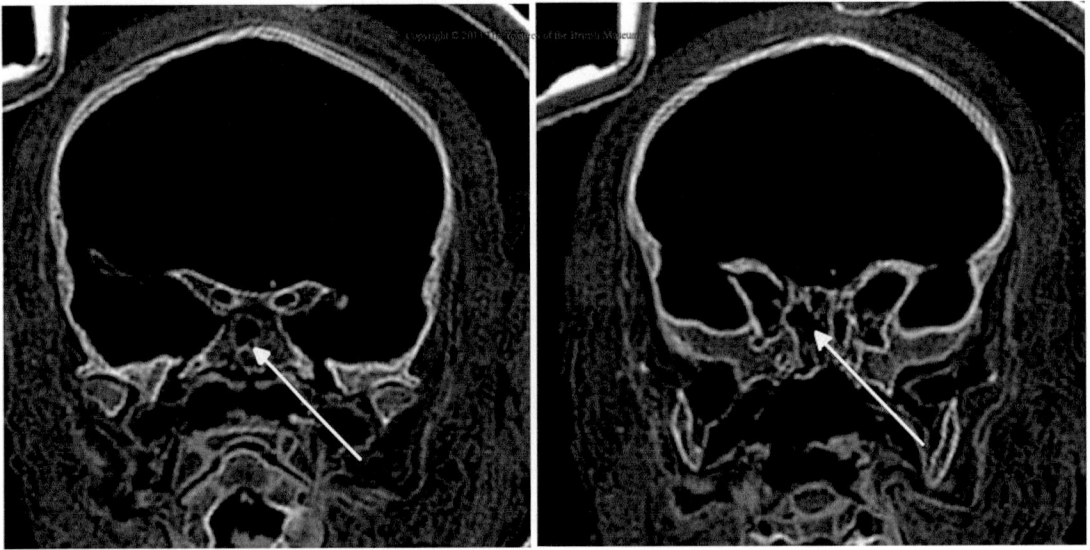

Fig. 4.84 Coronal view of skull - route of cranial perforation
Courtesy of the Trustees of the British Museum

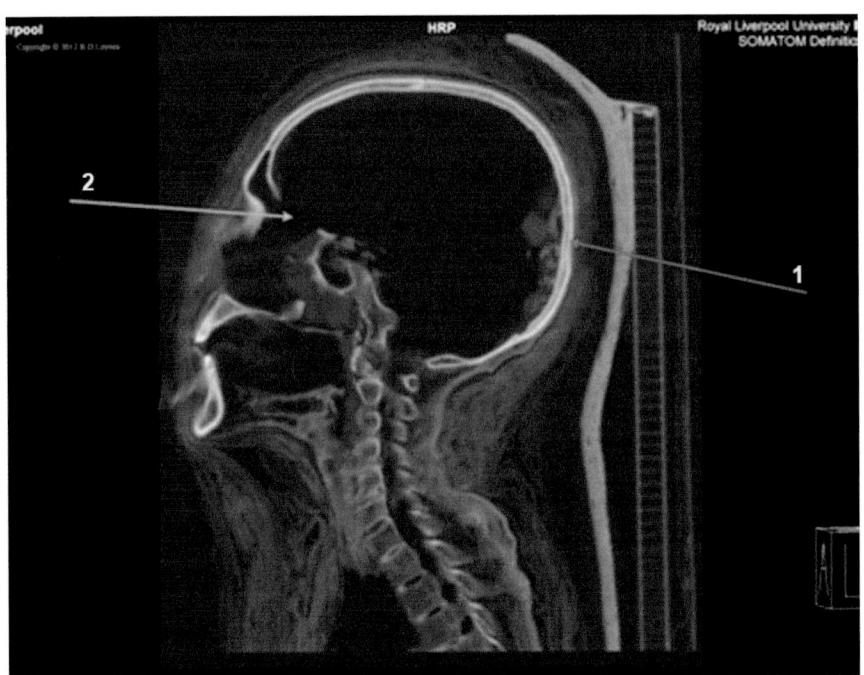

Fig. 4.85 Sagittal view of skull showing the excerebration route

RESULTS – THE HEAD

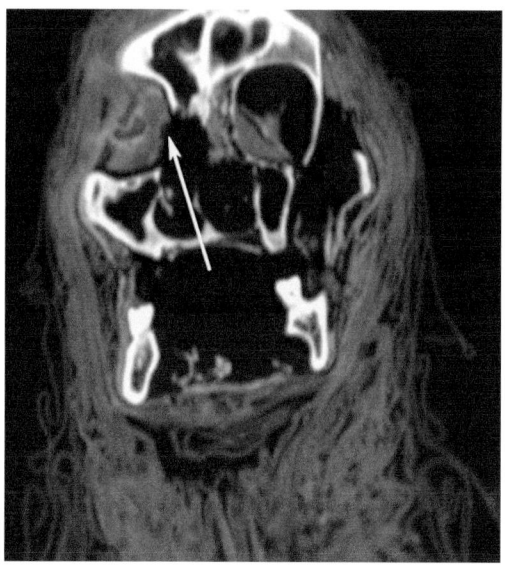

FIG. 4.86 CORONAL VIEW OF SKULL - EXCEREBRATION ROUTE IN ONE PLANE

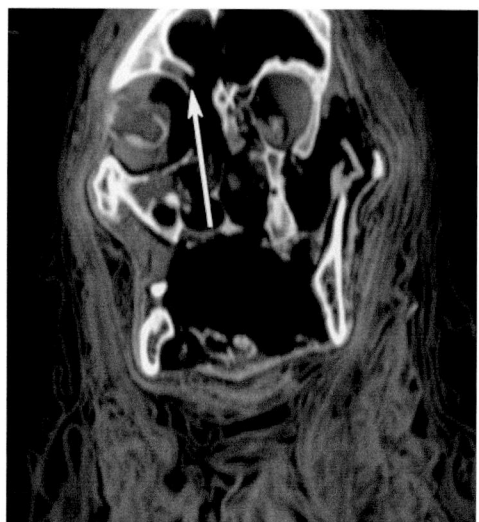

FIG. 4.87 CORONAL VIEW OF SKULL - EXCEREBRATION ROUTE IN SECOND PARALLEL PLANE

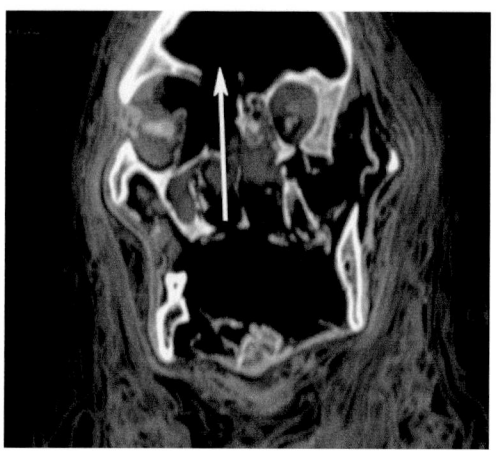

FIG. 4.88 CORONAL VIEW OF SKULL - EXCEREBRATION ROUTE IN THIRD PARALLEL PLANE

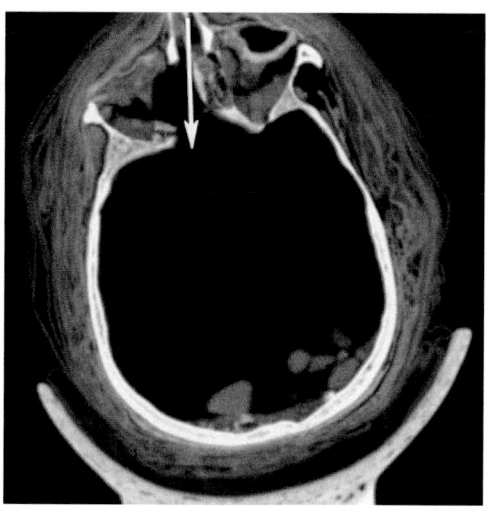

FIG. 4.89 AXIAL VIEW OF SKULL - EXCEREBRATION ROUTE

4.1.1.4 Trans-nasal/orbital perforation

There are two examples where the route used for excerebration has commenced in the nose, but has 'strayed' laterally to involve an orbit.

IX   Padiamunnebnesuttauwy - National Museums Liverpool (Accession No. M14050)

Head

The cranial cavity is empty of brain tissue but there is a small amount of material within the back of the cavity. As can be seen in Fig. 4.85, arrow 1 indicates this material that is a mixture of globular resin and a small amount of amorphous material.

Excerebration has been carried out through the trans-nasal route with removal of the cribriform plate (arrow 2, Fig. 4.85). However, the accuracy of the penetration of the skull is doubtful, as there is destruction of the medial wall of the right orbit as well as the cribriform plate (see Figs. 4.86 – 4.89).

XLVII.   Unnamed - Manchester Museum (Cat. No.MM1769)

Head

Excerebration has been performed via the nose, where the structures of the left nostril are damaged, passing laterally through the medial wall of the left orbit and through the superior orbital fissure into the cranial cavity (See Figs. 4.90 and 4.91 - black circles and Fig. 4.92).

There is a small amount of resin in the posterior cranial cavity (See Fig. 4.90 - arrow).

4.1.2 Trans-foraminal route

This route has been described by several authors (for example, Raven. Taconis., 2005: 58 and Wade, Nelson, Garvin, 2011: 250). Four instances of such an approach are found in this study. Whilst the fourth example, Number LVIII, is tentative the others are convincing.

VII Tahathor - Ipswich Museum (Cat. No. COLEM 1871.3.7)

Head

The cranial cavity contains amorphous granular material with a 'fluid level', indicating that it was probably fluid when placed within the skull, but subsequently became solid (See Fig. 4.93).

However, the position of the skull has changed since then. There are a variety of objects within the amorphous substance, which represent teeth and fragments of bone (See Fig. 4.94).

There are five teeth within the cranial cavity and seven teeth seen outside the skull, within the wrappings.

Returning to the description of the skull, whilst the cribriform plate is not actually visualised, the crista galli is seen and the internal structures of the nose are well preserved indicating that perforation of the cribriform plate had almost certainly not taken place. However, if the trans-nasal route has not been used for excerebration, there is evidence that the trans-foraminal route probably has. To support this, it is noteworthy that the dimensions of the foramen magnum are larger than normal. The anterior half of the foramen seems normal, whereas the posterior part is larger than normal as shown in Fig. 4.95 (41.08mms. as opposed to 34mms. as an approximate norm. in the sagittal plane and 44.47mms. as opposed to 25mms. in the transverse plane).

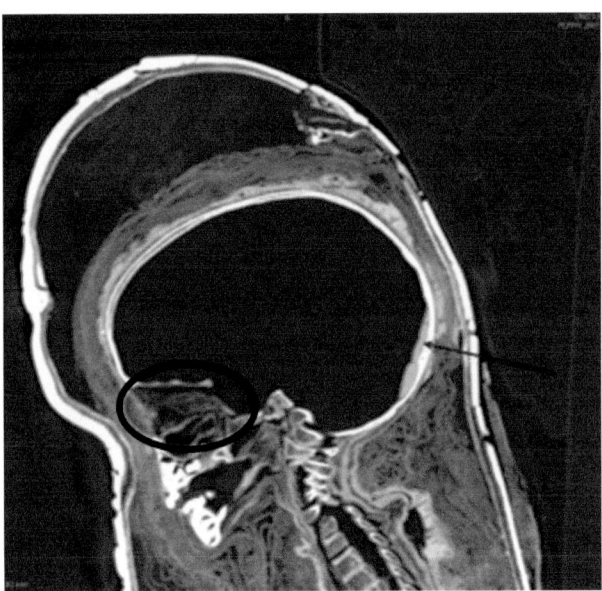

FIG. 4.90 SAGITTAL VIEW OF SKULL - TRANS-NASAL/ORBITAL ROUTE OF EXCEREBRATION

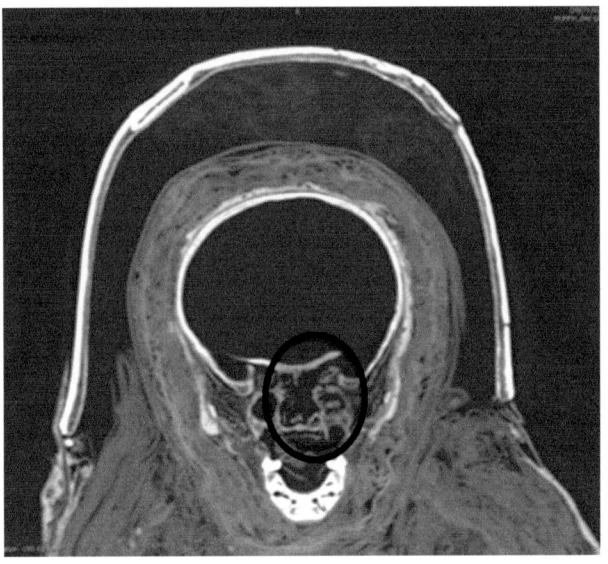

FIG. 4.91 CORONAL VIEW OF SKULL - TRANS-NASAL/ORBITAL ROUTE

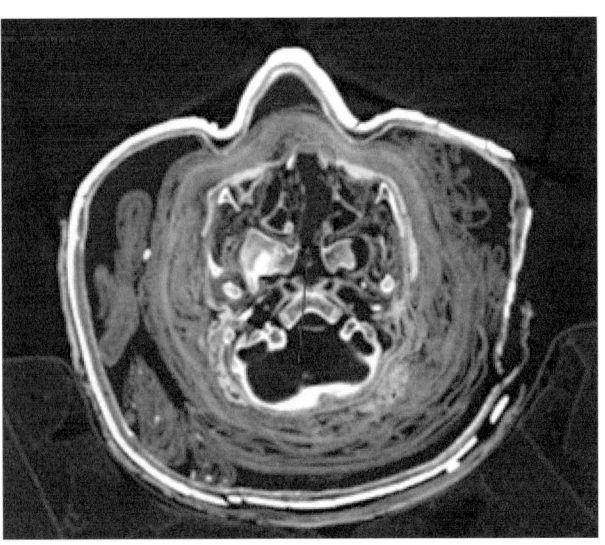

FIG. 4.92 AXIAL VIEW OF SKULL - TRANS-NASAL/ORBITAL ROUTE

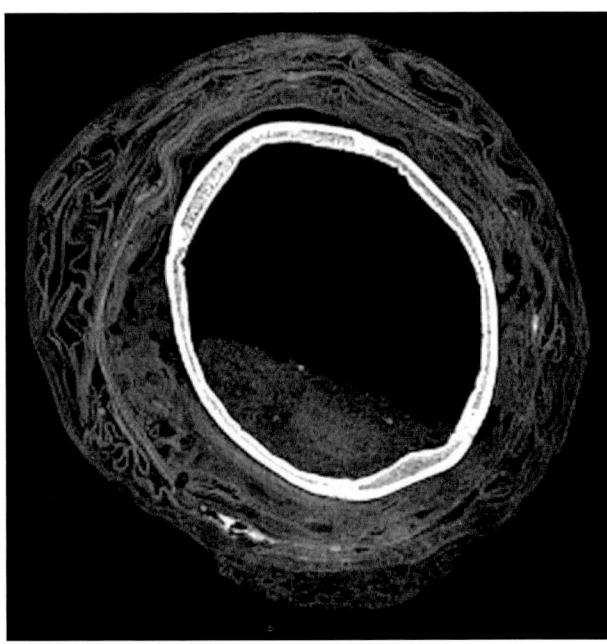

FIG. 4.93 AXIAL VIEW OF SKULL - GRANULAR MATERIAL

RESULTS – THE HEAD

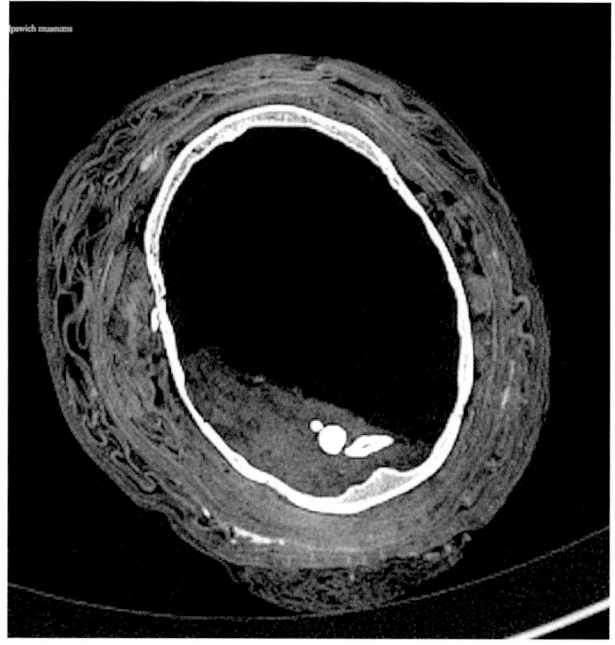

FIG. 4.94 AXIAL VIEW OF SKULL - TEETH IN GRANULAR MATERIAL

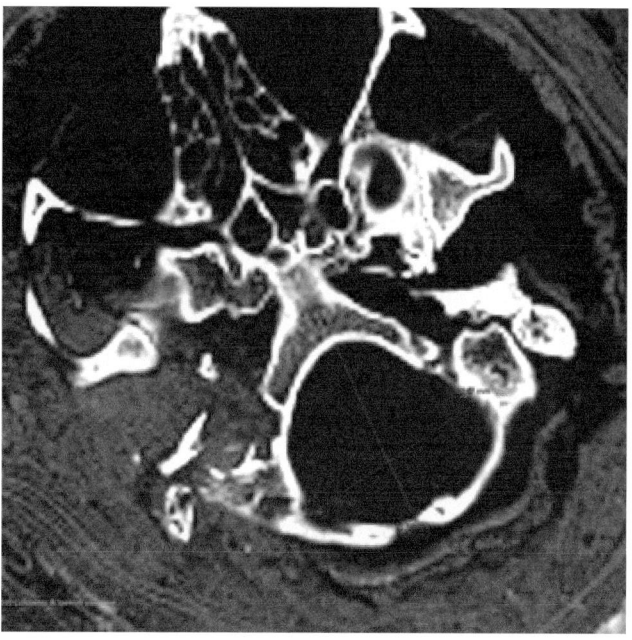

FIG. 4.95 AXIAL VIEW OF SKULL BASE - ENLARGED FORAMEN MAGNUM

Within the oral and naso pharynx there is the unusual appearance of the first cervical vertebra dislocated/translocated anteriorly (See Fig. 4.96).

More will be discussed regarding this feature in the next section on the cervical spine. There is some linen packing within the oropharynx. The images are dark and detail is lacking.

Neck

The main feature of the cervical spine is the complete disarticulation of the atlanto-occipital joint with translocation of the cervical spine anteriorly. There is no evidence of bony injury, indicating that this was achieved by 'sharp dissection'. In Figure 4.96 the lateral mass of the atlas is shown by the arrow 2 and the occipital facets by the arrow 1. No other abnormalities are seen in the cervical region other than the fact that the spinal canal has some granular material within it and the cervical spine is rotated in relationship to the skull.

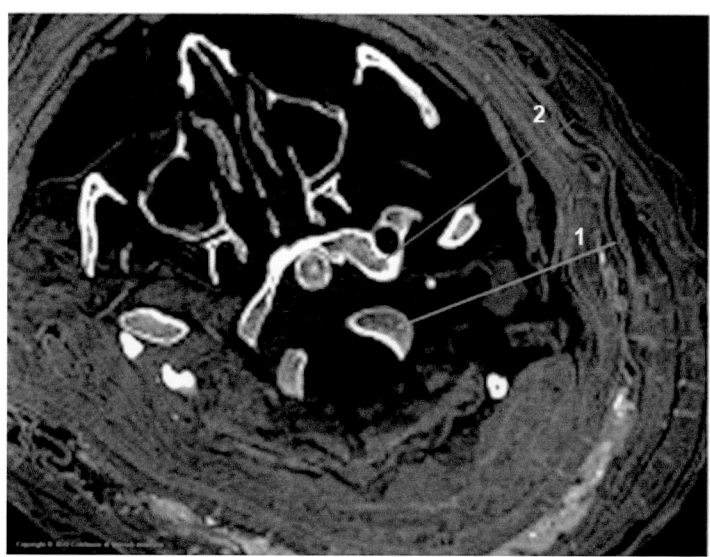

FIG. 4.96 AXIAL VIEW INFERIOR TO BASE OF SKULL - ANTERIORLY DISPLACED ATLAS

XV. Unnamed - National Museums Liverpool (Accession No. 13.10.11.25)

Head

Excerebration has been performed, there being no cerebral tissue present. There is a small amount of granular material in the posterior cranial fossa, more on the left than the right (arrow 1 in Fig. 4.97). This Figure also shows the foramen magnum - lines (5) and the posterior arch of the first cervical vertebra (Atlas) - arrow 3. It can be seen that the two structures lack the normal alignment. Also shown are the intact cribriform plate - arrows 4 and linen packing in the foramen magnum – arrow 2.

A coronal view shows displacement of the cervical spine to the right (See Fig. 4.98).

Axial views show rotation of the first cervical vertebra with respect to the foramen magnum. In Figs. 4.99 and 4.100, the midline of the skull is shown in 1 and the transverse axis of the foramen magnum and first cervical vertebra in 2.

This indicates that the cervico-occipital junction has been disturbed and is almost certainly the route of excerebration. A small amount of meninges has been retained in the left anterior fossa (See Fig. 4.101 - arrow 1).

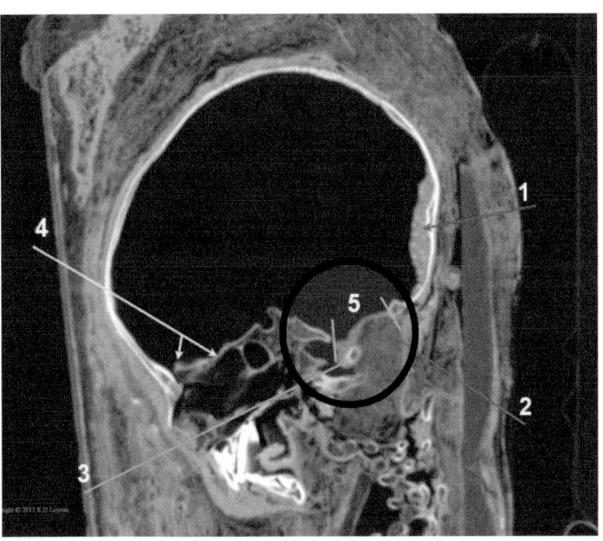

Fig. 4.97 Sagittal view of skull demonstrating trans-foraminal route

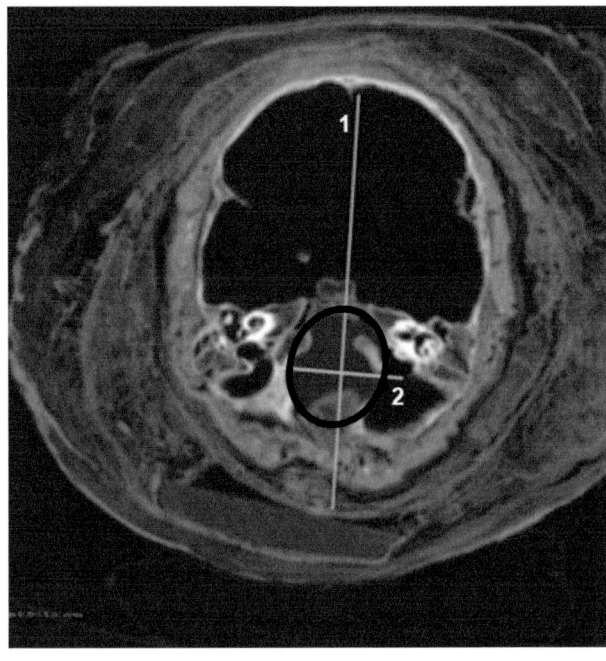

Fig. 4.99 Axial view close to skull base showing foramen magnum alignment

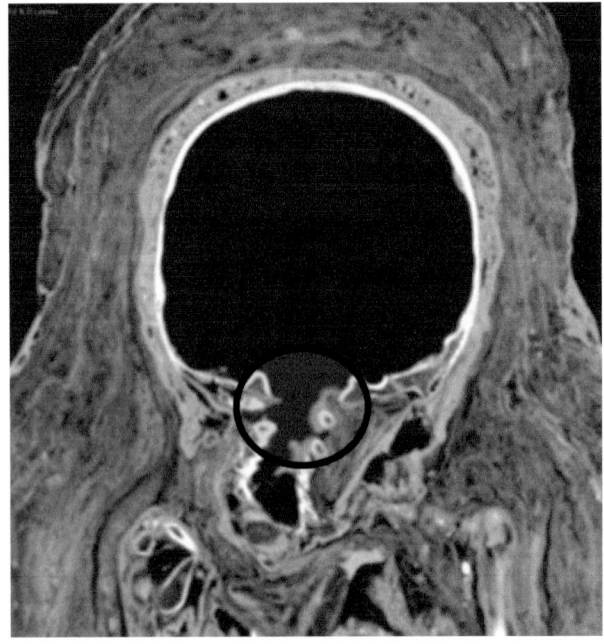

Fig. 4.98 Axial view of skull showing cervical spine displacement

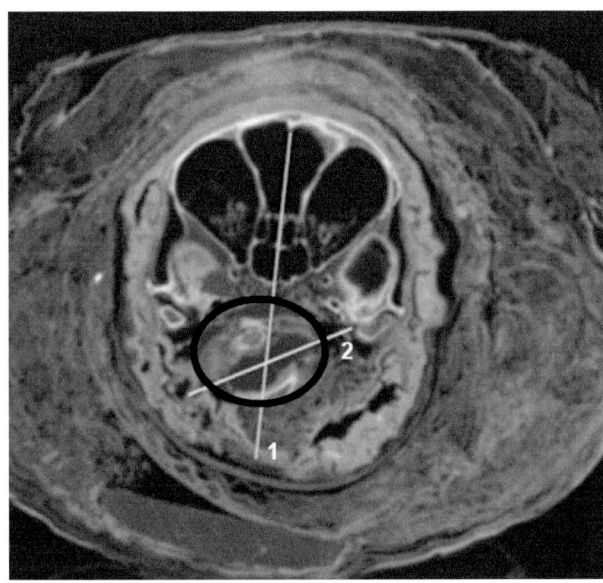

Fig. 4.100 Axial view close to skull base showing foramen magnum and atlas alignment

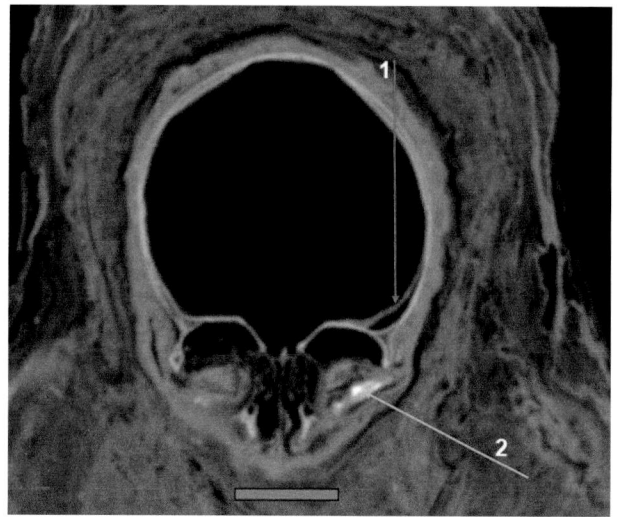

FIG. 4.101 CORONAL VIEW OF SKULL DEMONSTRATING MENINGES

XXXIX. Unnamed - St. Gallen (Cat. No.C3530)

Head

There is no evidence of perforation of the cribriform plate but the brain has been completely removed. A small amount of granular material is seen within the cranial cavity. There is no continuity between the cranium and the cervical spine, but this may well be post-mummification and have no bearing on the methods of mummification used, although the absence of a portal for excerebration in the usual place (cribriform plate) may well indicate use of the trans-foraminal route.

Neck

Severe disruption of the cervical spine is seen. Therefore, analysis cannot be made in this region (see Fig. 4.102).

LVIII. Unnamed - Manchester Museum (Cat. No. MM 13784)

Head

Excerebration has been performed, but there are intact ethmoid and sphenoid sinuses and cribriform plate (See Fig. 4.103 - arrow 1) with a moderately large amount of material in the posterior cranial fossa. This consists of two types of substance (See Fig. 4.103 - arrows 2 and 3) of which one may well be brain tissue (arrow 3). The presence of a fluid level as shown by the arrow 2 in Fig. 4.103 indicates the presence of a 'foreign' substance that was once liquid. The absence of the cervical spine prevents definite confirmation of a trans-foraminal excerebration, but it certainly cannot be excluded.

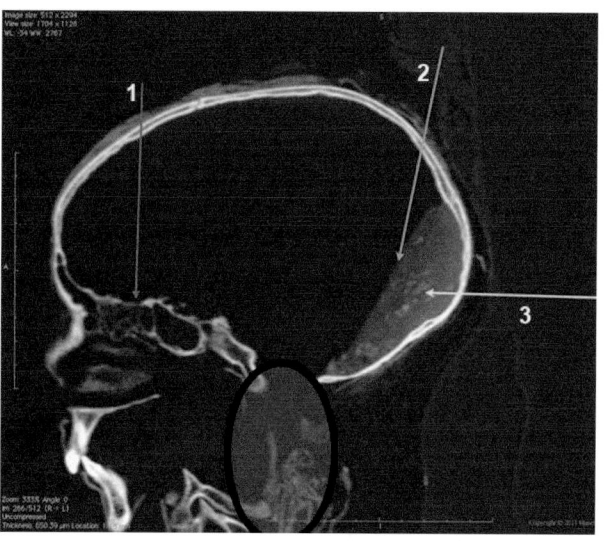

FIG. 4.103 SAGITTAL VIEW OF SKULL SHOWING A POSSIBLE TRANS-FORAMINAL ROUTE

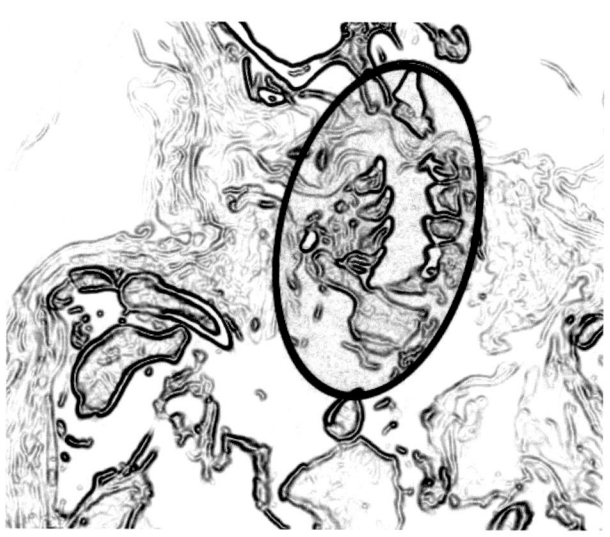

FIG. 4.102 CORONAL VIEW OF CERVICAL SPINE SHOWING MALALIGNMENT (AFTER IEM IMAGE)

4.1.3 Trans-basal route

This route has not been previously described in the literature. There is one such example in this study.

XXXII. Tjayasetimu - British Museum (Accession No.EA20744)

Head

The cranial cavity is almost empty, with only a small amount of brain tissue remaining. (See Fig. 4.104 - arrow 1). The cribriform plate is intact (arrow 2) and there is no disturbance of the posterior part of the neck in the region of the atlanto-occipital joint - arrow 3.

This leaves the question of identifying the route of excerebration. Further proof of an intact cribriform plate is seen in Fig. 4.105. The only obvious contender for this route would appear to be a large defect in the base of the skull, on either side of the basilar part of the occipital bone. This is seen in sagittal view in Fig. 4.106 (cf. the dotted arrow on the left and the intact bone seen in another mummy CT scan of the same area on the right). It is demonstrated in axial view in Fig. 4.107 (compare left Figure of this mummy with another on the right).

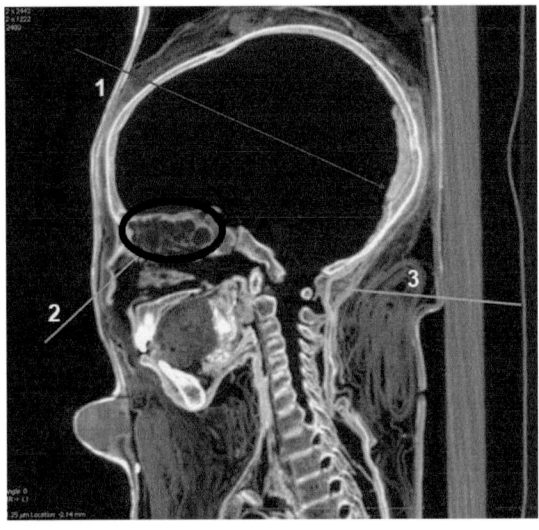

FIG. 4.104 SAGITTAL VIEW OF SKULL IN A MUMMY WHERE THE TRANS-BASAL ROUTE WAS USED WITH AN INTACT CRIBRIFORM PLATE AND A SMALL AMOUNT OF CEREBRAL TISSUE IN THE POSTERIOR CRANIAL FOSSA
COURTESY OF THE TRUSTEES OF THE BRITISH MUSEUM

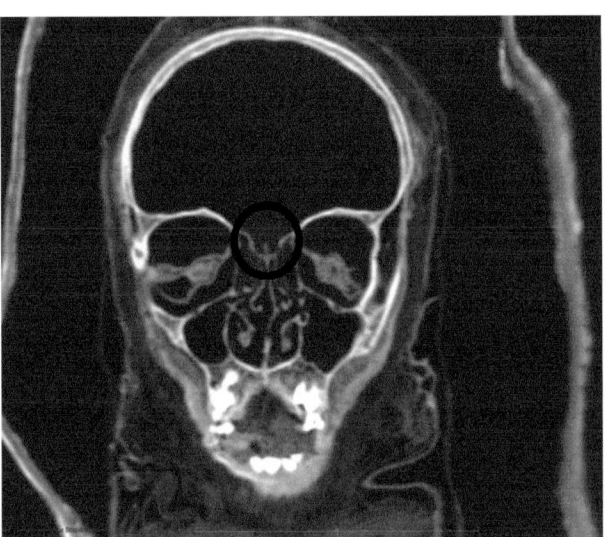

FIG. 4.105 CORONAL VIEW OF SKULL SHOWING THE TRANS-BASAL ROUTE WITH AN INTACT CRIBRIFORM PLATE
COURTESY OF THE TRUSTEES OF THE BRITISH MUSEUM

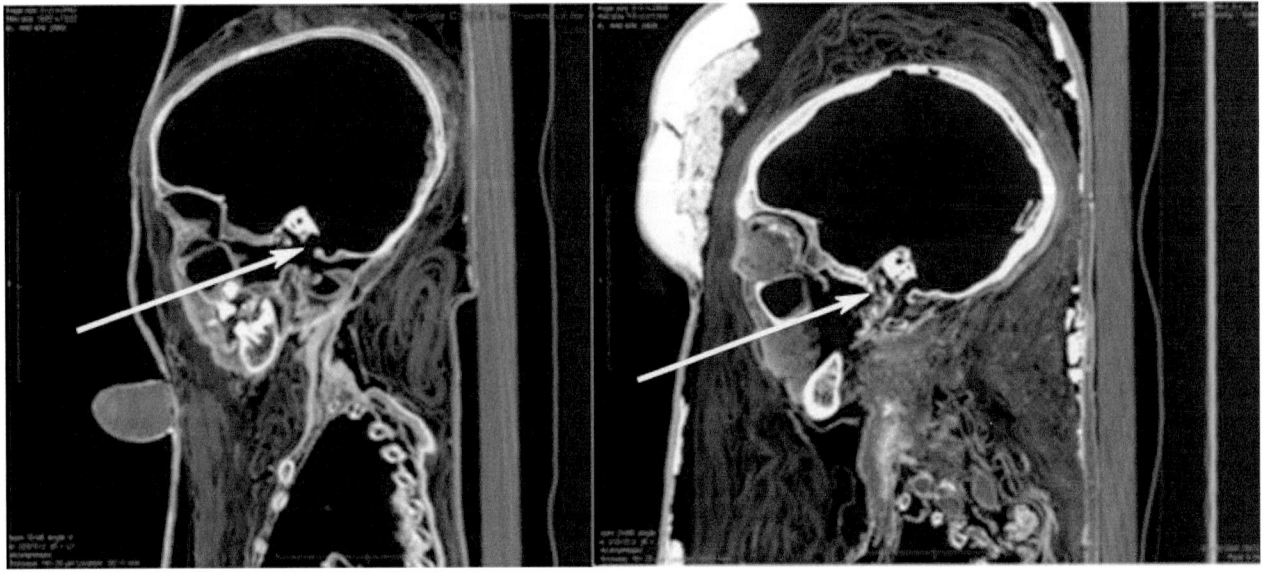

FIG. 4.106 SAGITTAL VIEW OF SKULL - TRANS-BASAL ROUTE
COURTESY OF THE TRUSTEES OF THE BRITISH MUSEUM

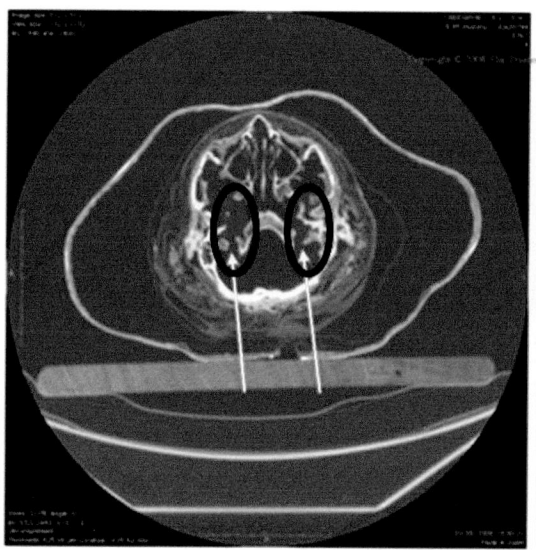
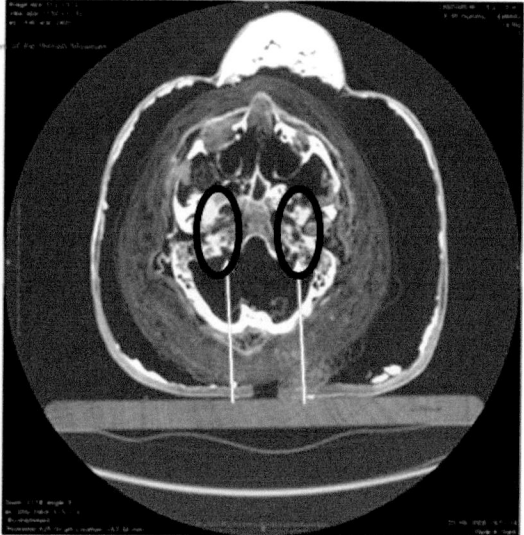

FIG. 4.107 AXIAL VIEW OF SKULL - TRANS-BASAL ROUTE
COURTESY OF THE TRUSTEES OF THE BRITISH MUSEUM

4.1.4 Trans-orbital route

Whilst the trans-orbital route has been mentioned in the past it is infrequent and refers to access commencing in the orbit and then perforating either the roof of the orbit (into the anterior cranial fossa) or perforating the medial wall of the orbit, the ethmoid sinuses and then the cribriform plate (Macke, Mache-Ribet and Connan, 2002: 73). The example below does not follow either of these routes but accesses the cranial fossa through the orbit and the superior orbital fissure. To achieve this the globe of the eye has been 'grooved' from the superior aspect to allow a direct passage to be created to the superior orbital fissure.

XIV Asru - Manchester University Museum (Accession No. MM1777)

Head

There is a small amount of material lying in the back of the cranial cavity (See Fig. 4.108). This material is hard as demonstrated by cracks in the lower third, in the occipital area. There is no evidence of brain material within the cranial cavity or of perforation of the cribriform plate nor is there evidence of a trans-foraminal approach. The only approach to the cranial cavity that can be detected is through the orbits. Here the remnants of the eyes can be seen desiccated and pushed aside. The superior orbital fissures appear larger than normal (See Fig. 4.109 and 4.110- arrows).

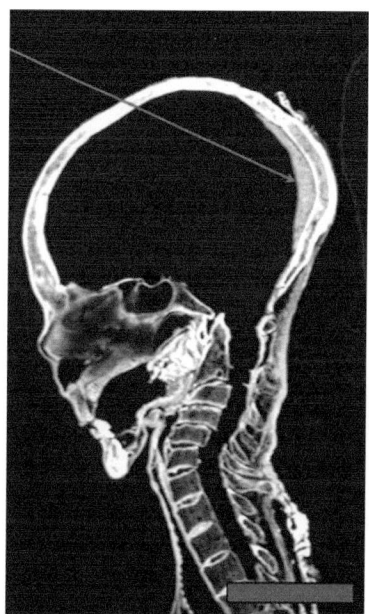
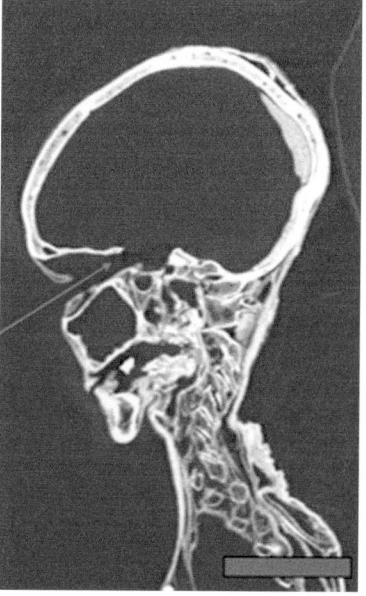
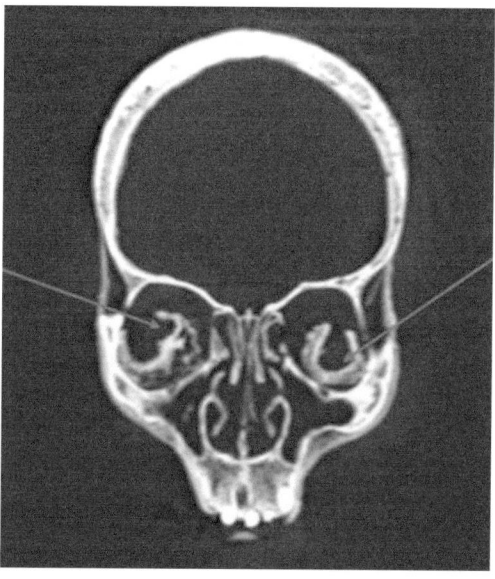

FIG. 4.108 SAGITTAL VIEW OF SKULL - FOREIGN MATERIAL IN POSTERIOR FOSSA

FIG. 4.109 SAGITTAL VIEW OF SKULL - TRANS-ORBITAL ROUTE

FIG. 4.110 CORONAL VIEW OF SKULL SHOWING DISTORTED EYES IN TRANS-ORBITAL ROUTE

4.1.5 No excerebration

There are six such cases.

II Namenkhetamun - BMAG (Cat. No.1966A23)

The skull is intact but slightly elongated with no evidence of perforation of the cribriform plate (See Fig. 4.111).

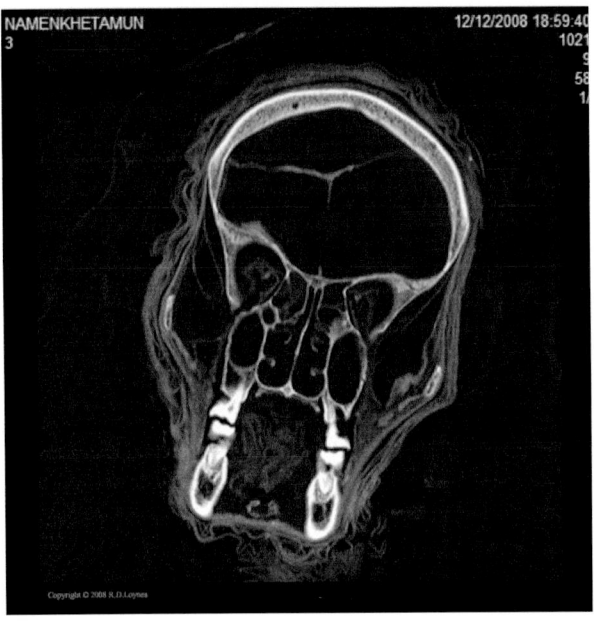

FIG. 4.111 CORONAL VIEW OF SKULL - INTACT CRIBRIFORM PLATE

As can also be seen in Fig. 4.111, the meninges are intact and are separated from the inner table of the skull in places. As expected, there is a significant amount of brain material present at the back of the skull (See Fig. 4.112).

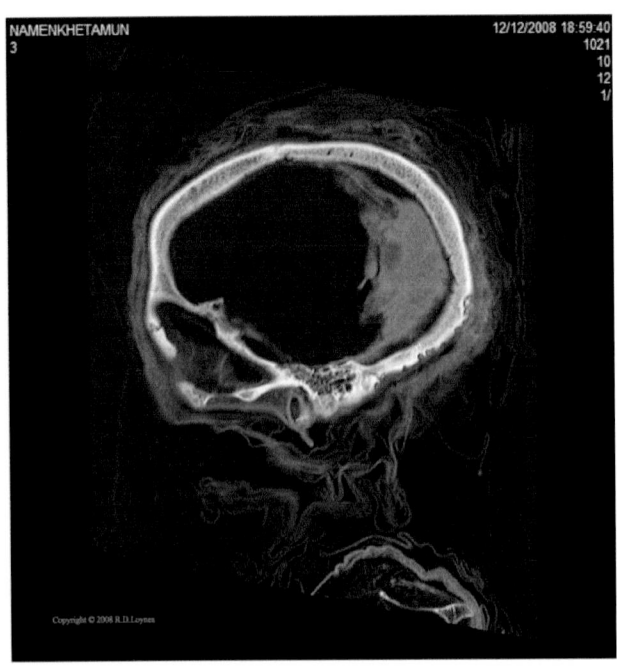

FIG. 4.112 SAGITTAL VIEW OF SKULL - CEREBRAL MATERIAL IN POSTERIOR CRANIAL CAVITY

XII Unnamed - Manchester University Museum (Accession No. MM1768)

Head

There is no evidence of penetration of the cranial cavity, the cribriform plate being intact (See Fig. 4.113, arrow 1). This Figure also shows that the desiccated brain tissue remains in the back of the skull (arrow 2).

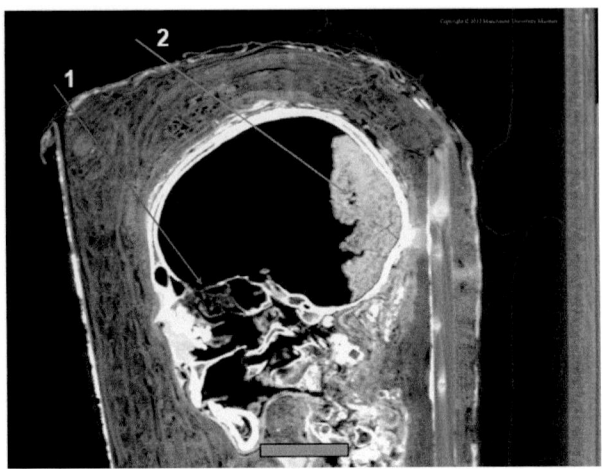

FIG. 4.113 SAGITTAL VIEW OF SKULL WITH INTACT CRIBRIFORM PLATE AND RETAINED BRAIN.

XIII Unnamed - Manchester University Museum (Accession No. MM1767)

Head

There is no evidence of penetration of the cribriform plate - Fig. 4.114 - arrow 1. The remnants of the brain lie in the posterior cranial fossa (Fig. 4.114 - arrow 2).

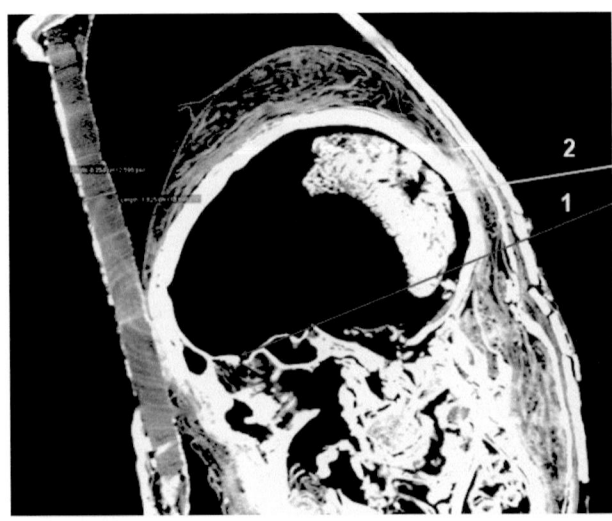

FIG. 4.114 SAGITTAL VIEW OF SKULL WITH INTACT CRIBRIFORM PLATE AND RETAINED BRAIN

XXIV. Unnamed – Basel Museum (Cat. No.BSAE.1030)

Head

There is no evidence of perforation of the cribriform plate (See Fig. 4.115 - arrow 2). The material within the cranial cavity could well be brain tissue, although it does look somewhat granular in places (1). There is also evidence of remnants of the meninges. All this lies in the posterior fossa (See Fig. 4.115).

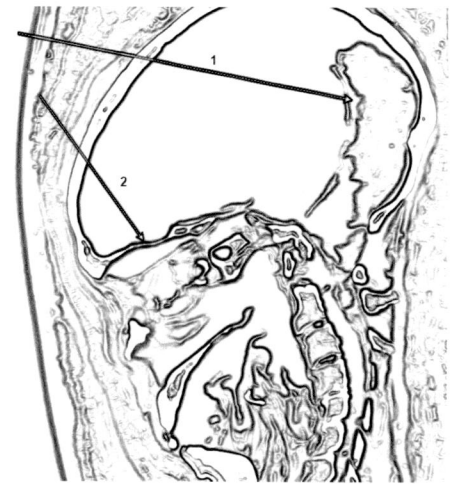

FIG. 4.115 SAGITTAL VIEW OF SKULL WITH INTACT CRIBRIFORM PLATE AND RETAINED BRAIN (AFTER IEM IMAGE)

LII. Unnamed child - Manchester Museum (Accession No. MM9319)

Head

There is no evidence of excerebration, with the desiccated brain lying in the posterior cranial cavity. There is no perforation of the cribriform plate and no disturbance of the atlanto-occipital region (See Fig. 4.116. - arrow 1 = cribriform plate; arrow 2 = brain; black circle = atlanto-occipital region).

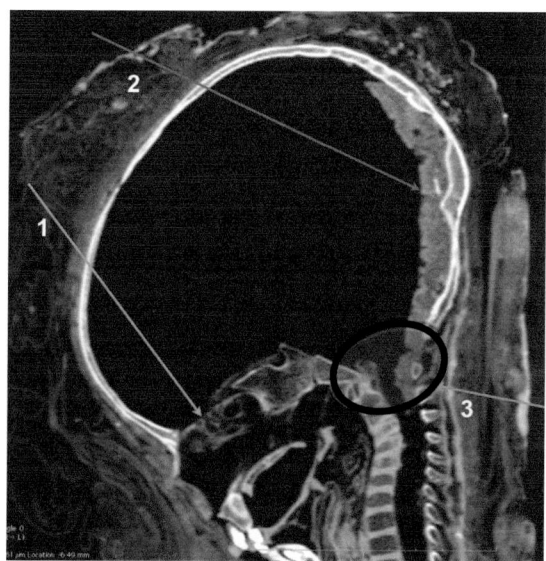

FIG. 4.116 SAGITTAL VIEW OF SKULL WITH INTACT CRIBRIFORM PLATE AND RETAINED BRAIN

LV. Unnamed child - Manchester Museum (Accession. No. MM 13011)

Head

The cribriform plate and ethmoid bone are undamaged (See Fig. 4.117) and there is evidence of desiccated brain tissue in the posterior cranial fossa (See Fig. 4.118 - arrow). Excerebration has not been performed.

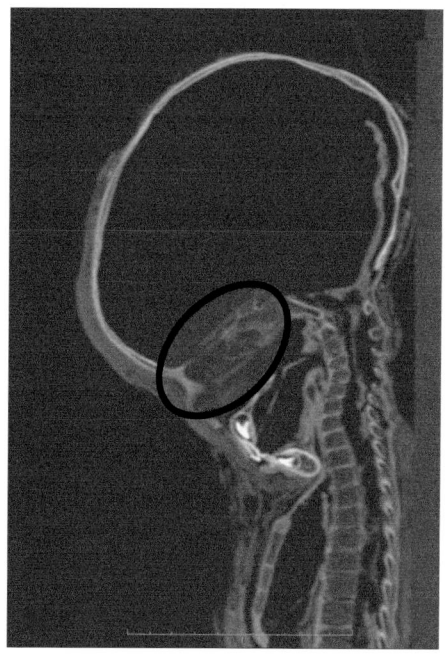

FIG. 4.117 SAGITTAL VIEW OF SKULL WITH INTACT CRIBRIFORM PLATE

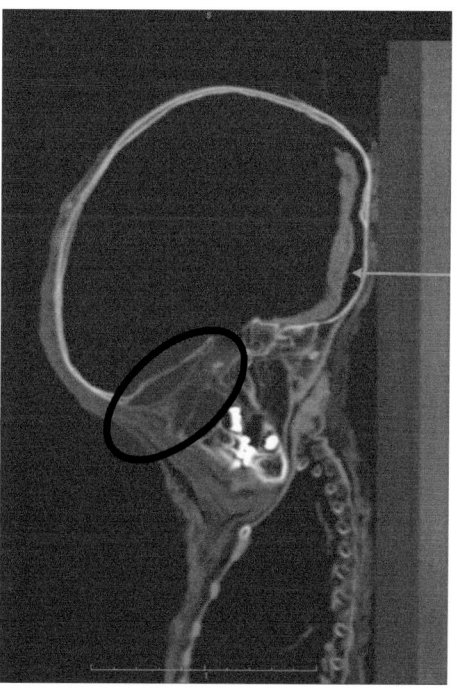

FIG. 4.118 SAGITTAL VIEW OF SKULL WITH BRAIN IN POSTERIOR CRANIAL FOSSA

4.2 Treatment of the eyes

The literature contains relatively few references to the treatment of the eyes by embalmers in ancient Egypt. Mention is made by some of the use of 'artificial' eyes – for example Gray, 1971: 125-126 and Aufderheide, 2010: 424; and Aufderheide and Rodriguez-Martin, 1998: 252. The term 'artificial eyes' refers to the use of plates of hard material laid over the desiccated globes, within the orbit. However, Aufderheide (2010 v.s.: 318) states, 'in view of their availability (preserved in 93%) little serious study of ancient eyes has been carried out'. The opportunity was, therefore, taken to record the treatment of the eyes in this series of mummy studies.

The X-rayed mummy in Exeter did not yield any evidence of the eyes (as would be expected) and in the case of one of the mummies in Sheffield (Mummy VI – Djedma'atiuesankh) the CT 'slices' did not show the orbits well enough to make comment. In the majority of the remaining fifty-eight cases it was possible to analyse the treatment of the eyes. The only exceptions were where there had been 'skeletonization' or disorganisation of the skull. This was found in six cases. The findings in the remaining fifty-two mummies will be reported below.

The methods of managing the eyes fall, broadly, into four groups. These are:

Removal
Desiccation
Packing the globe
The use of 'False Eyes' (Eye Plates)

4.2.1 Removal

There were four cases of removal, which in one case was supplemented by the inclusion of linen in the orbit and in a further case with the use of both linen in the orbit and the provision of 'eye plates' anteriorly.

NUMBER	ORIGIN	ERA	EYES
VII	Ipswich - Tahathor	D25	REMOVED
XIII	Manchester - MM1767	Roman	REMOVED REPLACED WITH LINEN
XXIII	Zurich - Yverdon - Nes-Shou - MY/3775	Ptolemaic	REMOVED
XXIX	BM - Hor - EA6659	D22	REMOVED, REPLACED LINEN and PLATES

TABLE 4.3 TREATMENT OF EYES BY REMOVAL

VII Tahathor - Ipswich Museum (Cat. No. COLEM 1871.3.7)

The contents of the orbits are difficult to see but there is a faint image of some structure within the orbits, but the detail is poor and may represent loose linen (See Fig. 4.95).

XIII Unnamed - Manchester University Museum (Accession No. MM1767)

The eyes do not appear to have been retained, but are replaced with linen packing superficially soaked in resin (See Fig. 4.119 - circle). There is no evidence of the use of eye plates.

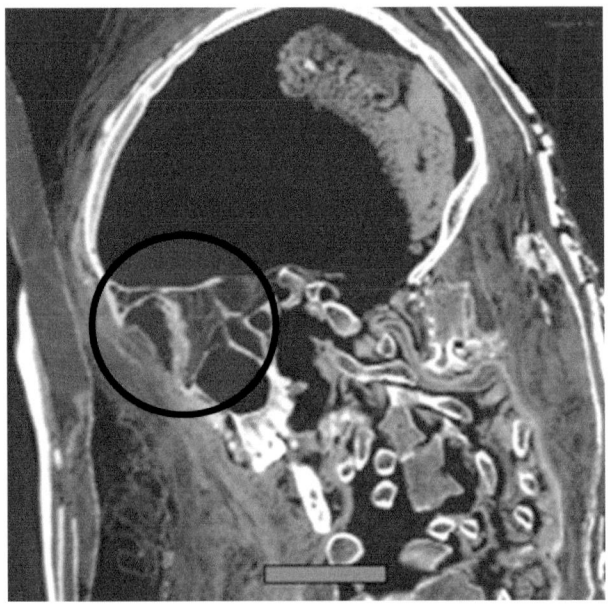

FIG. 4.119 SAGITTAL VIEW OF SKULL WITH EYE REPLACED BY RESIN-SOAKED LINEN

XXIII. Nes-Shou - Yverdon Museum (Accession No.MY/3775)

The eyes have been removed and not replaced. There is a little material remaining in the posterior parts of the orbits, but it is difficult to identify this substance.

XXIX. Hor - British Museum - (Accession No. EA 6659)

The eyes have been removed completely and replaced by a roll of resin-impregnated linen in each orbit. Eye plates (or 'false eyes') have been inserted into the orbits in front of the linen rolls. On the right side the linen roll and plate are found in the posterior aspect of the orbit (arrows 1 and 2 in Fig. 4.120). On the left side, the linen roll is in the posterior aspect of the orbit, but the plate is anterior, similar to the expected position of the eyelids (arrows 3 and 4 in Fig. 4.120).

Fig. 4.121 shows the roll of linen in the left orbit more clearly - arrow.

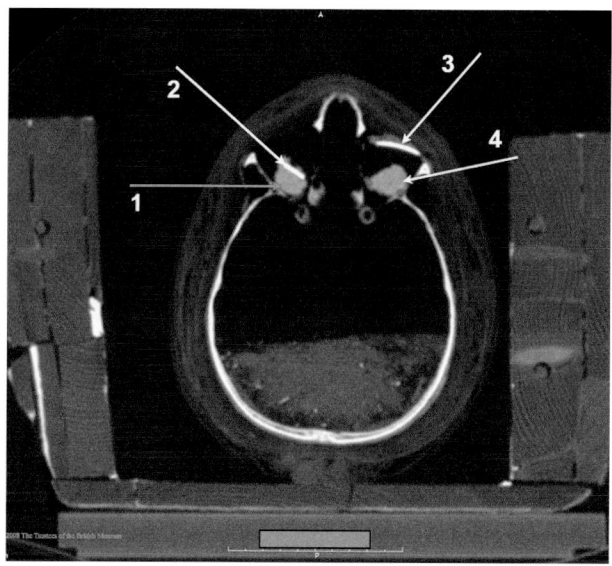

FIG. 4.120 AXIAL VIEW OF SKULL - LINEN ROLLS IN ORBITS AND EYE PLATES ANTERIORLY
COURTESY OF THE TRUSTEES OF THE BRITISH MUSEUM

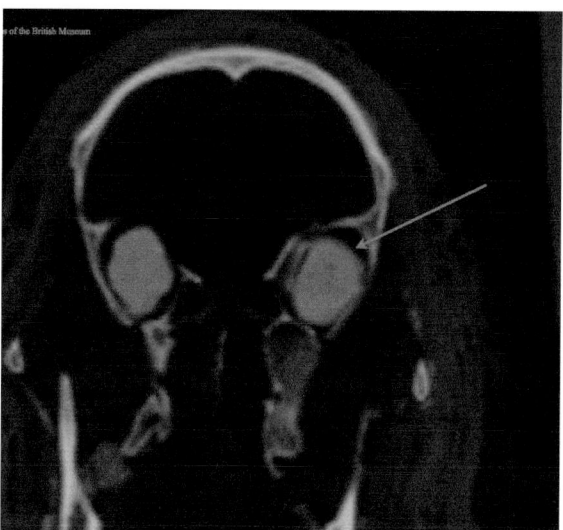

FIG. 4.121 CORONAL VIEW OF SKULL WITH LINEN ROLLS IN ORBITS
COURTESY OF THE TRUSTEES OF THE BRITISH MUSEUM

4.2.2 Desiccation

In twenty-one cases the eyes were left in situ and were desiccated. No additional procedures were performed. However, in a further nine cases the globes were enhanced by the addition of eye plates or linen anteriorly or by the insertion of linen or resin into the orbits. In three other cases, desiccation was accompanied by either loss of one of the eyes, collapse of the globes or emptying of the globes of the eyes.

NUMBER	ORIGIN	ERA	EYES
I	Birmingham - Graeco-Roman	Roman	DESICCATED
XII	Manchester - MM1768	Roman	DESICCATED
XVIII	Liverpool- M14048	Roman	DESICCATED
XXII	Zurich - Bern - 00/2	Unknown	DESICCATED
XXIV	Zurich - Basel - BSAE.1030	Roman	DESICCATED
XXVI	Zurich - Geneva - Infant	Unknown	DESICCATED
XXVII	Manchester - Demetria - MM11630	Roman	DESICCATED
XXVIII	Manchester - Sheri-Ankh – MM13783	D21	DESICCATED
XXXII	BM - EA20744	D22	DESICCATED
XXXVII	Zurich - Lenzburg - Sherit-Min	Ptolemaic	DESICCATED
XL	Zurich - Lausanne - 492	3IP	DESICCATED
XLI	Zurich - Lenzburg - K10351	Roman	DESICCATED
XLIV	Turin - Provv.610	Ptolemaic?	DESICCATED
XLVII	Manchester - MM1769	Roman	DESICCATED
LII	Manchester - MM9319 - child	Roman	DESICCATED
LIII	Manchester - MM1976.51a	D25	DESICCATED
LIV	Manchester - Salford 2	3IP	DESICCATED
LV	Manchester - MM13011	Ptolemaic	DESICCATED
LVI	Manchester - MM2109	Roman	DESICCATED
LVII	Manchester - MM1775 Artemidorus	Roman	DESICCATED
LIX	BM - EA 22108 Child	Roman	DESICCATED

TABLE 4.4 TREATMENT OF EYES BY DESICCATION ONLY

NUMBER	ORIGIN	ERA	EYES
III	Birmingham - Padimut	D20-21	DESICCATED + PLATES
IX	Liverpool - Padiamunnebnesuttauwy	D25	DESICCATED, RESIN IN ORBITS
X	Liverpool - Nesmin	Ptolemaic	DESICCATED ONLY - INF. RESIN
XV	Liverpool - 13.10.11.25	Roman	DESICCATED, PACKING IN FRONT
XIX	Zurich - Altdorf Child	Roman	DESICCATED. POST. ORBIT PACKING
XXXI	BM - Padiamunet - EA6682	D25	DESICCATED, PACKING IN FRONT
XXXIII	BM - EA22939	D22	DESICCATED, PACKING IN FRONT, PLATES
XXXVI	Zurich - Bern - AE9	Ptolemaic	DESICCATED, PADS IN FRONT
LX	BM - EA 6704	Roman	DESICCATED, LINEN BELOW

TABLE 4.5 TREATMENT OF EYES BY DESICCATION AND ENHANCEMENT BY USE OF PLATES/LINEN

The following cases had desiccation of the eye/s with the loss of one eye (presumably post-mortem), the complete collapse of the globe or emptying of the globe with a residual void.

XIV Asru - Manchester University Museum (Accession No. MM1777)

The only approach to the cranial cavity that can be detected is through the orbits. Here the remnants of the eyes can be seen desiccated and pushed aside. The superior orbital fissures appear larger than normal (See Fig. 4.109 and 4.110 - arrows). (P 63).

XLIII. Unnamed fromTebtynis - Turin (Cat. No. Suppl.19691)

The left eye remains in situ and is desiccated. There is no packing. The right eye has been lost. However, the presence of linen wrapping over the orbit suggests that the loss was prior to bandaging (See Fig. 4.122). No eye plates have been used.

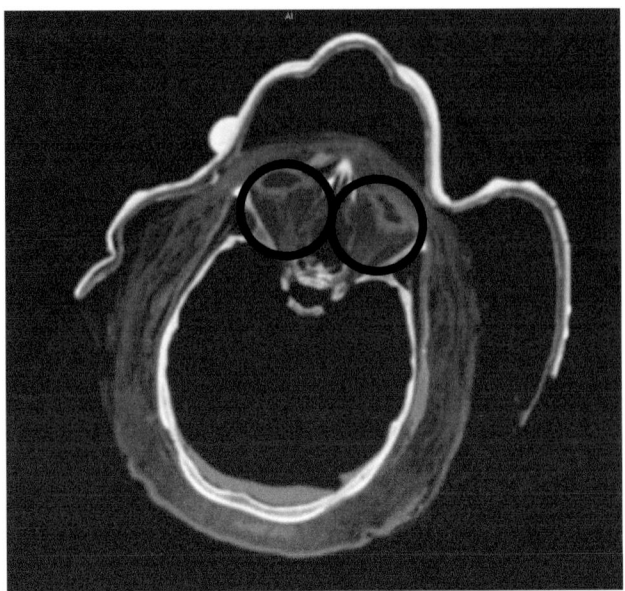

FIG. 4.123 AXIAL VIEW OF SKULL - REMNANTS OF THE GLOBES AND MUSCLES, BUT EMPTY GLOBES

It is useful to compare the structures of the desiccated eyeball (globe) in this case with those in the case of a desiccated globe where the contents have not been evacuated. Compare the desiccated globe – arrow 1 in Fig. 4.124 with the arrow 1 in Fig. 4.125. The arrows 2 in the two figures show the anterior compartments of the eyes. The much larger solid remnant of globe can be seen in Fig. 4.125, where the anterior compartment is much smaller.

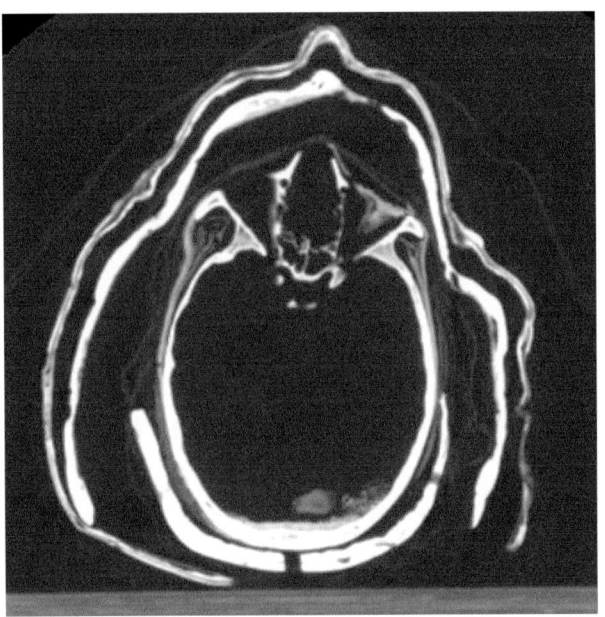

FIG. 4.122 AXIAL VIEW OF SKULL - DESICCATION OF LEFT EYE AND LOSS OF RIGHT EYE.

XLV. Unnamed - Manchester Museum (Cat. No.MM1766)

The eyes have been left in situ and are desiccated. The optic nerves and orbital muscles can be seen clearly. The globes of the eyes have been emptied but no packing introduced (See Fig. 4.123).

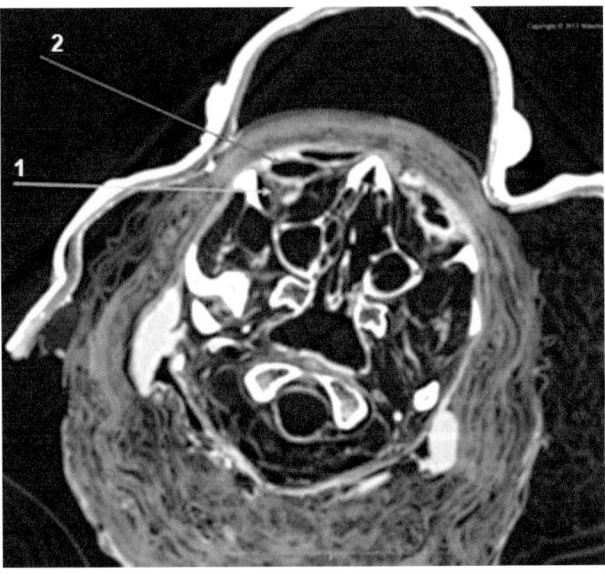

FIG. 4.124 AXIAL VIEW OF SKULL WITH LARGE REMAINING CAVITY IN EYEBALL IN MUMMY XLV

RESULTS – THE HEAD

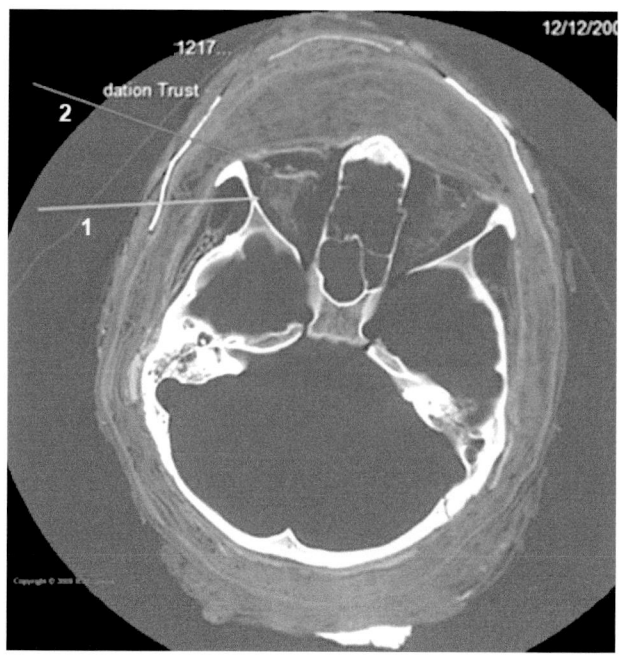

FIG. 4.125 AXIAL VIEW OF SKULL. SMALL ANTERIOR COMPARTMENT – RED ARROW. LARGE REMNANT OF SOLID EYE – BLUE ARROW IN MUMMY I

4.2.3 Packing

In fourteen cases the eyes were opened and packed with material. The material used was linen. On some occasions the linen was soaked in resin. Plates have been added in front of the packed globes in five cases.

NUMBER	ORIGIN	ERA	EYES
II	Birmingham - Namenkhetamun	D26	OPENED, PACKED,
V	Sheffield - Nesitanebetasheru	D25	OPENED, PACKED, PLATES
VIII	Liverpool - Padiamun - 53.72a	D22	OPENED, PACKED,
XI	Liverpool - Padiamun - M14003	D26	OPENED, PACKED, PLATES
XVI	Liverpool - M13997a	Roman	OPENED, PACKED,
XVII	Liverpool - Ankhesenaset - M 14000	3IP	OPENED, PACKED, PLATES
XXV	Zurich - Geneva - TjesMoutPert - D0242	D22-25	OPENED, PACKED,
XXX	BM - Pef-Tjau-Emawy-Khonsu- EA6681	D25	OPENED, PACKED, PLATES
XXXIV	BM - EA25258	D22	OPENED, PACKED, PLATES
XXXVIII	Zurich – St. Gallen – Shepenese	D26	OPENED, PACKED
XLII	Turin – Taaset – Suppl. 9480	Ptolemaic	OPENED, PACKED
IL	Manchester - MM5053.a - Perenbast	D22	OPENED, PACKED
L	Perth - 23/1936	D26	OPENED, PACKED
LI	Manchester - MM9354a - Khary	D19-Ptolemaic	OPENED, PACKED

TABLE 4.6 EYES OPENED AND PACKED – SOME WITH THE USE OF EYE PLATES ('FALSE EYES')

Examples of packing within the eye globe are given below. It can be seen that the amount of packing varied considerably.

II Namenkhetamun (BMAG - Cat. No.1966A23)

The orbits contain the eyes that can be seen along with their muscles and the optic nerves. However, the globes of the eyes have been opened and packed with material. There are no false eyes or eye plates present (see Fig. 4.126).

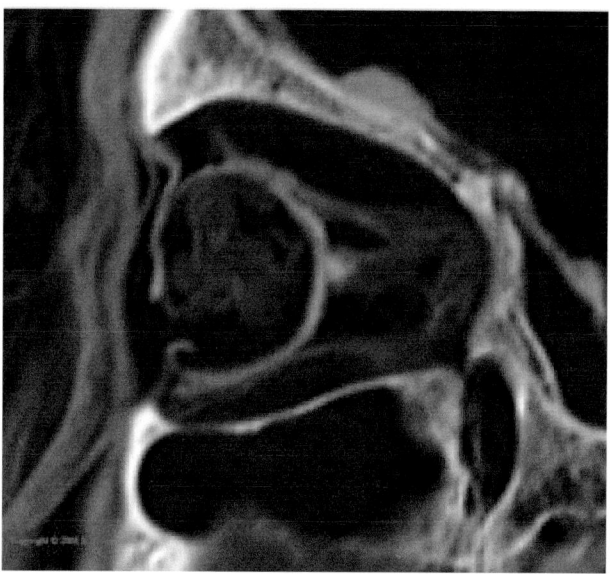

FIG. 4.126 SAGITTAL VIEW OF ORBIT - LINEN PACKING WITHIN THE GLOBE OF THE EYE

VIII Padiamun - National Museums Liverpool (Accession No. 53.72a)

The eyes have been retained, but with packing of a mixture of amorphous material and linen bandages (see Fig. 4.127). There is damage to the anterior aspect of the left eye as can be seen in Fig. 4.129.

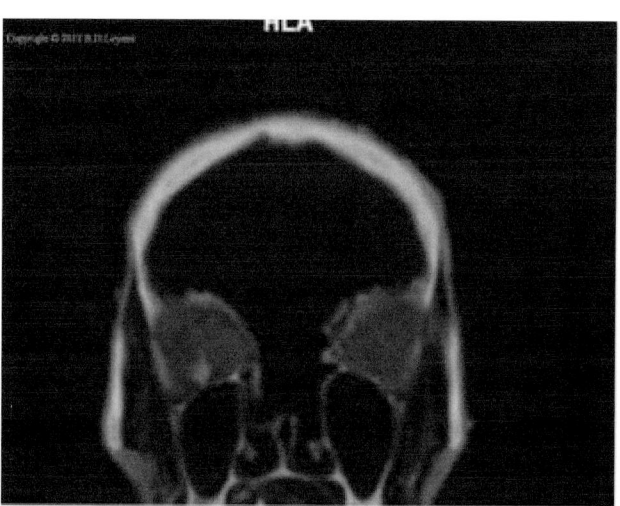

FIG. 4.127 CORONAL VIEW OF SKULL - EYES TIGHTLY PACKED WITH LINEN

The outer layer of the eyeball can be seen clearly in Fig. 4.128 (See arrow). The packing lies within this layer.

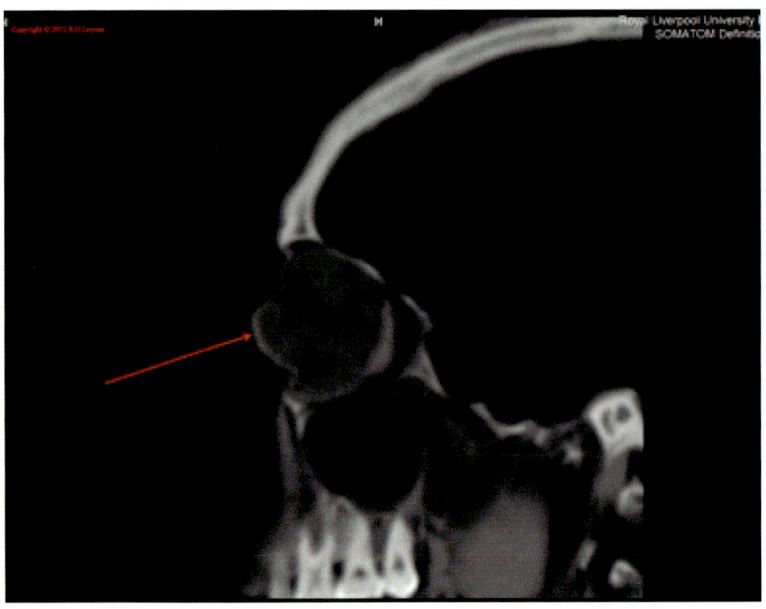

Fig. 4.128 Sagittal view of orbit demonstrating outer layer of the eye (sclera and cornea)

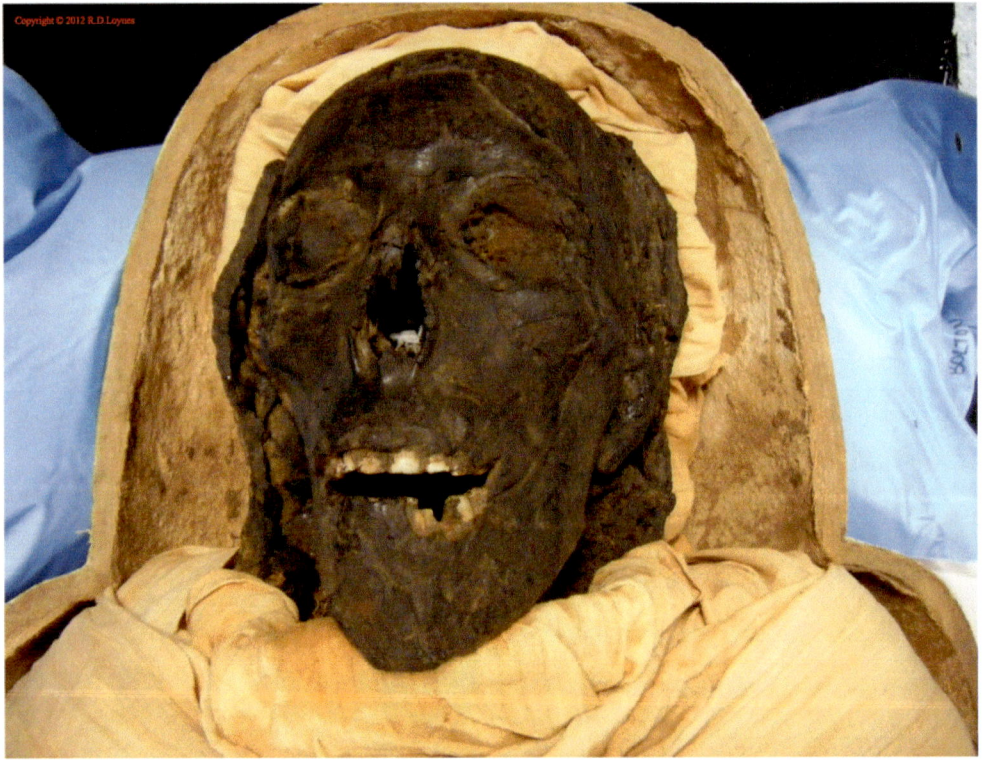

Fig. 4.129 External appearance of the damaged left eye

XVI. Unnamed - National Museums Liverpool (Accession No. M13997a)

The eyes have been left in situ and the desiccated remains of the globes, muscles and optic nerves can be clearly seen along with incision of the globe and the insertion of a small amount of linen (See Figs. 4.130 and 4.131). There is no evidence of the use of eye plates or false eyes.

RESULTS – THE HEAD

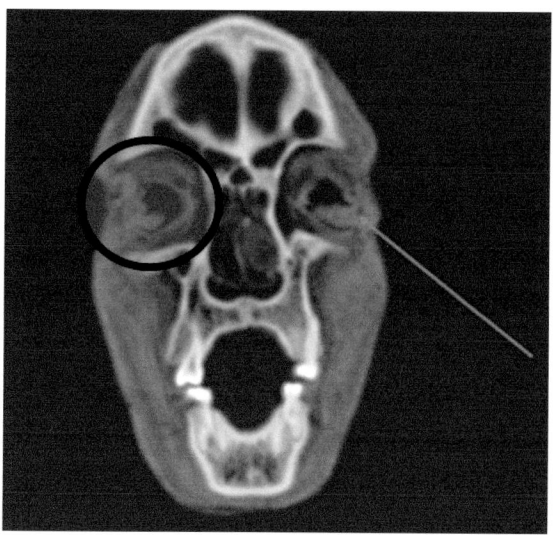

FIG. 4.130 CORONAL VIEW OF SKULL - LOOSELY PACKED EYES

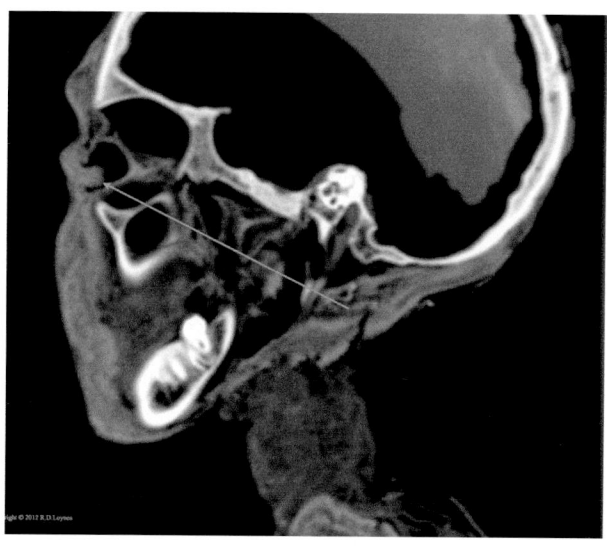

FIG. 4.131 SAGITTAL VIEW OF ORBIT WITH SMALL AMOUNT OF PACKING THROUGH ANTERIOR WALL OF GLOBE

XXV. TjesMoutPert - Geneva Museum (Cat. No.D0242)

The eye on the right has been retained and packed with linen. There is a radio-dense object at the front of the eye globe. On the left the eye has also been packed with a very radio-dense object, again with linen within it. It appears to be resin soaked linen around other less heavily soaked linen (See Figs. 4.132, 4.133 and 4.134).

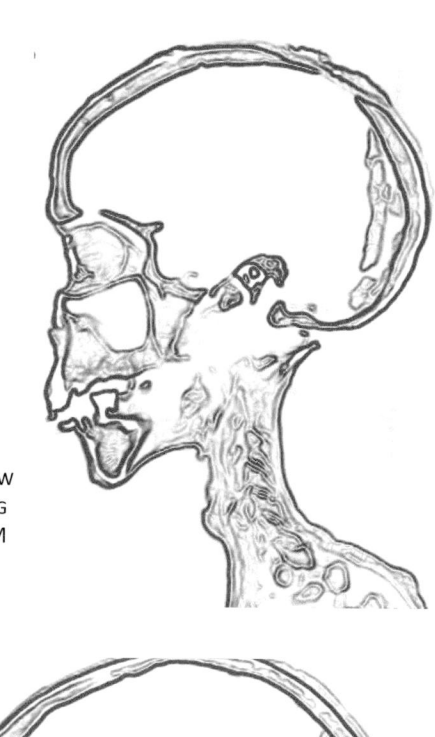

FIG. 4.133 SAGITTAL VIEW OF SKULL - LINEN PACKING OF RIGHT EYE (AFTER IEM IMAGE)

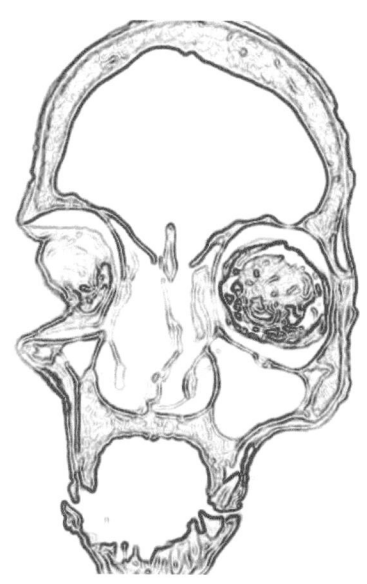

FIG. 4.132 CORONAL VIEW OF SKULL SHOWING BOTH PACKED EYES (AFTER IEM IMAGE)

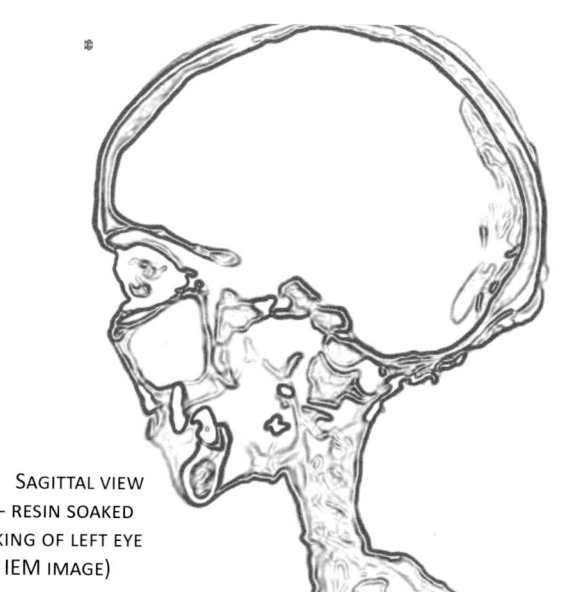

FIG. 4.134 SAGITTAL VIEW OF SKULL - RESIN SOAKED LINEN PACKING OF LEFT EYE (AFTER IEM IMAGE)

IL. Perenbast - Manchester University Museum (Accession No. MM5053.a)

The eyes have been left in situ opened anteriorly and packed with linen (See Figs. 4.135 and 4.136). No eye plates have been used in this case.

L. Ta-Kr-Hb - Perth Museum and Art Gallery (Cat. No. 23/1936)

The eyes have been retained in situ, desiccated and moderately tightly packed with linen (see Figs. 4.137 and 4.138).

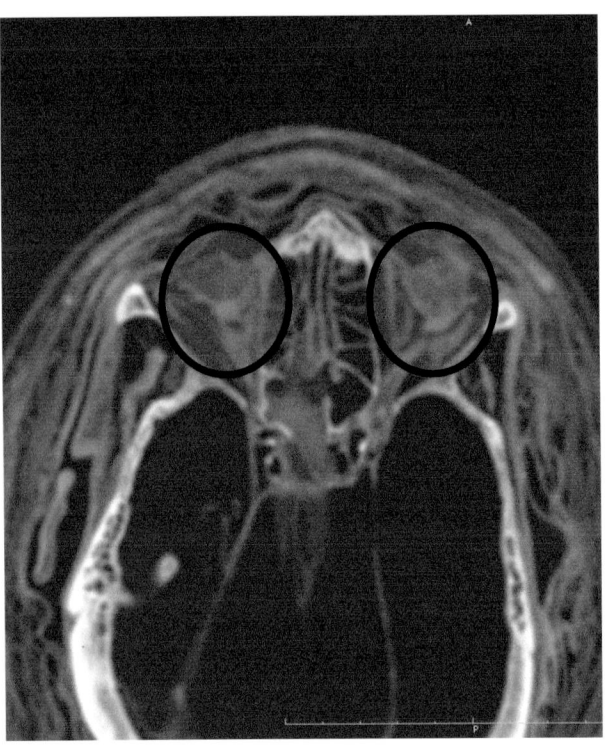

FIG. 4.135 AXIAL VIEW OF SKULL - EYES PACKED FROM ANTERIOR INCISIONS

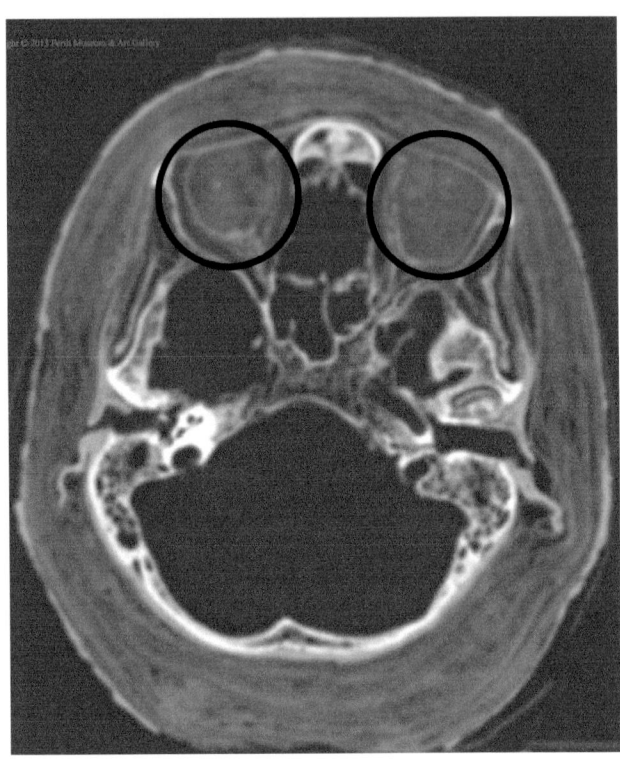

FIG. 4.137 AXIAL VIEW OF SKULL - TIGHT PACKING OF LINEN INTO GLOBES

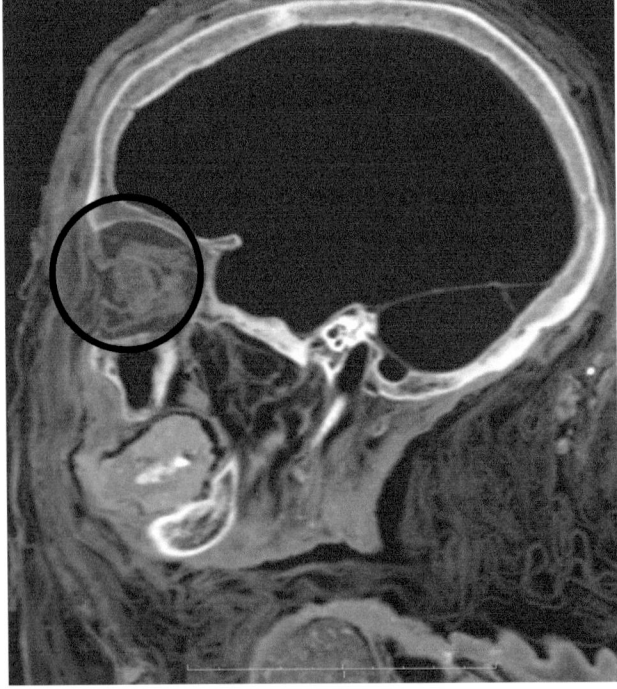

FIG. 4.136 SAGITTAL VIEW OF ORBIT - EYES PACKED FROM ANTERIOR INCISIONS

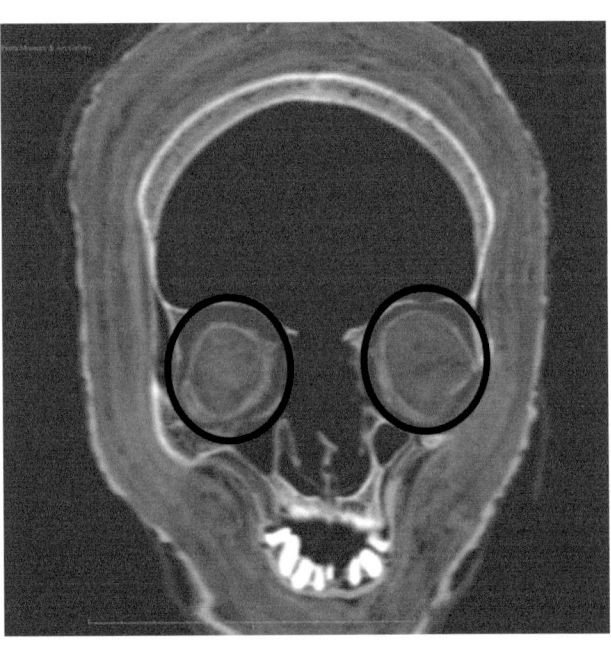

FIG. 4.138 CORONAL VIEW OF ORBITS SHOWING TIGHT PACKING OF LINEN INTO GLOBES

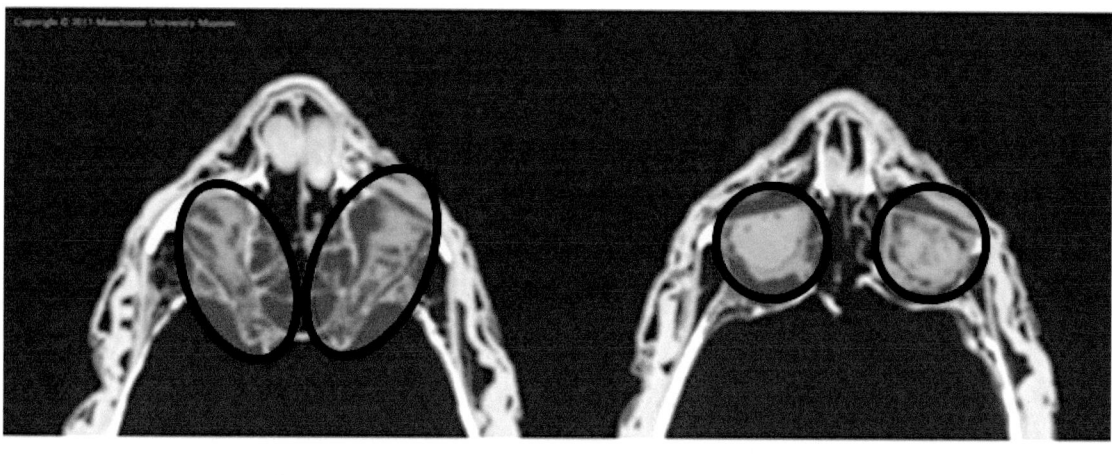

FIG. 4.139 AXIAL VIEW OF SKULL - PACKED EYES. MORE RESIN IN THE LINEN ON THE RIGHT THAN THE LEFT

LI. Khary - Manchester Museum (Accession No. MM9354a)

The eyes have been retained and are desiccated as seen in the left (I) of Fig. 4.139. In the right orbit a heavily resin-soaked pack has been inserted. On the left a less heavily resin-soaked pack of linen has been inserted within the globe (See II of Fig. 4.139). Eye plates have not been used to cover the eyes.

4.2.4 Eye Plates – 'False Eyes'

The following cases are those where 'false eyes' or eye plates have been used.

V Nesitanebetasheru - Sheffield Museum (Cat. No. J93.1283)

Whilst the images are not absolutely clear, there is good evidence of the treatment of the eyes that have been opened, packed with linen and covered at the front with eye plates (See Fig. 4.140).

XI. Padiamun - National Museums Liverpool (accession No. M14003)

The eyes are retained. The globes of the eyes have been opened, packed with linen (See Fig. 4.141, arrow 2) and eye plates inserted at the front of the opened globe (arrow 1). The optic nerves are seen passing through the optic foramina (3). The eye-plates are clearly seen in Figs. 4.142 and 4.143.

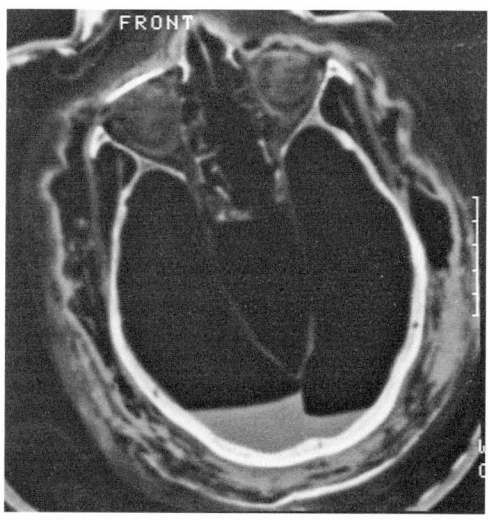

FIG. 4.140 AXIAL VIEW OF SKULL SHOWING PACKED EYES AND EYE PLATE OVER RIGHT EYE

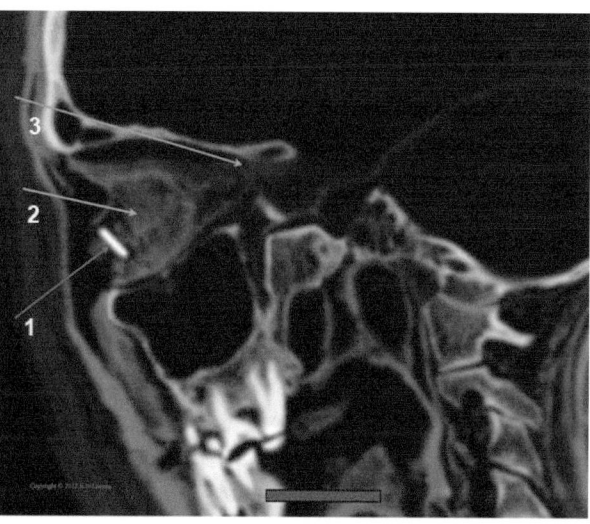

FIG. 4.141 SAGITTAL VIEW OF ORBIT - PACKED EYE WITH EYE PLATE

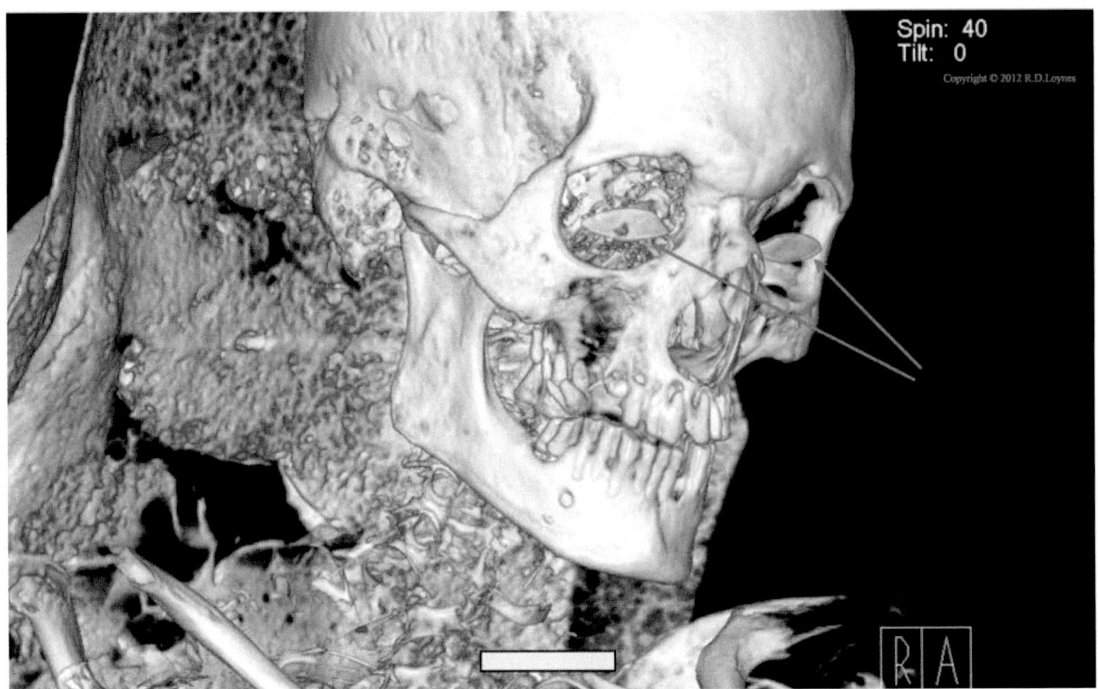

FIG. 4.142 3D RECONSTRUCTION SHOWING EYE PLATES

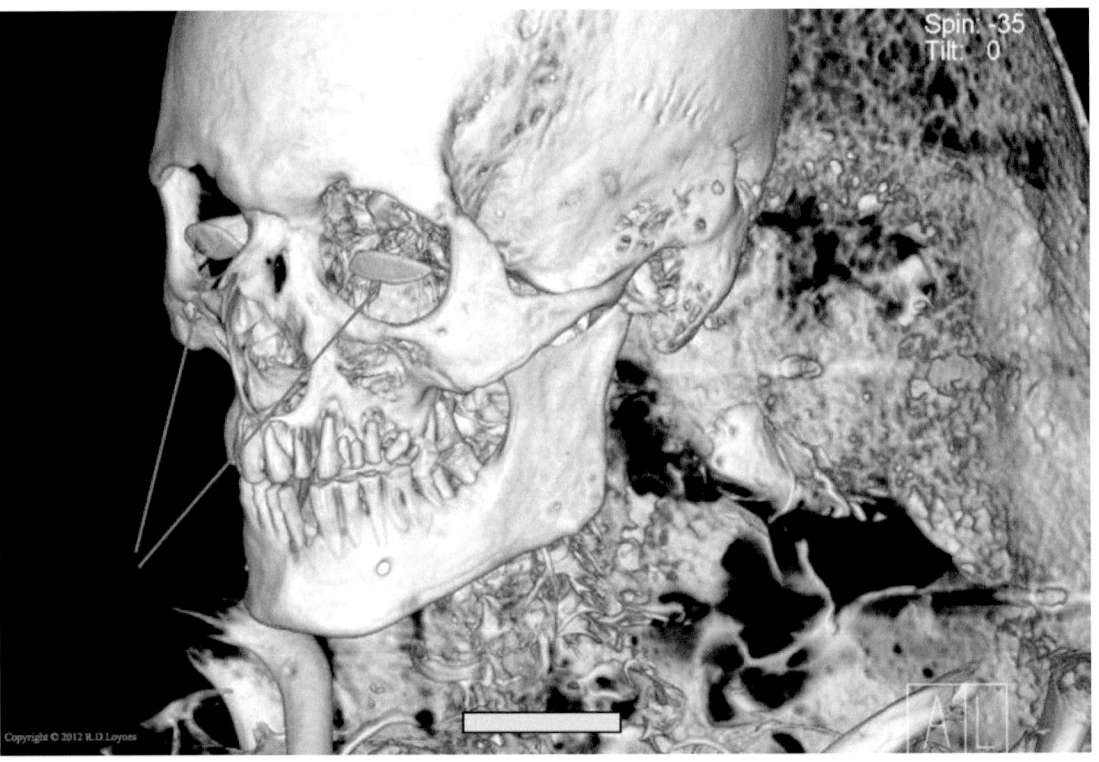

FIG. 4.143 3D RECONSTRUCTION SHOWING EYE PLATES

XVII. Ankhesenaset - National Museums Liverpool (Accession No. M14000)

The eyes are in situ and the globes packed with linen. Small eye plates have been inserted over the front of the globes (See Figs. 4.144 and 4.145- Remnants of ocular muscles and optic nerves = arrows 1; remnants of wall (sclera) of eyes = arrows 2; packing within the eyes = arrows 3; eye plates = arrows 4).

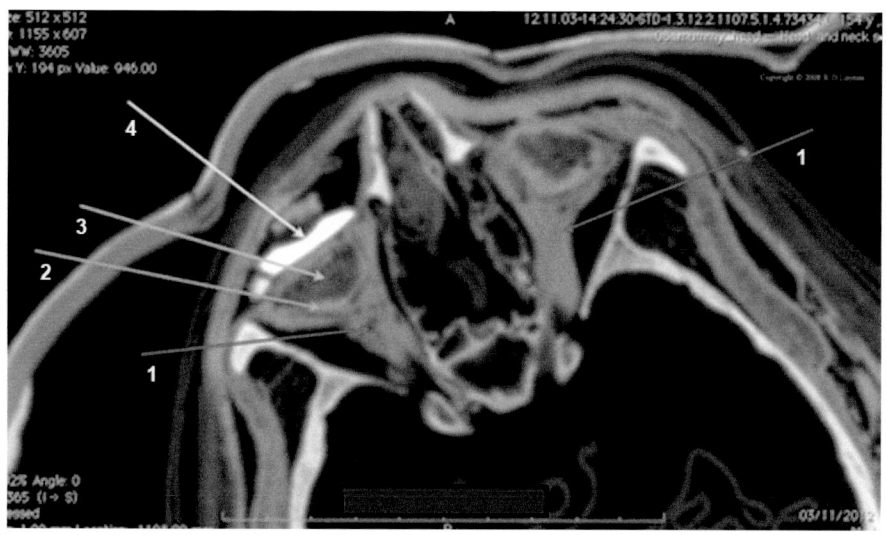

FIG. 4.144 AXIAL VIEW OF ORBITS SHOWING DETAIL OF THE EMBALMING PROCESS OF THE EYES

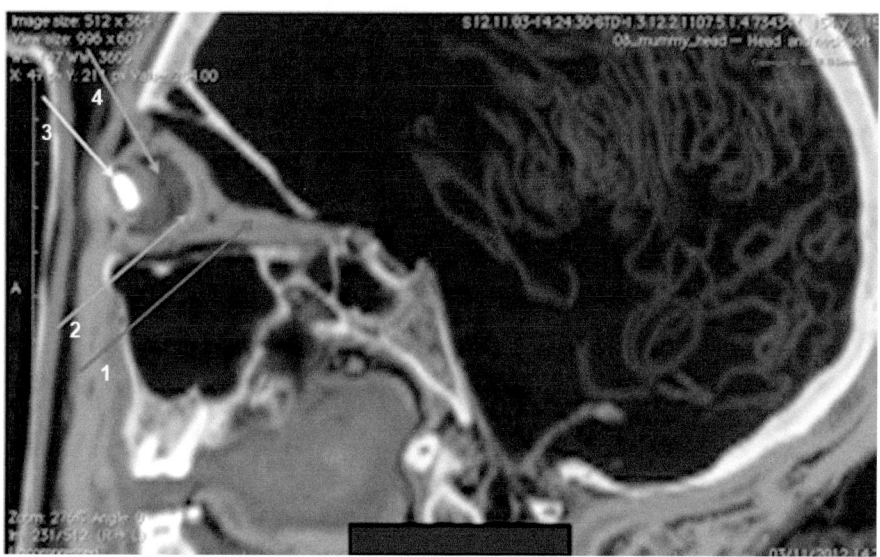

FIG. 4.145 SAGITTAL VIEW OF ORBITS SHOWING DETAIL OF THE EMBALMING PROCESS OF THE EYES

XXX. Pef-Tjau-Emawy-Khonsu - British Museum - (Accession No. EA 6681)

The eyes have been retained, opened, packed with linen and eye plates inserted over the front of the eyes (See Figs. 4.146 and 4.147 - arrows). It can be seen from the remains of the optic nerves and orbital muscles that the eye globes themselves have been retained (See Fig. 4.148 - arrows).

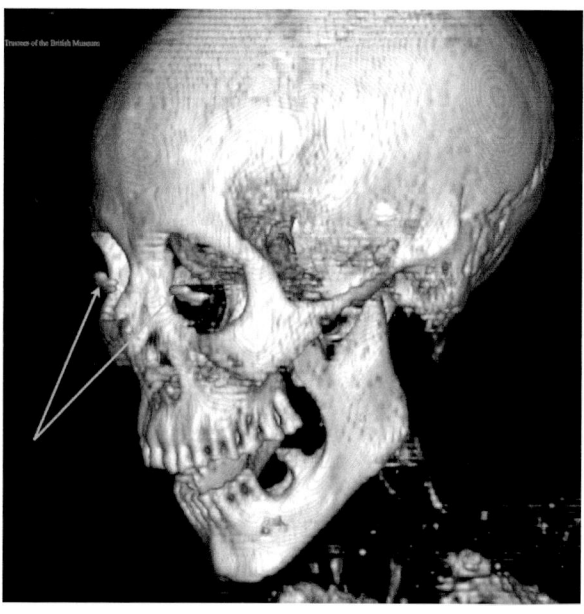

FIG. 4.146 EYE PLATES IN 3D IMAGE

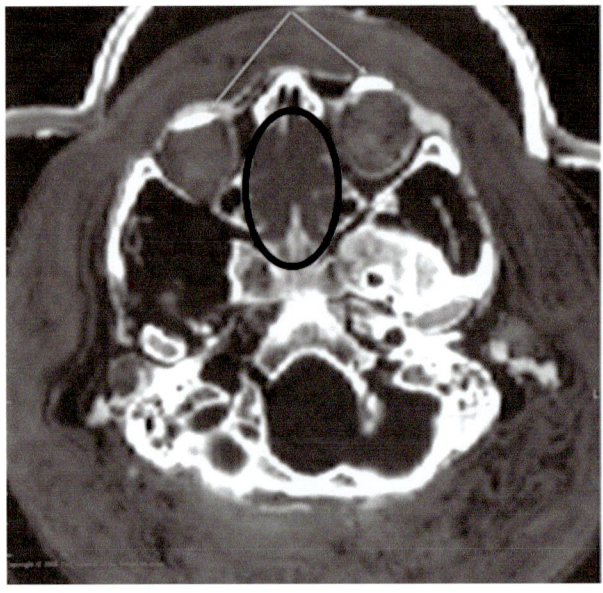

FIG. 4.147 AXIAL VIEW OF SKULL - EYE PLATES – ARROWS

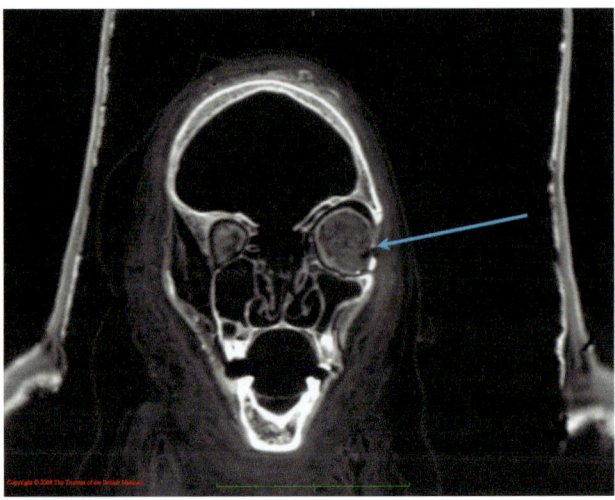

FIG. 4.149 CORONAL VIEW OF SKULL DEMONSTRATING PACKED EYES
COURTESY OF THE TRUSTEES OF THE BRITISH MUSEUM

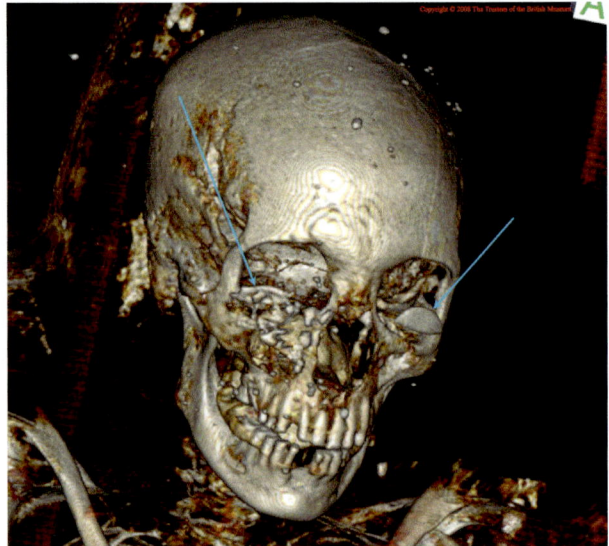

FIG. 4.150 3D RECONSTRUCTION SHOWING EYE PLATES
COURTESY OF THE TRUSTEES OF THE BRITISH MUSEUM

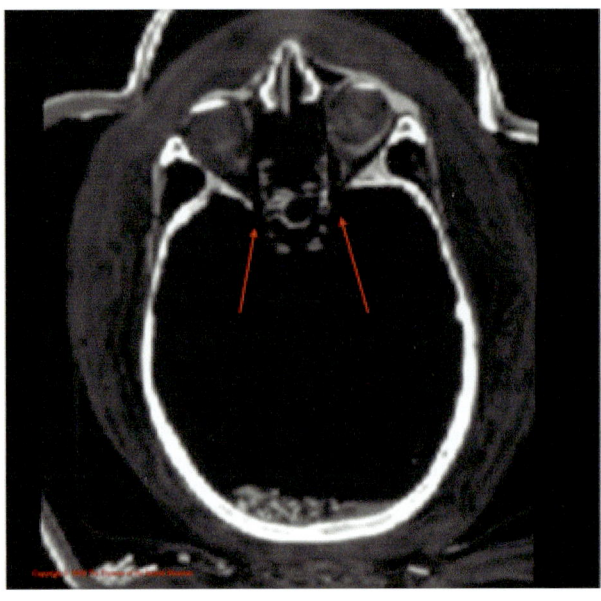

FIG. 4.148 AXIAL VIEW OF SKULL - EYE PLATES AND PACKED EYES

XXXIV. Unnamed - British Museum - (Accession No. EA 25258)

The eyes have been retained, desiccated and packed with linen (See Fig. 4.149 - arrow). Eye plates (false eyes) have also been inserted anterior to the anatomical globe. (Also see Fig. 4.149 and Fig. 4.150 - arrows and Fig. 4.151). The eye plate on the left is easily recognisable, but that on the right has been covered in a material that looks like molten metal splatter.

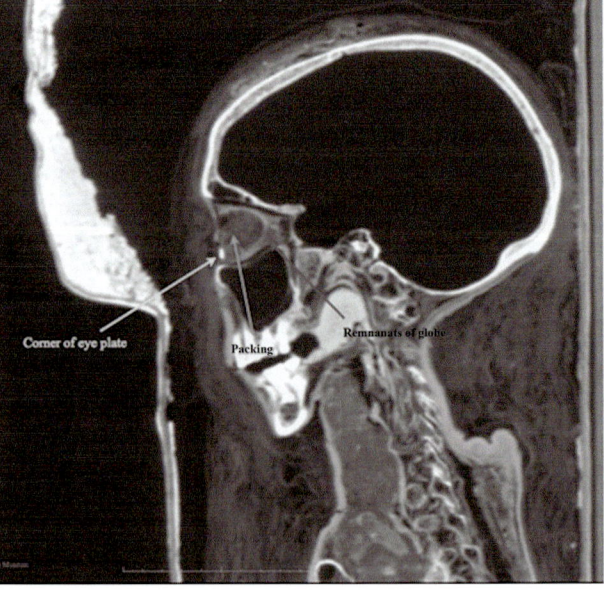

FIG. 4.151 SAGITTAL VIEW OF ORBITS - EMBALMING METHOD FOR EYES
COURTESY OF THE TRUSTEES OF THE BRITISH MUSEUM

4.3 Treatment of the mouth

The Opening of the Mouth Ceremony was not exclusively targeted at the mouth but was intended to 're-awaken' all the senses (Budge, 1899: 189,192,196 and197; Taylor, 2010: 88; Ikram and Dodson, 1998: 16) and to restore the 'life force' to the mummy and associated funerary statues (David, 2002: 121). It appears, therefore, that the mouth held a special significance to the ancient Egyptian embalmer and associated priesthood. Its treatment during mummification/embalming is therefore of some importance.

There are eight mummies where there is no evidence of the treatment of the mouth due to disruption, a lack of CT detail or the presence of a 'false mummy'. The remaining fifty-two cases break down into seven groups as follows:

Empty
Linen packing
Linen + Resin
Linen + Granular material (possibly clay)
Granular material only
Resin only
A Gold Plate over the tongue

4.3.1 Empty mouth

The group of mummies with empty mouths contains twenty-two subjects as shown in Table 4.7. In these cases there has been no attempt to fill the mouth. The tongue does remain in situ and is desiccated.

An example of a typical appearance of the mouth in such cases is shown in Fig. 4.152.

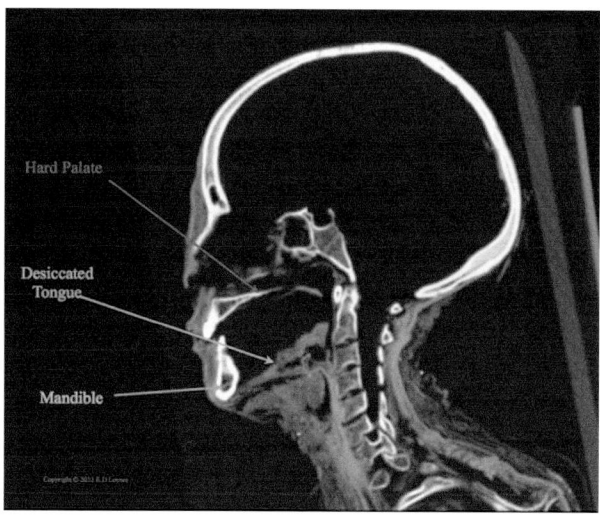

FIG. 4.152 SAGITTAL VIEW OF SKULL SHOWING EMPTY MOUTH WITH DESICCATED TONGUE

4.3.2 Linen packing

There are thirteen mummies in which the mouth has been packed with linen alone. These are shown in Table 4.8. In eleven of the thirteen mummies the oral packing is loose, as is seen in the three examples shown in Figs 4.153, 4.154 and 5.155.

In contrast, there is linen tightly packed into the mouth in only two cases – that is in mummies XXXI and XLV. They are illustrated in Figs. 4.156, 4.157 and 4.158. It is, however, interesting that these mummies come from significantly different era – namely Dynasty 25 and the Roman era. In the case of the Dynasty 25 mummy, there is tight packing of linen within the cheeks as well. The arrows in Fig. 4.157 show this.

NUMBER	ORIGIN	ERA
I	Birmingham - Graeco-Roman	Roman
IX	Liverpool - Padiamunnebnesuttauwy	D25
X	Liverpool - Nesmin	Ptolemaic
XIII	Manchester - M1767	Roman
XVIII	Liverpool- M14048	Roman
XIX	Zurich - Altdorf Child	Roman
XXIV	Zurich - Basel - BSAE.1030	Roman
XXVI	Zurich - Geneva - Infant	Unknown
XXVII	Manchester - Demetria - 11630	Roman
XXVIII	Manchester – Ta-Sheri-Ankh – MM13783	Ptolemaic
XXX	BM - Ankh-Unen-Nefer - EA6681	D25
XXXVII	Zurich - Lenzburg - Sherit-Min	Ptolemaic
XL	Zurich - Lausanne - 492	3IP
L	Perth - 23/1936	D26
LI	Manchester - M9354a - Khary	D19/Ptolemaic
LII	Manchester - M9319 - child	Roman
LIV	Manchester - Salford 2	3IP
LV	Manchester - MM13011	Ptolemaic
LVI	Manchester - MM2109	Roman
LVII	Manchester - MM1775 - Artemidorus	Roman
LVIII	Manchester - MM13784	Middle Kingdom
LIX	BM - EA 22108 Child	Roman

TABLE 4.7 MUMMIES WITH EMPTY MOUTHS

NUMBER	ORIGIN	ERA
II	Birmingham - Namenkhetamun	D26
VII	Ipswich - Tahathor	D25
XI	Liverpool - Padiamun - M14003	D26
XXII	Zurich - Bern - 00/2	Unknown
XXIII	Zurich - Yverdon - Nes-Shou - MY/3775	Ptolemaic
XXV	Zurich - Geneva - TjesMoutPert - D0242	D22-D25
XXXI	BM - Padiamunet - EA6682	D25
XXXVI	Zurich - Bern - AE9	Ptolemaic
XLIII	Turin - (Tebtynis) - Suppl.19691	Ptolemaic?
XLIV	Turin - Provv.610	Ptolemaic?
XLV	Manchester - M1766	Roman
XLVII	Manchester - M1769	Roman
LIII	Manchester - MM1976.51a	D25

TABLE 4.8 MOUTH PACKING WITH LINEN ONLY

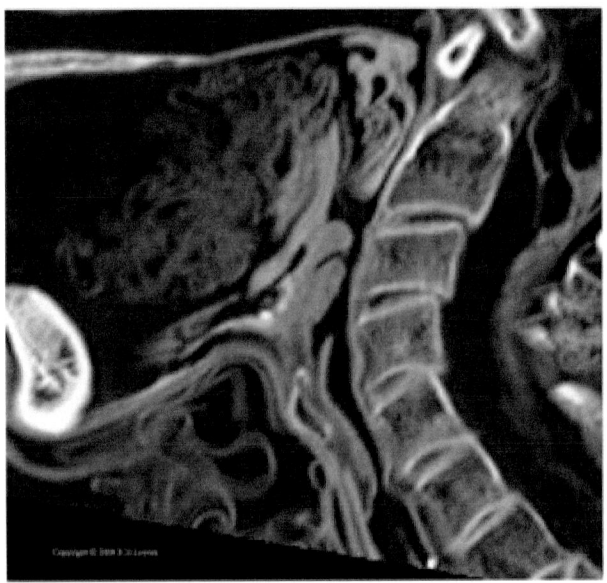

Fig. 4.153 Sagittal view of pharynx - loose linen packing within the mouth.

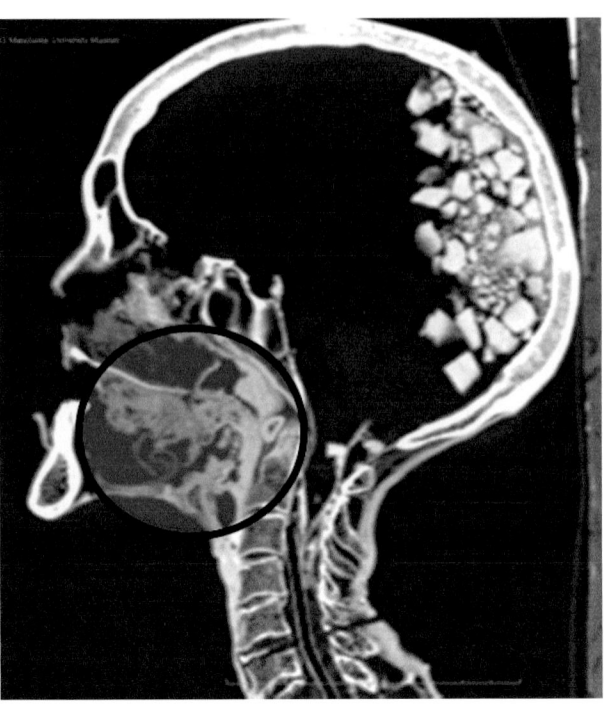

Fig. 4.155 Sagittal view of skull - loose linen packing within the mouth.

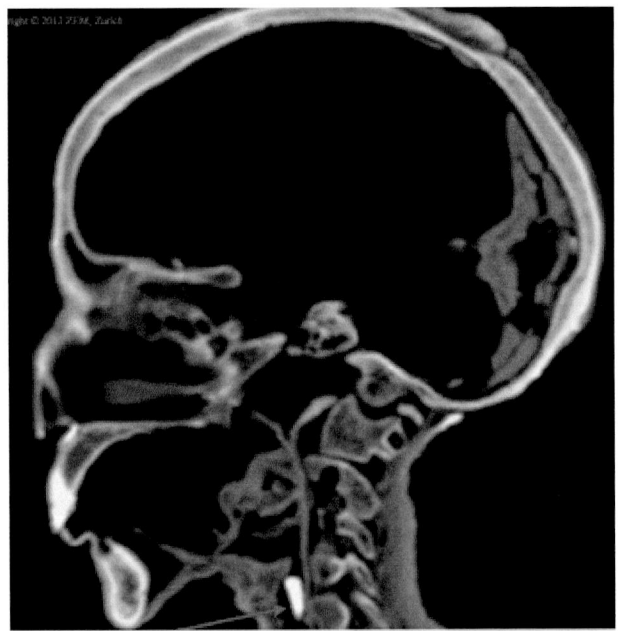

Fig. 4.154 Sagittal view of the skull - loose linen packing within the mouth.

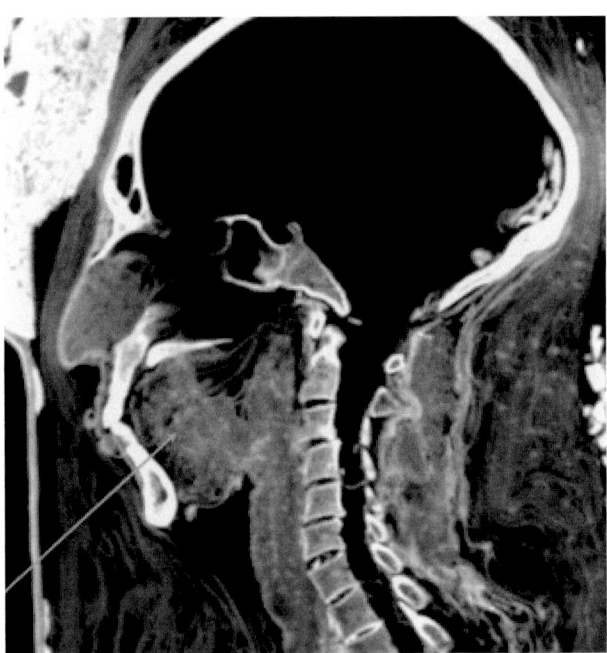

Fig. 4.156 Sagittal view of skull - tight linen packing within the mouth in Mummy XXXI

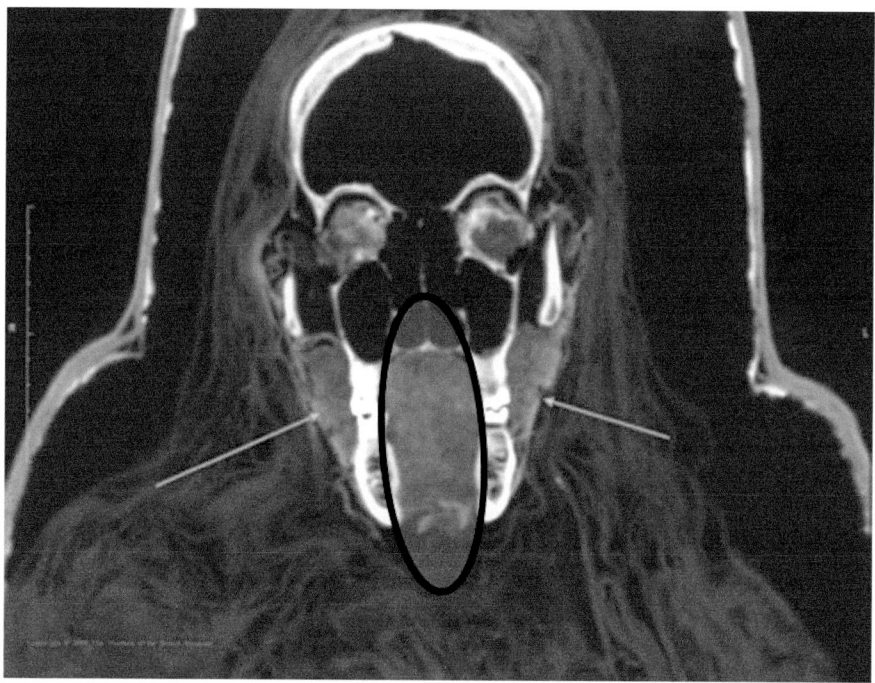

FIG. 4.157 CORONAL VIEW OF SKULL - TIGHT LINEN PACKING WITHIN THE MOUTH IN MUMMY XXXI. ALSO SHOWN IS THE LINEN WITHIN THE CHEEKS.

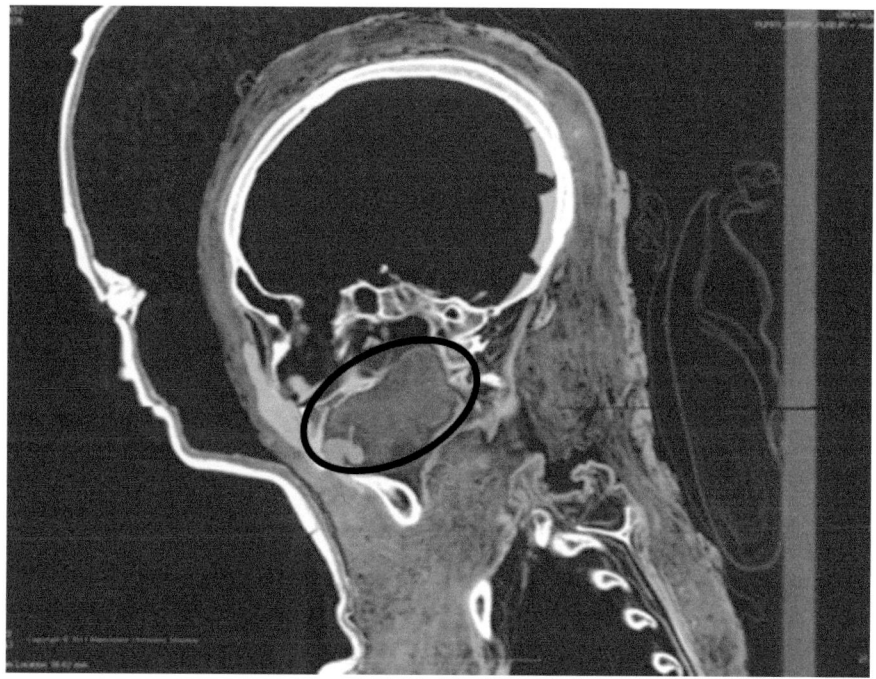

FIG. 4.158 SAGITTAL VIEW OF SKULL - TIGHT LINEN PACKING IN THE MOUTH – MUMMY XLV

4.3.3 Linen plus resin

There are only three cases of the use of resin with linen packing. They are mummies VIII, XLI and XLII from Dynasty 22, the Roman era and the Ptolemaic era respectively.

VIII Padiamun - National Museums Liverpool (Accession No. 53.72a)

The floor of the mouth along with the tongue, has been pushed upwards by packing of the neck (see next section). The cavity contains some resin posteriorly and, in front of this, some linen packing. There are two dense opacities lying in the anterior layers of the linen, which appear to be the damaged teeth (See Fig. 4.159. - arrows 1). The arrow 2 shows sub-cutaneous packing in the neck.

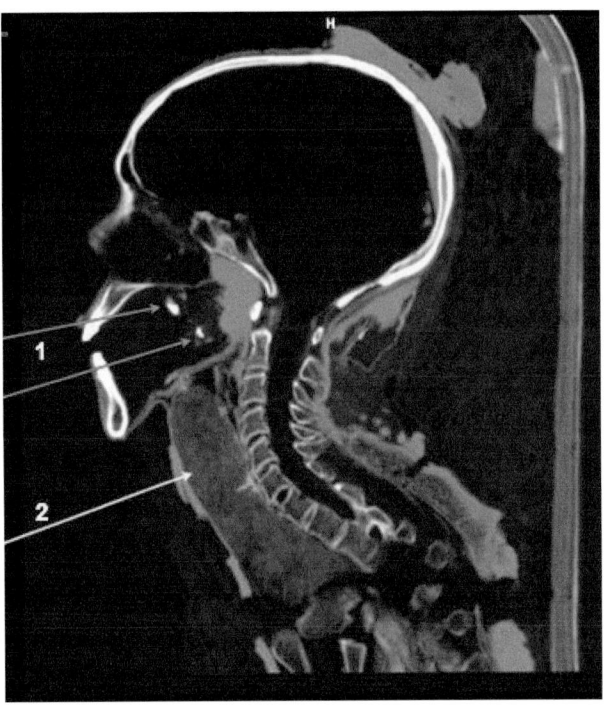

FIG. 4.159 SAGITTAL VIEW OF SKULL SHOWING THE USE OF RESIN AND LINEN IN THE MOUTH

XLI. Unnamed child - Lenzburg (Cat. No.K-10351)

The mouth contains some resin and linen packing.

XLII. Ta-aset - Turin (Cat. No. Suppl. 9480)

The mouth has been loosely packed with linen posteriorly and resin anteriorly. There are 4 loose teeth in the back of the pharynx.

4.3.4 Linen plus 'granular material' – possibly clay

Again, there are only three cases in this category: Mummies V, XXXII and LX dating to Dynasty 25, Dynasty 22 and the Roman era respectively. An example of this technique is shown in the case of Mummy LX.

LX. Name - Unnamed - British Museum (Cat. No. EA 6704)

The mouth is partly open and a linen pack inserted anterior to other material - probably clay or a mixture of resin and sawdust (See Fig. 4.160 and 4.161 - arrows 2 = linen, arrows 1 = resin mix).

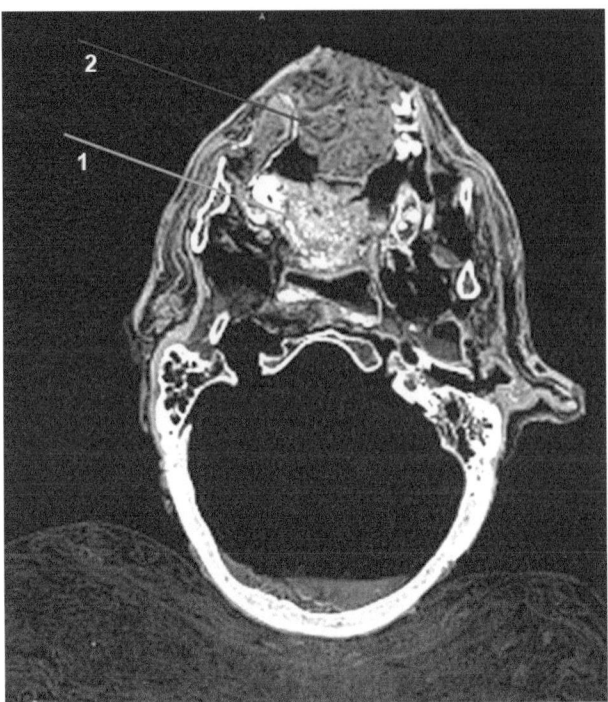

FIG. 4.160 AXIAL VIEW OF SKULL DEMONSTRATING THE USE OF BOTH LINEN AND 'GRANULAR' MATERIAL
COURTESY OF THE TRUSTEES OF THE BRITISH MUSEUM

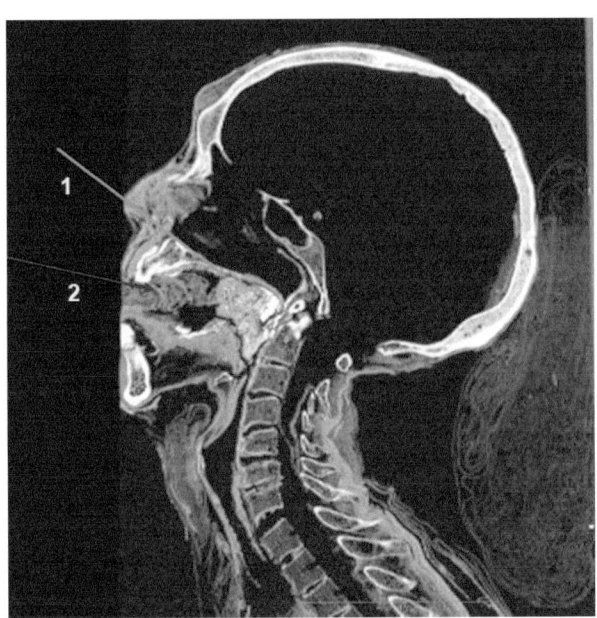

FIG. 4.161 SAGITTAL VIEW OF SKULL - USE OF BOTH LINEN AND 'GRANULAR' MATERIAL
COURTESY OF THE TRUSTEES OF THE BRITISH MUSEUM

4.3.5 Granular material alone (possibly clay)

Such a technique was found in five cases. These are shown in Table 4.9. Some examples are shown below.

NUMBER	ORIGIN	ERA
III	Birmingham - Padimut	D20-21
XIV	Manchester – MM1777 - Asru	D26
XVII	Liverpool - Ankhesenaset	3IP
XXXIII	BM - EA22939	D22
IL	Manchester - MM5053.a - Perenbast	D22

TABLE 4.9 GRANULAR MATERIAL IN THE MOUTH

III Padimut (BMAG – Cat. No. 1991W1)

Examination of the mouth reveals not only dental and periodontal disease but also a significant amount of granular material within the oral cavity. This material has been packed in to the extent that the teeth are forced apart slightly. Also seen in the lower part of Fig. 4.162 is evidence of granular material packed into the neck below the lower jaw (See Fig. 4.162).

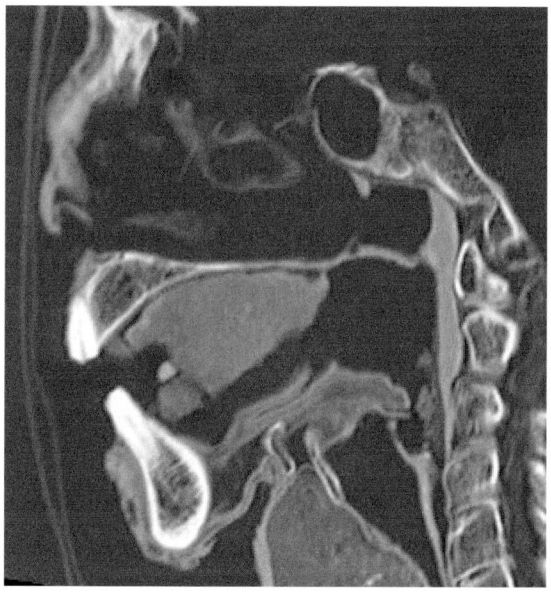

FIG. 4.162 SAGITTAL VIEW OF PHARYNX - PACKING IN MOUTH AND NECK

XVII. Ankhesenaset - National Museums Liverpool (Accession No. M14000)

As can be seen in Fig. 4.163 the mouth has been tightly stuffed with granular material resulting in the teeth being forced open.

It is of interest to note that in only one of these cases was sub-cutaneous packing of the neck omitted. That is in the case of Mummy XIV, Asru, from the Late Period (Dyn.26).

4.3.6 Resin alone

Again there are five cases in this category. They are shown in Table 4.10.

NUMBER	ORIGIN	ERA
XII	Manchester - M1768	Roman
XVI	Liverpool - M13997a	Roman
XXIX	BM - Hor - EA6659	D22
XXXIV	BM - EA25258	D22
XXXVIII	Zurich - St. Gallen - Shepenese	D26

TABLE 4.10 TREATMENT OF THE MOUTH - RESIN ONLY

In the cases of Mummies XII, XVI and XXIX there is only a small amount of resin used in the mouth. However, in the case of the remaining two mummies (XXXIV and XXXVIII) a large amount of resin has been forced into the mouth. These are shown below.

XXXIV. Unnamed - British Museum - (Accession No. EA 25258)

The mouth has had the floor depressed, the tongue pushed backwards and radio-dense packing (possibly resin) inserted (See Fig. 4.164). In this case there is also subcutaneous packing within the neck.

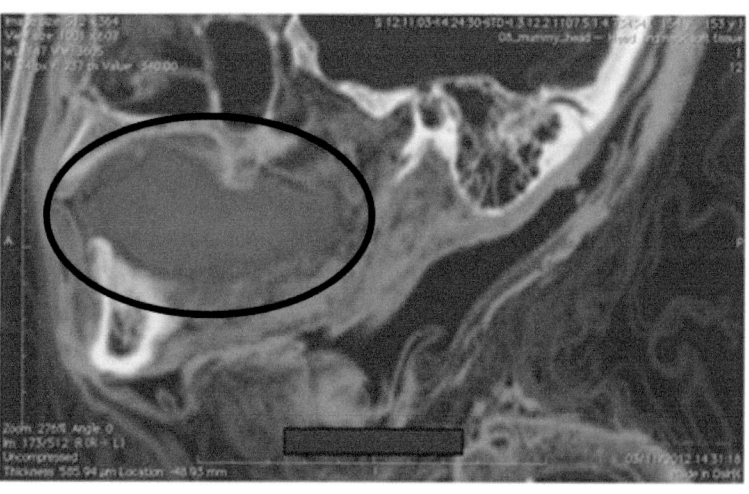

FIG. 4.163 SAGITTAL VIEW OF PHARYNX – EXCESS AMORPHOUS MATERIAL IN THE MOUTH CAUSING THE TEETH TO BE FORCED APART.

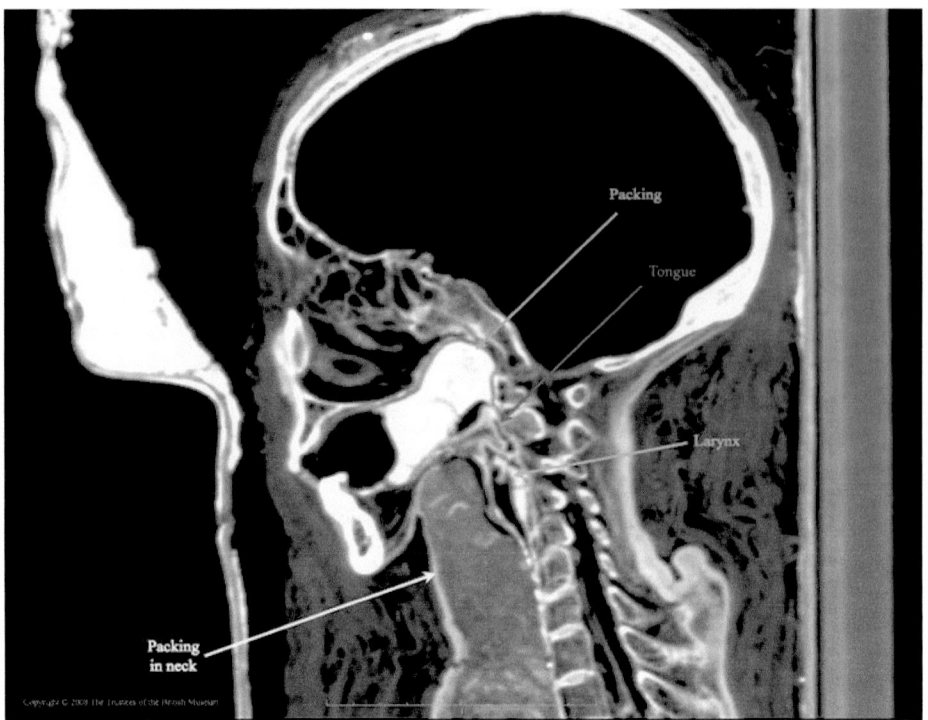

FIG. 4.164 SAGITTAL VIEW OF SKULL - RESIN IN THE MOUTH AND PACKING IN THE NECK
COURTESY OF THE TRUSTEES OF THE BRITISH MUSEUM

XXXVIII. Shepenese - St. Gallen (no Number)

The mouth has been packed with resin (See Fig. 4.165 - arrow 2). The tongue remains in situ. Parts of the larynx are also preserved (See Fig. 4.165 - arrow 1). In this case there is no sub-cutaneous packing in the neck.

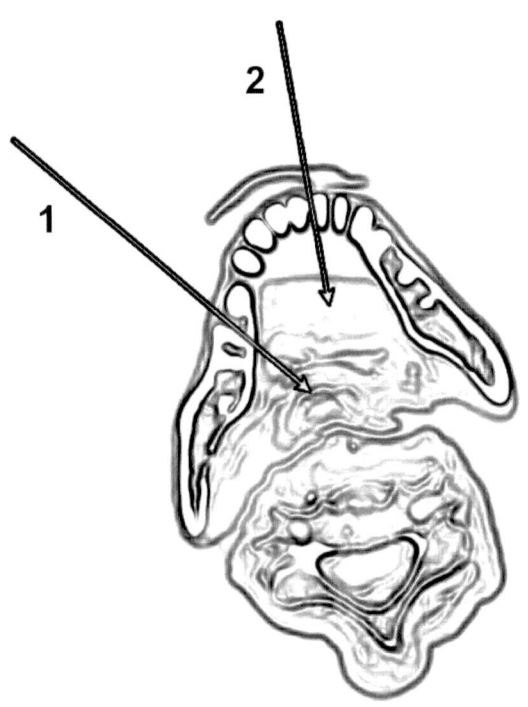

FIG. 4.165 AXIAL VIEW AT LEVEL OF MANDIBLE - RESIN PACKING WITHIN THE MOUTH (AFTER IEM IMAGE)

4.3.7 A metal plate over the tongue (possibly gold)

This technique was found in a child from the Roman era, Mummy XV.

XV. Unnamed - National Museums Liverpool (Accession No. 13.10.11.25)

In the pharynx there is a plate of radio-dense material (it has been suggested that this is gold) overlying the tongue. As can be seen in Figs. 4.166, 4.167 and 4.168, this is folded at the edges. Abd al-Latif al-Baghdadi, a twelfth century Arab writer is quoted by Pettigrew as referring to the use of a gold plate placed on the tongue. (Pettigrew, 1834: 63).

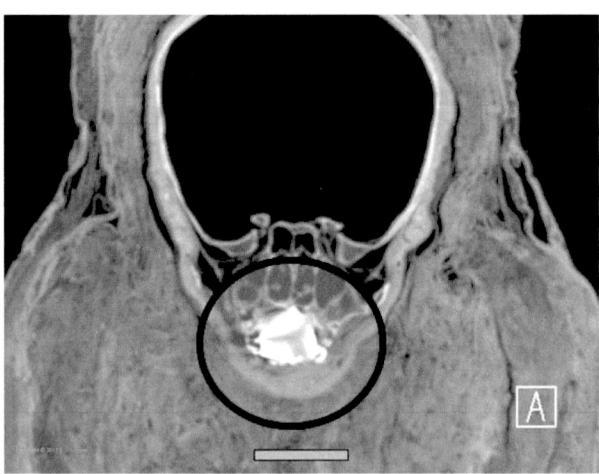

FIG. 4.166 CORONAL VIEW OF SKULL - METAL PLATE OVER THE TONGUE (POSSIBLY GOLD)

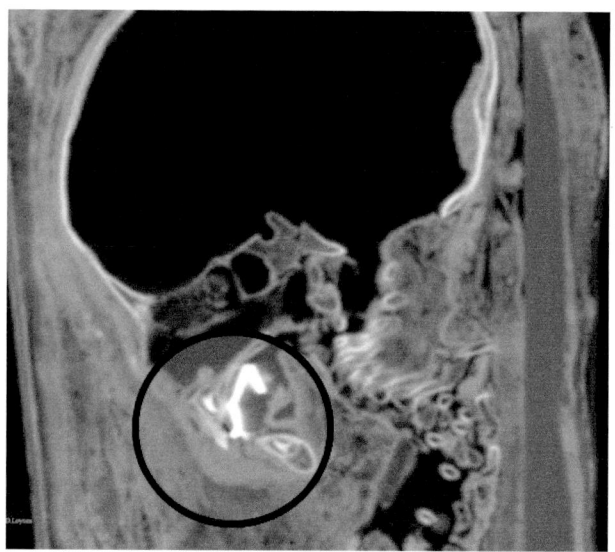

Fig. 4.167 Sagittal view of skull - metal plate over the tongue (possibly Gold)

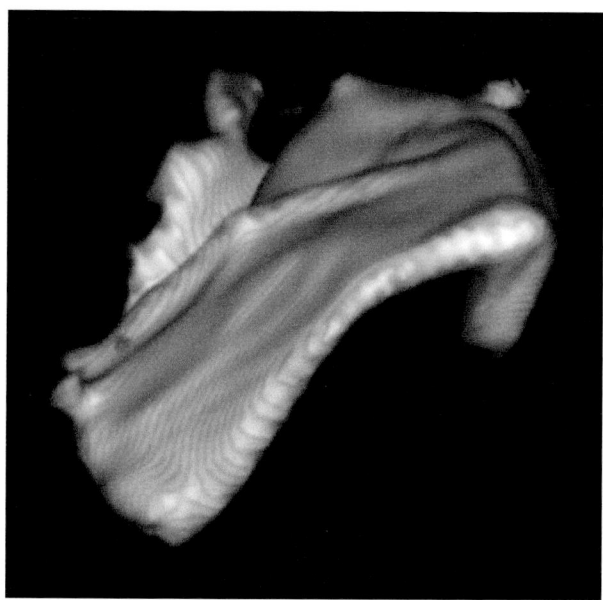

Fig. 4.168 3D reconstruction of metal plate lying over tongue

4.4 Treatment of the ears

Initially it was intended to record the treatment of the ears – that is, were they blocked or 'open'. However, there were too many cases in which the ears were either not visible or damaged to allow a proper demonstration of the frequency of a particular treatment. This particular aspect of investigation was therefore abandoned.

Chapter Five

Results – The Trunk

5.1 Introduction

Taking the descriptions of Herodotus and Diodorus Siculus (v.s.) as a starting point, it would be expected that some form of evisceration would have been attempted on many of the bodies of the deceased. Herodotus describes 'the most perfect process' as including excerebration, evisceration via a left flank incision and desiccation in 'natrum'.

However, analysis of the mummies in this study reveals that this is not always the case. Also, where evisceration has been performed, the techniques and results are variable. However, Herodotus' description of a 'second process' involving a lytic enema to dissolve the viscera but without surgical opening of the abdomen would have been expected to result in both the absence of a flank incision (or perineal approach) and the absence of viscera within the abdominal cavity. His 'third method' involving the use of an enema which cleanses the lower bowel followed by desiccation could explain some of the findings discussed in section 5.2.4.5 (P 174).

It should be noted here that the presence of an abdominal incision is all that is noted. The length, exact placement and direction of the incision has not been analysed as the distortion of the body wall by desiccation and, on occasions, packing through the incision as well as packing within and therefore distention of the wall of the abdomen makes analysis difficult and often spurious. In some case the body wall, although present, is not complete. For these reasons a more detailed analysis of the incision itself has not been performed in this project.

5.2 Grouping

The results will be considered in groups as follows:

- The use of an abdominal incision
- The use of a perineal approach
- No incision visible
- The extent of visceral clearance
- The use of canopic packages
- The use of inserted materials

However, it should be noted that of the fifty-nine mummies CT scanned, one scan in analogue form provided no useful information, four mummies were sufficiently disorganized to provide no information on the trunk and one showed a linen pack shaped as if it had been in an abdominal incision but with a disorganized body. The remaining fifty-three mummies provided the following information.

5.2.1 Abdominal incision

Those mummies with a definite or almost certain abdominal incision are shown in Table 5.1.

NUMBER	ORIGIN	ERA
I	Birmingham - Graeco-Roman	Roman
II	Birmingham - Namenkhetamun	D26
III	Birmingham - Padimut	D20-21
V	Sheffield - Nesitanebetasheru	D25
VI	Sheffield - Djedma'atiuesankh	D26
VII	Ipswich - Tahathor	D25
VIII	Liverpool - Padiamun - 53.72a	D22
IX	Liverpool - Padiamunnebnesuttauwy	D25
X	Liverpool - Nesmin	Ptolemaic
XI	Liverpool - Padiamun - M14003	D26
XIV	Manchester – MM1777 - Asru	D26
XVI	Liverpool - M13997a	Roman
XVII	Liverpool - Ankhesenaset - 14000	3IP
XVIII	Liverpool- M14048	Roman
XIX	Zurich - Altdorf Child	Roman
XXII	Zurich - Bern - 00/2	Unknown
XXIII	Zurich - Yverdon - Nes-Shou - MY/3775	Ptolemaic
XXV	Zurich - Geneva - TjesMoutPert - D0242	D22-25
XXVI	Zurich - Geneva - Infant	Unknown
XXVII	Manchester - Demetria - MM11630	Roman
XXVIII	Manchester – Ta-Sheri-Ankh – MM13783	Ptolemaic
XXIX	BM - Hor - EA6659	D22
XXX	BM - Pef-Tjau-Emawy-Khonsu - EA6681	D25
XXXI	BM - Padiamunet - EA6682	D25
XXXII	BM - EA20744	D22
XXXIII	BM - EA22939	D22
XXXIV	BM - EA25258	D22
XXXVI	Zurich - Bern - AE9	Ptolemaic
XXXVIII	Zurich - St. Gallen - Shepenese	D26
XXXIX	Zurich - St. Gallen - C3530	D21
XL	Zurich - Lausanne - 492	3IP
XLI	Zurich - Lenzburg - K10351	Roman
XLIII	Turin - (Tebtynis) - Suppl.19691	Ptolemaic ??
XLIV	Turin - Provv.610	Ptolemaic ??
XLVIII	Manchester - MM3496	D18
XLIX	Manchester - MM5053.a - Perenbast	D22
LIII	Manchester - MM1976.51a	D25
LX	BM - EA 6704	Roman

TABLE 5.1 MUMMIES WITH AN ABDOMINAL INCISION

The relevant reports follow.

I The Graeco-Roman Mummy in Birmingham (Cat. No. 1894A15)

Thorax

The thoracic cage comprising of the ribs, spine, sternum and costo-vertebral junctions, shows significant asymmetry. This is the result of posterior dislocation of the left 6th to 10th ribs inclusive and subluxation of the left 4th and 5th ribs. There is also dislocation of the right 8th, 9th and 10th ribs, all at the costo-vertebral joints. Finally there are dislocations of the left 2nd, 3rd and 4th costo-chondral junctions (See Figs. 5.1 and 5.2).

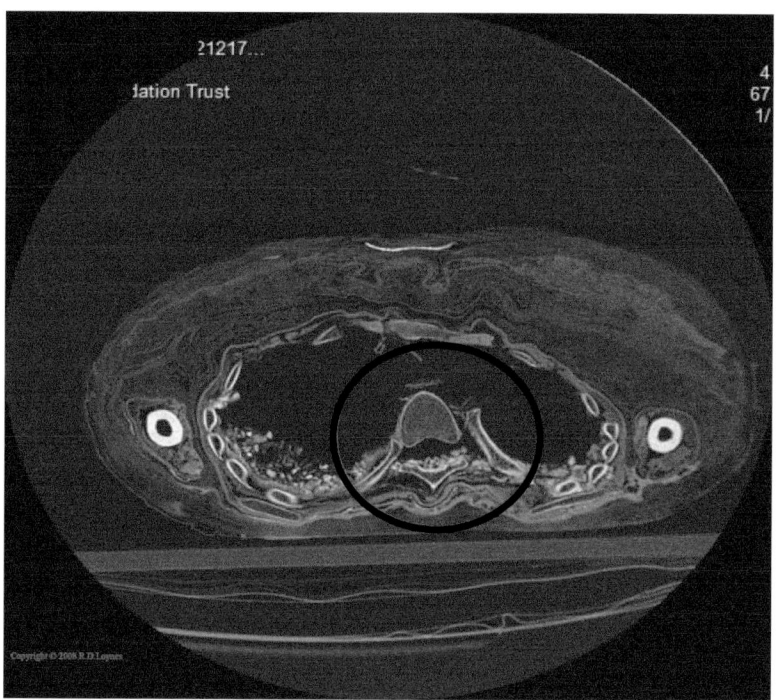

Fig. 5.1 Axial view of thorax showing costo-vertebral dislocation

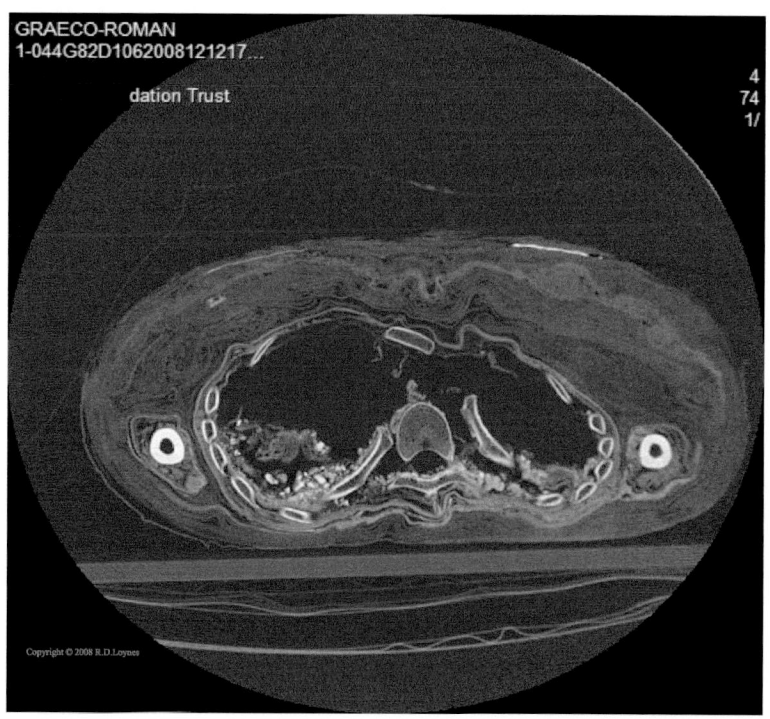

Fig. 5.2 Axial view of thorax showing costo-vertebral dislocation

There is, however, no evidence of bony damage associated with these dislocations/subluxations. It takes a significant force to cause dislocations of the costo-vertebral joints and it would be very unlikely to happen, as the result of trauma, in the absence of bony damage. It seems more likely, therefore, that the damage to the costo-vertebral joints took place after death, i.e. during the mummification process. This could be achieved by dissecting the costo-vertebral joints from the inside of the thoracic cavity, accessed from the incision in the abdomen. However, the necessary 'surgery' to divide the costo-transverse ligaments (following disruption of the costo-vertebral joints) to allow this degree of movement of the ribs, would be extremely difficult to perform blind with access only through the abdomen! To re-enforce the concept of a trans-abdominal/thoracic approach it is noted that there is no convincing evidence of an incision through the skin of the posterior wall of the thorax. There is a continuous extension of the granular material from the thoracic cavity to the para-vertebral and sub-scapular spaces on the left side (opposite the dislocated ribs) and to a lesser extent on the right side.

Why this was performed remains a matter of conjecture, but it is noticeable that the afore-mentioned dislocations are accompanied by an attempt at compression of the left rib cage, making the thorax somewhat smaller. Unfortunately, this has resulted in asymmetry that has been corrected in the final form of the mummy by padding out the resultant defect! (See Fig. 5.3 and 5.4).

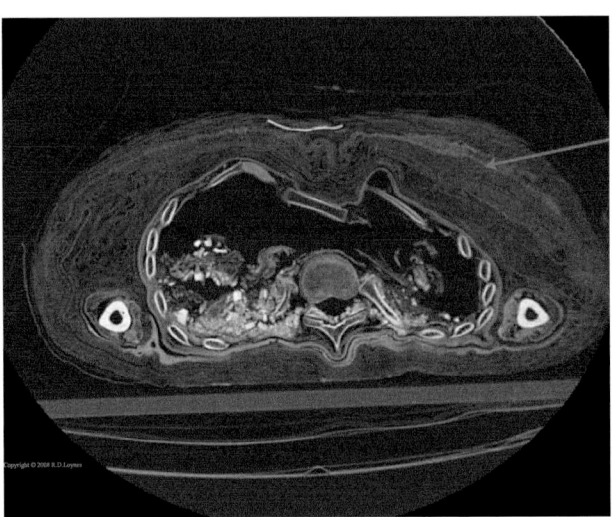

FIG. 5.3 AXIAL VIEW OF THORAX - ASYMMETRY WITH ANTERIOR PADDING ON LEFT

The thoracic cavity itself is loosely 'filled' with a mixture of granular material and body tissues – probably bowel (certainly the appearance is tubular). The granular material is of varying density with both high and low radio-dense constituents. The cavity contains only a modest amount of material with more on the right than the left side. There is no evidence of layers of material or of fluid levels, such as would be associated with the use of resins (See Fig. 5.5).

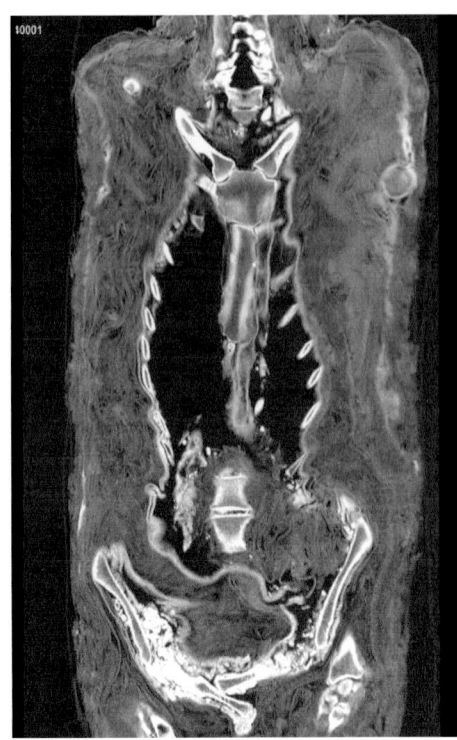

FIG. 5.4 CORONAL VIEW OF THORAX - ASYMMETRY WITH ANTERIOR PADDING ON LEFT

There is no evidence of the diaphragm remaining and presumably it was removed during the evisceration process, allowing easier access. There is little convincing evidence of the presence of the heart, which is surprising.

Abdomen

The anterior abdominal wall contains a left sided incision that runs from the upper abdomen laterally to the lower abdomen in the region of the symphysis pubis in or near the mid line. The incision has not been closed and there is evidence of the material used for wrapping crossing from the outside to the inside of the abdomen through this incision (See Fig. 5.6).

The abdominal cavity contains a mixture of granular, radio-dense material similar to that seen in the thorax (presumably 'mummification material' - packing) and material that appears tubular and is therefore likely to be human tissue such as bowel. As in the thorax, the abdomen is loosely packed. There is also a significant amount of material (possibly linen) within the thoracic/abdominal cavity that is in continuity with that passing through the abdominal embalming incision. Finally, there is the presence, in the trunk cavity, of two packages that might represent canopic packages (although normally four in number, it is conjecture that the other two may have disintegrated and not be readily visible as entities).

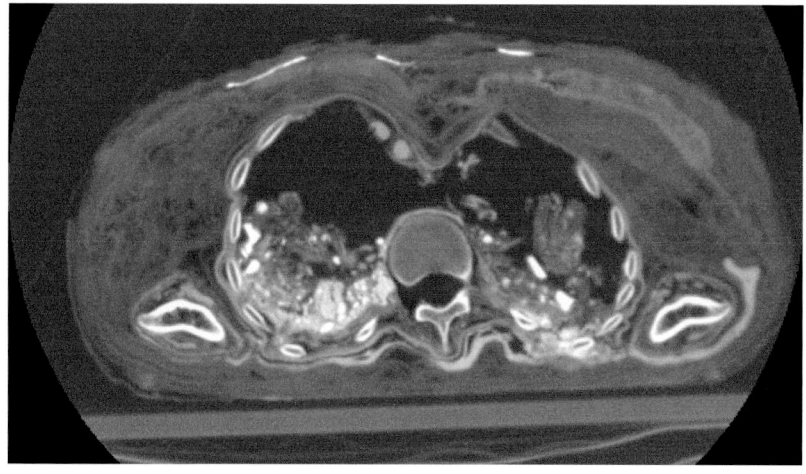

FIG. 5.5 AXIAL VIEW OF THORAX SHOWING CHEST CONTENTS

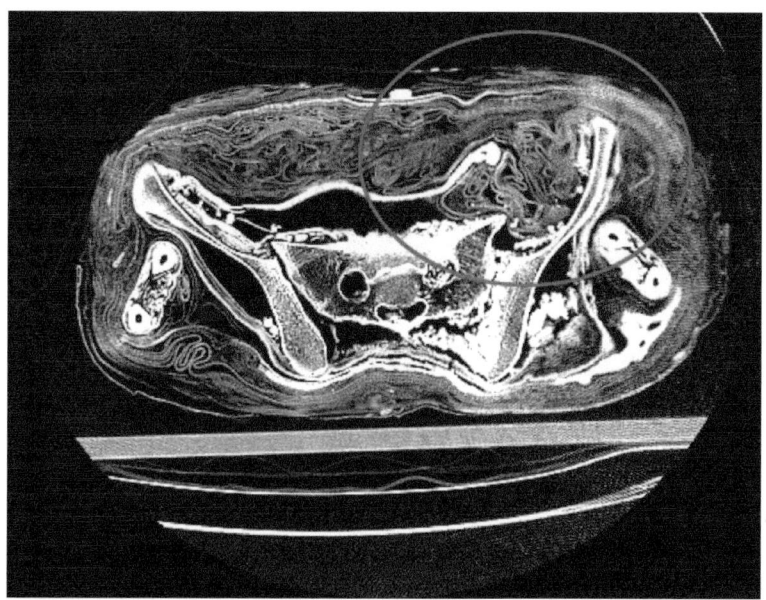

FIG. 5.6 AXIAL VIEW OF LOWER ABDOMEN - LEFT FLANK INCISION

II Namenkhetamun (BMAG - Cat. No.1966A23)

Thorax

The body wall (sternum, ribs and thoracic spine) and shoulder girdle are intact and symmetrical, except for the left lower posterior thoracic wall, where there is a hole (See Fig. 5.7 and 5.8).

It is noted that fragments of the body wall have been projected into the body cavity, indicating that the wall was in a hard, brittle state when the hole was made. There is an indication that the hole has been 'closed' with a plug of material (See Fig. 5.9).

Examination of the thorax reveals that the pleura and mediastinum remain in situ (See Fig. 5.10) but there is no evidence of the heart being present despite clear evidence of the great vessels and trachea. The diaphragm on both sides is intact anteriorly but breeched through the posterior half of the muscle via a hole in the posterior body wall on the left side in the paraspinal region at the level of T11 to L1.

The body cavity contains a small amount of granular material posteriorly along with some 'biological' tissue. The nature of the latter tissue is difficult to ascertain but could be tubular, that is bowel. No fluid levels are seen in the thorax, indicating the absence of the use of resin within the cavity of this mummy.

Abdomen

The abdominal incision lies on the left side in the posterolateral position behind the line of the arm. A small amount of linen crosses through the incision and hangs posteriorly, in the upper part of the incision. Over all, the incision appears small (See Figs. 5.11 and 5.12).

The abdominal cavity is flattened and contains a couple of flat packs of amorphous material.

The rectum, bladder, urethra and male genitalia are readily seen in situ. The other abdominal organs appear to have been removed and probably returned to the thoracic cavity.

There is no evidence of canopic packages.

Pelvis and Hips

There is no evidence of damage to the bony structures of the pelvis or the hip joints.

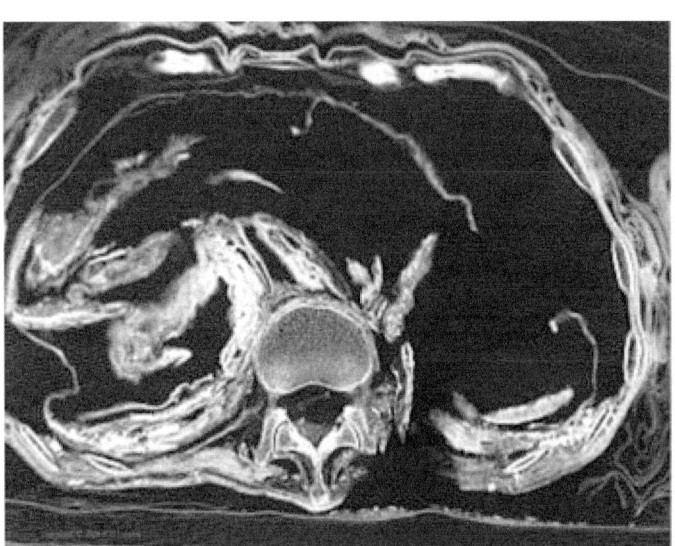

FIG. 5.7 AXIAL VIEW OF LOWER THORAX - PERFORATION IN POSTERIOR WALL.

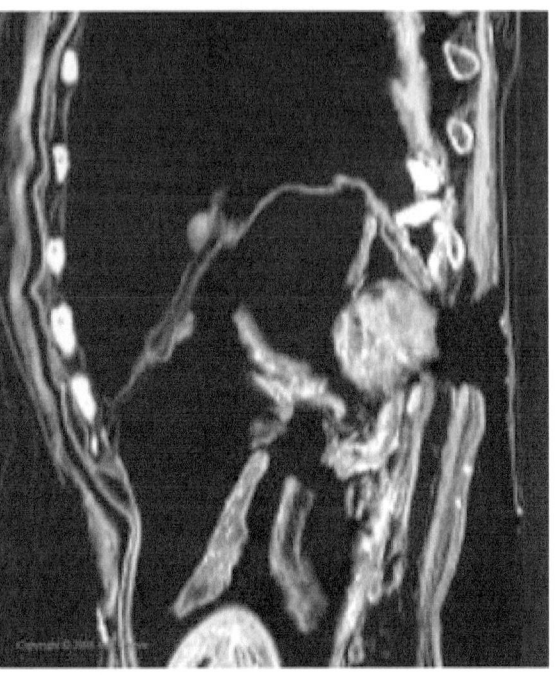

FIG. 5.9 SAGITTAL VIEW OF LOWER THORAX – PLUG OF MATERIAL IN PERFORATION

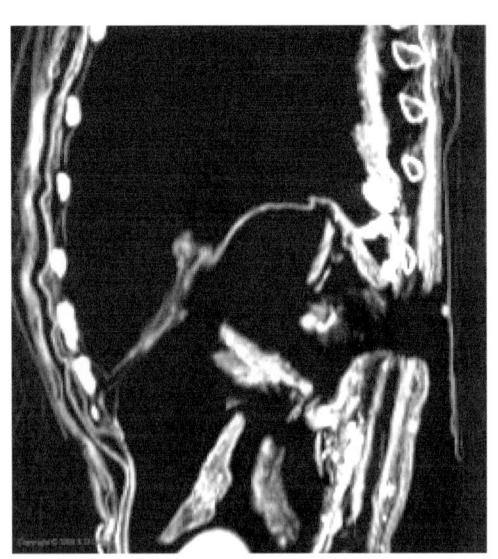

FIG. 5.8 SAGITTAL VIEW OF LOWER THORAX - PERFORATION IN POSTERIOR WALL.

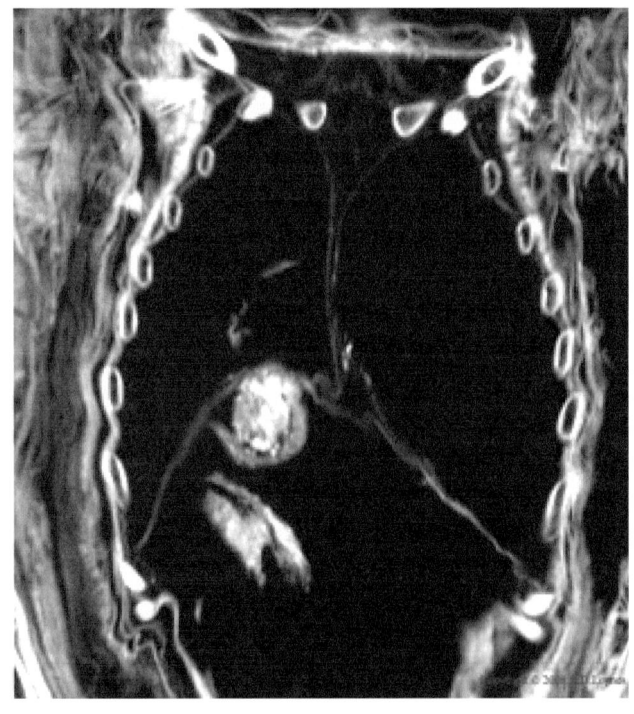

FIG. 5.10 CORONAL VIEW OF THORAX SHOWING REMNANTS OF PLEURA AND MEDIASTINUM

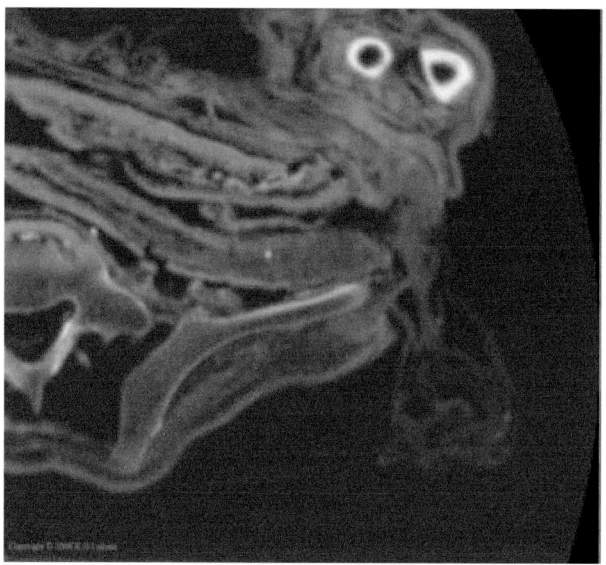

FIG. 5.11 AXIAL VIEW OF LOWER ABDOMEN - MATERIAL HANGING FREE FROM ABDOMINAL INCISION

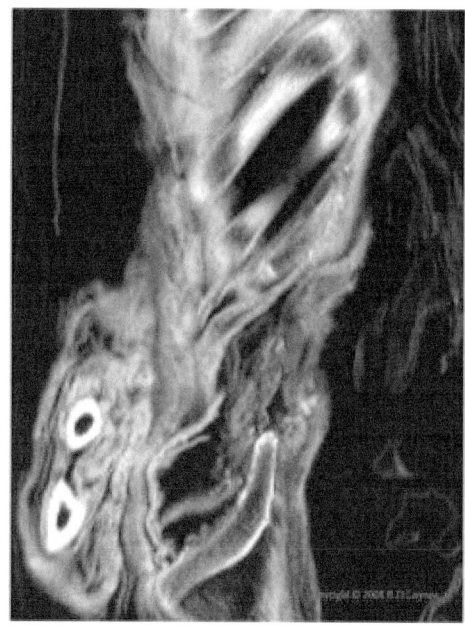

FIG. 5.12 SAGITTAL VIEW OF ABDOMEN - MATERIAL IN ABDOMINAL INCISION

III Padimut (BMAG – Cat. No. 1991W1)

Thorax

Both shoulder joints are congruent. There is a hole in the right rib cage anteriorly from the level of the lower sternum caudally; otherwise the rib cage is intact. The thoracic cavity contains radio-dense material lying posteriorly throughout the full extent of the cavity. There are two fluid levels in this material, indicating the introduction of the substance on two occasions with time allowed after the first introduction for it to become solid. It is presumed that this substance is resin (See Fig. 5.13).

There is also other material within this cavity that is likely to be biological in origin and probably represents organs such as intestines returned to the cavity after mummification. Remnants of the diaphragm are visible anteriorly but absent posteriorly.

There are structures within the mediastinum, including an entity containing chambers which is almost certainly the heart – somewhat distorted by desiccation. However, the point of interest is that it has not been removed from its normal position within the mediastinum (See Figs. 5.14 and 5.15).

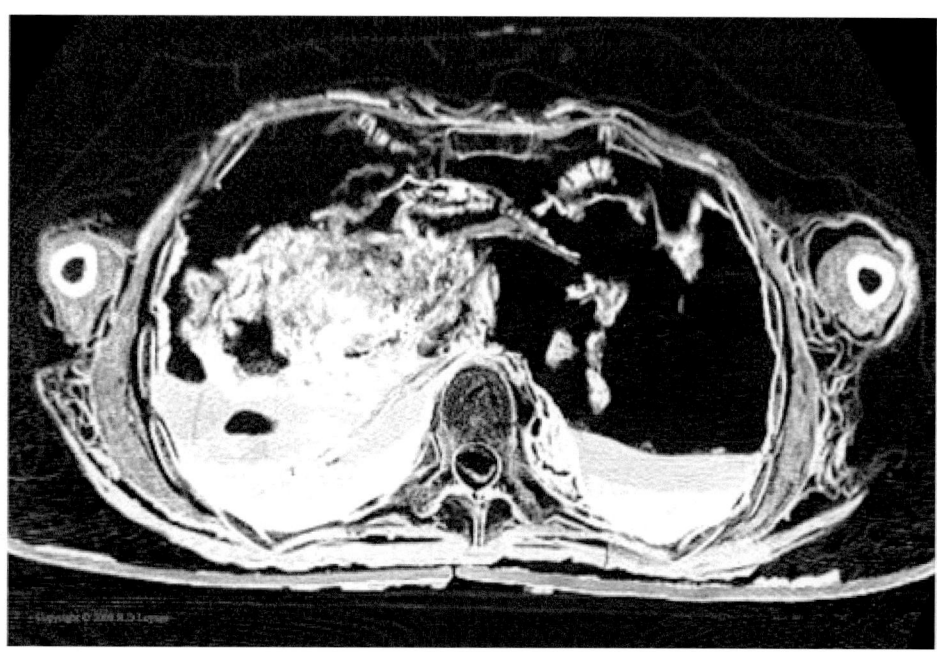

FIG. 5.13 AXIAL VIEW OF THORAX - FLUID LEVELS IN 'RESIN'

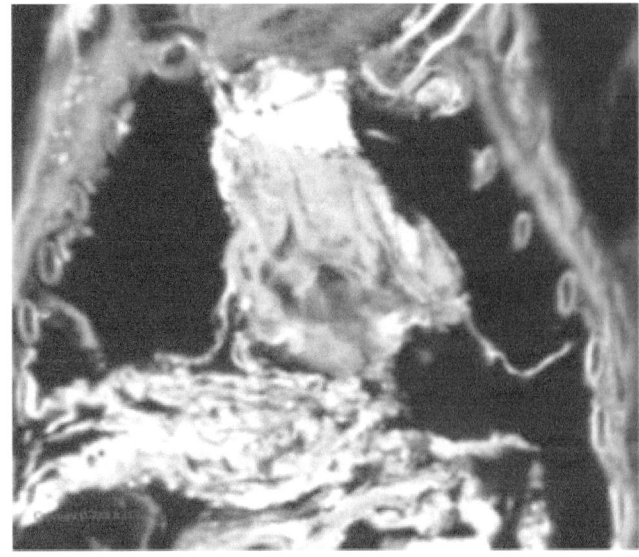

Fig. 5.14 Coronal view of thorax - heart in mediastinum

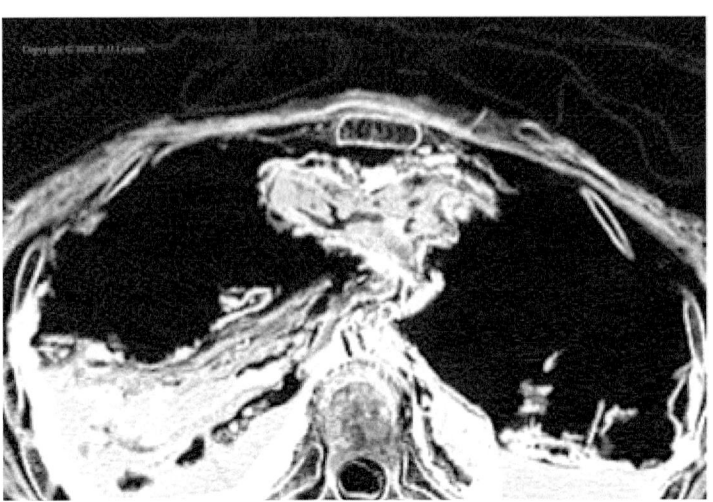

Fig. 5.15 Axial view of thorax - heart in mediastinum

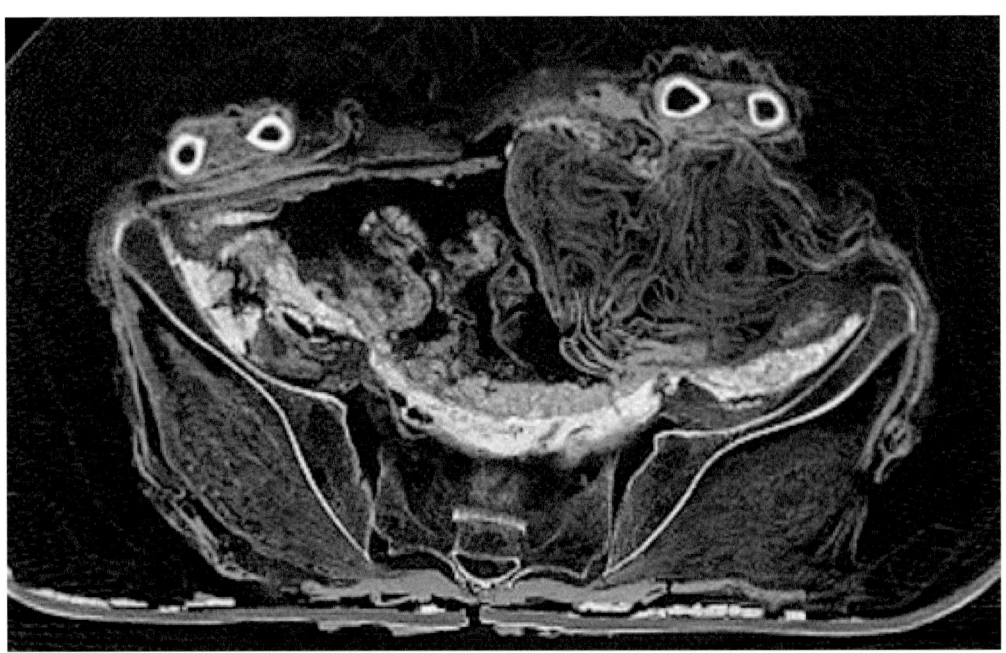

Fig. 5.16 Axial view of lower abdomen showing contents

Abdomen

There is an incision in the left wall of the abdomen. This has not been closed and there is abundant material – presumably linen – crossing this incision and packing most of the left side of the abdominal cavity.

Whilst there is a small amount of material resembling the 'resin' in the thorax, most of the substance in the abdomen is either granular or biological and is mostly on the right side. On the left, the majority of packing is linen (See Fig. 5.16).

The intestines, with the exception of the rectum, have been removed. The returned organs in the abdomen are randomly arranged without any convincing evidence of canopic packages.

Pelvis and Hips

Whilst the sacro-iliac joints are not completely congruous, there is no evidence of true dislocation or disruption. This is also the case with the pubic symphysis. The hip joints are congruous to a point that is probably within the norm for 3000 year old mummies. There are breaches in and loss of some of the soft tissues overlying the hip joints and the possibility that this occurred during unwrapping cannot be ruled out.

V Nesitanebetasheru - Sheffield Museum (Cat. No. J93.1283)

Thorax

The thoracic cavity is asymmetrical superiorly with a layer of granular material lying posteriorly with a fluid level that has cracked in several places. The asymmetry has resulted in bandaging with different styles of packing outside the chest wall on each side. No abnormality of the costo-vertebral joints is seen (See Figs. 5.17 and 5.18).

No mediastinal structures have been retained and the viscera have been returned to the body cavity. The arrangement of the viscera is somewhat random but there is a suggestion of packages seen in one image (See Fig. 5.19).

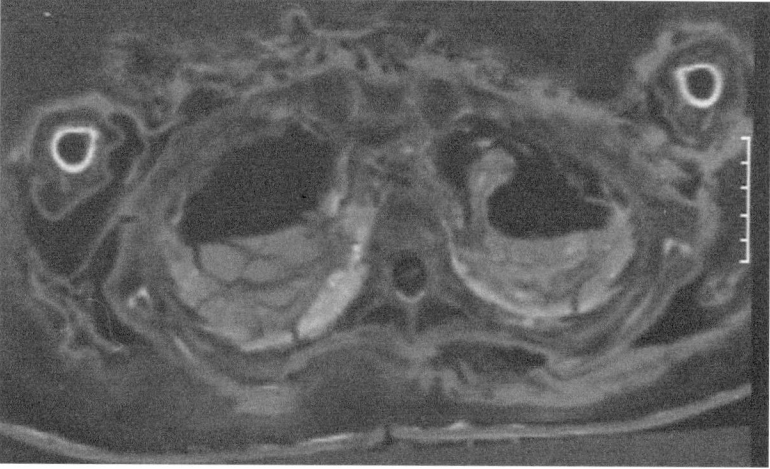

FIG. 5.17 AXIAL VIEW OF THORAX SHOWING PACKING

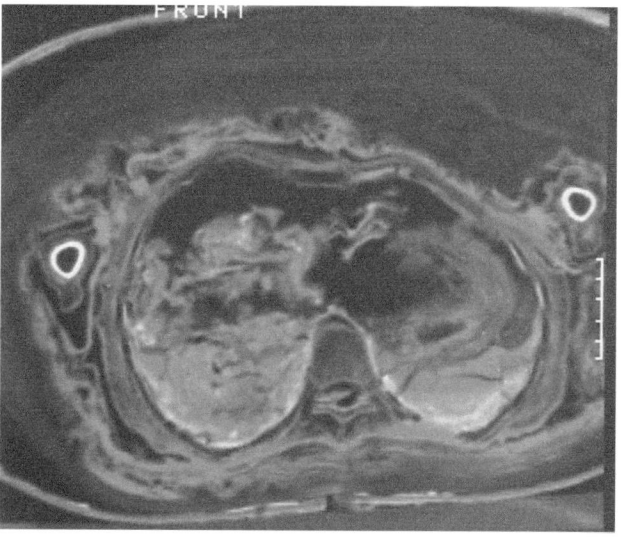

FIG. 5.18 AXIAL VIEW OF THORAX DEMONSTRATING ASYMMETRICAL CHEST WALL AND EXTERIOR PACKING.

PREPARED FOR ETERNITY

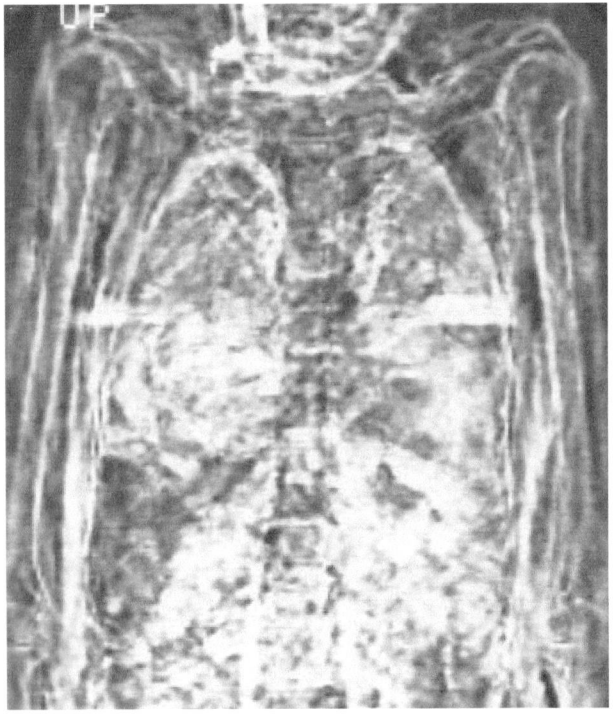

FIG. 5.19 CORONAL VIEW OF THORAX - PROBABLE CANOPIC PACKAGES

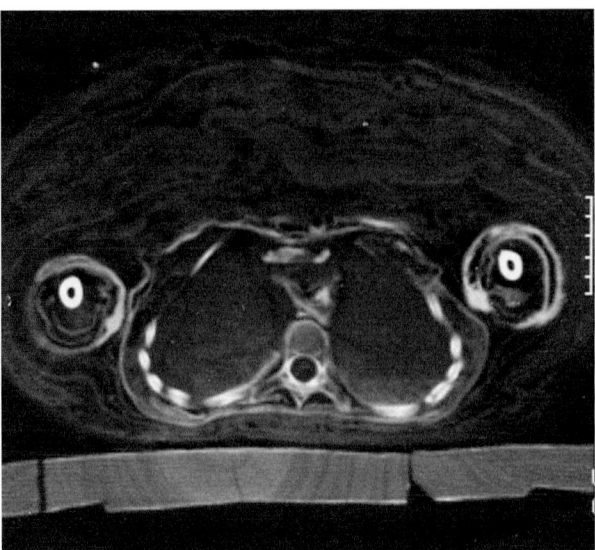

FIG. 5.20 AXIAL VIEW OF THORAX INCLUDING THE MEDIASTINUM.

Abdomen

There is only one axial image of the abdomen that does not confirm an abdominal incision (nor refute one). The forearms are seen lying on the anterior abdominal wall.

Pelvis and Hips

The images are not clear enough to determine the state of the hip joints with regard to arthritis, but they do appear to be in joint and congruous.

VI Djedma'atiuesankh - Sheffield Museum (Cat. No. J93.1284)

Thorax

The thorax is symmetrical and the wall intact. The midline structures are preserved throughout the thoracic cavity, indicating that the mediastinum has been retained (probably including the heart). The two thoracic cavities are filled completely with granular material that contains cracks (See Fig. 5.20).

Abdomen

There is an incision in the left flank that has not been closed. The abdominal cavity is filled with the same

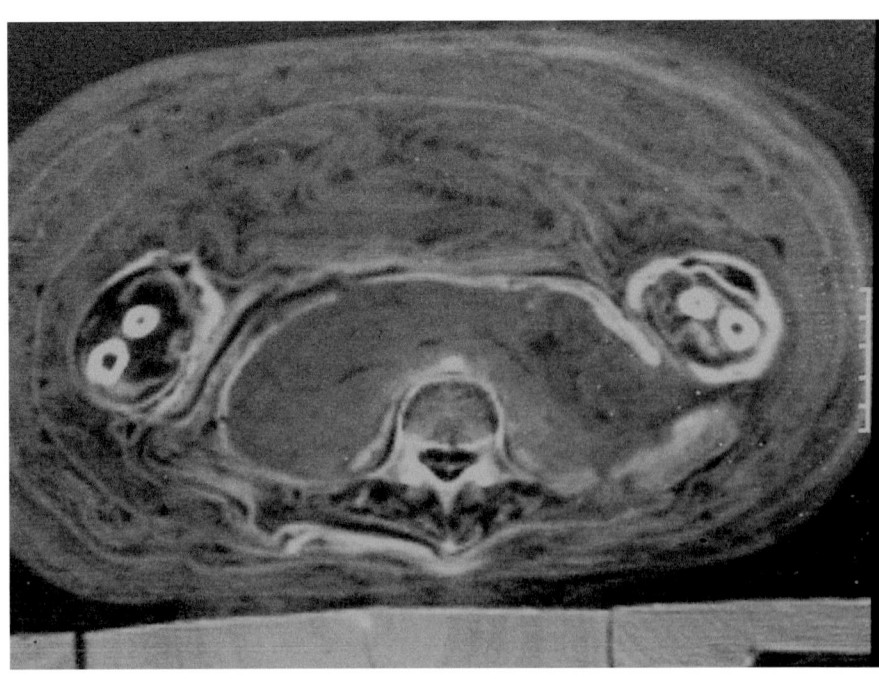

FIG. 5.21 AXIAL VIEW OF ABDOMEN.

granular material as in the thorax. The anterior abdominal wall is flattened with linen material crossing through the incision into the abdominal cavity and viscera have not been returned to the thoracic or abdominal cavity (See Figs. 5.20 and 5.21).

Pelvis and Hips

The pelvic ring is intact and the hips congruous with the upper femoral epiphysis visible on the right side. Within the pelvic cavity, there are two types of filling but what this represents is uncertain as the demonstrated extent is only 6 cms and the pelvis is not fully demonstrated. The material other than the granular matter is regular and round in cross section. It may be a package of viscera or a packed rectum (See Fig. 5.22).

VII   Tahathor - Ipswich Museum (Cat. No. COLEM 1871.3.7)

Thorax and Shoulders

There are a variety of fractures of the scapulae including bilateral fractures of the lateral ends of the scapular spine as it broadens to form the acromion. See Fig. 5.23 showing the fracture on the right and at least three fractures of the blade of the right scapula as seen in Fig. 5.24.

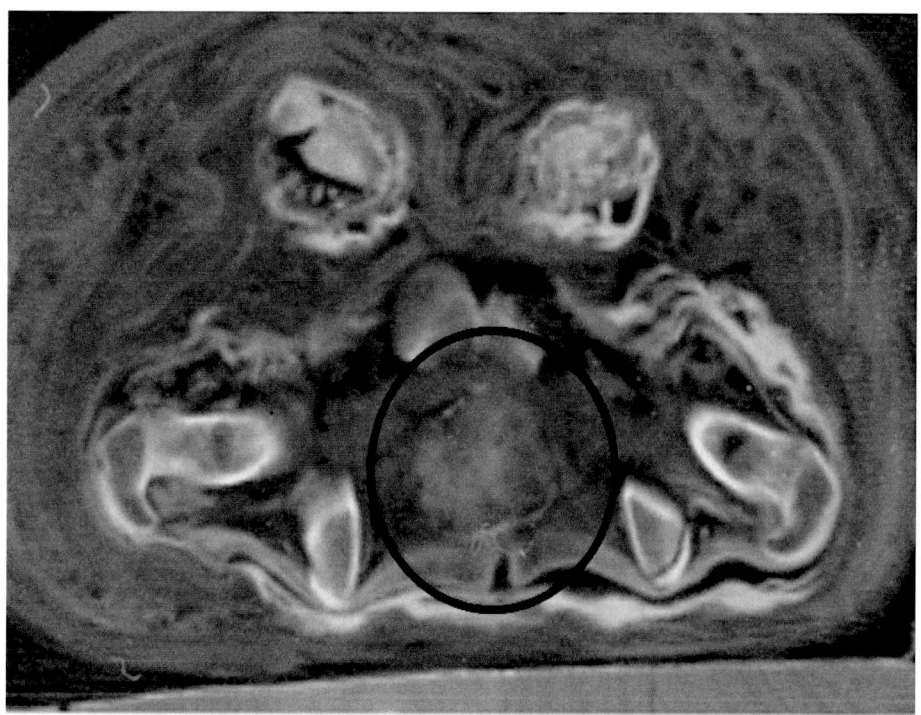

FIG. 5.22 AXIAL VIEW OF PELVIS SHOWING CONTENTS.

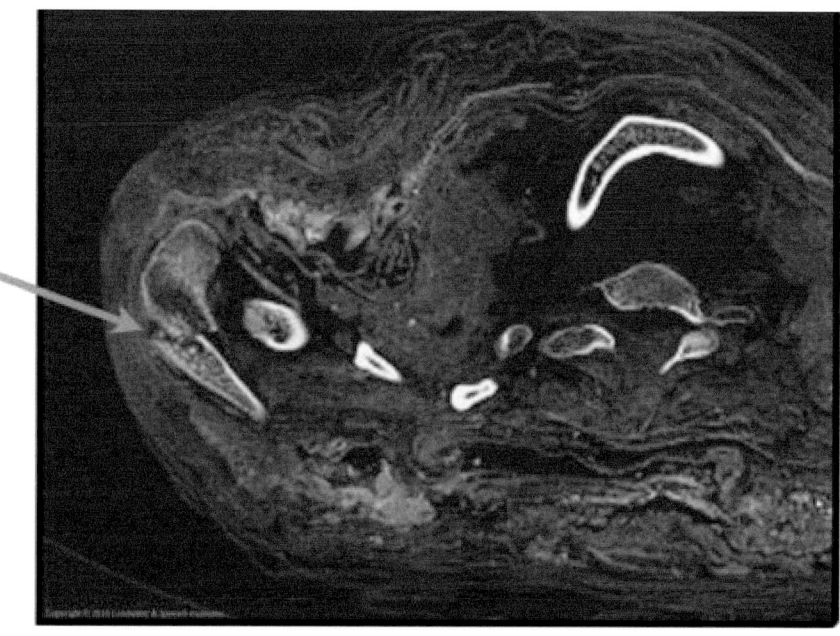

FIG. 5.23 AXIAL VIEW OF RIGHT SHOULDER - FRACTURED ACROMION

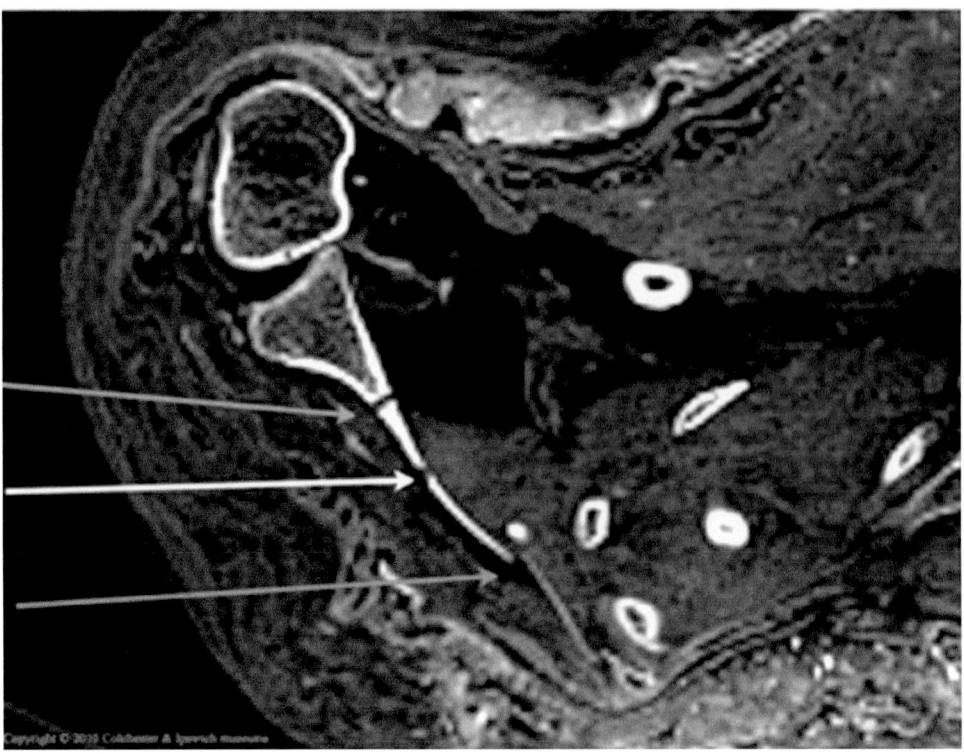

Fig. 5.24 Axial view of right shoulder - scapular fractures

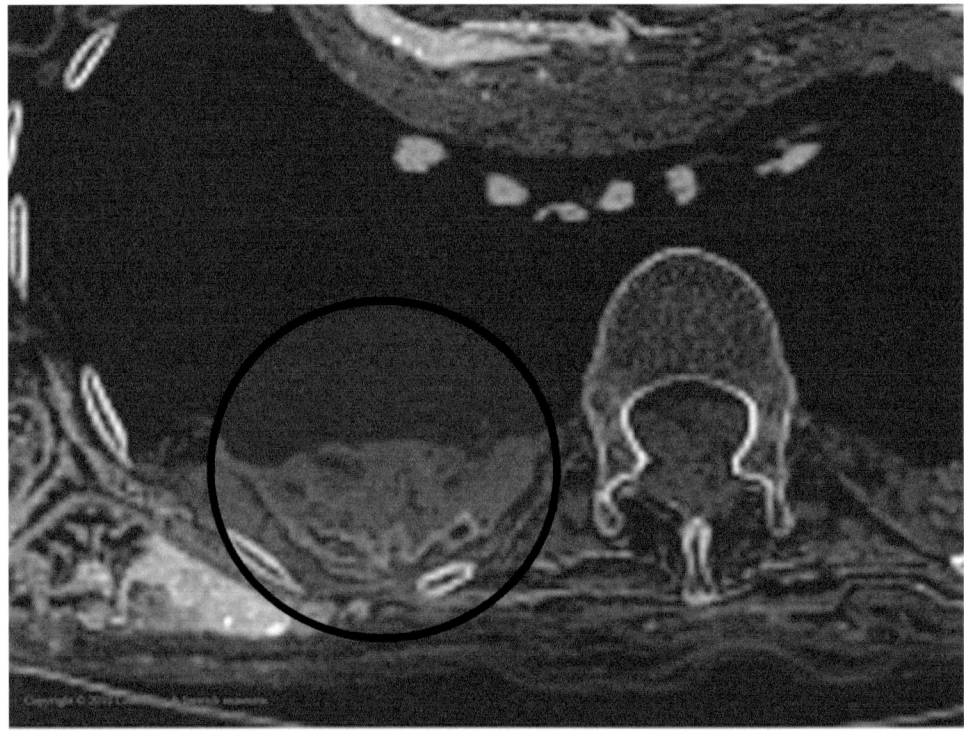

Fig. 5.25 Axial view of thorax showing viscera

There is a further, similar but single fracture of the blade of the left scapula. Finally, in the right scapula there is a fracture of the neck, detaching the glenoid. Both acromio-clavicular joints and clavicles are intact. Although the right sterno-clavicular joint remains intact there is separation of the medial end of the left clavicle from the manubrium sterni but no dislocation of the gleno-humeral joints.

The rib cage is intact but the left side is of smaller volume due to considerable antero-posterior compression in the lower part. The cavity of the thorax contains granular material in both sides, there being significantly more in the right than the left. There are no fluid levels and in the right side there are contained structures at the T9 to L2 levels including teeth (as mentioned above) and other structures which are either returned bowel or possibly liver (See Fig. 5.25).

There is no evidence of a mediastinum or any of the midline organs such as heart or great vessels and no evidence of a diaphragm.

Abdomen

As the body cavity continues into the abdomen and pelvis, the body wall (specifically on the left) is difficult to see clearly and may even have disintegrated. Therefore, it is impossible to be definite about the presence of an abdominal incision, but, on balance, there is one. However, it can be said that the abdominal organs are not evident and appear to have been removed. In fact, there is very little within the abdominal cavity except the odd tooth.

Pelvis and Hips

Within the pelvis, at the level just inferior to the coccyx, there are the outlines of thin structures that probably represent pelvic organs (See Fig. 5.26).

However, at the level of the symphysis pubis, there are two distinct tubular structures that could be the vagina and rectum (see Fig. 5.27).

With regard to the bony pelvis, there is a certain amount of separation of the sacro-iliac and pubic symphysis joints. The latter being seen in Fig. 5.27 (arrowed). The hip joints are well contained and show no evidence of arthritis.

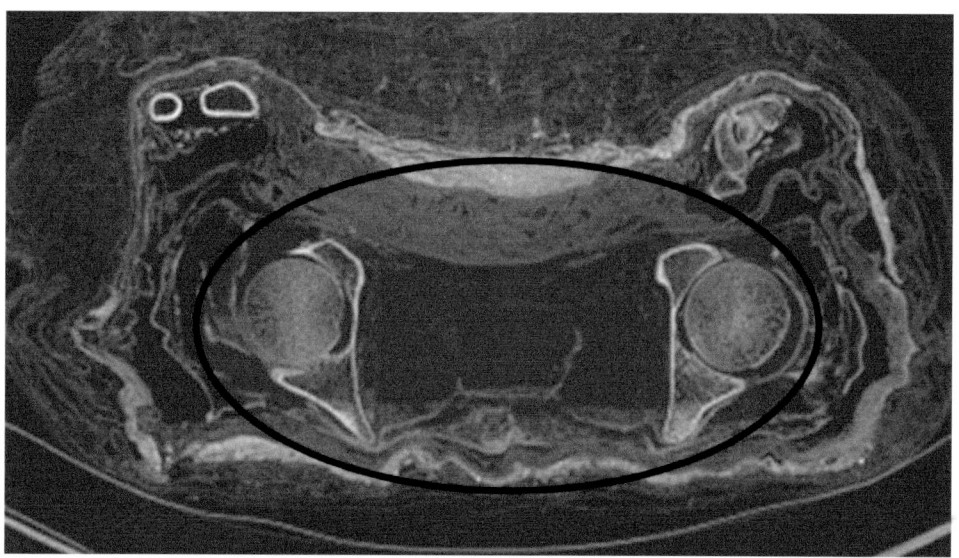

FIG. 5.26 AXIAL VIEW OF PELVIC ORGANS

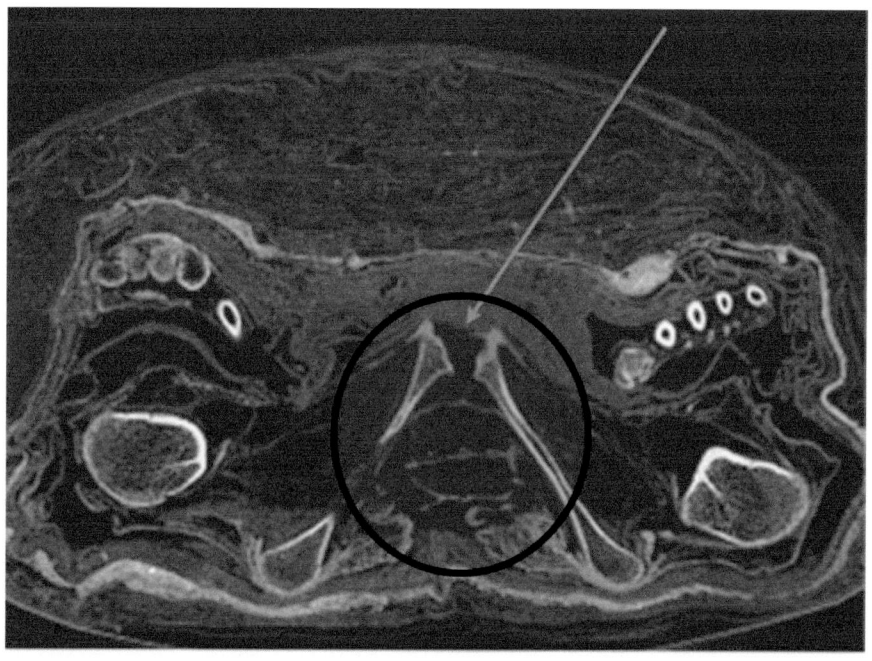

FIG. 5.27 AXIAL VIEW OF PELVIS SHOWING TUBULAR STRUCTURES AND DIASTASIS OF SYMPHYSIS PUBIS

VIII Padiamun - National Museums Liverpool (Accession No. 53.72a)

Thorax

The thorax has been subjected to significant damage to the anterior wall. The manubrium and body of the sternum are separated and lying free within the chest cavity along with some of the structures of the anterior wall. Fig. 5.28 shows the parts of the sternum lying on the resin at the back of the thoracic cavity. 1 = manubrium and 2 = body of the sternum.

In Fig. 5.29, the anterior wall (1) and body of sternum (2) are shown lying on the resin layer.

The upper part of this anterior thoracic wall disruption corresponds to the total disruption of the torso at the junction of the third and fourth thoracic vertebrae.

There may be returned organs within the thoracic cavity but no clear evidence of mediastinal structures. The thorax contains a mixture of resin and granular material, with cracks and cavities within the resin layer. Fig. 5.30 shows a solid organ containing vascular structures (circle). Fig. 5.31 shows one of several tubular structures within or on the resin layer - arrow.

Abdomen

Loss of the abdominal wall down to the level of the upper sacrum excludes any definite assertion that there was a trans-abdominal evisceration. However, it is clear that evisceration has been carried out and there are no other routes indicated by the images. Therefore, an abdominal incision has to be assumed.

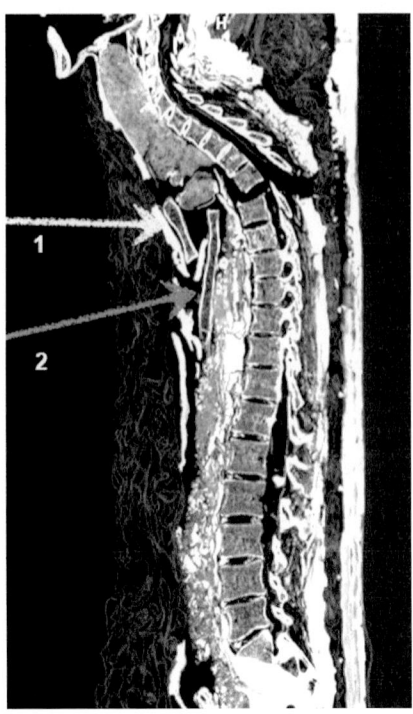

FIG. 5.28 SAGITTAL VIEW OF TRUNK – COMPRESSED ANTERIOR THORACIC WALL

The pelvis has been cleared to a large extent, but some structure still exists which is constraining the flow of resin and granular material (See Fig. 5.32).

Arrow 1 indicates the bony pelvis and arrow 2 the structure constraining the resin and particularly the granular material. The perineum itself is not clearly shown (and the phallus not seen at all), but there is a structure at the site of the anatomical perineum restraining the resin that has been introduced from above.

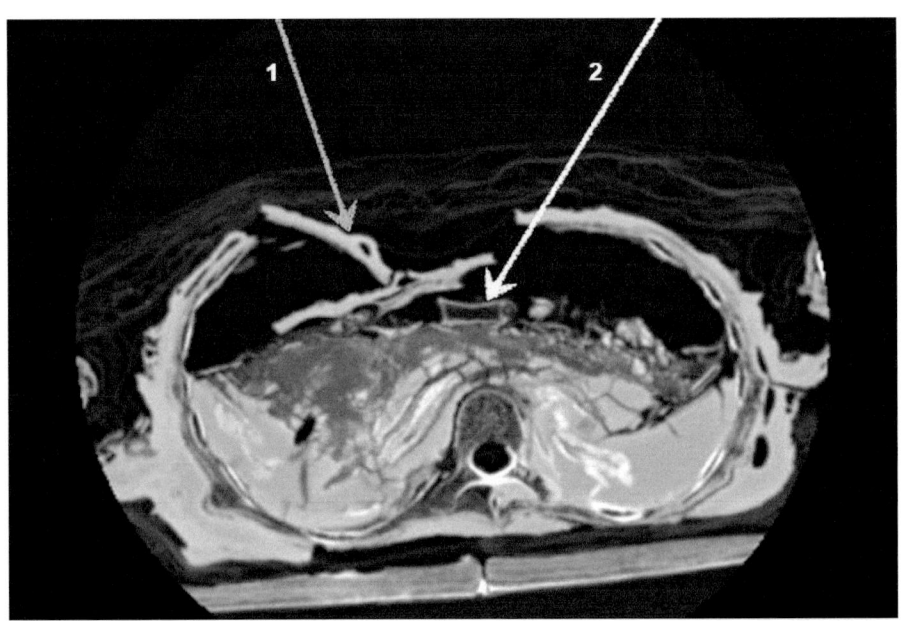

FIG. 5.29 AXIAL VIEW OF THORAX - POSITION OF STERNUM

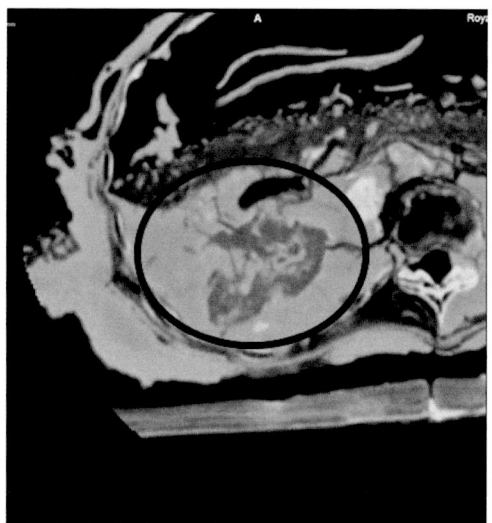

Fig. 5.30 Axial view of right lower thorax - organ containing vascular structures

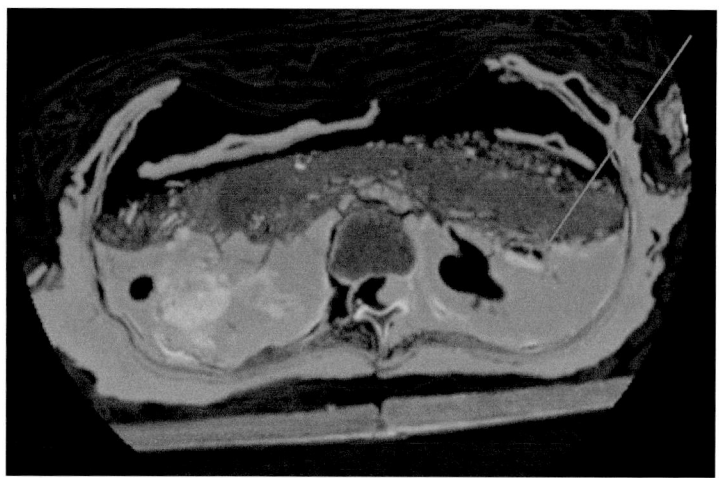

Fig. 5.31 Axial view of lower thorax - tubular structures within resin

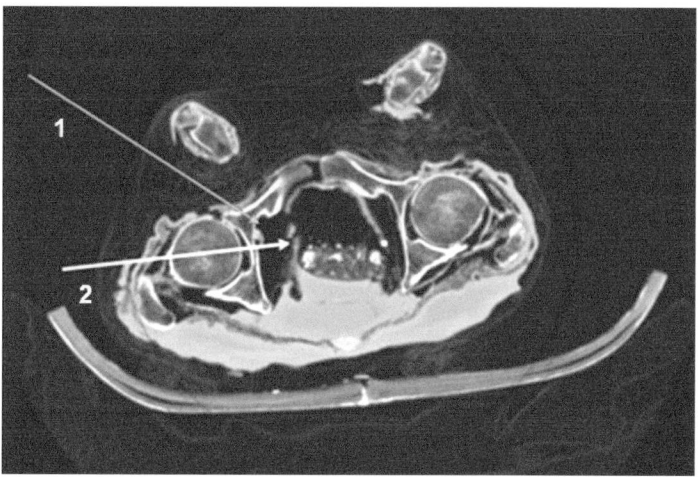

Fig. 5.32 Axial view of pelvis - constraining structures within pelvis

IX Padiamunnebnesuttauwy - National Museums Liverpool (Accession No. M14050)

Thorax

The chest wall is symmetrical, but the sternum has been disconnected from the left rib cage and lies posterior and towards the right (See Fig. 5.33), where the circle indicates the remaining connection between sternum and costal cartilages. Arrows 1 show the fractured costal cartilage on the left. The diaphragm is visible bilaterally (See Fig. 5.34).

Overlying the spine and on the right side of the thorax there is a 'mesh' like structure overlain by a layer of clay which could well represent desiccated intra-thoracic structures such as lung (arrow 2 in Fig. 5.33). There is a similar appearance on the left, but with a thinner layer of both structures but there is no evidence of the mediastinum and, in particular, the heart.

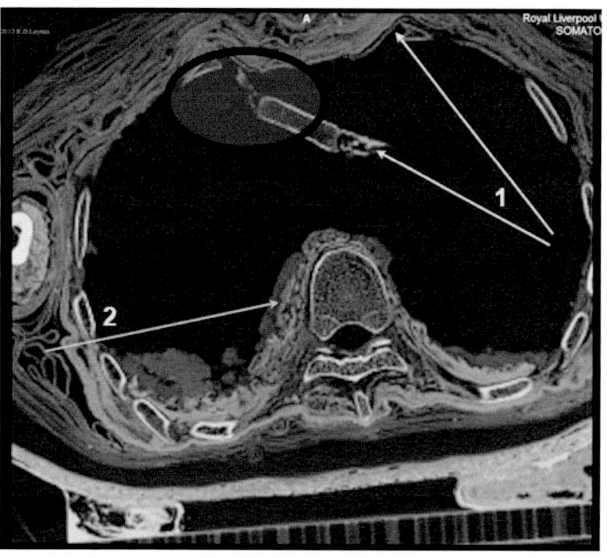

Fig. 5.33 Axial view of thorax - intra-thoracic viscera and 'loose' sternum

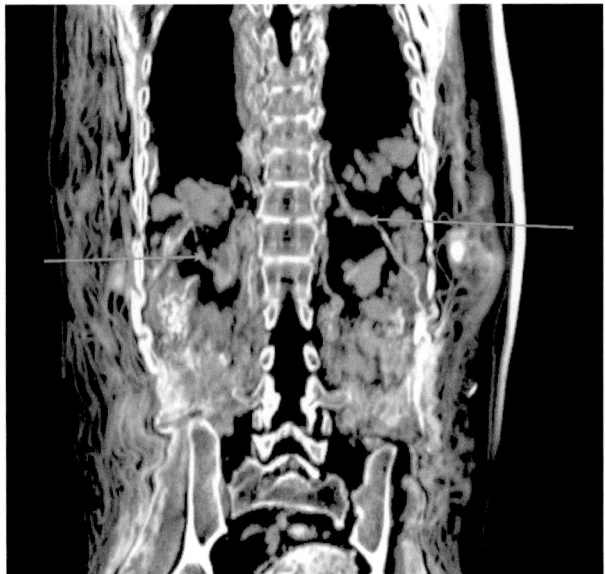

FIG. 5.34 CORONAL VIEW OF TRUNK- REMNANTS OF DIAPHRAGM

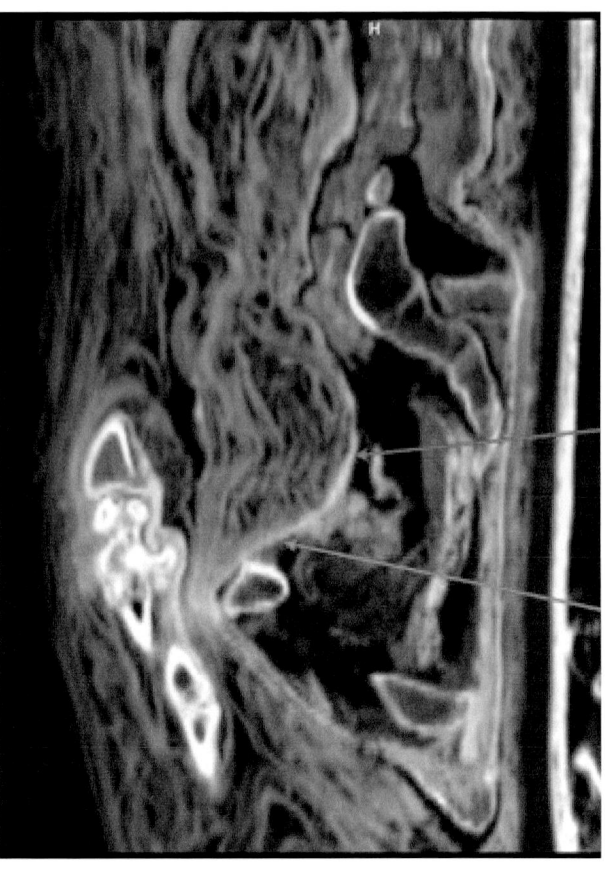

FIG. 5.35 SAGITTAL VIEW OF ABDOMEN SHOWING INTACT ABDOMINAL WALL

Abdomen

The abdominal cavity is a continuation of the thoracic cavity with an incomplete diaphragm. Evidence of both viscera and foreign material is seen within the abdomen but there is no evidence of the 'classical' left lateral abdominal wall incision. A transverse incision in the supra-pubic area is seen on the sagittal views (See Figs. 5.35 and 5.36).

In Fig. 5.36, the arrows 1 indicate the margins of the abdominal wall, that is the edges of the incision. Arrow 2 indicates the gap between the margins of the incision and the area within the circle indicates the packing (linen) which has crossed from outside into the pelvic cavity. The pelvic cavity contains a small amount of material - possibly returned viscera.

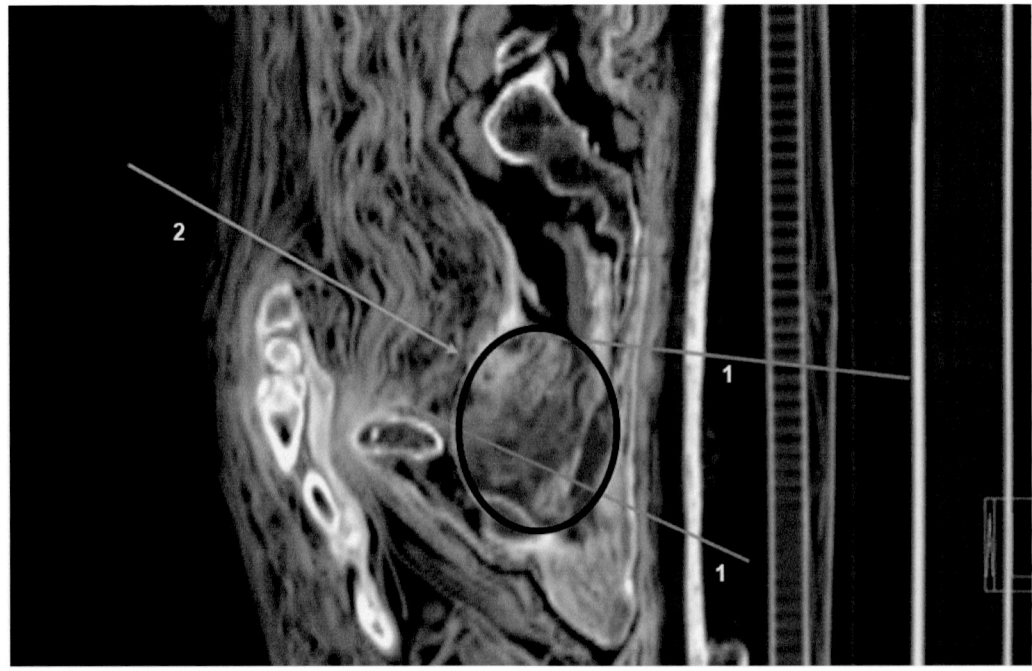

FIG. 5.36 SAGITTAL VIEW OF ABDOMEN SHOWING INCISION

X. Nesmin- National Museums Liverpool (Accession No. 56.22.79a)

Thorax

The trachea can be traced from the neck down as far as the level of T4, that is just above the level of its bifurcation into the two bronchi, behind the manubrium sterni.

The thoracic cage is intact and symmetrical. The remnants of the mediastinum (1) and the diaphragm close to the mid-line (2) are seen in Fig. 5.37.

No evidence of any visceral contents is seen, either retained or returned but there is a common level of resin in the thoracic cavity in continuity with that in the abdomen. It is clearly seen in the paravertebral gutters and laterally, with the surface being level with the anterior margin of the body of T10. On the left side there is a roll of material, impregnated with resin which lies obliquely with its superior part embedded in the resin and the inferior half protruding forwards. The superior border is at the level of T10 and the inferior border level with L2 (See Figs. 5.38 and 5.39 - arrow 1).

Where the superior end of the protruding roll lies within the resin, its appearance is very similar to two other structures that may be two other rolls of linen (See Fig. 5.40 for location and Fig. 5.41 for the original scan picture).

Although remnants of the mediastinum are visible (arrow 3 Fig. 5.37 and arrow Fig 5.42), no mediastinal structures are in evidence and almost total thoracic evisceration has been accomplished.

One of the most impressive features in the thorax is the recent fractures of the left 8th, 9th and 10th ribs (see Fig. 5.43. arrows). There are, also, old healed fractures of the right 9th, 10th and 11th ribs.

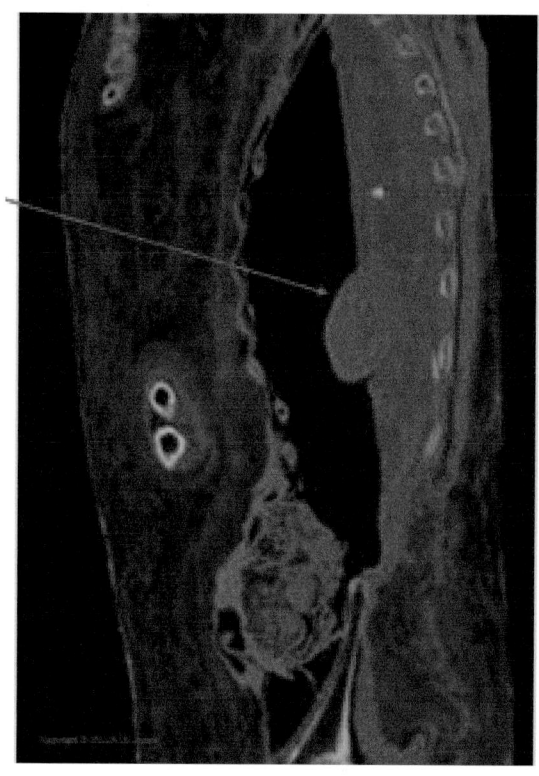

FIG. 5.38 SAGITTAL VIEW OF TRUNK - CANOPIC PACKAGE

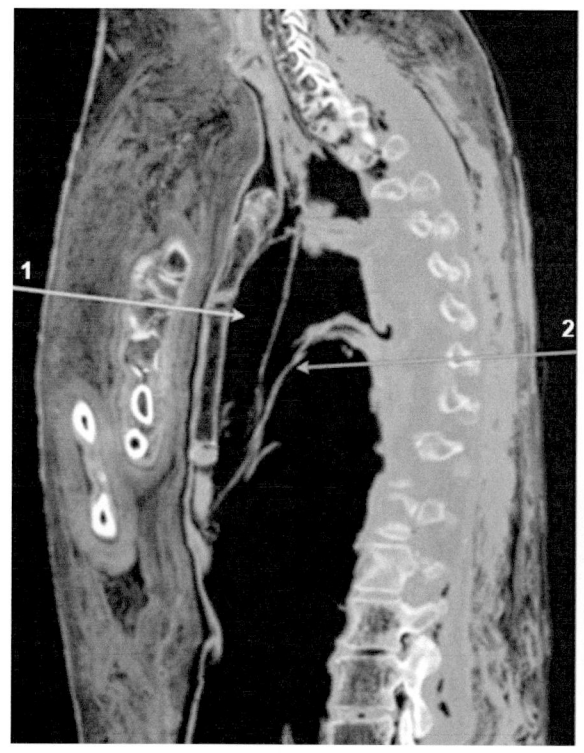

FIG. 5.37 SAGITTAL VIEW OF THORAX - MEDIASTINUM AND DIAPHRAGM

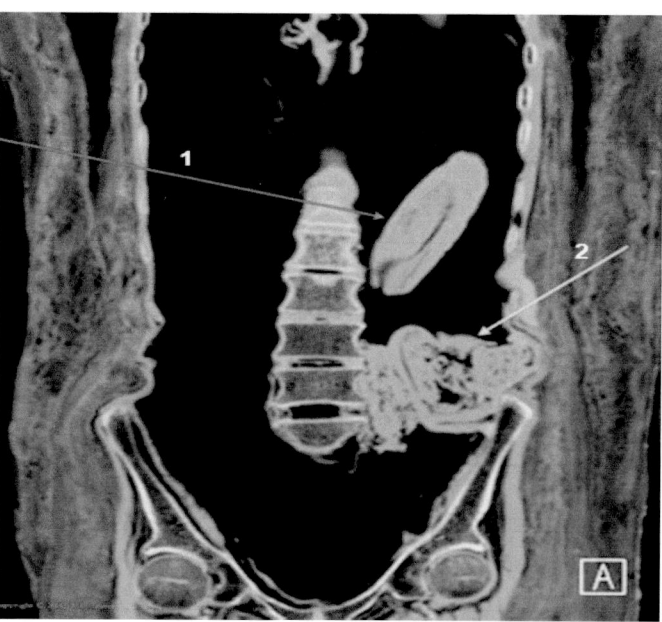

FIG. 5.39 CORONAL VIEW OF TRUNK - CANOPIC PACKAGE

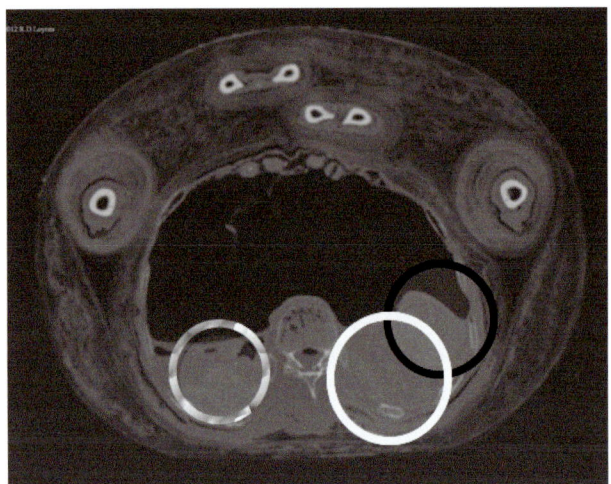

FIG. 5.40 AXIAL VIEW OF LOWER THORAX - POSITION OF PACKAGES

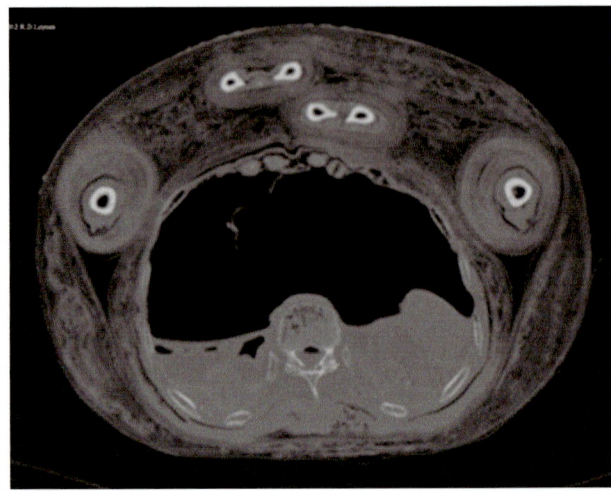

FIG. 5.41 AXIAL VIEW OF LOWER THORAX - POSITION OF PACKAGES - ORIGINAL IMAGE

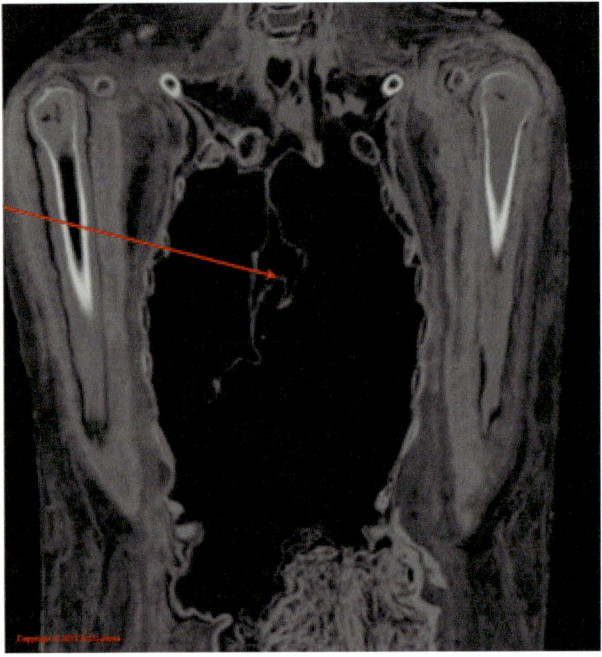

FIG. 5.42 CORONAL VIEW OF THORAX – MEDIASTINUM

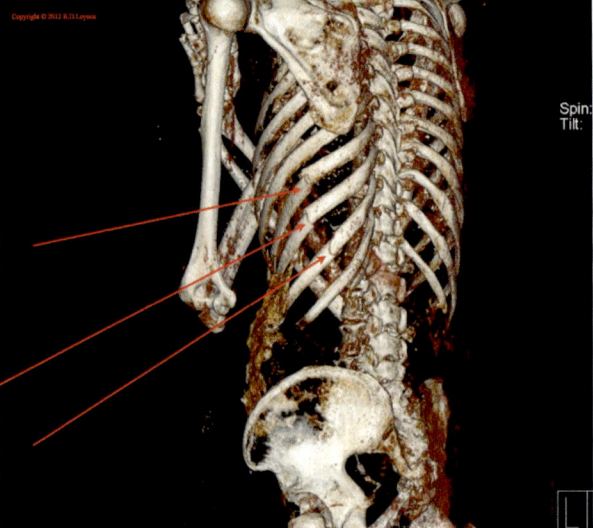

FIG. 5.43 3D RECONSTRUCTION SHOWING FRACTURED LEFT RIBS

Abdomen

There is a short left flank incision with linen packed through the incision into the abdominal cavity reaching as far as the right margin of the lumbar vertebral bodies (See Fig. 5.44).

Pelvis and Hips

Complete evisceration of the pelvis has been performed with a little resin in the posterior part. The external genitalia are clearly seen but the overall structure is a little odd, with a double structure at one level (See Fig. 5.45) and a single one more distally (Fig.5.46). This may well represent a false phallus. There is a suggestion that the perineum has been removed and a linen pack arranged just superficial to the position of the pelvic floor and resin inserted from above (with a little leakage).

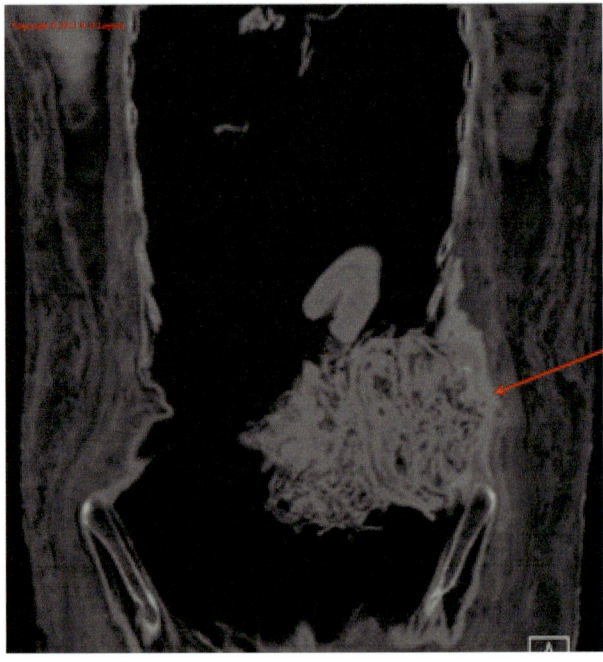

FIG. 5.44 CORONAL VIEW OF ABDOMEN - PACK IN ABDOMINAL INCISION

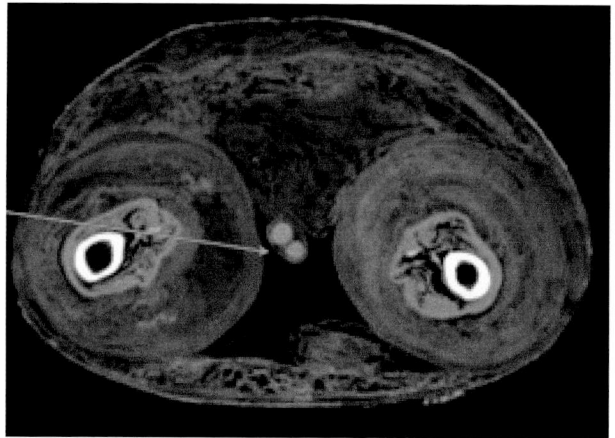

FIG. 5.45 AXIAL VIEW INFERIOR TO PELVIS - DOUBLE STRUCTURE OF PHALLUS

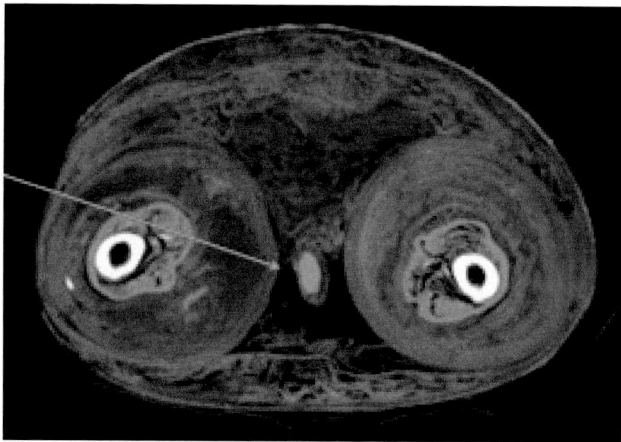

FIG. 5.46 MORE DISTAL AXIAL VIEW INFERIOR TO PELVIS – SINGLE STRUCTURE OF PHALLUS

XI. Padiamun - National Museums Liverpool (accession No. M14003)

Thorax

The rib cage is grossly intact and symmetrical. However, there are un-displaced fractures of the left 1st, 2nd, 3rd and 4th ribs and of the right 1st, 2nd, 3rd, 4th, 5th, 6th, 7th, 8th and 9th ribs with evidence of fractures of some of the upper costal cartilages. As there is no sign of healing all of these fractures could well be associated with the disruption at the cervico-thoracic junction previously described. The right sterno-clavicular joint is also dislocated - again possibly associated with the disruption at the cervico-thoracic junction. There is a healed fracture of the medial end of the right clavicle.

The thoracic cavity is in continuity with the abdominal cavity and the diaphragm has been completely removed. There are biological tissues in the position of the upper mediastinum, from T2 to T4. See Fig. 5.47. arrow 2. The thoracic and abdominal cavities are almost completely filled with amorphous granular material – possibly clay (See Fig. 5.48 arrow 1).

The exception to this statement is the presence of two rolls containing radio-dense material (probably resin) in the right upper thorax (See Fig. 5.47 - arrow 1 and Fig. 5.49 - arrows and bandages which have been inserted into the abdominal incision (See Fig. 5.48 - arrow 2). The two rolls of material in the thorax may represent canopic packages or they may have been used to plug a gap in the suprapleural membrane. The filling of the thoracic cavity can be seen to be so complete that it is limited only by the suprapleural membrane (Sibson's fascia) – (See Fig. 5.50).

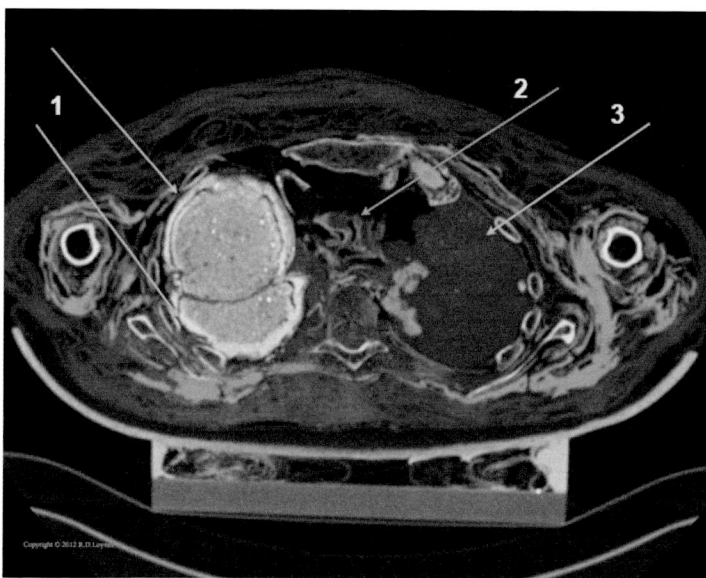

FIG. 5.47 AXIAL VIEW OF THORAX

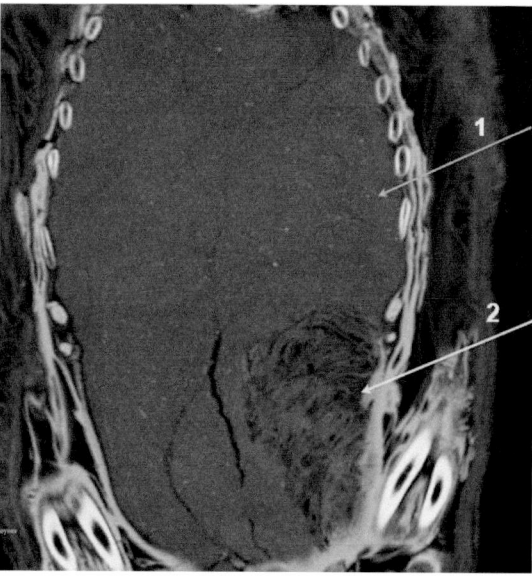

FIG. 5.48 CORONAL VIEW OF TORSO

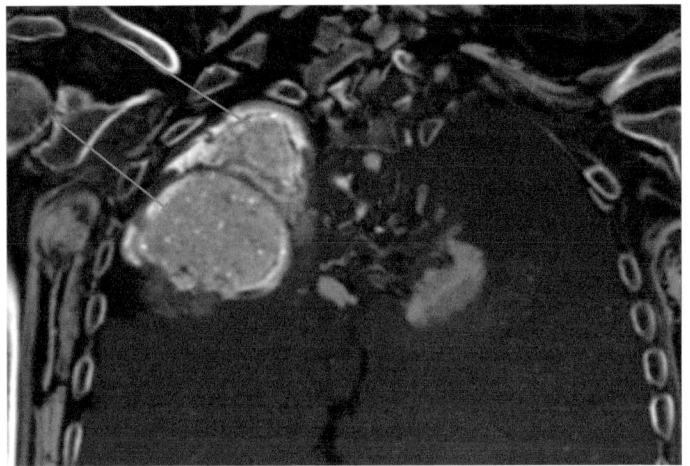

FIG. 5.49 CORONAL VIEW OF UPPER THORAX- ROLLS OF MATERIAL ON THE RIGHT

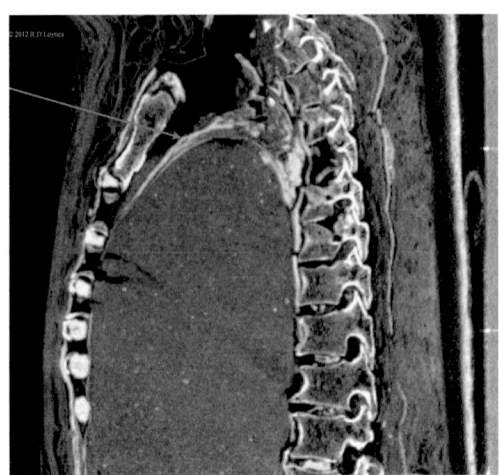

FIG. 5.50 SAGITTAL VIEW OF THORAX - SIBSON'S FASCIA

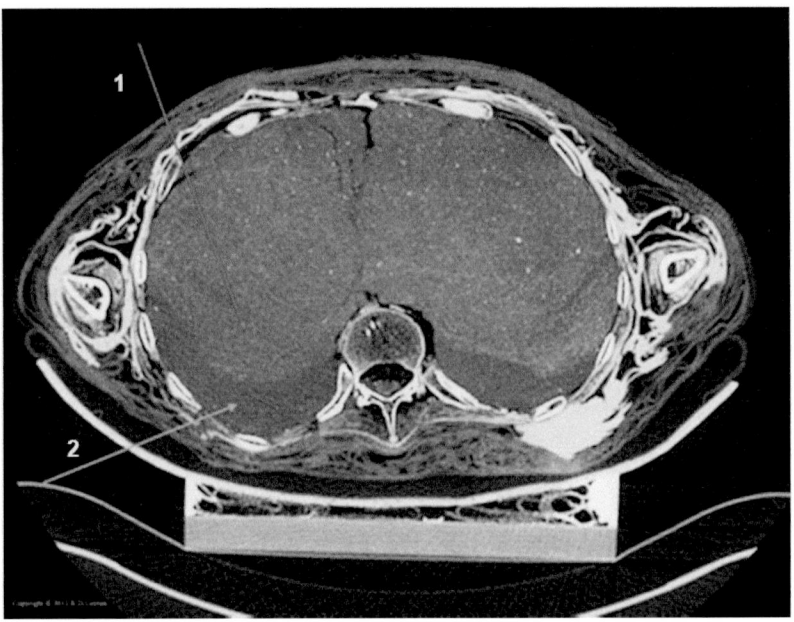

FIG. 5.51 AXIAL VIEW OF THORAX SHOWING TWO LAYERS OF MATERIAL

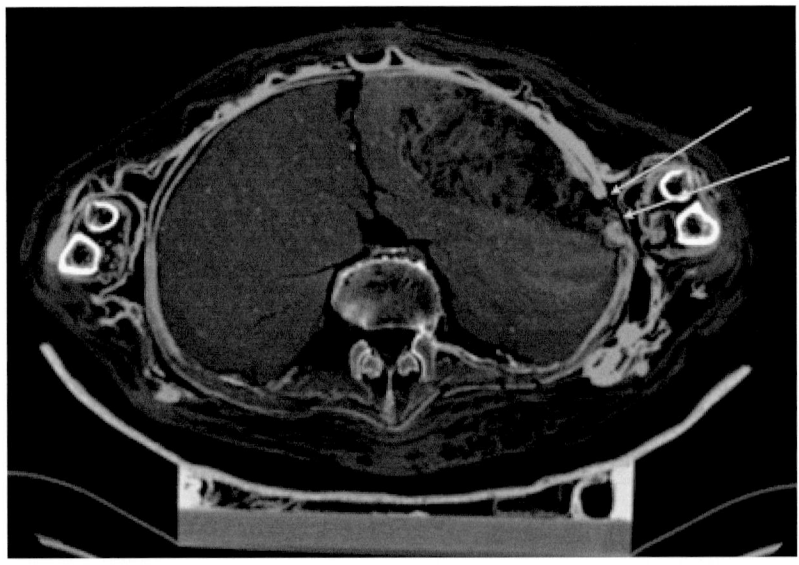

FIG. 5.52 AXIAL VIEW OF ABDOMEN - EXTENT OF ABDOMINAL INCISION

Whilst this material seems to be amorphous, examination of the axial views, in the thoracic region, reveals that there are two distinct layers of material (See Fig. 5.51, arrows 1 and 2).

The mediastinum and contents is absent except for the area of the great vessels.

Abdomen

The abdominal cavity and its filling are continuous with the cavity of the thorax. There are bandages within the upper left quadrant of the abdomen (See Fig. 5.48 - arrow 2). These appear to have been inserted through a left flank incision that has been, largely, closed. A very short residual incision is seen - shown between the the arrows in Fig. 5.52.

Whilst the body cavity, including the abdomen is almost completely filled with the amorphous granular material, this is limited inferiorly/distally by a membrane, presumably the peritoneum (See Fig. 5.53 - arrow 2). This figure also shows radio-dense material in the upper rectum - arrow 1 - and the air filled rectum and anal canal - arrow 3.

Anterior to the peritoneal filling is a space that could represent an air filled bladder. There is no evidence of the viscera being returned to the abdominal cavity.

Pelvis and Hips

See above description related to Fig. 5.53 for the review of internal organs. The hip joints are congruous and there is no evidence of arthritis. There is an undisplaced fracture of the posterior half of the left iliac crest (See Fig. 5.54 - black circle). This may have been post-mortem.

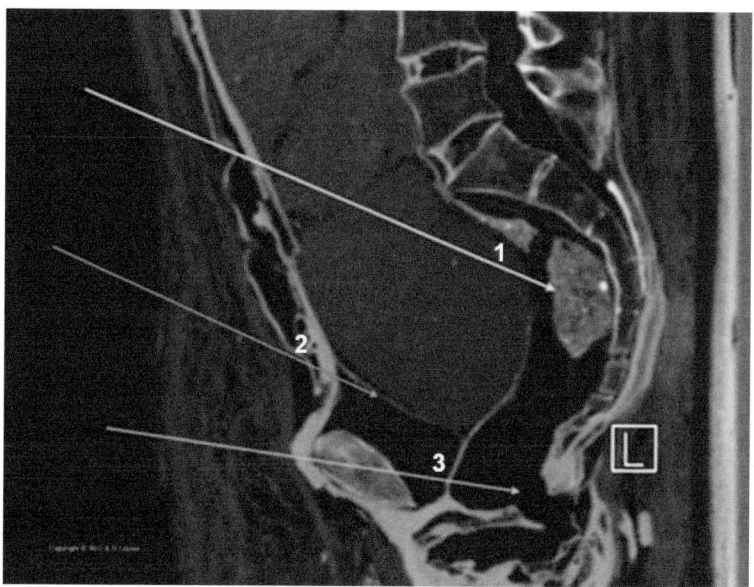

FIG. 5.53 SAGITTAL VIEW OF PELVIS SHOWING STRUCTURES

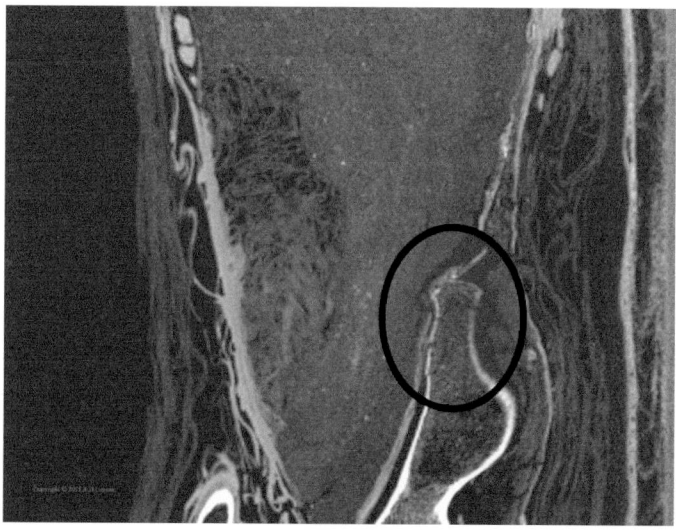

FIG. 5.54 SAGITTAL VIEW OF LOWER ABDOMEN - FRACTURED ILIAC CREST

XIV Asru - Manchester University Museum (Accession No. MM1777)

Thorax

The trachea continues into the thorax, with its bifurcation lying at the upper level of the manubrium sterni. This is, normally at the level of the lower border of the manubrium in the recumbent body and up to two inches lower than this in the erect body, in full inspiration (Last, 1966: 336) (See Fig. 5.55; 1 = trachea and its bifurcation. 2 = upper border of manubrium sterni. 3 = empty mediastinum. 4 = remains of diaphragm).

The chest wall is symmetrical and the ribs are in joint posteriorly and exhibit no fractures. The costal cartilages are calcified. There is a small remnant of biological tissue in the left posterior sulcus of the thorax (See Fig. 5.56; 1 = remains of mediastinum. 2 = remains of biological tissue - possibly lung) and a hole in the posterior wall of the thorax on the left (1.5 cms. in diameter) - 3 in Fig. 5.56. but no evidence of packing of the cavity.

Fig. 5.57 shows the remains of the great vessels, in the superior mediastinum - 1, the empty pericardium - 2 and the remains of the diaphragm - 3. The diaphragm is deficient posteriorly.

Abdomen

There is evidence of a left flank incision, seen on the axial views. Compare arrow 3 on the left with arrow 1 on the right in Fig. 5.58.

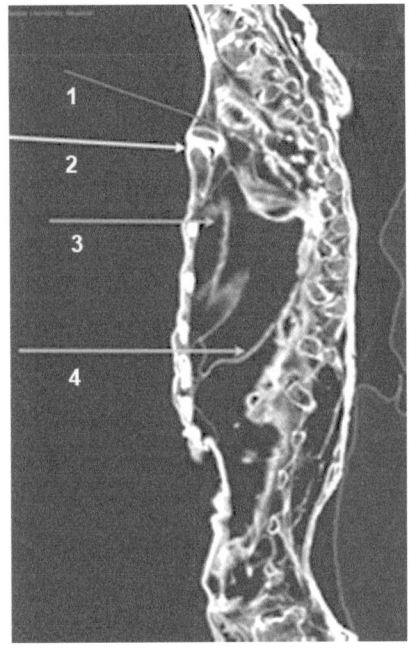

FIG. 5.55 SAGITTAL VIEW SHOWING THORACIC STRUCTURES

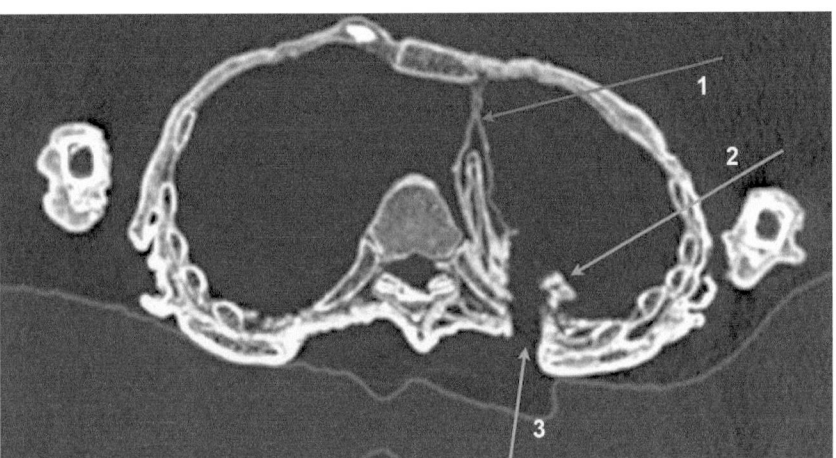

FIG. 5.56 AXIAL VIEW LOWER THORAX - MEDIASTINUM AND POSTERIOR DEFECT

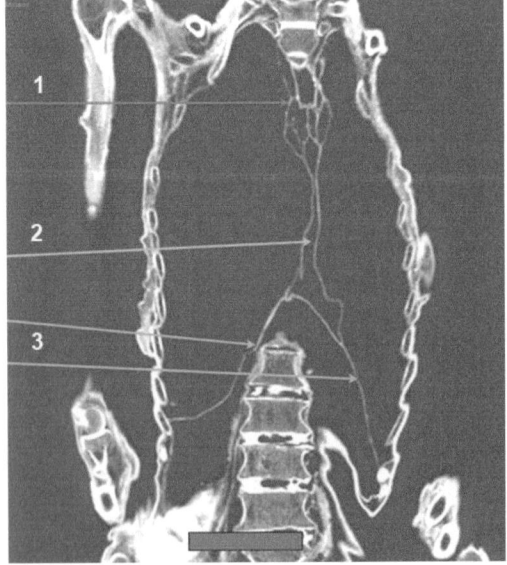

FIG. 5.57 CORONAL VIEW THORAX - GREAT VESSELS, MEDIASTINUM AND DIAPHRAGM

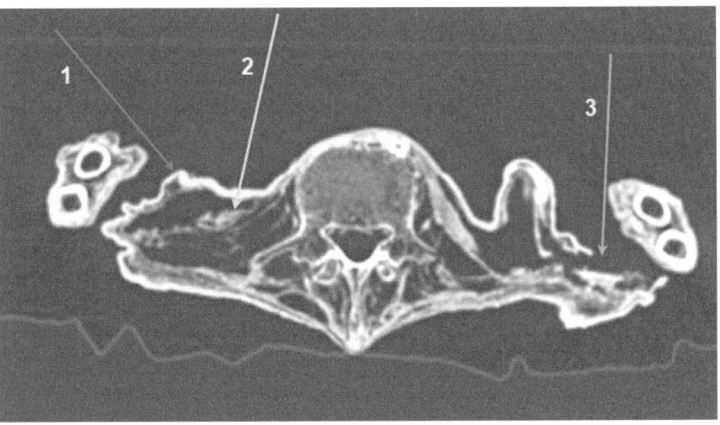

FIG. 5.58 AXIAL VIEW OF LOWER ABDOMEN - ABDOMINAL INCISION

This figure also shows evidence of peritoneal and other abdominal biological tissues - 2. There is no packing within the abdomen and the cavity has collapsed.

Pelvis and Hips

The pelvic ring is intact, with only slight incongruity of the sacro-iliac joints.

There is evidence of the expected intra-pelvic organs, namely the bladder, vagina and rectum.

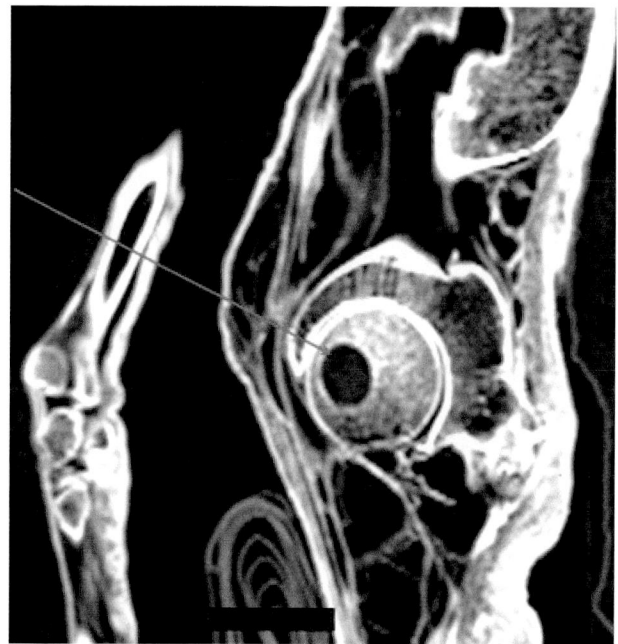

FIG. 5.59 SAGITTAL VIEW OF PELVIS SHOWING FEMORAL HEAD BIOPSY

The hips joints and, in particular the right femoral head and neck, are of interest. The right femoral neck has been the site of a recent biopsy with a large bone biopsy trephine (See Figs. 5.59 and 5.60). As can be seen in Fig. 5.60, the subsequent defect has been filled with packing - possibly linen. It can also be seen that the floor of the acetabulum has been perforated by the instrument - arrow 2.

There is no evidence of arthritis in the hip joints.

XVI. Unnamed - National Museums Liverpool (accession No. M13997a)

Thorax

The overall rib cage contour is normal but with many rib fractures (without healing). Some of these fractures are illustrated in Fig. 5.61, the right 1st, 2nd, 4th, 5th, 6th, 7th, 8th, 9th, and 10th ribs and the left 1st, 4th, 5th, 6th, 7th, 8th, and 9th ribs are fractured but the costo-vertebral joints are intact. The sternum is depressed, with distortion of the costal cartilages. There is a fracture at the junction of the middle and outer thirds of the right clavicle and undisplaced fractures of both scapular blades.

Remnants of the diaphragm are present bilaterally, but there is no evidence of the mediastinum or its structures. In other words, evisceration has been thorough. A small amount of resin is present in the posterior 'gutter' on both sides of the thoracic cavity. The resin is crazed in several places. On the left side of the lower thoracic cavity there is a canopic package containing returned organs. It extends from T10 to L3 (See Fig. 5.62).

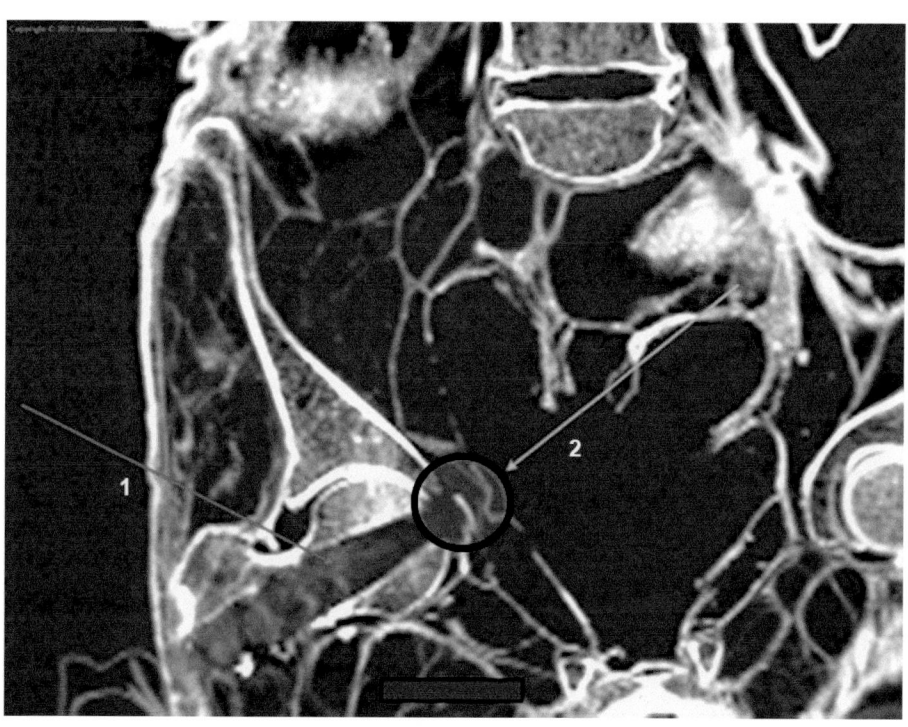

FIG. 5.60 CORONAL VIEW OF PELVIS SHOWING FEMORAL HEAD BIOPSY

Abdomen

There is a left flank incision with linen packed through it (See Fig. 5.63). Lines indicate the edges of the incision.

The resin lying on the posterior wall of the thorax continues down into the abdomen and pelvis. There is a further pack of tissue - probably returned organs with some resin, lying on the front of the lumbar spine (See Fig. 5.64 - black circle).

Pelvis and Hips

The bony pelvis is complete with intact sacro-iliac joints and symphysis pubis.

There are no organs remaining within the pelvis with the exception of the rectum and vagina inferiorly. The perineum has been used as a route to eviscerate and a plug of linen has then been inserted. Fig. 5.65 shows this perineal plug - 4. The pool of resin is shown by arrow 3 and the lower extremity of the abdominal linen by the arrow 1. Within the resin is a filamentous structure, which may be linen - arrow 2.

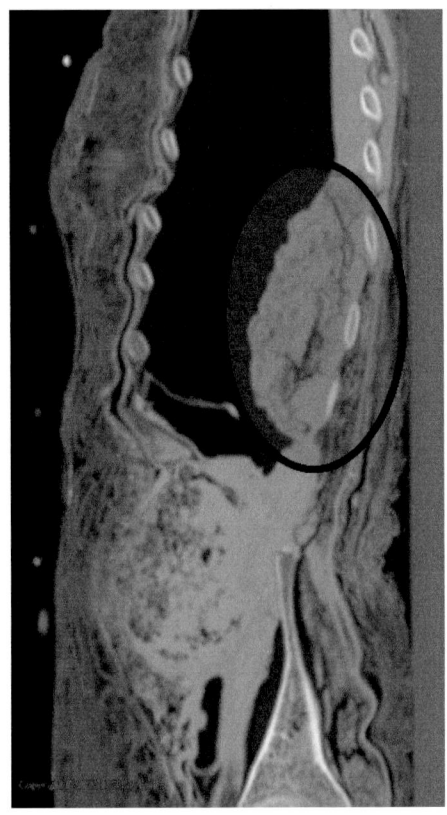

FIG. 5.62 SAGITTAL VIEW OF TRUNK - RETURNED VISCERA

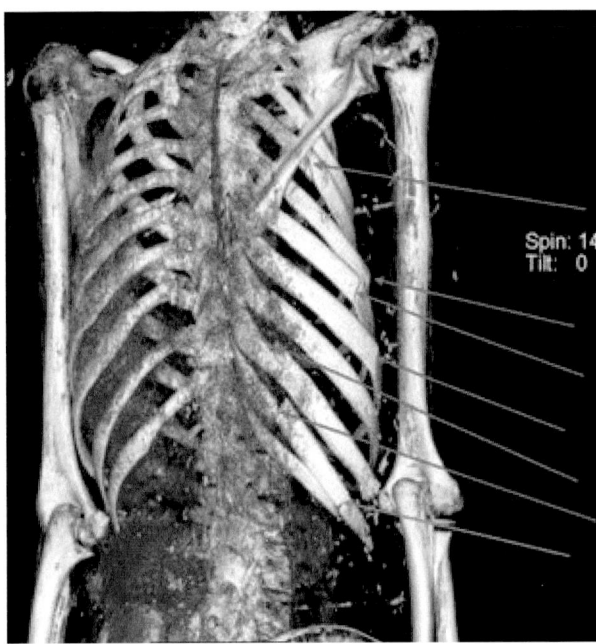

FIG. 5.61 3D RECONSTRUCTION - RIGHT FRACTURED RIBS – POSTERIOR VIEW

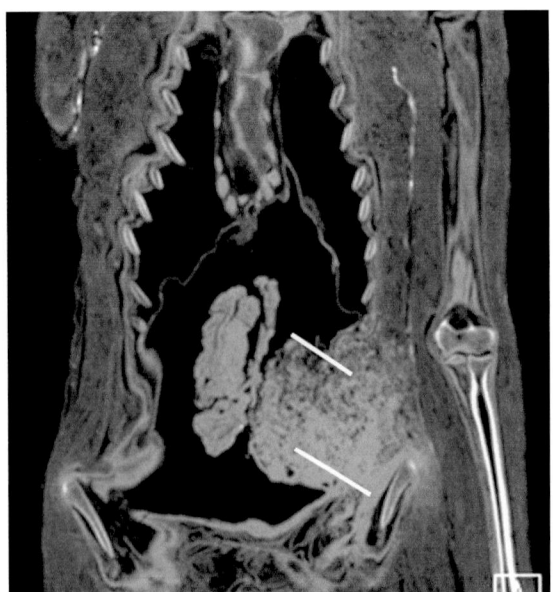

FIG. 5.63 CORONAL VIEW OF TRUNK - LINEN IN ABDOMINAL INCISION

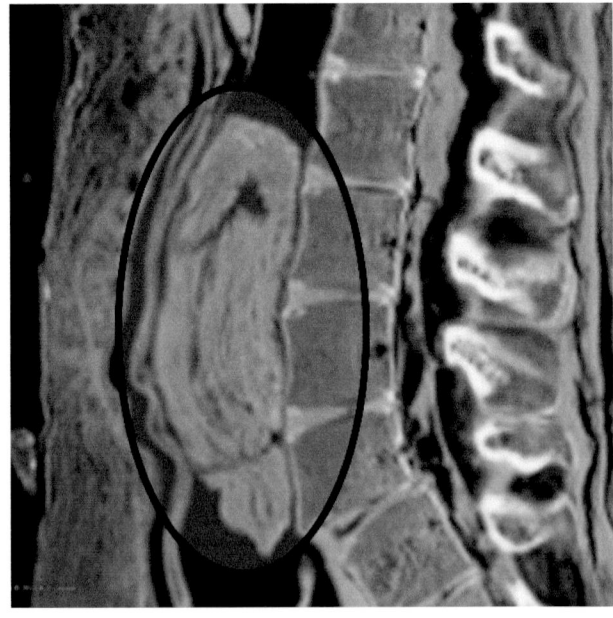

FIG. 5.64 SAGITTAL VIEW OF LOWER ABDOMEN - VISCERAL PACKAGE

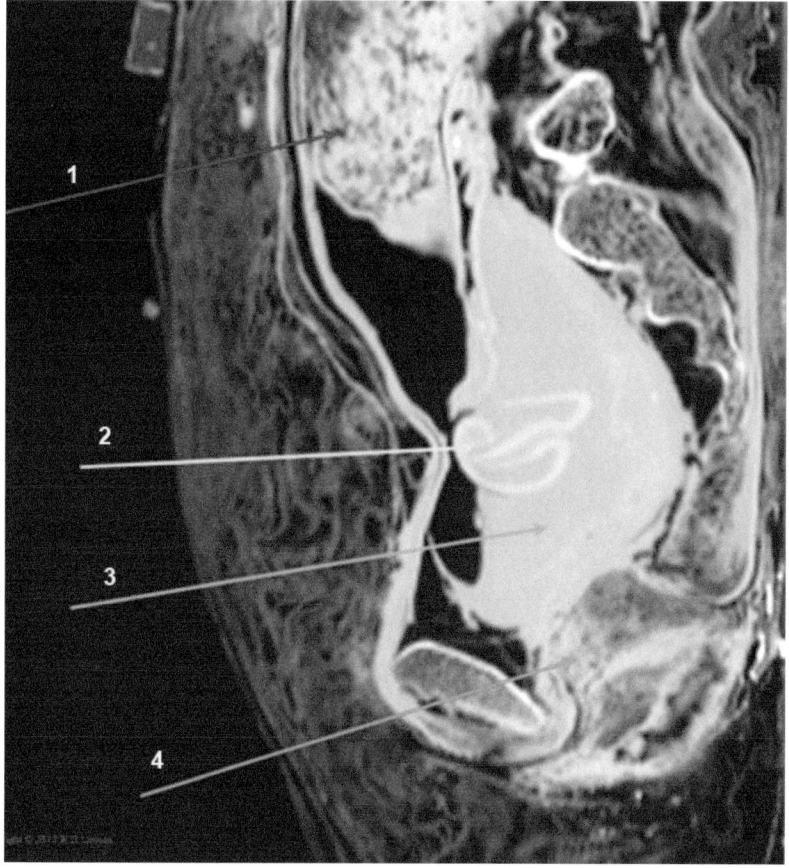

FIG. 5.65 SAGITTAL VIEW OF PELVIS - PERINEAL PLUG, RESIN AND LINEN IN ABDOMEN

XVII. Ankhesenaset - National Museums Liverpool (Accession No. M14000)

Thorax

There has been complete evisceration of the thoracic cavity with several canopic packages within the thorax and abdomen, as can be seen in Fig. 5.66 - black circle. The actual number of packages is difficult to determine as they are curved and twisted around one another. Some of these packages contain viscera that may be tubular, but at least one package contains a radio-dense solid organ, which may represent liver or lung (See Fig. 5.67 - black circle).

There is some granular material in the posterior aspect of the thorax (and pelvis) - arrows 1 in Fig. 5.68 and some resin in the posterior part of the thorax (See Fig.5.68 - arrow 2).

The rib cage is intact and of a normal shape with no evidence of the mediastinum or heart.

Abdomen

Evisceration is via a left flank incision, as is clearly seen in Fig. 5.69 - black box. This incision can be traced across and slightly downwards over the abdominal wall but there is no evidence of linen crossing the incision. As has previously been noted the abdominal cavity has been filled with canopic packages and some granular material.

Pelvis and Hips

The bony pelvis is intact with no evidence of hip arthritis. The perineum is intact and shows female characteristics.

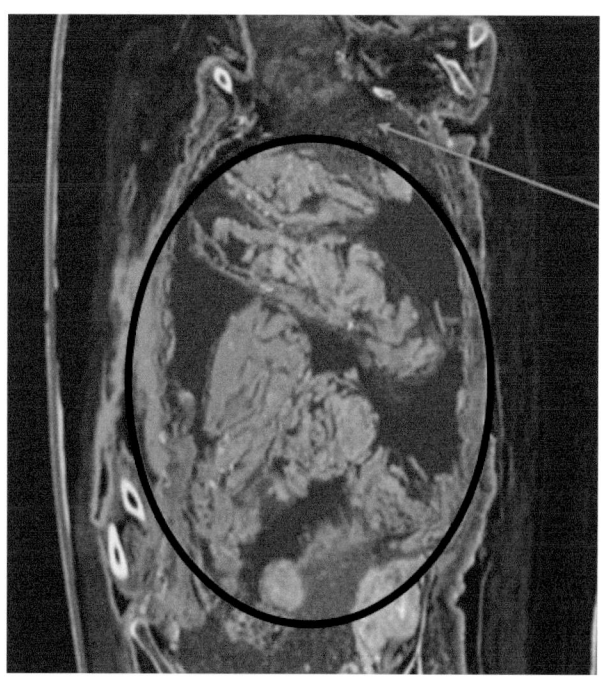

FIG. 5.66 CORONAL VIEW OF TRUNK - CANOPIC PACKAGES

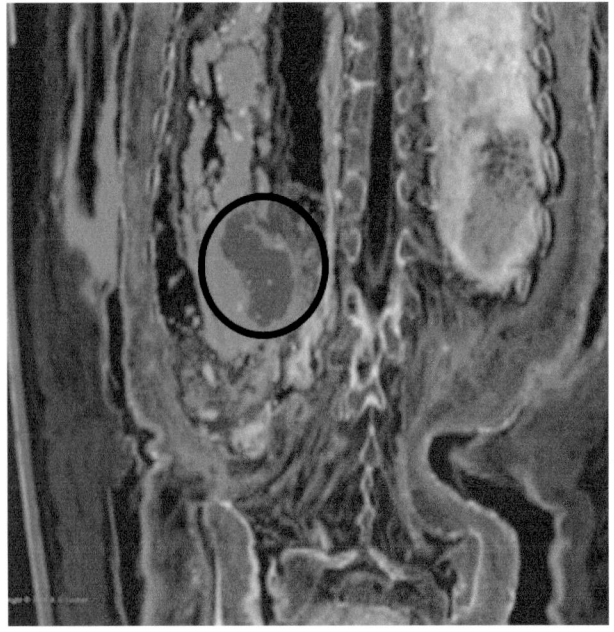

FIG. 5.67 CORONAL VIEW OF ABDOMEN - SOLID ORGAN – POSSIBLY LIVER

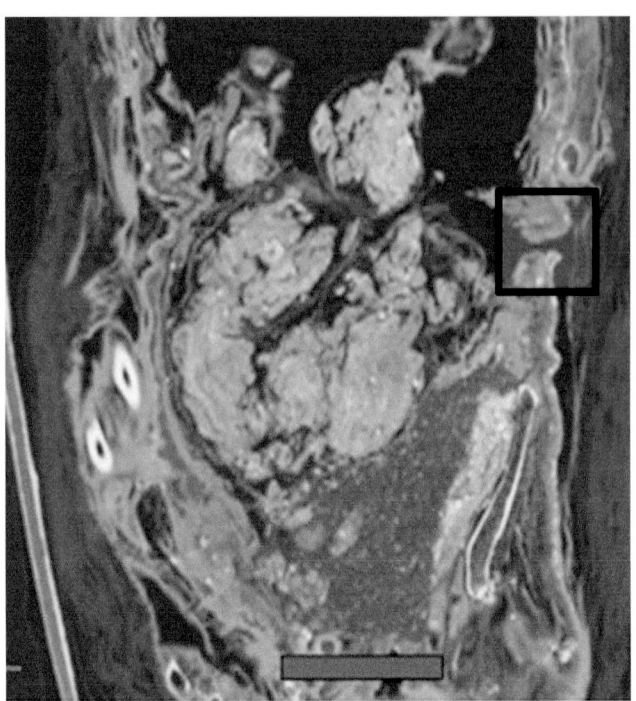

FIG. 5.69 CORONAL VIEW OF ABDOMEN –LEFT FLANK INCISION

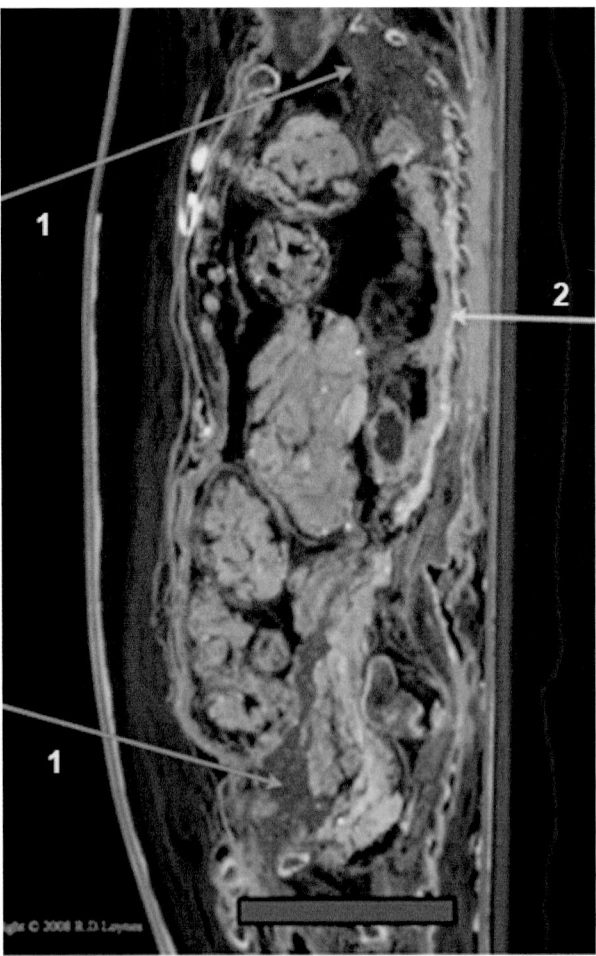

FIG. 5.68 SAGITTAL VIEW OF TRUNK - GRANULAR MATERIAL AND RESIN

XVIII. Unnamed - National Museums Liverpool - (AccessionNo. M14048)

Thorax

There is severe disruption of the rib cage, worse on the left than the right side, as can be seen in Figs. 5.70 and 5.71. Given the severe displacement of some of the ribs, it would appear that this disruption has occurred postmortem. Evidence that this occurred prior to wrapping is shown in Fig. 5.72, where the addition of a false breast in the wrappings can be seen alongside the distorted rib cage on the left.

There has been complete evisceration of the thorax and abdomen. Five canopic packages have been returned to the body cavity. Sections through these packages can be seen in Fig. 5.73 - arrows.

Whilst the detail of the contents of these packages is difficult to determine, because of their infiltration with resin, it is probable that they contain viscera. For the sake of clarity it should be stated that there is no evidence of retention of the mediastinum or heart.

Abdomen

There is a left flank incision (between lines), through which some of the evisceration has been performed (See Fig. 5.74). Linen has been packed through this incision.

A further incision has been made in the perineum to enhance the evisceration process. As a result, the perineum and its structures have been completely destroyed (See Fig. 5.75).

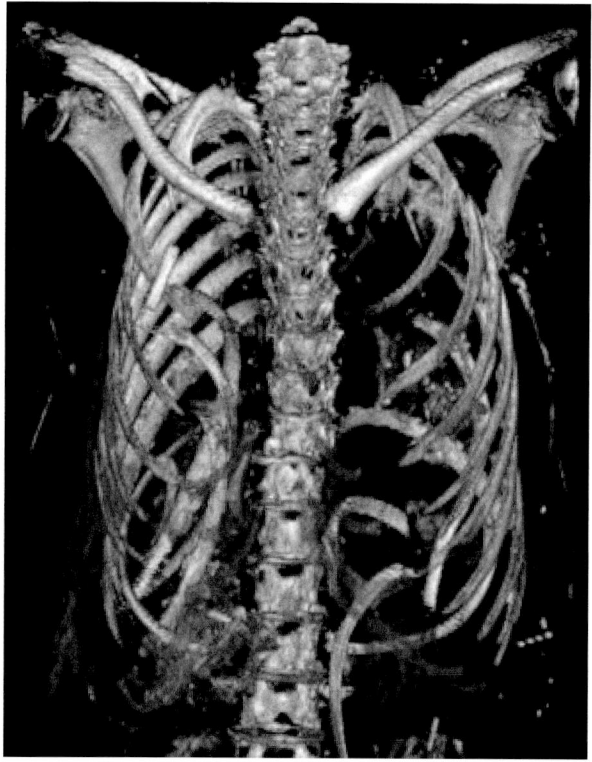

FIG. 5.70 3D RECONSTRUCTION SHOWING DISRUPTION OF RIB CAGE – ANTERIOR ASPECT

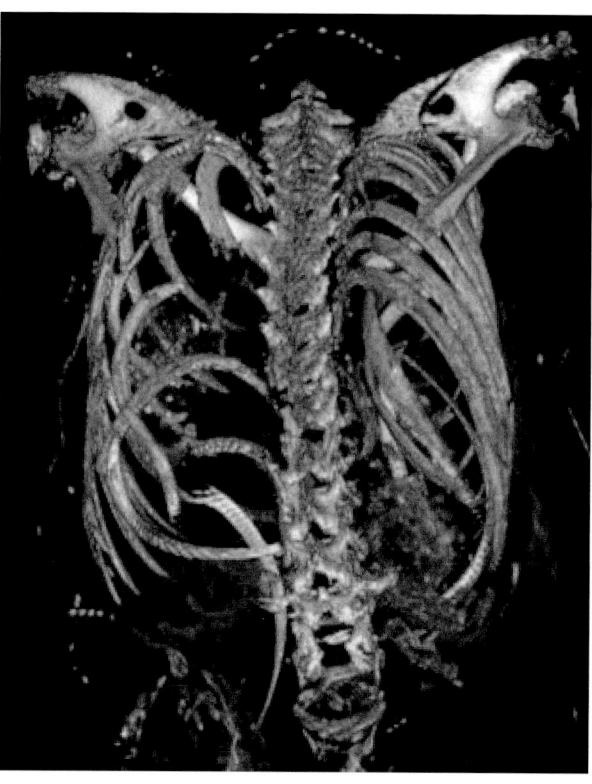

FIG. 5.71 3D RECONSTRUCTION SHOWING DISRUPTION OF RIB CAGE – POSTERIOR ASPECT

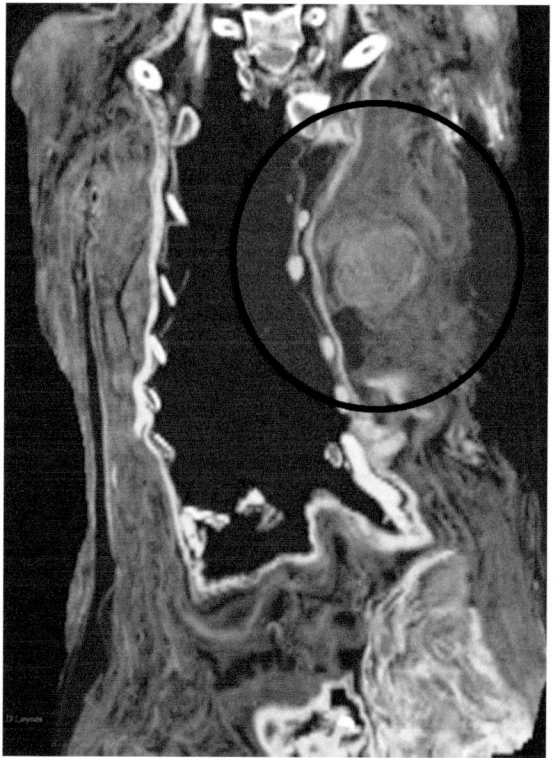

FIG. 5.72 CORONAL VIEW OF TRUNK - FALSE BREAST IN WRAPPINGS

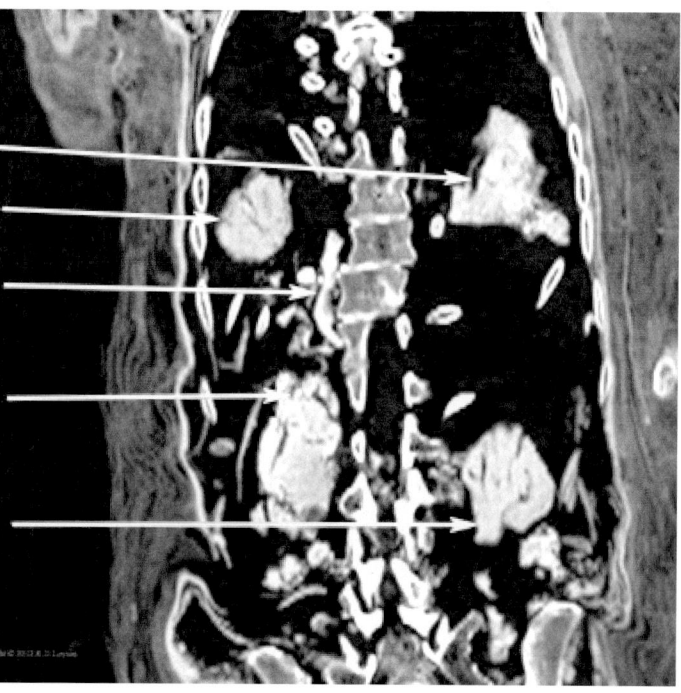

FIG. 5.73 CORONAL VIEW OF TRUNK - CANOPIC PACKAGES

In this figure the arrow 5 shows the perineal pack. Arrow 4 indicates the overlapping, dislocated pubic rami. Arrow 3 indicates the linen introduced from above. Arrow 2 indicates some high radio-dense material, which is probably resin with another substance mixed within it, also introduced from above. Arrow 1 indicates further returned viscera that are un-packaged.

Pelvis and Hips

There is significant disruption of the bony pelvis, with dislocation of both sacro-iliac joints and the symphysis pubis (See Figs. 5.76 and 5.77).

There are fractures of the left inferior pubic ramus - Fig. 5.78, and the left acetabulum - Fig. 5.79.

As already noted, a perineal approach has been used to aid complete evisceration of the pelvis (See Fig. 5.75). The hip joints are intact and show no evidence of arthritic change.

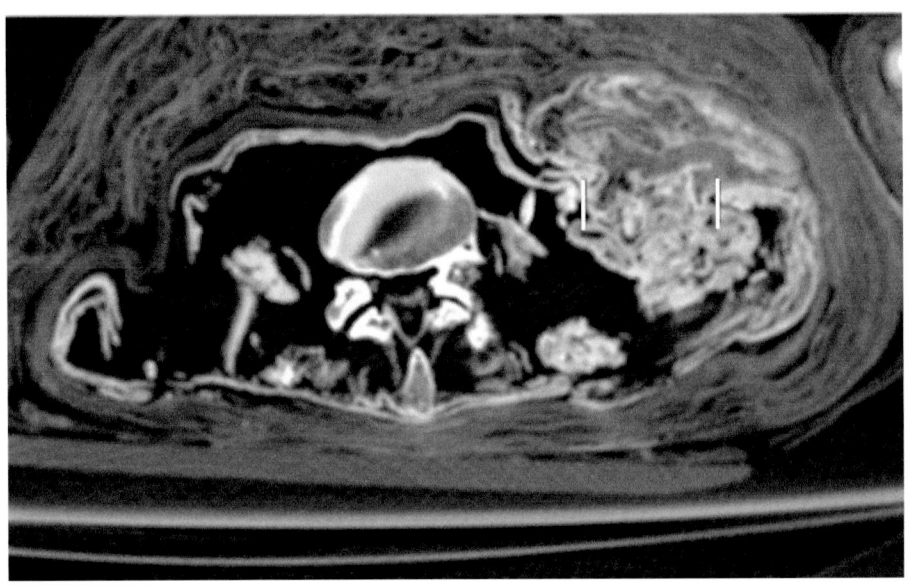

FIG. 5.74 AXIAL VIEW OF ABDOMEN - LEFT FLANK INCISION

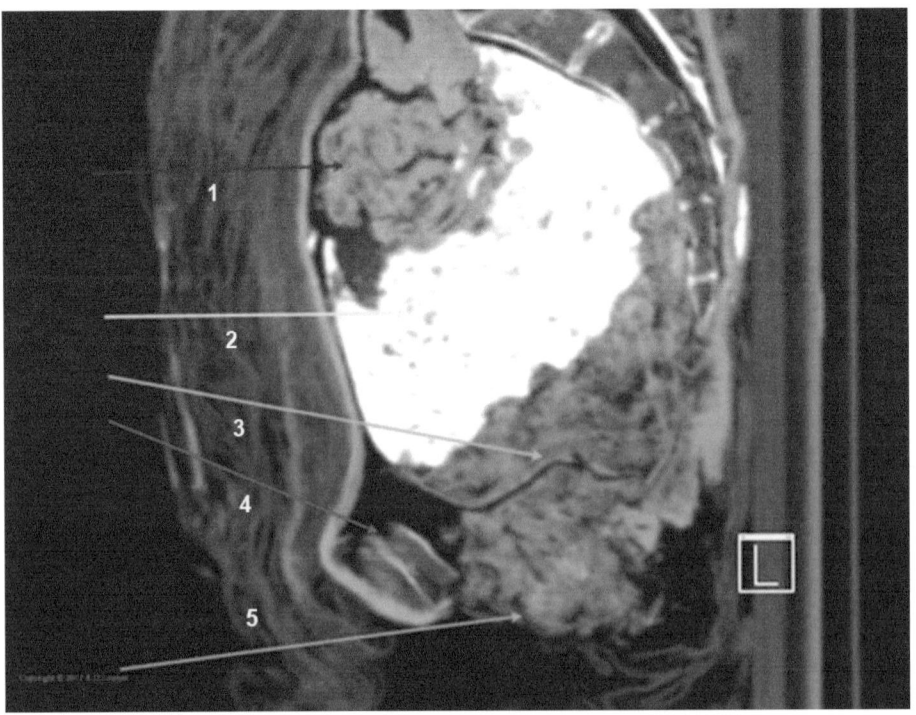

FIG. 5.75 SAGITTAL VIEW OF PELVIS - DESTROYED, FEATURELESS PERINEUM

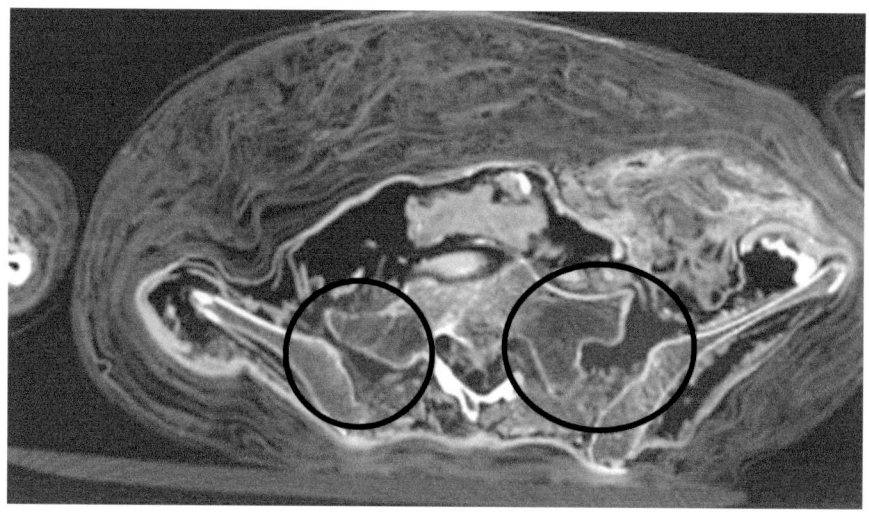

Fig. 5.76 Axial view of pelvis - disorganised sacro-iliac joints

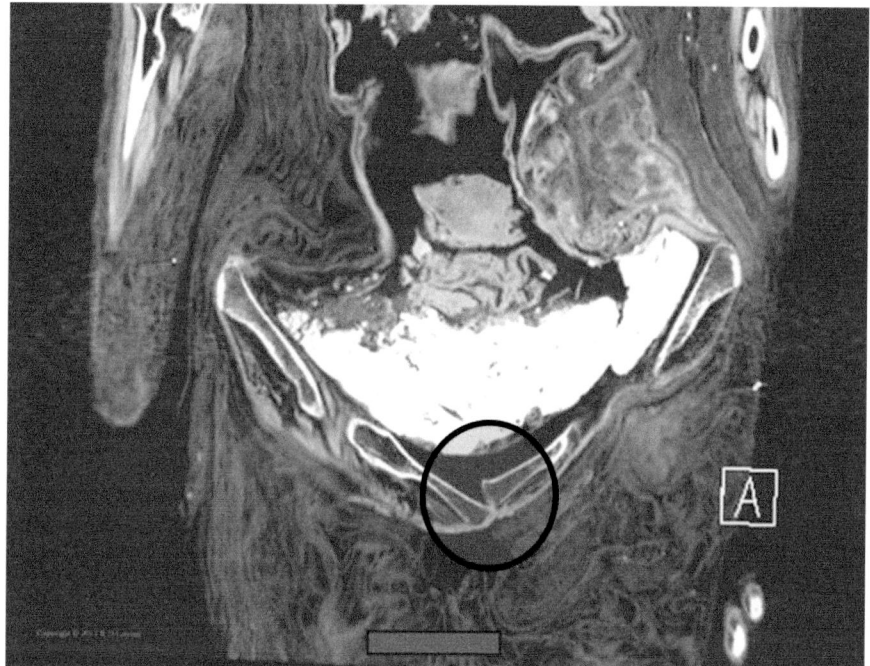

Fig. 5.77 Coronal view of pelvis - dislocated symphysis pubis

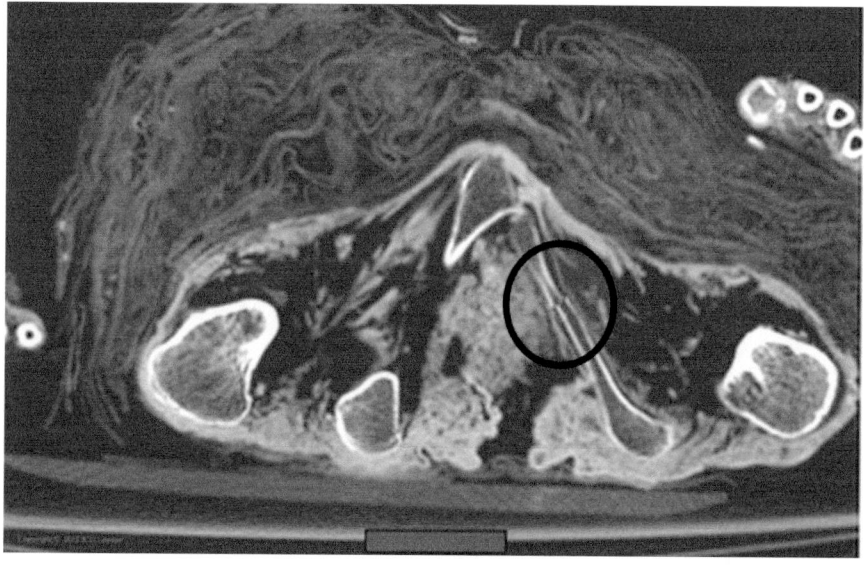

Fig. 5.78 Axial view of pelvis - fractured inferior pubic ramus

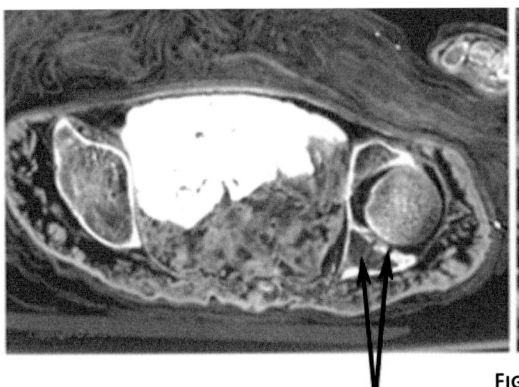
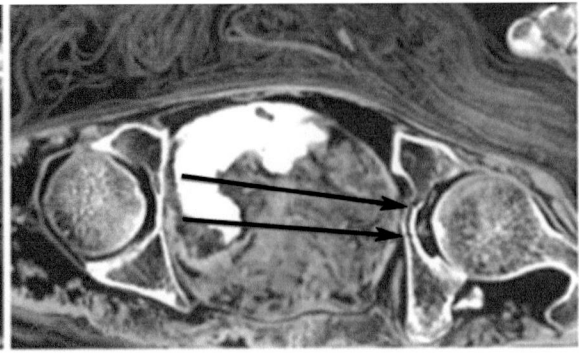

FIG. 5.79 Axial view of pelvis - acetabular fractures

XIX. Unnamed (Child) - Altdorf Museum

Thorax

The rib cage is a normal shape with no evidence of collapse or compression.

The upper part is packed with linen - from T1 to T5 but is otherwise empty - with complete evisceration and no evidence of the mediastinum or its contents (See Fig. 5.80). The sternum is intact.

Abdomen

There is an incision (more like a massive hole) in the left flank (lateral abdominal wall) with complete evisceration. However there are two packages lying in the left paraspinal gutter. These are of different radio-densities, the upper posterior one being denser. It is possible that this more dense package is of resin soaked linen and the other of biological material, that is returned viscera. These may represent canopic packages (See Fig. 5.81).

Pelvis and Hips

The pelvis is intact and the hips congruent. There is material of different radio-densities within the lower pelvis. Again this may represent some packing and some retained tissue such as the rectum (See Fig. 5.82).

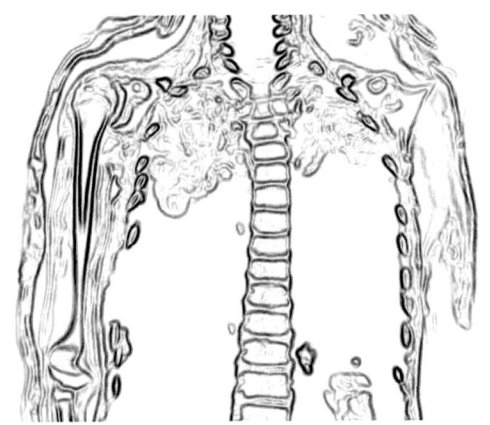

FIG. 5.80 Coronal view of thorax - empty apart from linen packs (After IEM image)

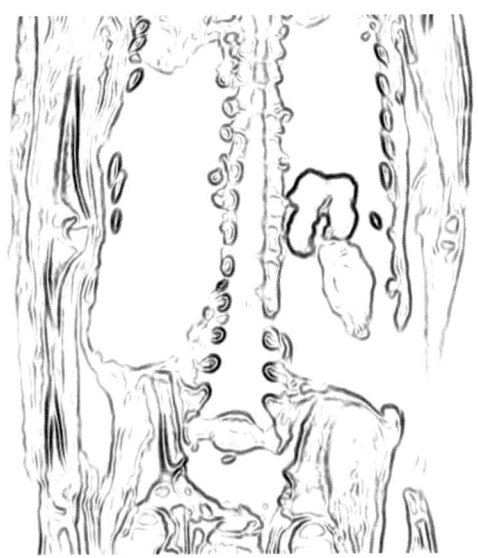

FIG. 5.81 Coronal view of trunk - canopic packages in abdomen (After IEM image)

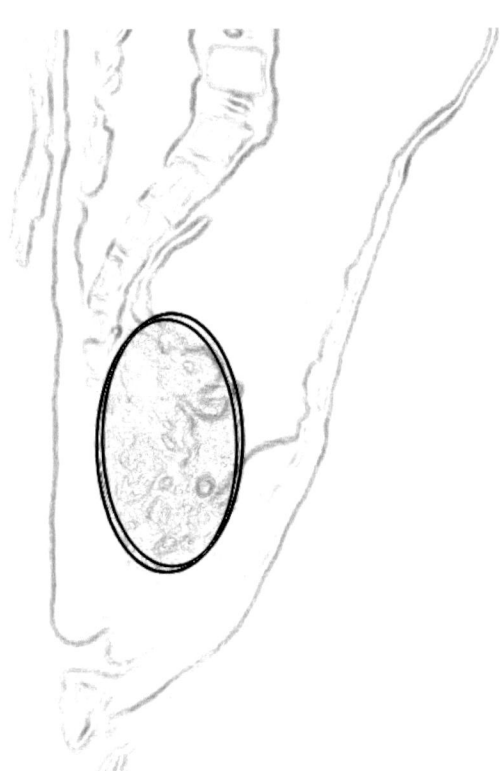

FIG. 5.82 Sagittal view of lower abdomen - material in lower pelvis (After IEM image)

XXII. Unnamed - Bern Museum - Cat. No. AE 1

Thorax

The rib cage is symmetrical and intact without any evidence of dislocation of the costo-vertebral joints or fractures.

The mediastinum remains and there is evidence of retention of the heart (Fig. 5.83. 2: mediastinum. 3: heart). However, there is no evidence of retention of the diaphragm. Resin has been inserted into the thorax on both sides (Fig. 5.83 - 1) along with evidence of biological tissue posteriorly on both sides of the thorax. Fig. 5.84 shows the tissue on the right - arrow 1 and two rolled linen packs. The one on the left (Fig. 5.84 arrow 3) has an object in it (possibly a *Wadjet* eye seen in Fig. 5.85 - black circle). The other is lower down, anteriorly in the mid-line and is in continuity with the packing in the abdomen, which is also in continuity with that coming from the site of the incision. (Fig. 5.86 - 1). The mass of biological material in the right para-spinal gutter is not wrapped and could represent returned viscera.

Abdomen

In the abdomen, there is a clearly visible left flank incision (Fig.5.86 lines 2) with linen packed through it into the abdominal and lower thoracic cavities. The previously noted mass of biological material in the thorax continues into the right side of the abdomen. There is also some resin mixed into this mass.

Overlying the left inguinal region (but, in fact, just medial to and in the same plane as the left wrist - see Fig.5.87) there is an object, which could well be an amulet, in that it has definite shape (see Fig. 5.87 and 5.88 - circle).

Pelvis and Hips

The pelvis is intact and the hips are congruous. There is loss of joint space in the hips, but this could well be secondary to mummification.

The perineum has been completely destroyed and there is no linen pack but there is a plaque of resin over the perineum and a void where the pelvic organs would be normally found. The pelvis tends towards the female shape (See Fig. 5.89).

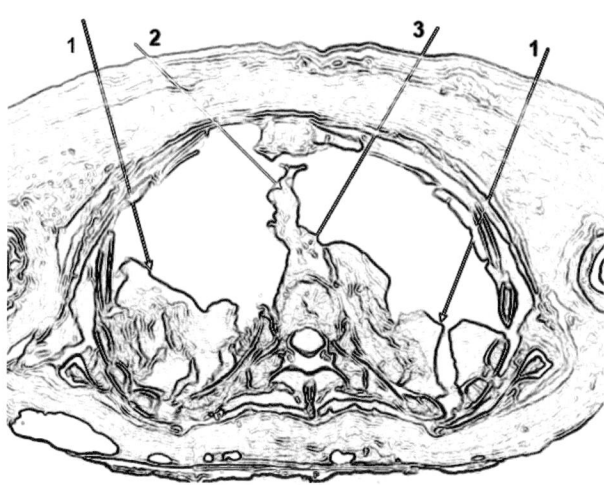

FIG. 5.83 AXIAL VIEW OF THORAX - MEDIASTINUM, HEART AND RESIN (AFTER IEM IMAGE)

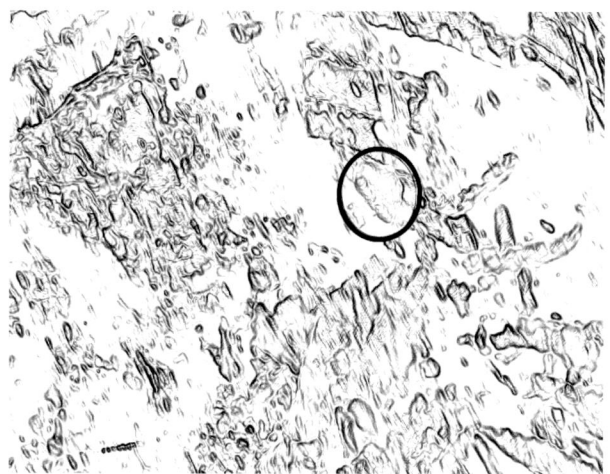

FIG. 5.85 3D RECONSTRUCTION OF OBJECT POSSIBLY WADJET EYE (AFTER IEM IMAGE)

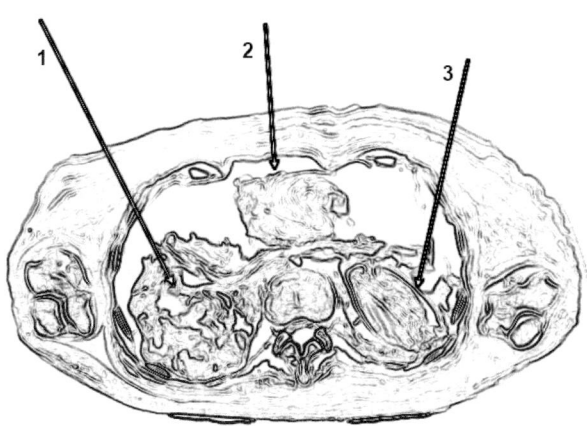

FIG. 5.84 AXIAL VIEW OF LOWER THORAX WITH RETURNED VISCERA (AFTER IEM IMAGE)

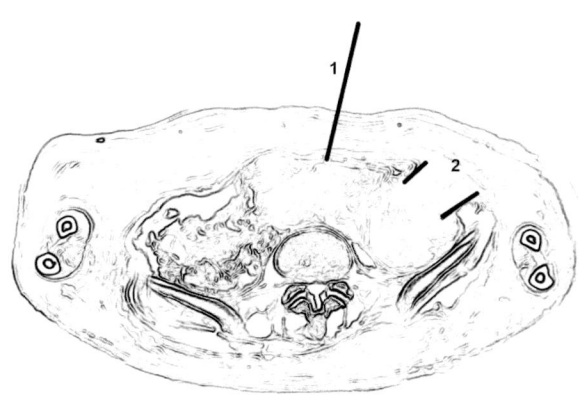

FIG. 5.86 AXIAL VIEW LOWER ABDOMEN – LEFT FLANK INCISION AND PACKING (AFTER IEM IMAGE)

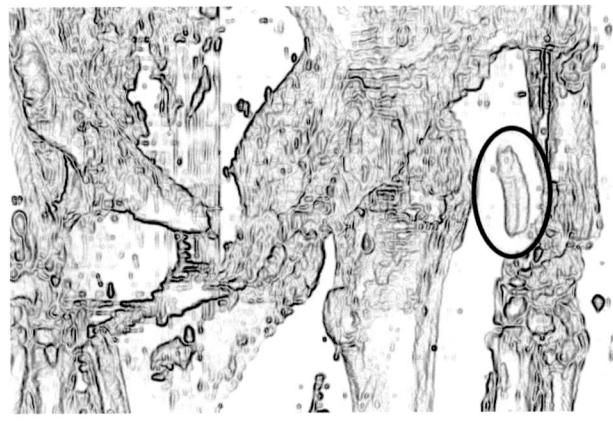

Fig. 5.87 3D RECONSTRUCTION AT LEVEL OF PELVIS SHOWING POSSIBLE AMULET (AFTER IEM IMAGE)

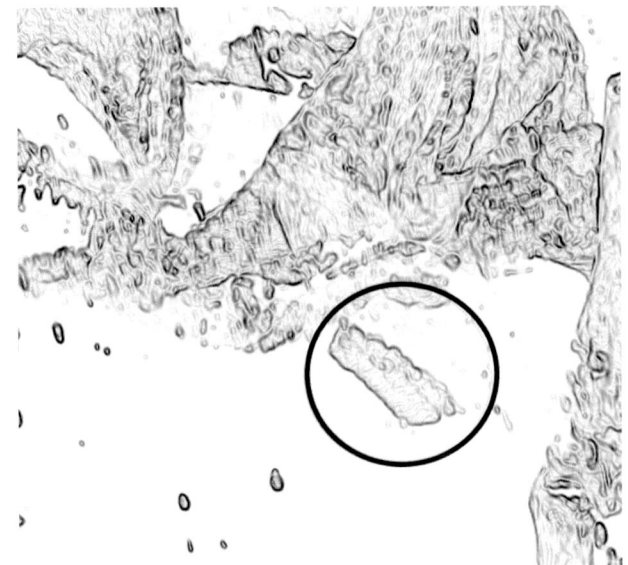

Fig. 5.88 3D RECONSTRUCTION AT LEVEL OF PELVIS SHOWING POSSIBLE AMULET (AFTER IEM IMAGE)

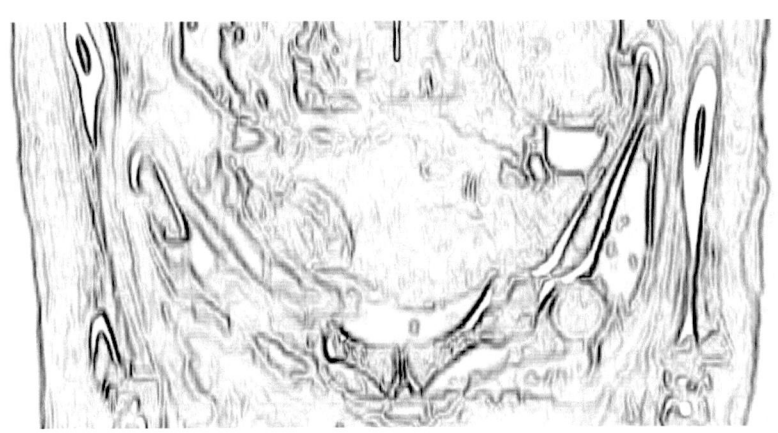

Fig. 5.89 CORONAL VIEW OF PELVIS SHOWING FEMALE SHAPE OF THE PELVIS (AFTER IEM IMAGE)

XXIII. Nes-Shou Yverdon - Museum (Accession No.MY/3775).

Thorax

The chest wall is symmetrical with no evidence of damage to the ribs. The trachea discontinues at the level of the manubrium sterni. There has been complete evisceration of the thoracic cavity with no evidence of the mediastinum or any of its structures. Resin is seen in the posterior 'gutters' of the thoracic cavity, which has set with a 'fluid level'. There is a thin layer of resin over the anterior aspect of the spinal vertebral bodies. It is interesting to note that there has been escape of the resin through the posterior thoracic wall into the subcutaneous tissues and through to the posterior layers of bandages (See Fig. 5.90 - arrow 2). Within the resin, on the left, is a heart scarab (See Fig. 5.90 - arrow 3 and Fig. 5.91). There are two canopic packages lying within the resin, in the thoracic region, on the right (See Fig. 5.90 - arrows 1).

Abdomen

There is a left sided flank incision and linen packing penetrates the incision (Fig.5.92 - arrow), which is covered by an amulet (See Fig. 5.92 - black circle). This amulet is in the shape of a *Sistrum* with head of Hathor at the neck (See Fig. 5.93).

Complete evisceration of the abdomen has been performed and a canopic package is seen within the right iliac fossa. In common with those in the thorax it consists of rolled linen soaked in resin, and contains some granular material. Fig. 5.94.

Pelvis and Hips

The bony pelvis is intact. Although an abdominal incision has been used, a trans-perineal evisceration has also been performed. The external genitalia have been removed and replaced by a false phallus. Fig. 5.95. Fig. 5.96 shows the amulet (*Sistrum*) - arrow and the false phallus.

RESULTS – THE TRUNK

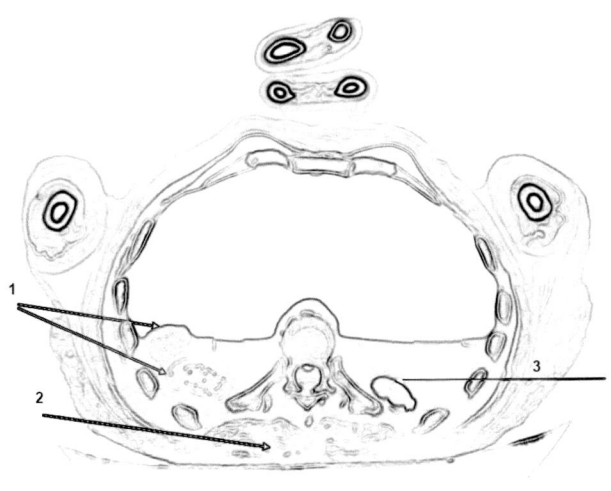

FIG. 5.90 AXIAL VIEW OF THORAX SHOWING CONTENTS (AFTER IEM IMAGE)

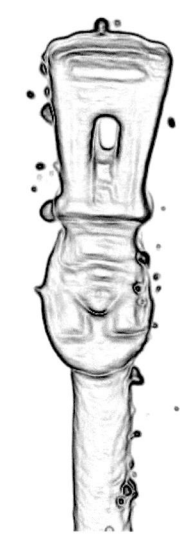

FIG. 5.93 3D RECONSTRUCTION OF SISTRUM SHAPED AMULET (AFTER IEM IMAGE)

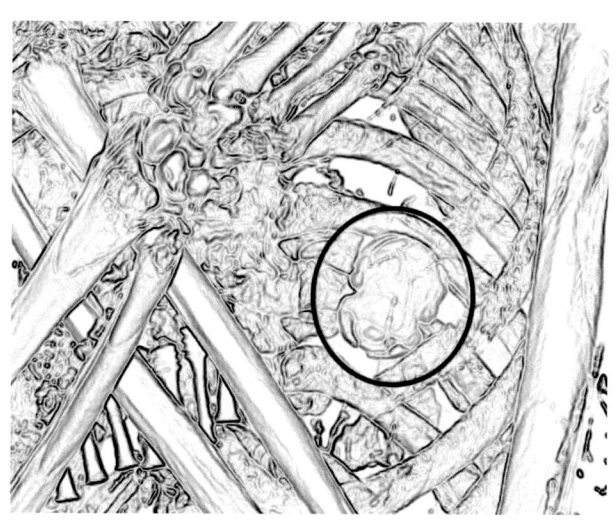

FIG. 5.91 3D RECONSTRUCTION OF HEART SCARAB (AFTER IEM IMAGE)

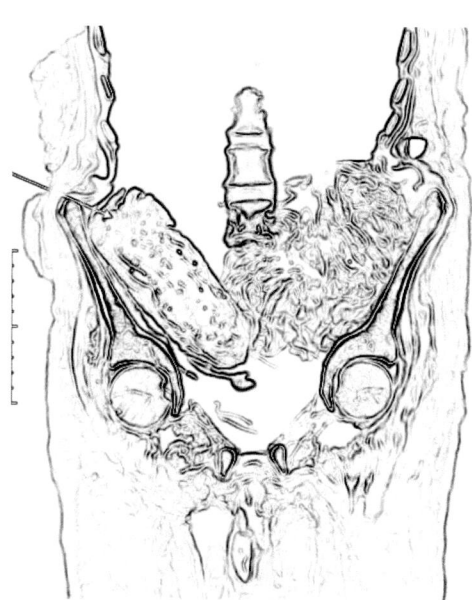

FIG. 5.94 CORONAL VIEW OF PELVIS - CANOPIC PACKAGE (AFTER IEM IMAGE)

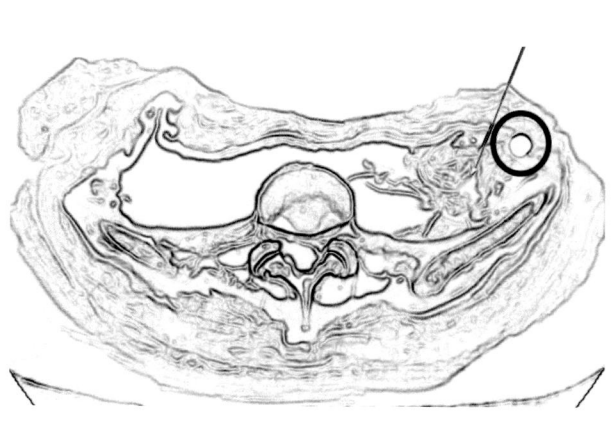

FIG. 5.92 AXIAL VIEW SHOWING ABDOMINAL INCISION AND AMULET (AFTER IEM IMAGE)

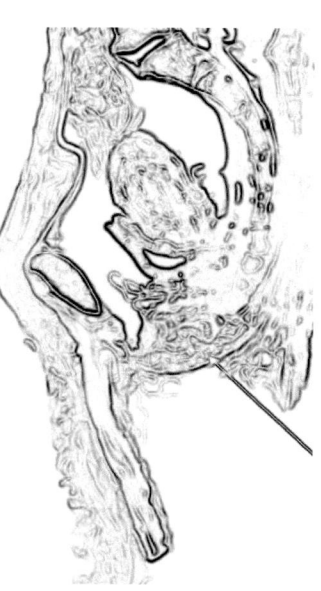

FIG. 5.95 SAGITTAL VIEW OF PELVIS - PERINEUM AND FALSE PHALLUS (AFTER IEM IMAGE)

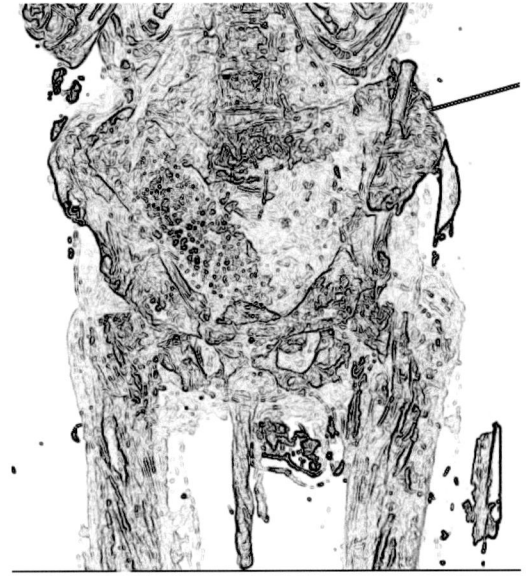

FIG. 5.96 3D RECONSTRUCTION OF FALSE PHALLUS AND AMULET (AFTER IEM IMAGE)

XXV. TjesMoutPert - Geneva Museum (Cat. No.D0242)

Thorax

The rib cage is normal and symmetrical. The mediastinum and its contents, including the heart, have been retained. Both hemi-diaphragms are present but are perforated. The lungs have been removed (See Fig. 5.97).

There is a small amount of resin within both sides of the thorax but no canopic packages.

Abdomen

There is a left flank incision (See Fig. 5.98 - arrow). Evisceration has been complete with no evidence of returned viscera or canopic packages. The shape of the abdominal wall indicates that, in the absence of flattening, the abdomen may well have contained something that has been robbed out in the past. There is a certain amount of resin in the posterior part of the abdominal cavity.

Pelvis and Hips

The bony pelvis is intact. The hips are congruous with no evidence of arthritis. The remains of the rectum, vagina and urethra are clearly visible.

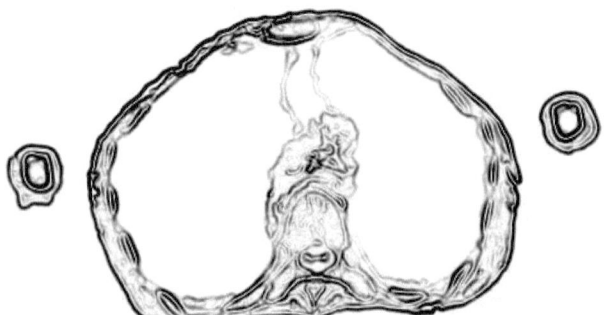

FIG. 5.97 AXIAL VIEW OF THORAX AND MEDIASTINUM

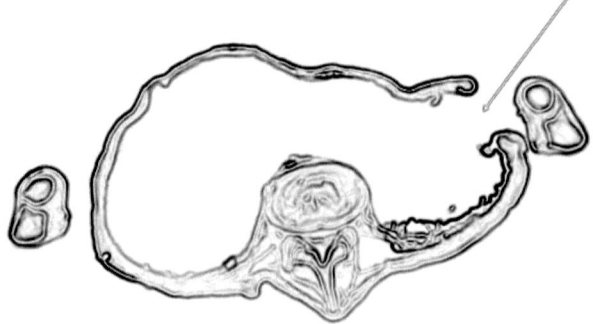

FIG. 5.98 AXIAL VIEW OF ABDOMINAL INCISION (AFTER IEM IMAGE)

XXVI. Unnamed - Geneva Museum Cat. No. D404

Thorax

The rib cage is normal, intact and symmetrical. The chest has not been compressed.

The mediastinum has been retained. Although the outlines of other mediastinal structures are clear, there is no definitive evidence of the heart. However, its presence cannot be absolutely excluded (See Fig. 5.99 - arrow 2). There is some biological tissue present on both sides of the spine as well as resin in the para-spinal gutters (Fig.5.99 - arrows 1 and 3). Both hemi-diaphragms are present, but perforated posteriorly.

Abdomen

There is a left flank incision with linen passing through it into the abdominal cavity (See Fig. 5.100 - arrow 2). Two rolls of resinous material are seen in the right side of the abdomen and probably represent canopic packages (Fig. 5.100 - arrow 1). A small amount of resin is seen posteriorly on both sides of the abdomen.

Pelvis and Hips

Whilst the sacro-iliac joints are intact, there is some disruption and overlapping at the pubic symphysis (See Fig. 5.101 - black circle).

The hips are congruous. However, the posterior third of the left femoral head epiphysis is unusually radio-dense, which probably indicates avascularity (See Fig. 5.102).

On the other hand, the right femoral capital epiphysis seems to be slipping slightly posteriorly (See Fig. 5.103).

There is a suggestion of the outline of male external genitalia. Arrow 2- Fig. 5.104. This figure also shows the radio-density of the left femoral epiphysis - black circle.

RESULTS – THE TRUNK

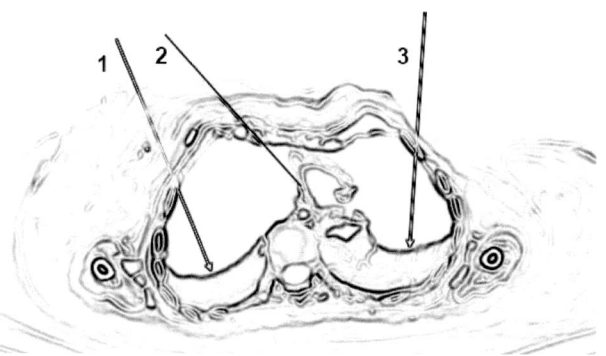

FIG. 5.99 AXIAL VIEW OF THORAX - MEDIASTINUM AND RESIN (AFTER IEM IMAGE)

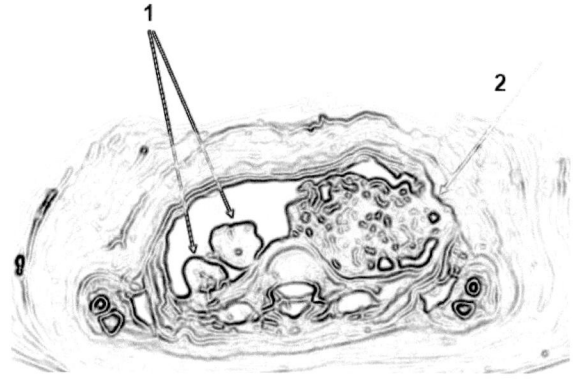

FIG. 5.100 AXIAL VIEW OF ABDOMINAL INCISION AND CANOPIC PACKAGES (AFTER IEM IMAGE)

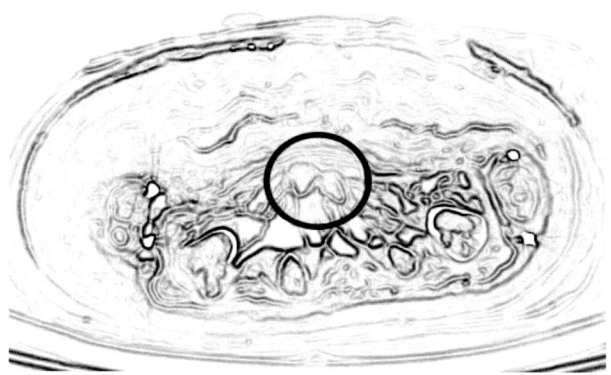

FIG. 5.101 AXIAL VIEW OF PELVIS – PUBIC SYMPHYSIS (AFTER IEM IMAGE)

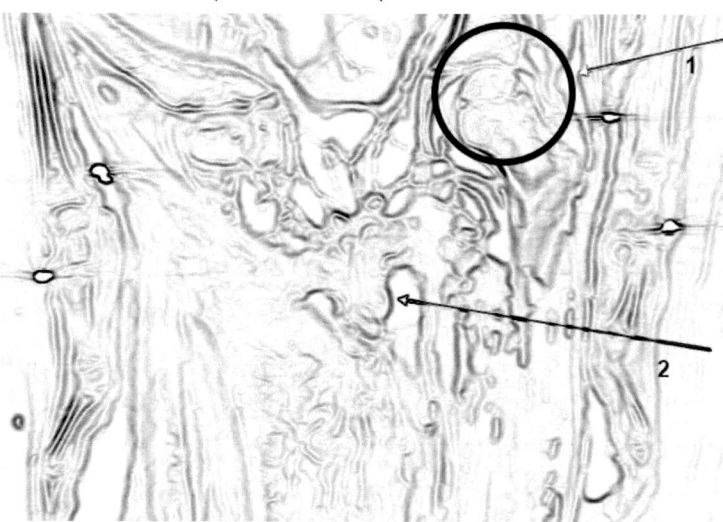

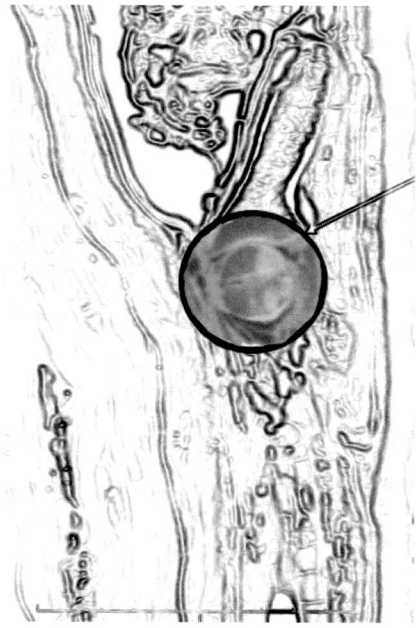

FIG. 5.102 SAGITTAL VIEW OF PELVIS - LEFT FEMORAL HEAD (AFTER IEM IMAGE)

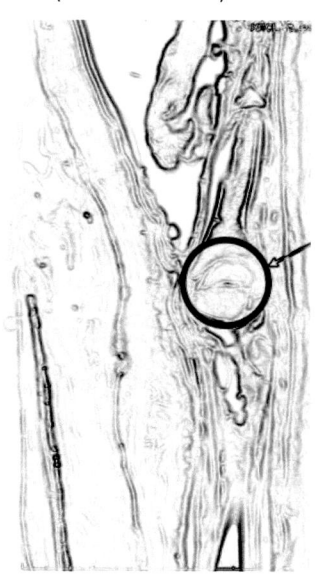

FIG. 5.103 SAGITTAL VIEW OF PELVIS - RIGHT FEMORAL HEAD (AFTER IEM IMAGE)

FIG. 5.104 CORONAL VIEW OF PELVIS - EXTERNAL GENITALIA AND LEFT FEMORAL HEAD (AFTER IEM IMAGE)

XXVII. Demetria - Manchester Museum (Cat. No.MM11630)

Thorax

There is compression of the rib cage with costo-vertebral dislocation of the left 5th to 12th ribs and right 5th to 11th ribs (See Fig. 5.105; 8th ribs and compare with Fig. 5.106). This compression can also be seen in Figs. 5.107 and 5.108.

The mediastinum is absent, but there is 'biological' tissue overlying the thoracic vertebrae (arrows 1 in Fig. 5.109). In Fig.5.109 arrow 3 indicates the thoracic vertebral body and the arrow 2 the sternum. Resin has not been used to pack the thoracic cavity.

Abdomen

There is so much folding of the abdominal wall that a flank incision cannot be confirmed or excluded (See Fig. 5.110). Evisceration has been thorough, with little or no return of the viscera to the body cavity.

Pelvis and Hips

Both sacro-iliac joints and the symphysis pubis are dislocated but there are no fractures of the pelvis (See Fig. 5.111 and 5.112 - where the pubic bones indicated with arrows should be opposite one another). The pelvic cavity is empty. The perineum is difficult to see because of the distorted pelvis, but there is a strong suggestion of a rectum - Fig. 5.113, arrow 2 and a vagina, arrow 1.

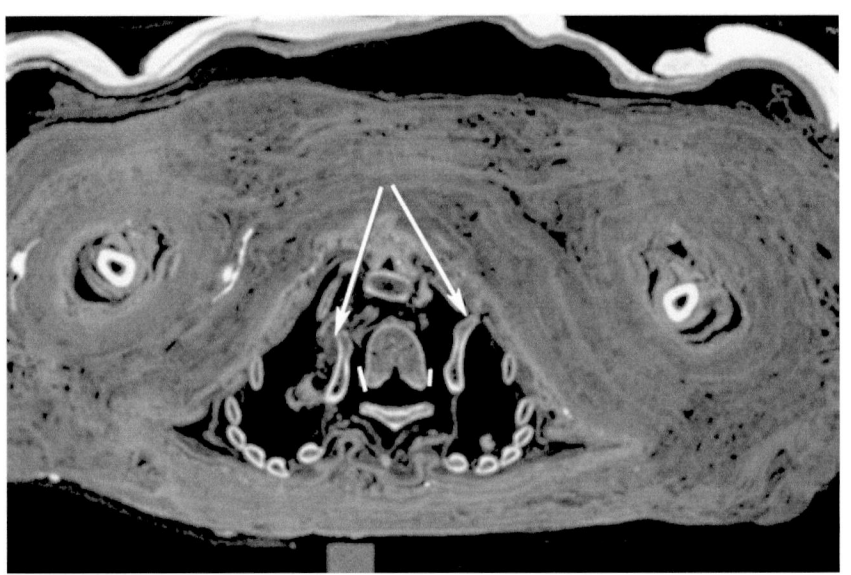

FIG. 5.105 AXIAL VIEW OF THORAX - DISLOCATED COSTO-VERTEBRAL JOINTS

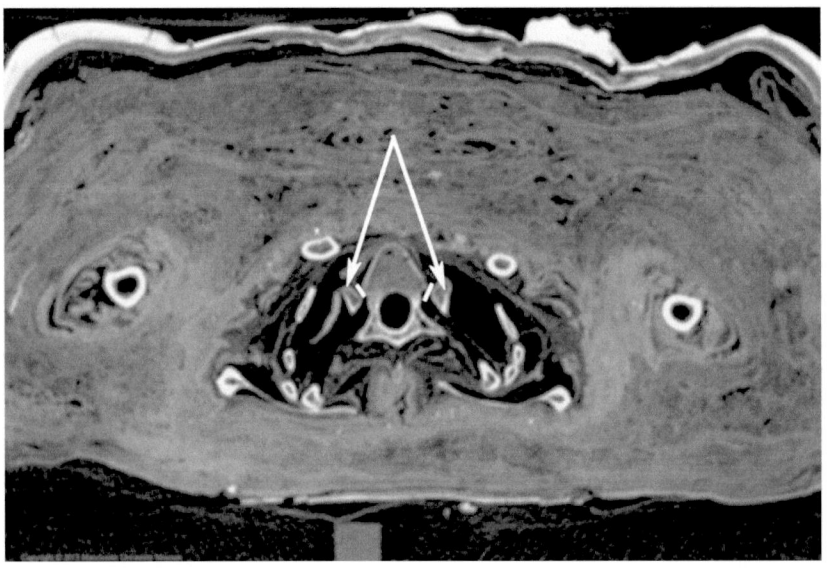

FIG. 5.106 AXIAL VIEW OF THORAX - INTACT COSTO-VERTEBRAL JOINTS

RESULTS – THE TRUNK

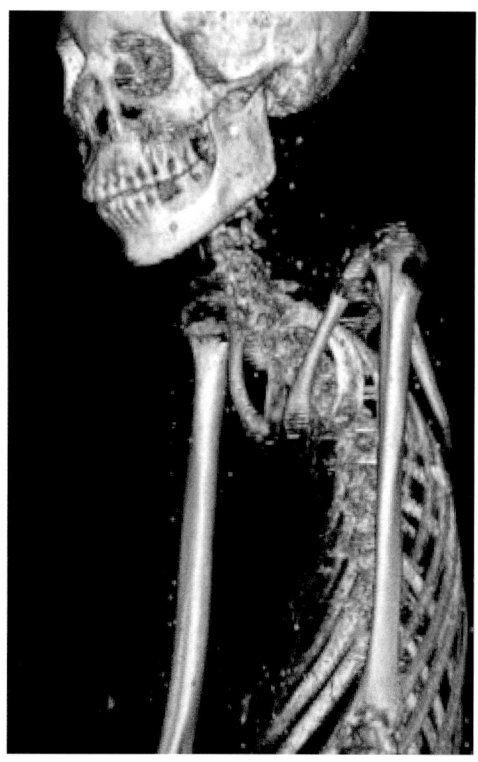

FIG. 5.107 3D RECONSTRUCTION OF COMPRESSED RIB CAGE

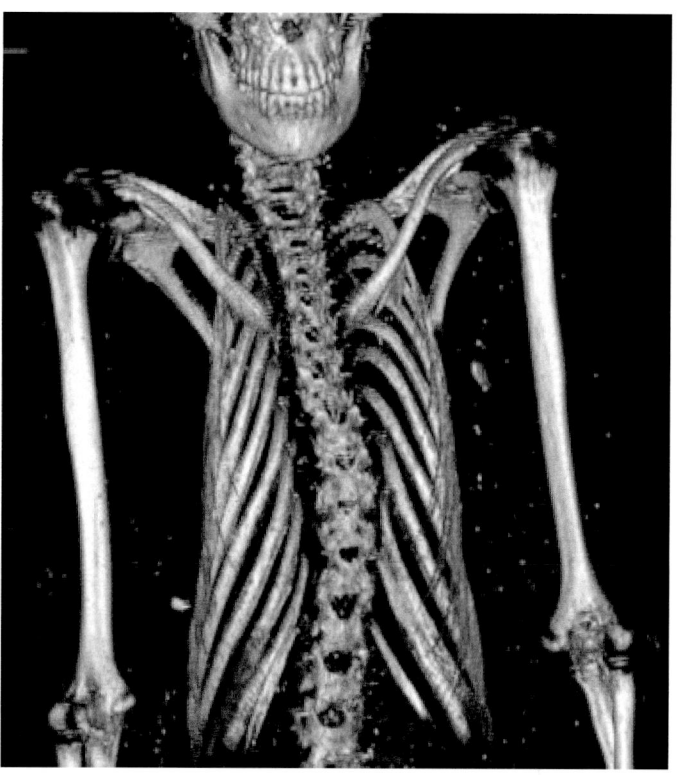

FIG. 5.108 3D RECONSTRUCTION OF COMPRESSED RIB CAGE

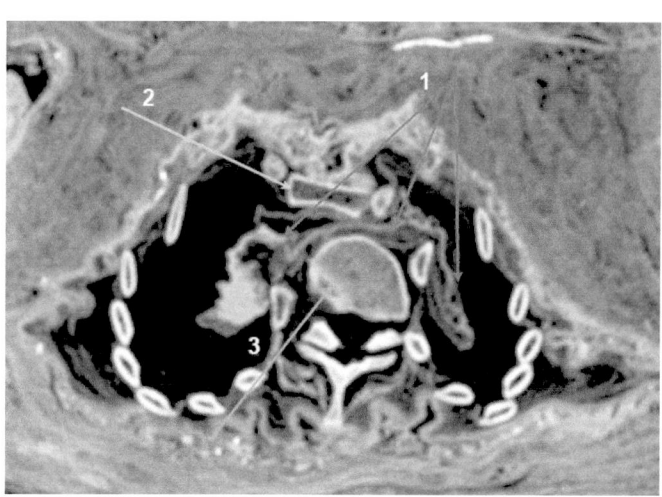

FIG. 5.109 AXIAL VIEW OF COMPRESSED THORAX

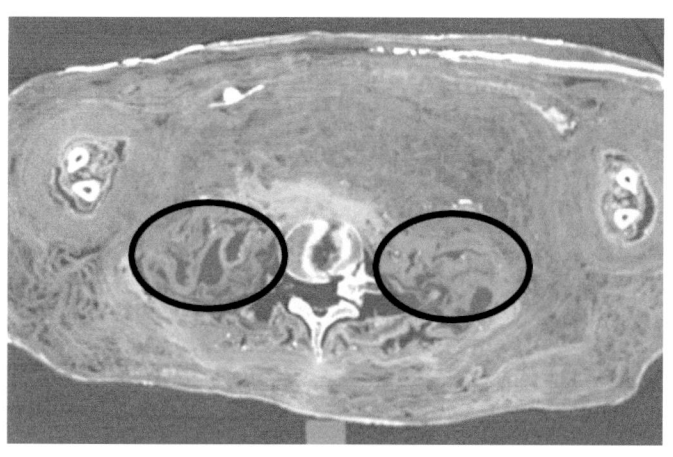

FIG. 5.110 AXIAL VIEW OF LOWER ABDOMEN SHOWING FOLDS IN ABDOMINAL WALL

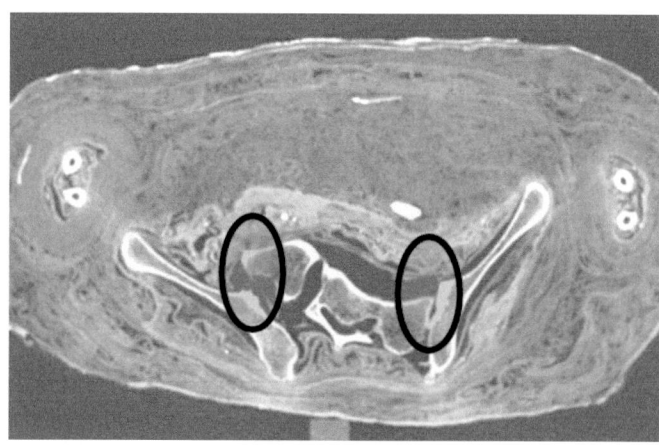

FIG. 5.111 AXIAL VIEW OF PELVIS - DISLOCATED SACRO-ILIAC JOINTS (SIJ)

119

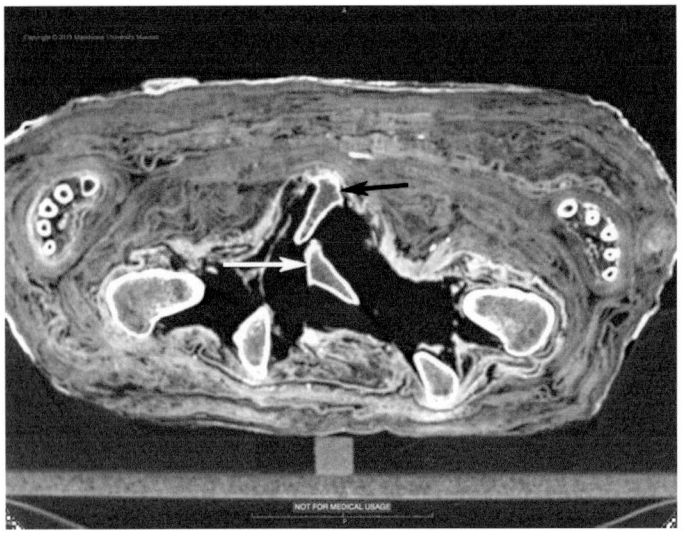

FIG. 5.112 AXIAL VIEW OF PELVIS - DISLOCATED SYMPHYSIS PUBIS

XXVIII. Ta-Sheri-Ankh - Manchester Museum - (Cat. No. MM13783)

Thorax

The thorax has sustained damage anteriorly, as can be seen in Fig. 5.114 - the line indicates a sharp intersection between the damaged and non-damaged areas. That part of the rib cage that is intact appears to be normal in shape. Whilst this damage is extensive, the left upper arm remains in situ, although there is dislocation of the left elbow and detachment of both hands at the wrists (See Figs. 5.115 and 5.116, where the measured lines show the relative positions of the left distal radius and the left carpus - normally articulating with the radius).

Despite the damage, the thorax contains three canopic packages. The one on the right and the more medial one on the left may well contain viscera. The third appears to

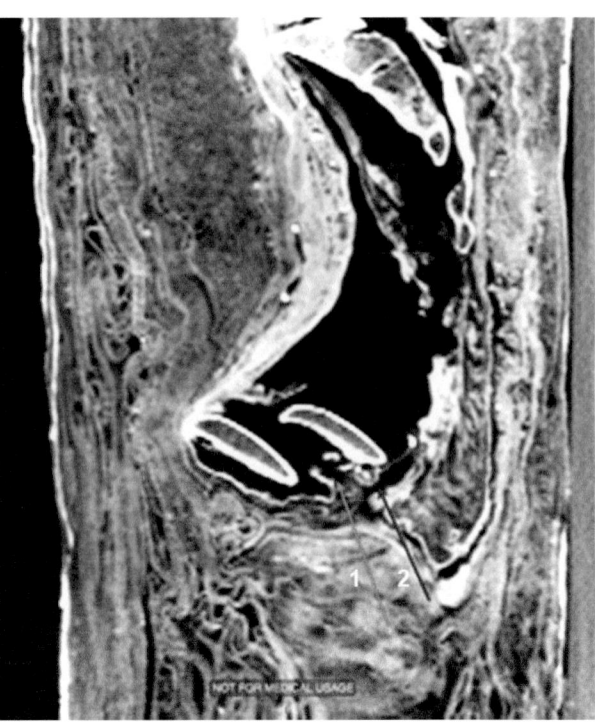

FIG. 5.113 SAGITTAL VIEW OF PELVIS - PERINEAL STRUCTURES

be of resin soaked linen (See Fig. 5.117). The thorax also contains the debris from the damaged anterior thoracic wall. No mediastinal contents or other viscera are seen in the thoracic cavity.

There is a layer of resin in the thorax that has pooled in the concavity of the normal thoracic kyphosis and has infiltrated several of the thoracic vertebral bodies. It has soaked through all the posterior tissues as far as the bandages (See Fig. 5.118).

Abdomen

There is a left flank incision - seen in Fig. 5.119 (black lines) with linen crossing the incision, into the abdominal cavity.

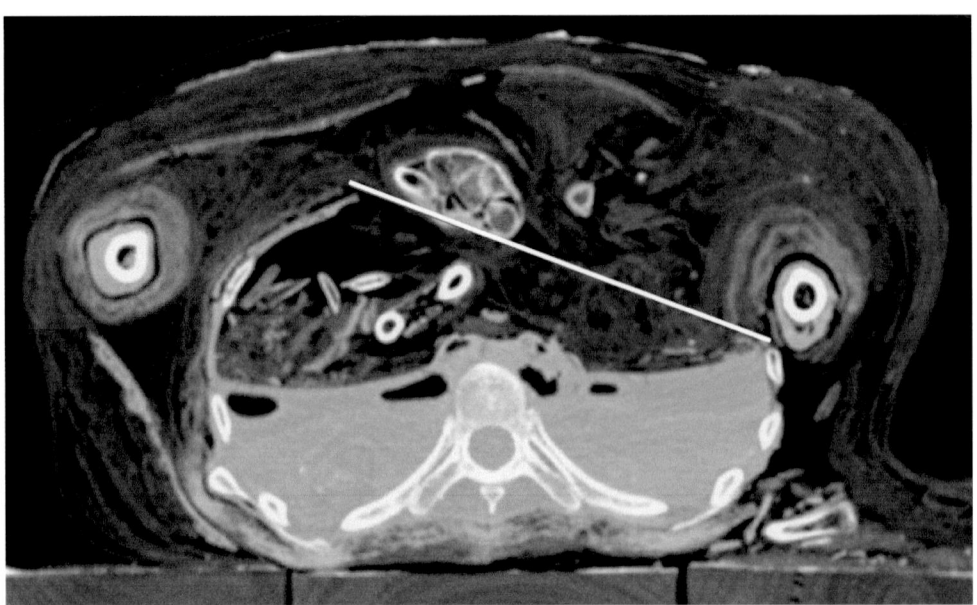

FIG. 5.114 AXIAL VIEW OF THORAX - ANTERIOR THORACIC WALL DAMAGE

Although the three above-mentioned canopic packages encroach into the abdomen, there are no additional ones in this region.

The right side of the lower abdominal wall has fragmented and fallen into the cavity (See Fig. 5.120).

Pelvis and Hips

The bony pelvis is intact and the hip joints congruous showing no signs of arthritis.

There are no viscera within or returned to the pelvic cavity. External genitalia are not seen.

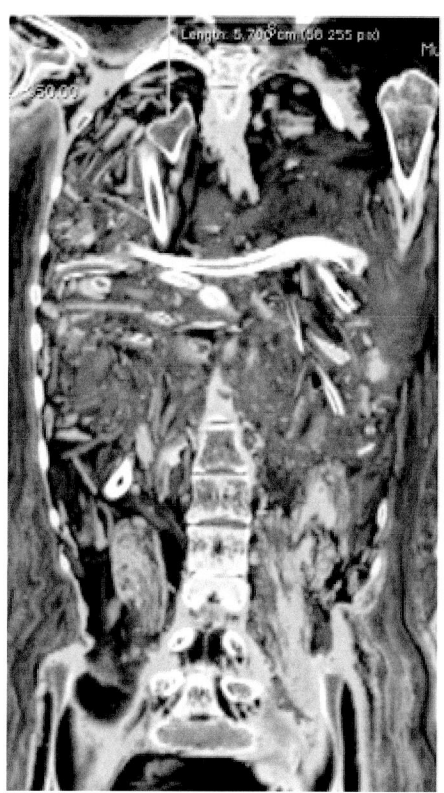 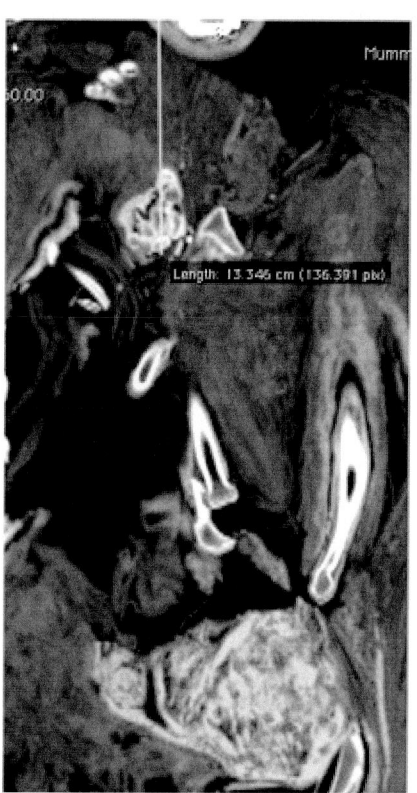

FIG. 5.115 CORONAL VIEW OF TRUNK SHOWING POSITION OF CARPUS

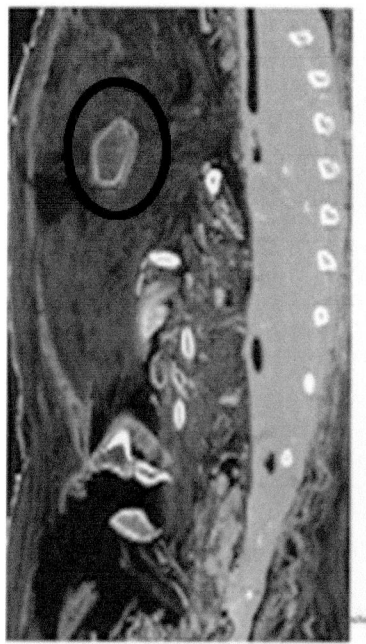 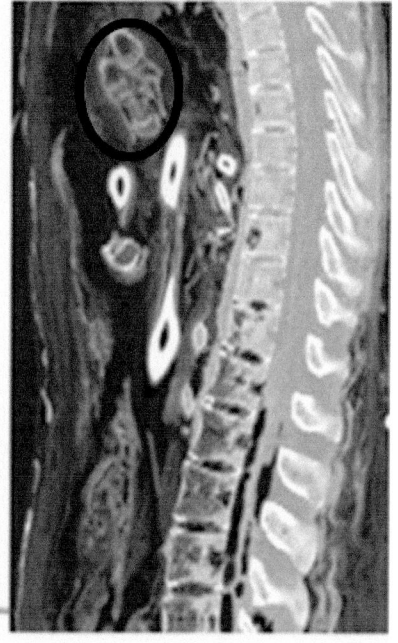

FIG. 5.116 SAGITTAL VIEW OF TRUNK SHOWING POSITION OF CARPUS

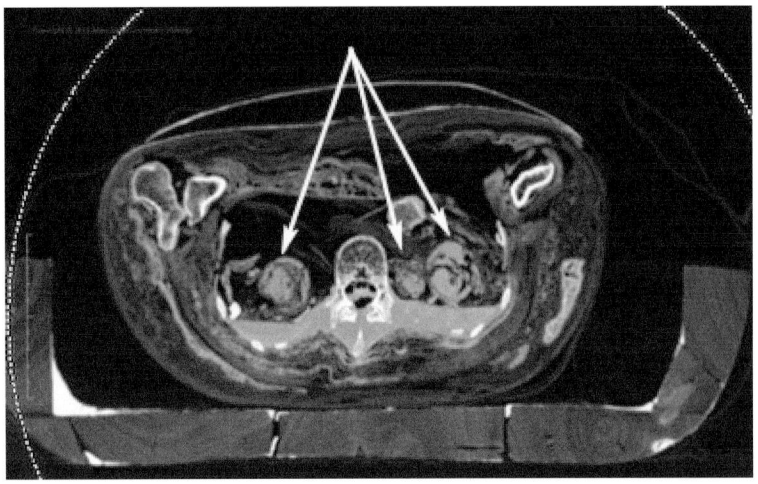

FIG. 5.117 AXIAL VIEW OF LOWER THORAX - CANOPIC PACKAGES

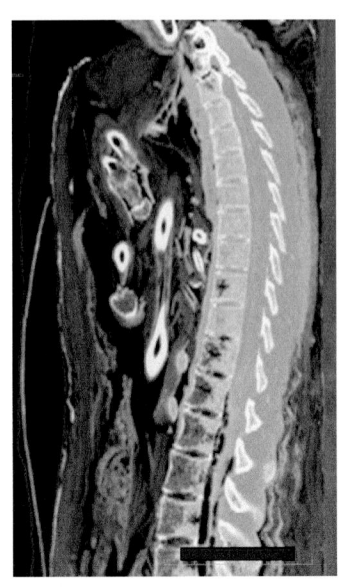

FIG. 5.118 SAGITTAL VIEW OF TRUNK SHOWING POSTERIOR PENETRATION OF RESIN

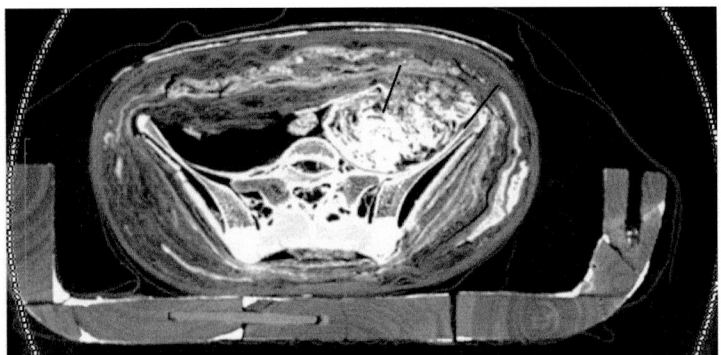

FIG. 5.119 AXIAL VIEW OF LOWER ABDOMEN SHOWING LEFT FLANK INCISION

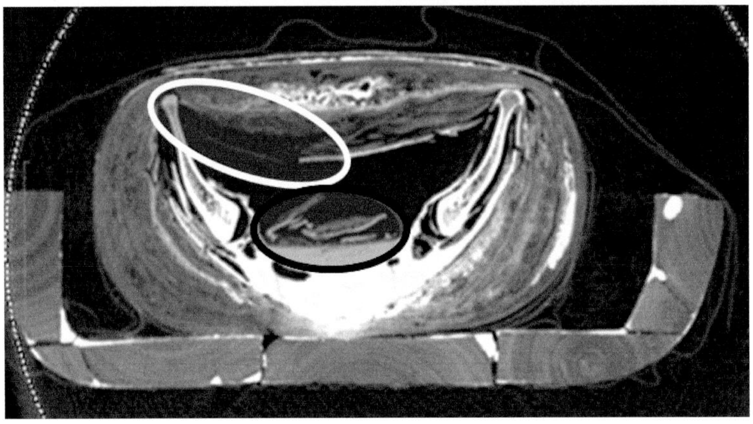

FIG. 5.120 AXIAL VIEW OF LOWER ABDOMEN SHOWING DAMAGE TO ANTERIOR ABDOMINAL WALL

XXIX. Hor - British Museum - (Accession No. EA 6659)

Thorax

The rib cage is largely intact, although the left 2nd rib is lying free within the thorax (See Fig. 5.121). There are fractures of the left 6th rib (Fig. 5.122) and of the right 6th, 7th and 8th ribs (Fig. 5.123).

The mediastinum, its contents and the diaphragms have been removed. There is a haphazard mix of linen (2), clay (granular) and returned viscera (1) within the cavity of the torso (See Fig. 5.124). The more radio-dense material may be resin.

Abdomen

There is a left flank incision as shown in Fig. 5.125 (lines). As has been described in the thorax, the packing in the abdomen (following evisceration) consists of a mix of linen, clay and returned viscera.

Pelvis and Hips

The bony pelvis is intact, with intact sacro-iliac joints and symphysis pubis but there is an un-displaced fracture of the right iliac bone (See Fig. 5.126).

The perineum is intact with a visible rectum (2) and well-demonstrated external genitalia (1) (See Fig. 5.127).

RESULTS – THE TRUNK

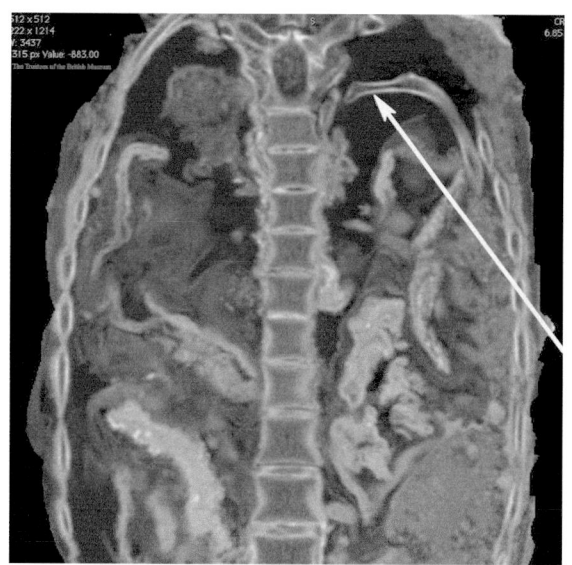

FIG. 5.121 CORONAL VIEW OF THORAX – POSITION OF LEFT 2ND RIB
COURTESY OF THE TRUSTEES OF THE BRITISH MUSEUM

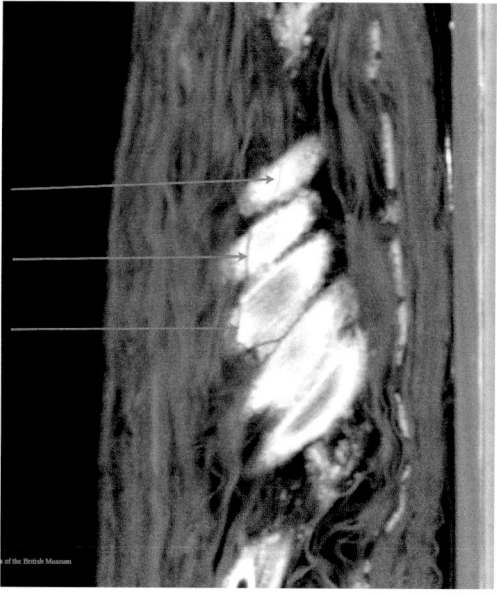

FIG. 5.123 SAGITTAL VIEW OF THORAX - FRACTURED RIGHT RIBS
COURTESY OF THE TRUSTEES OF THE BRITISH MUSEUM

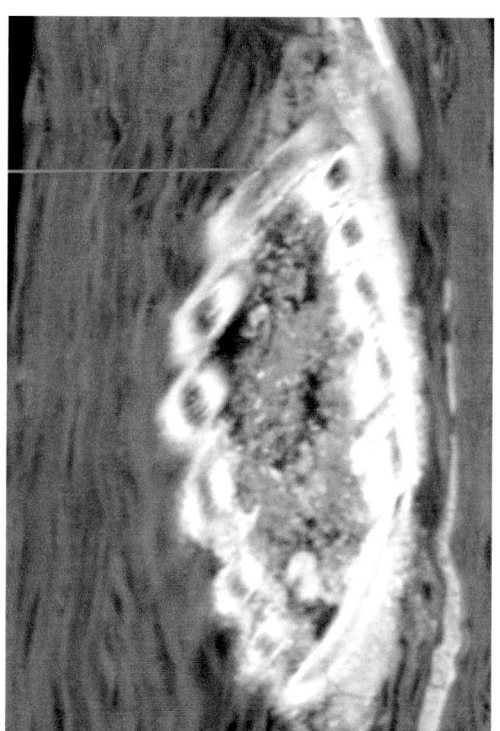

FIG. 5.122 SAGITTAL VIEW OF THORAX - LEFT 6TH RIB FRACTURE
COURTESY OF THE TRUSTEES OF THE BRITISH MUSEUM

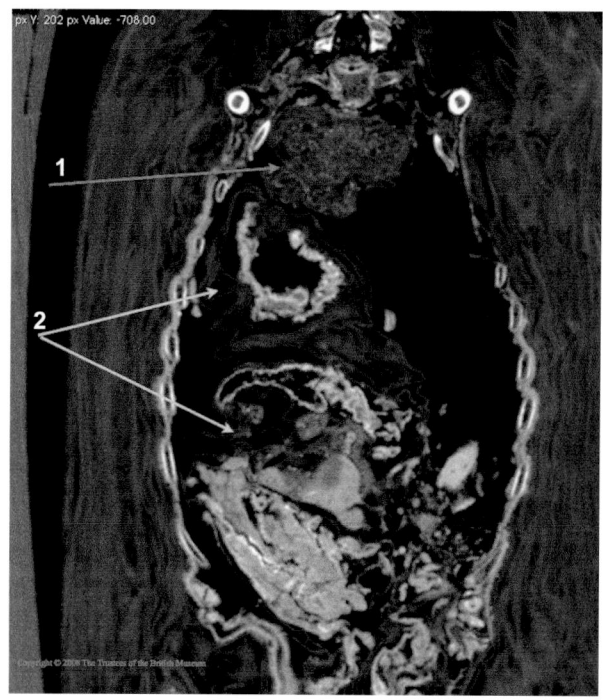

FIG. 5.124 CORONAL VIEW OF TRUNK - CONTENTS OF TORSO
COURTESY OF THE TRUSTEES OF THE BRITISH MUSEUM

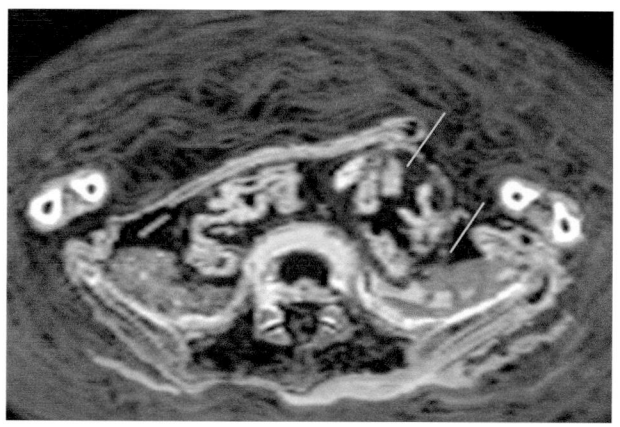

FIG. 5.125 AXIAL VIEW OF LOWER ABDOMEN – LEFT FLANK INCISION
COURTESY OF THE TRUSTEES OF THE BRITISH MUSEUM

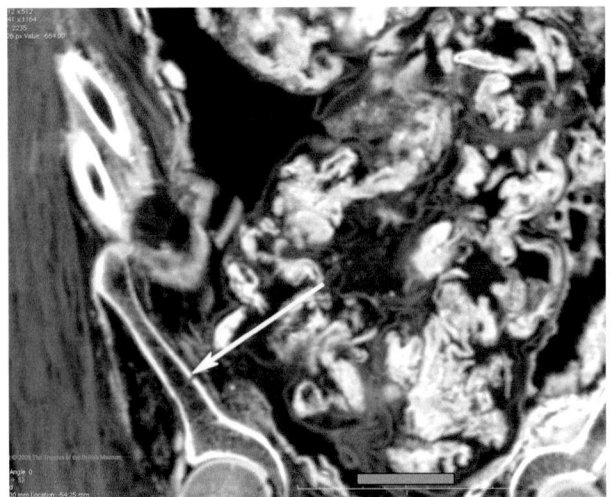

FIG. 5.126 CORONAL VIEW OF PELVIS - FRACTURED RIGHT ILIAC BONE
COURTESY OF THE TRUSTEES OF THE BRITISH MUSEUM

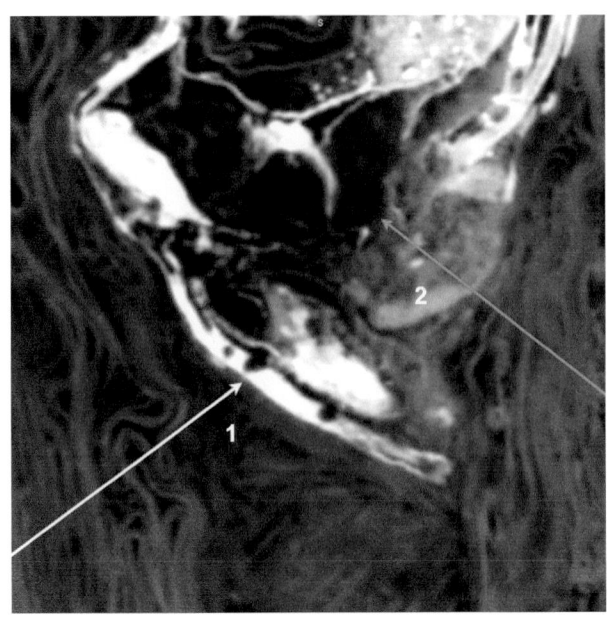

FIG. 5.127 SAGITTAL VIEW OF PERINEUM
COURTESY OF THE TRUSTEES OF THE BRITISH MUSEUM

XXX. Pef-Tjau-Emawy-Khonsu - British Museum - (Accession No. EA 6681)

Thorax and Abdomen

The thorax has, to a large extent, been destroyed. The vertebral bodies from C3 caudally have been removed. There are five vertebral bodies lying within the abdominal cavity (four of these are shown in Fig. 5.130 - arrows) that appear to be lumbar vertebrae, as judged by the antero-posterior orientation of the posterior joint facets. The rib cage is absent, although there is a certain amount of debris within the thorax, which consists of small parts of ribs (See Fig. 5.128 - white circle and Fig. 5.129 - black circle). Parts of the body of the sternum are shown in Fig. 5.128 - black circles and in Fig. 5.129 - arrow. In the space where one would expect to find the thoracic spine and ribs there are two resin 'casts' which were originally within the rib cage as can be seen by their cross sectional shape (Fig. 5.129) and the rib indentations (arrows 2 in Figs. 5.130 and 5.131).

Although the original abdominal wall has been lost through fragmentation, a linen pack of the expected shape is seen in the usual position of a left flank incision, (Fig. 5.132 - circle.)

Pelvis and Hips

The bony pelvis has been completely disrupted, with dislocation of the sacro-iliac joints (Fig. 5.133 - circles) and pubic symphysis (Fig. 5.134 - circle).

Two canopic packages are seen but no biological material within the pelvis (Fig. 5.135). One package contains resin soaked linen (white circle) the other appears granular and may be of clay and resin (black circle). The hip joints are congruous and show no sign of arthritis.

There is a mid-line structure, below the perineum, which is either the real phallus or a false phallus. It is difficult to be dogmatic as the structure is soaked in resin and has fractured in several places but is wrapped separately and does extend up to the perineum.

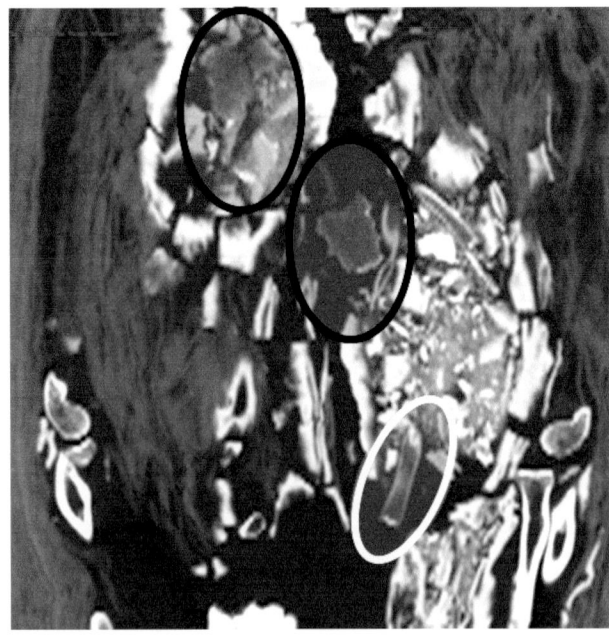

FIG. 5.128 CORONAL VIEW OF TRUNK - FRAGMENTS OF RIBS AND STERNUM

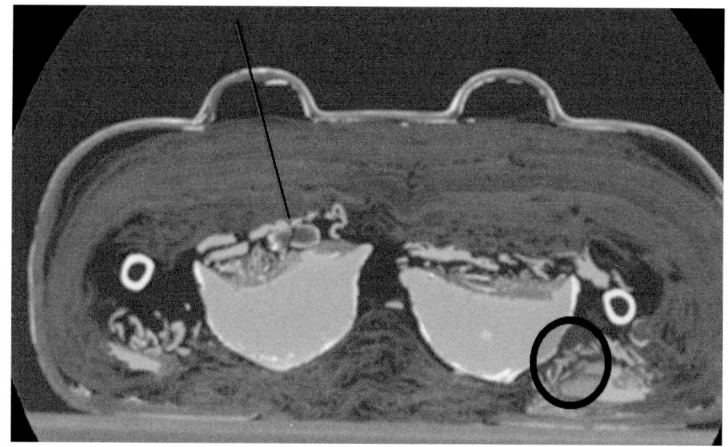

Fig. 5.129 Axial view of thorax - rib fragments and resin casts

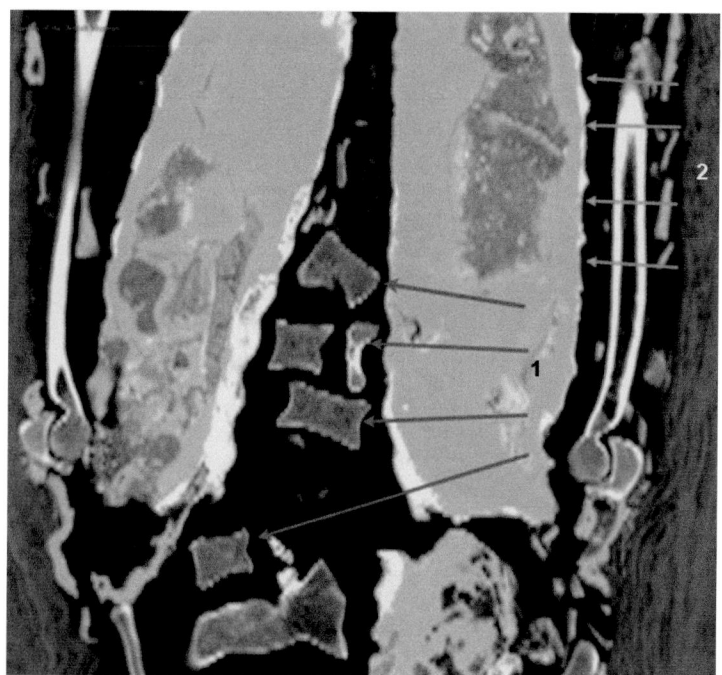

Fig. 5.130 Coronal view of thorax - vertebrae and resin casts

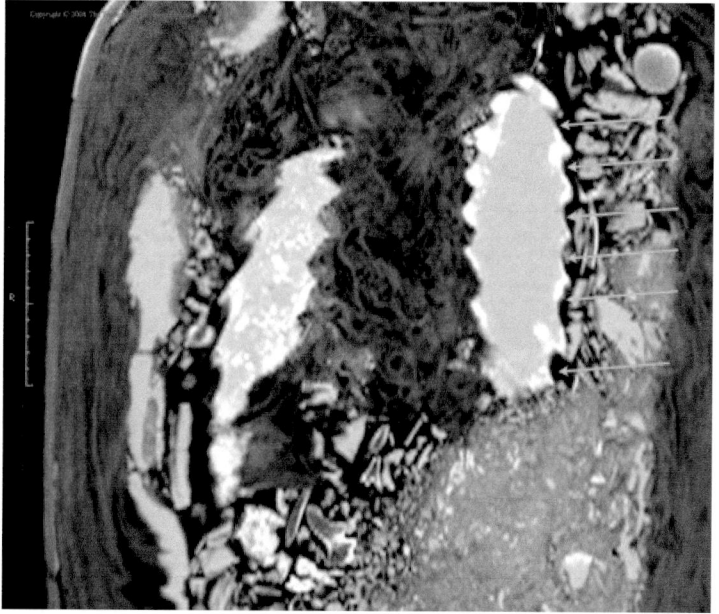

Fig. 5.131 Coronal view of thorax – indentations in the resin cast

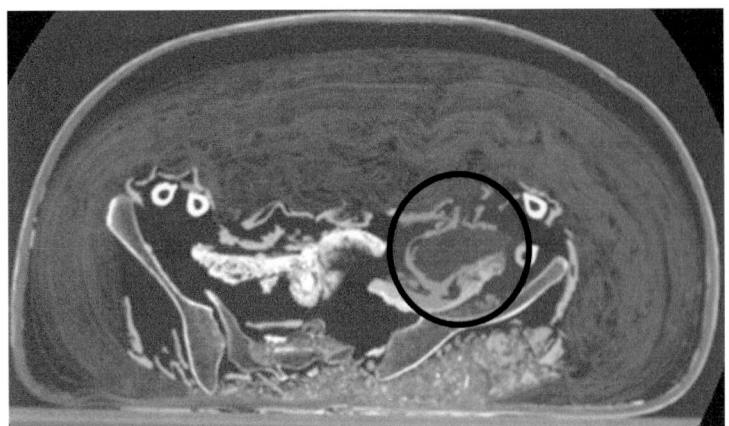

FIG. 5.132 AXIAL VIEW LOWER ABDOMEN - SHAPE OF LINEN FROM ABDOMINAL INCISION

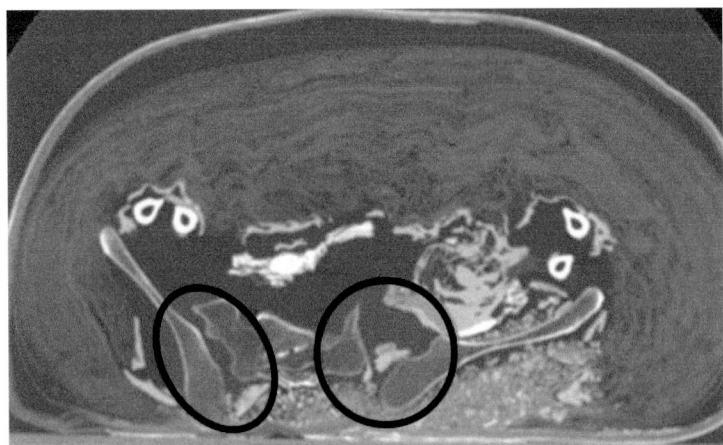

FIG. 5.133 AXIAL VIEW OF PELVIS - DISLOCATED SIJS

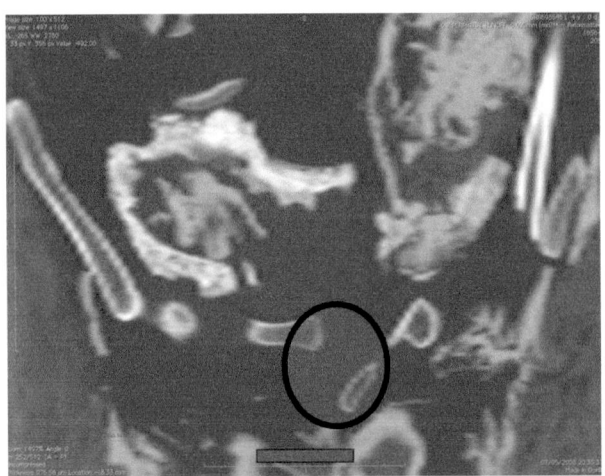

FIG. 5.134 CORONAL VIEW OF PELVIS - DISLOCATED SYMPHYSIS PUBIS

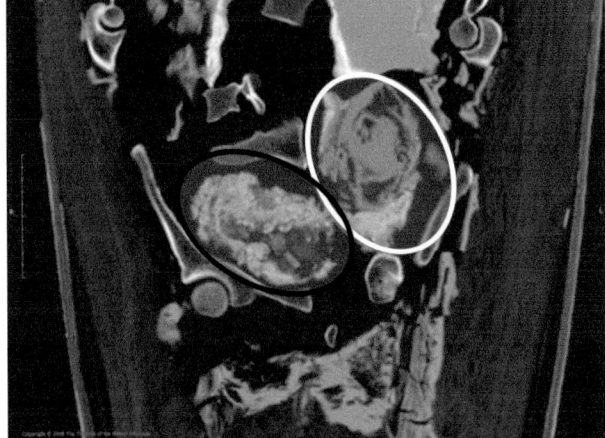

FIG. 5.135 CORONAL VIEW OF PELVIS AND LOWER ABDOMEN - CANOPIC PACKAGES

XXXI. Padiamunet - British Museum - (Accession No.EA6682)

Thorax

The thoracic wall, i.e. the rib cage, is largely intact. The left 1st rib has been removed from its normal position and lies free in the thorax (See Fig. 5.136). The sternum lies free within the thorax and is intact (See Fig. 5.137).

Within the thoracic cavity there is radio-dense, granular material bilaterally (Fig. 5.138 - arrows 2) which may be clay. There is, also, some lesser radio-dense material on top of this (See Fig. 5.138 - arrows 1). Finally, there is some material on the left side, which may well be biological in origin, i.e. viscera, (See Fig. 5.138 - arrow 3). Evidence of the superior mediastinum and the great vessels is seen (See Figs. 5.139 and 5.140) but there is no evidence of the heart.

Abdomen

There is a left flank incision as seen in Fig. 5.141 (between the lines). Further radio-dense material, which appears to be a mixture of clay and debris from the body wall, is present in the left side of the abdomen. The body wall itself has fragmented and fallen away from the inner surface of the bandaging (See Fig. 5.142 - 2 = body wall and 1 = inner surface of bandaging).

Pelvis and Hips

The bony pelvis is intact apart from a right SIJ subluxation that has occurred prior to the completion of mummification, as there is granular material within the joint (See Fig. 5.143). The hip joints are congruous with no evidence of arthritic change. The pelvic cavity contains resin and radio-dense material but no evidence of pelvic organs. The perineum is intact and a phallus can be clearly seen.

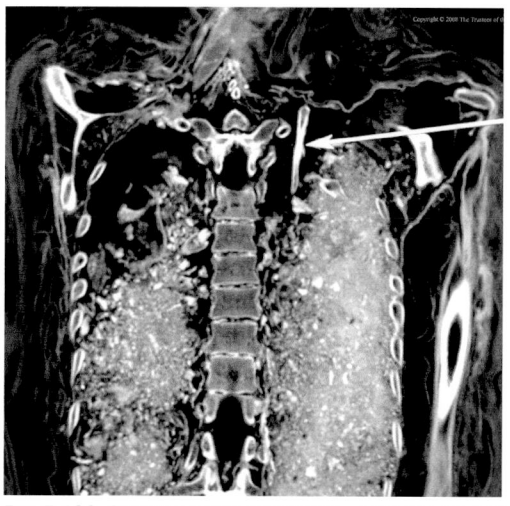

FIG. 5.136 CORONAL VIEW OF THORAX - LEFT 1ST RIB LYING FREE
COURTESY OF THE TRUSTEES OF THE BRITISH MUSEUM

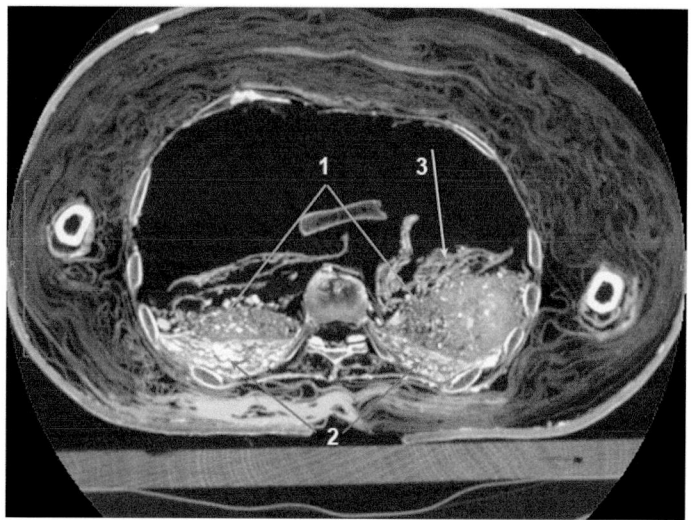

FIG. 5.138 AXIAL VIEW SHOWING MATERIAL WITHIN THE THORAX
COURTESY OF THE TRUSTEES OF THE BRITISH MUSEUM

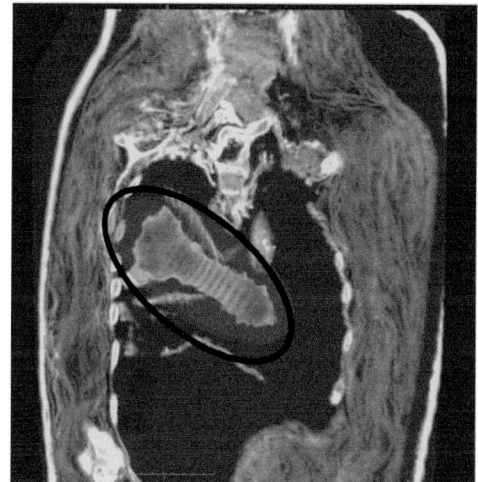

FIG. 5.137 CORONAL VIEW OF STERNUM LYING FREE WITHIN THE THORAX
COURTESY OF THE TRUSTEES OF THE BRITISH MUSEUM

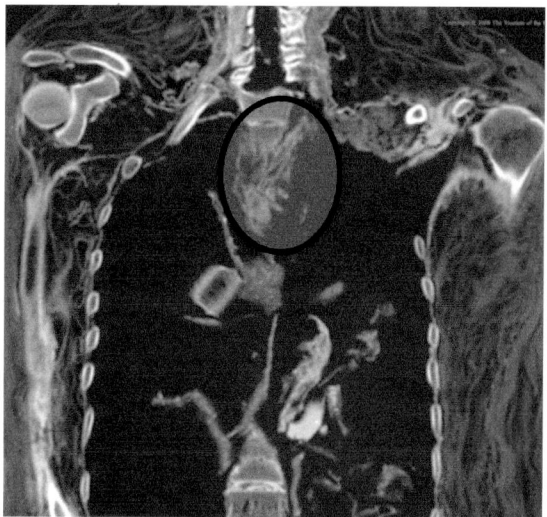

FIG. 5.139 CORONAL VIEW OF SUPERIOR MEDIASTINUM
COURTESY OF THE TRUSTEES OF THE BRITISH MUSEUM

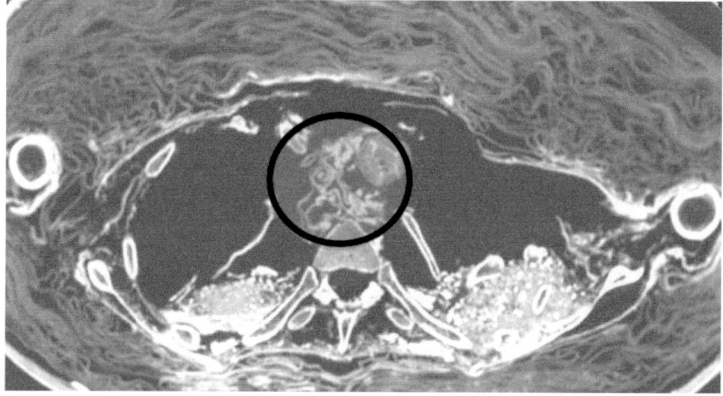

FIG. 5.140 AXIAL VIEW OF SUPERIOR MEDIASINUM
COURTESY OF THE TRUSTEES OF THE BRITISH MUSEUM

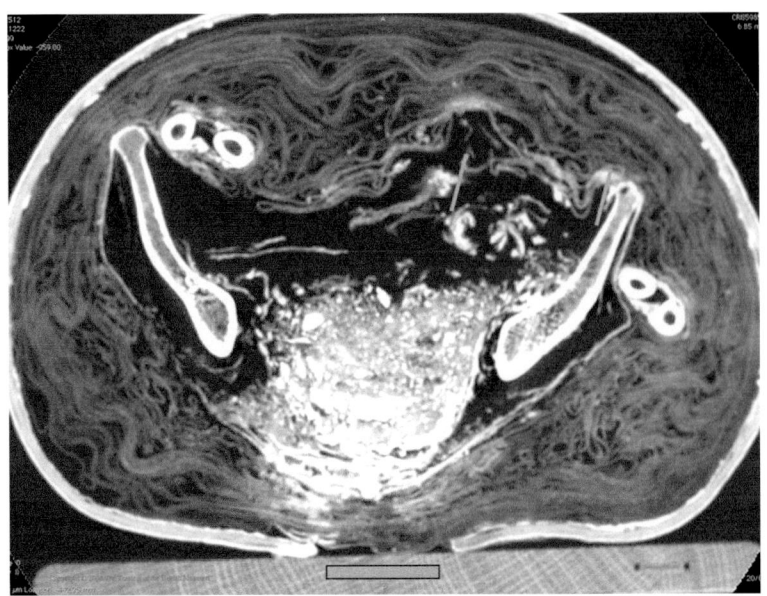

Fig. 5.141 Axial view of abdominal incision
Courtesy of the Trustees of the British Museum

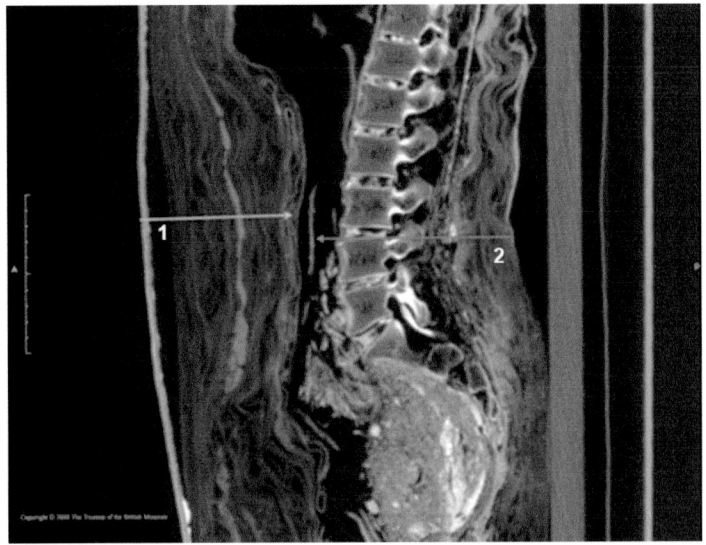

Fig. 5.142 Sagittal view of trunk showing compressed abdomen
Courtesy of the Trustees of the British Museum

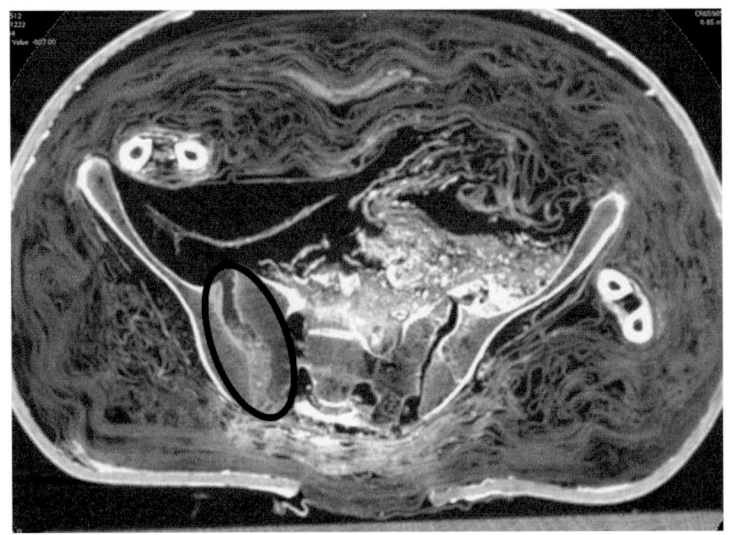

Fig. 5.143 Axial view of pelvis - subluxed right SIJ
Courtesy of the Trustees of the British Museum

XXXII. Tjayasetimu - British Museum (Accession No.EA20744)

Thorax

The thoracic wall is symmetrical and a normal shape with no evidence of fracture or dislocation of the ribs. The cavity is largely empty but remnants of the pleura and lungs are seen, the latter being desiccated, flattened and lying on the posterior wall (See Fig. 5.144). The diaphragm is also easily seen (See Fig. 5.145).

Abdomen

There is a left flank incision, through which linen has been packed (See Figs. 5.146 and 5.147). The abdomen has been eviscerated and the viscera returned as a package infiltrated with resin - circle in Fig. 5.149. A granular substance (possibly a mixture of resin and sawdust) fills the posterior abdominal cavity and loose viscera are seen lying anteriorly in the lower abdomen within the resin (See Figs. 5.148 and 5.149 arrows and Fig. 5.150).

Pelvis and Hips

The bony pelvis is intact with no disturbance of the sacro-iliac joints or symphysis pubis.

The pelvic cavity is almost empty, the abdominal packing having terminated at the pelvic brim. However there are a few outlines of organs in the cavity with the most prominent being a structure that is almost certainly the uterus (See Fig. 5.151).

The perineum is intact and has not been used as an evisceration route.

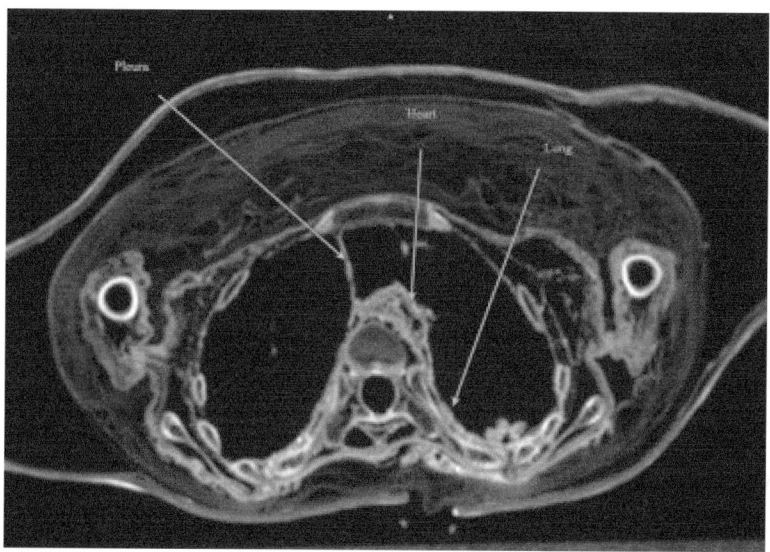

FIG. 5.144 AXIAL VIEW OF THORAX -REMNANTS OF VISCERA
COURTESY OF THE TRUSTEES OF THE BRITISH MUSEUM

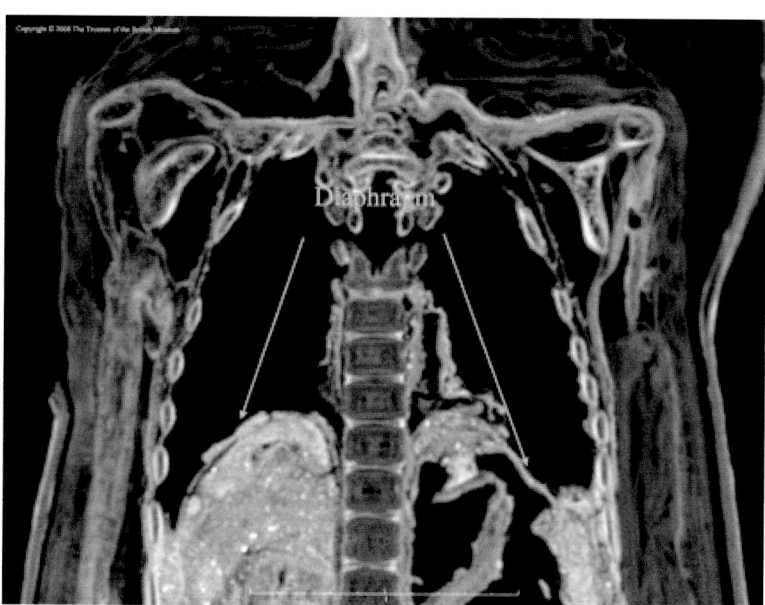

FIG. 5.145 CORONAL VIEW OF THORAX SHOWING DIAPHRAGMS
COURTESY OF THE TRUSTEES OF THE BRITISH MUSEUM

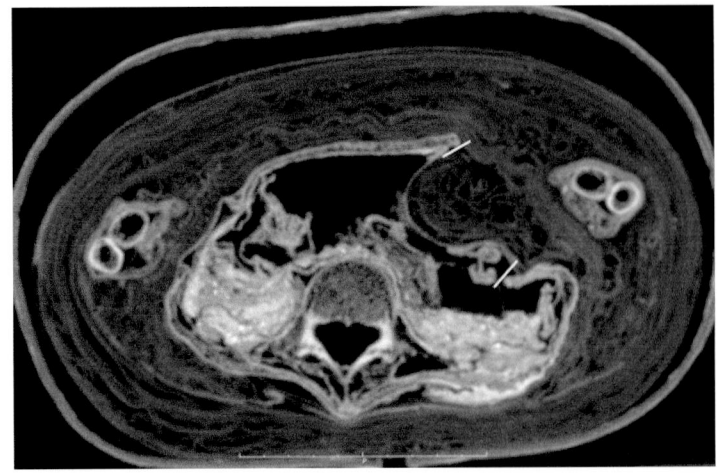

Fig. 5.146 Axial view showing abdominal incision
Courtesy of the Trustees of the British Museum

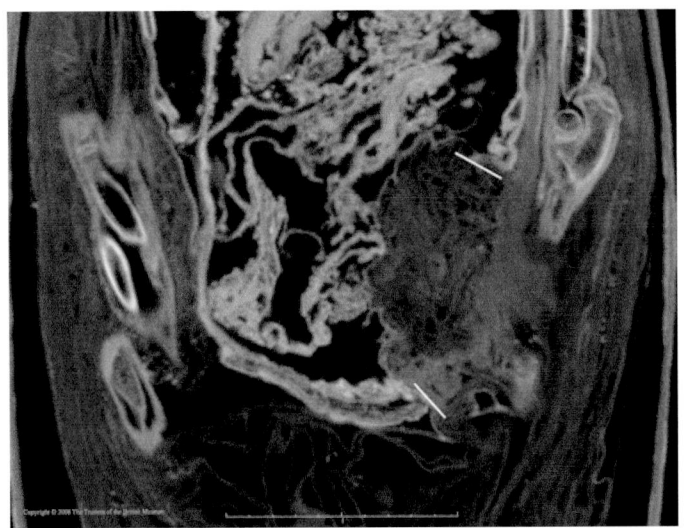

Fig. 5.147 Coronal view of abdominal incision
Courtesy of the Trustees of the British Museum

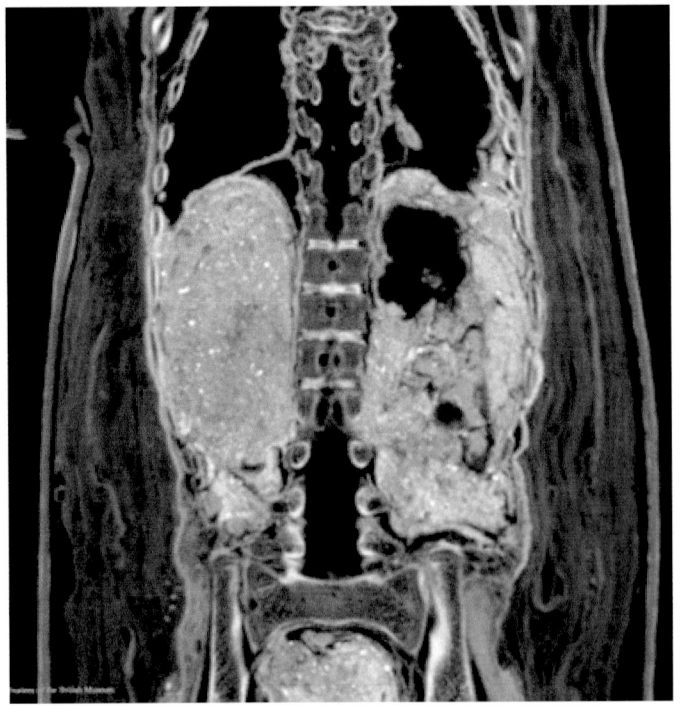

Fig. 5.148 Coronal view showing material within abdomen
Courtesy of the Trustees of the British Museum

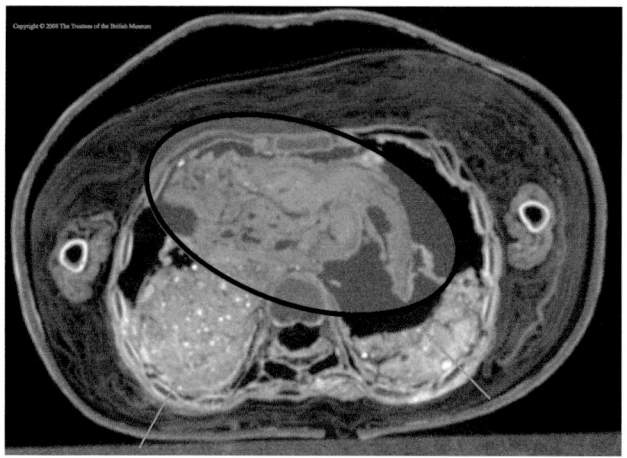

FIG. 5.149 AXIAL VIEW SHOWING MATERIAL WITHIN ABDOMEN
COURTESY OF THE TRUSTEES OF THE BRITISH MUSEUM

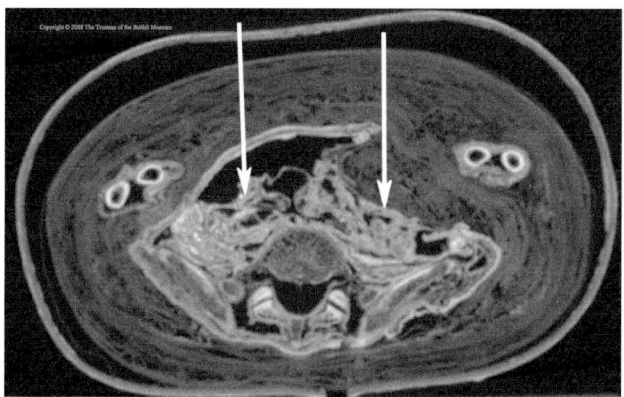

FIG. 5.150 AXIAL VIEW OF LOWER ABDOMEN - VISCERA
COURTESY OF THE TRUSTEES OF THE BRITISH MUSEUM

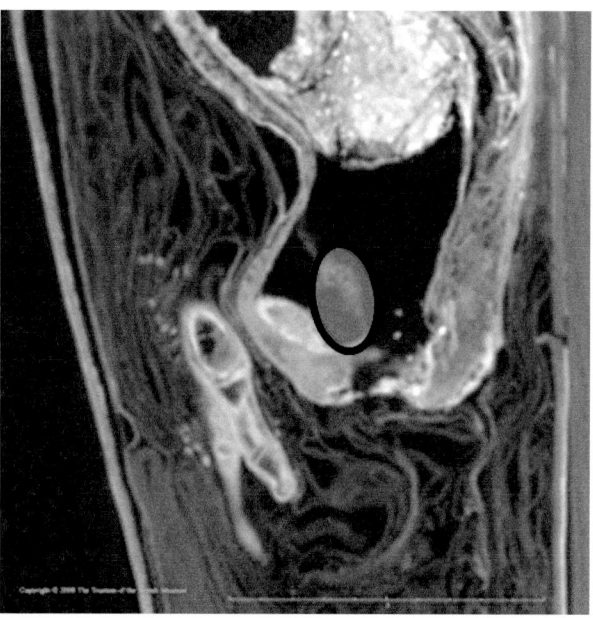

FIG. 5.151 SAGITTAL VIEW SHOWING AN ORGAN WITHIN PELVIS
- POSSIBLY UTERUS
COURTESY OF THE TRUSTEES OF THE BRITISH MUSEUM

XXXIII. Tjenmutengebtiu - British Museum - (Accession No. EA 22939)

Thorax

The chest wall is intact and symmetrical with no dislocations of the posterior ends of the ribs. There are, however, undisplaced postero-lateral fractures of the right 3rd to 8th ribs. No sign of healing of these fractures is observed, indicating that they occurred either shortly before death or post-mortem. Fig. 5.152 shows the fractures of the 6th, 7th and 8th ribs – arrows.

Evisceration of the thorax has been thorough, with no remaining evidence of the mediastinum or its contents. The thoracic viscera along with those of the abdomen have been returned to the body cavity in five canopic packages (See Fig. 5.153). The package in the right upper thorax contains facetted amorphous objects measuring approximately 1.5 to 2.0 cms in diameter. There are nine or ten such objects - possibly gall stones (See Fig. 5.154 and 5.155).

The diaphragm is absent.

Abdomen

There is a left flank incision, which has been covered with a metal plate (See Fig. 5.156 - arrow). Linen passes through the incision into the abdominal cavity (See Fig. 5.156 – lines).

Abdominal evisceration has been thorough and the viscera returned to the body cavity in canopic packages, as mentioned in the section on the thorax. As with several places in the thorax, there is a thin layer of granular radio dense material on the posterior wall of the abdomen (See Fig. 5.157).

Pelvis and Hips

The bony pelvis is intact with normal sacro-iliac joints and pubic symphysis. The hip joints are normal with a reasonably good covering of articular cartilage on the femoral head (Fig. 5.158 - arrow 2) and the acetabulum (Fig. 5.158 - arrow 1). The pelvic cavity is largely empty, the linen from the abdomen stopping approximately at the pelvic brim (Fig. 5.159 - arrow 1). There are a few folds of linen within the pelvis (Fig. 5.159- arrow 2) and a metal amulet over the perineum (Fig. 5.159 - arrow 3). The soft tissues of the perineum remain in situ. The perineal route has not been used for evisceration.

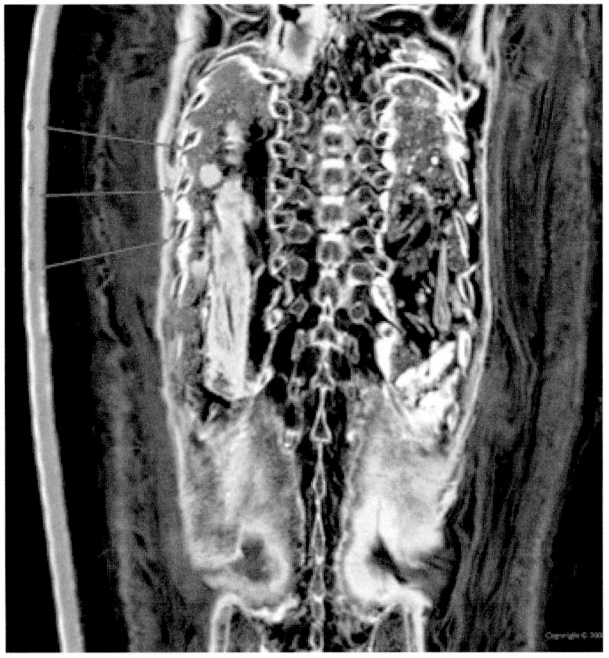

Fig. 5.152 Coronal view of trunk - fractured right ribs
Courtesy of the Trustees of the British Museum

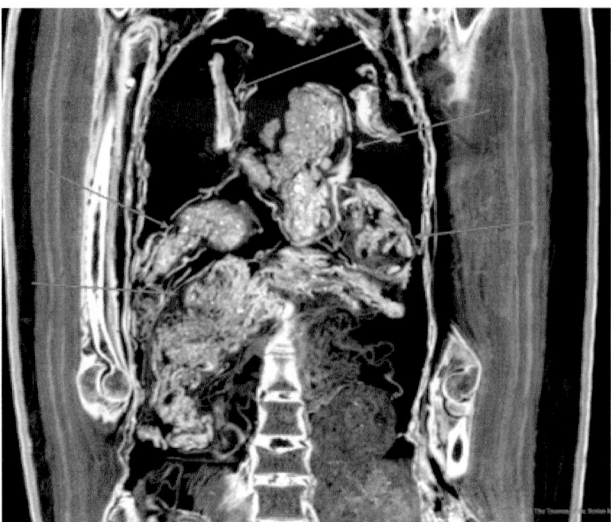

Fig. 5.153 Coronal view of trunk - canopic packages
Courtesy of the Trustees of the British Museum

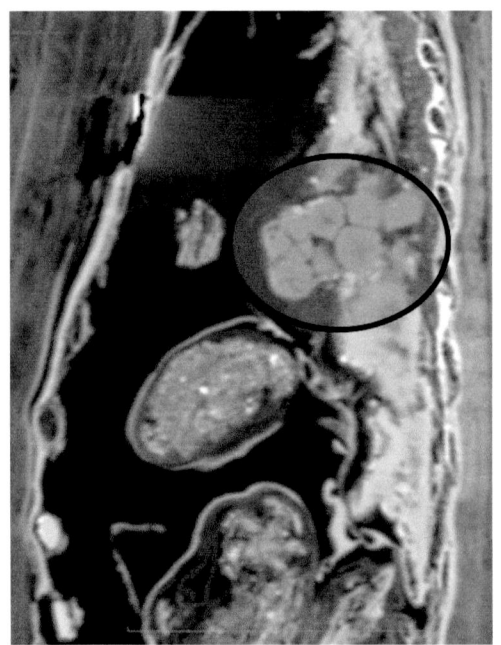

Fig. 5.154 Sagittal view of thorax - facetted objects – probably gallstones
Courtesy of the Trustees of the British Museum

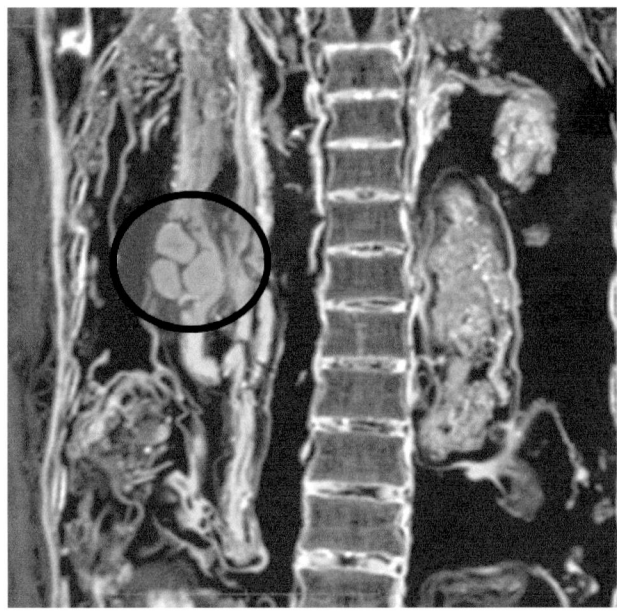

Fig. 5.155 Coronal view of thorax - facetted objects – probably gallstones
Courtesy of the Trustees of the British Museum

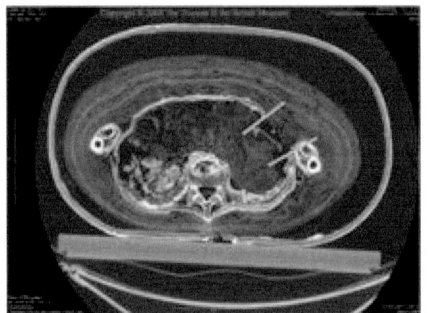

Fig. 5.156 Axial view showing abdominal incision and incision plate
Courtesy of the Trustees of the British Museum

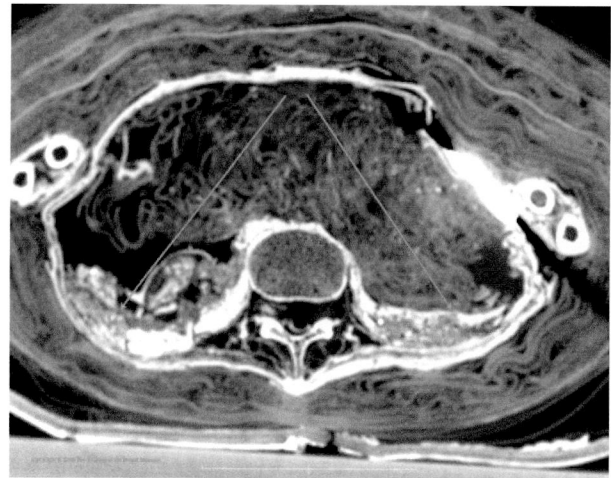

FIG. 5.157 Axial view of abdomen demonstrating material on posterior wall

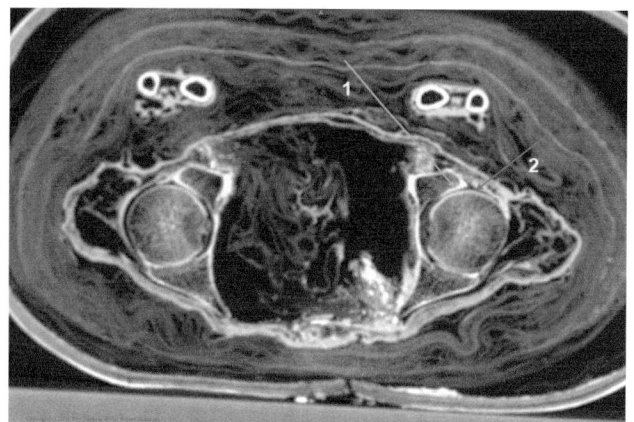

FIG. 5.158 Axial view of pelvis - left hip joint articular cartilage

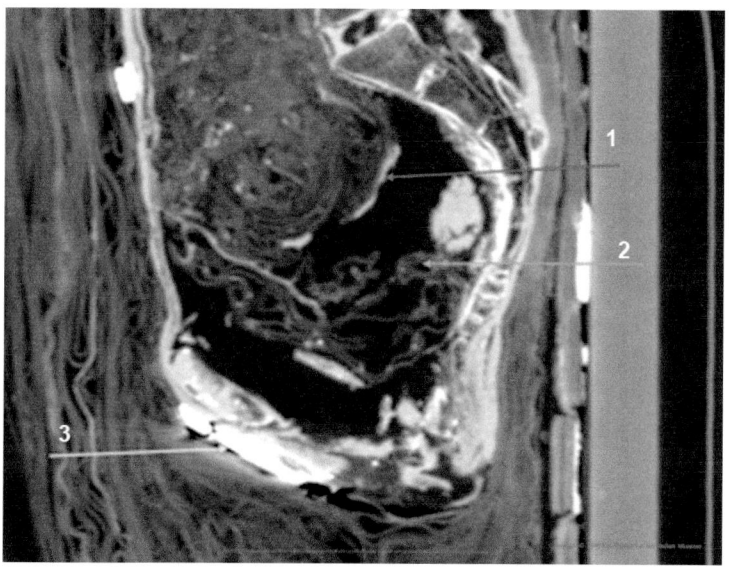

FIG. 5.159 Sagittal view showing pelvic contents and plate over perineum
Courtesy of the Trustees of the British Museum

XXXIV. Unnamed - British Museum - (Accession No. EA 25258)

Thorax

There has been complete evisceration of the thorax with removal of the mediastinum and its contents. A small amount of radio dense material remains lying on the posterior wall of the thorax, which may be resin. The viscera have been returned but are not in discreet packages.

The rib cage is intact. There is no evidence of the diaphragm.

Abdomen

There is a left flank incision, through which linen crosses. This incision is partly closed with a pack of granular material, possibly clay (See Fig. 5.160). As stated above, evisceration has been thorough and the viscera have been returned to the body cavity without packaging.

Pelvis and Hips

Slight subluxation of the left sacro-iliac joint is seen, but this is almost certainly post-mortem. The bony pelvis is abnormal in that there are fractures of the superior margins of the acetabula (Fig. 5.161) and both inferior pubic rami (Fig. 5.162). The pubic symphysis is intact.

The pelvic cavity has been eviscerated and packed with material of two different radio densities. The pelvic floor (i.e. the perineum) is intact.

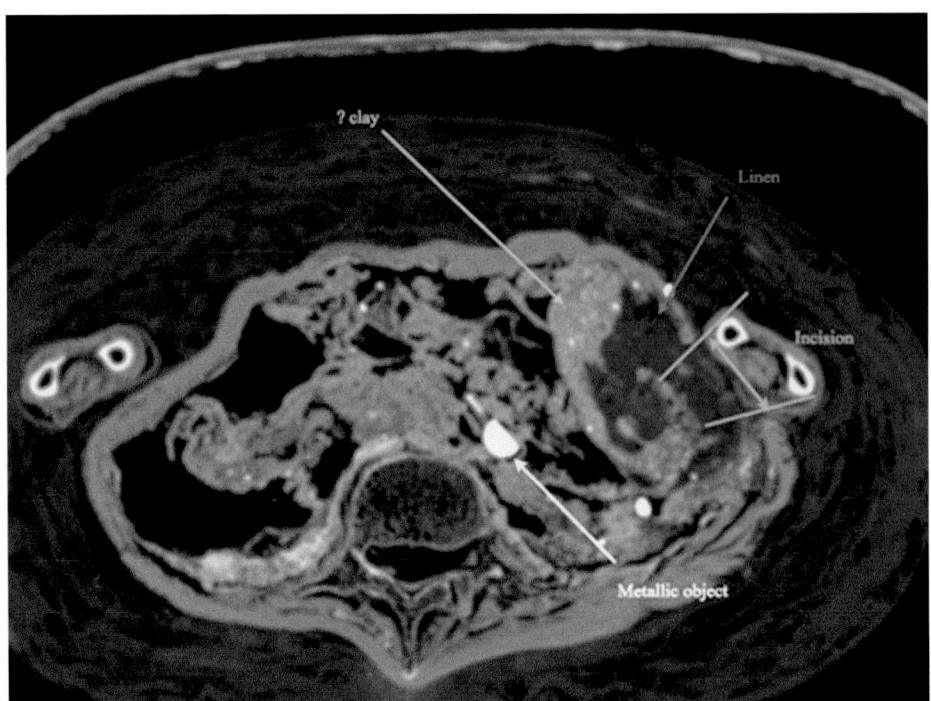

Fig. 5.160 Axial view showing abdominal incision and contents
Courtesy of the Trustees of the British Museum

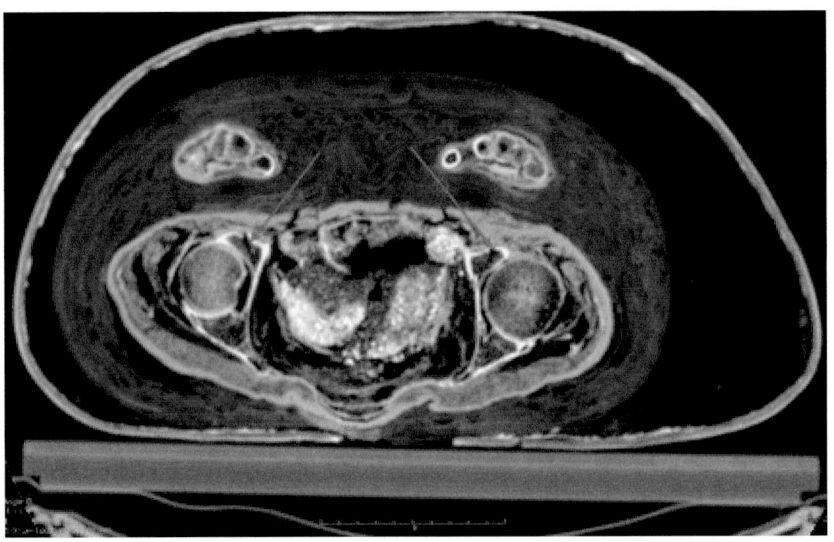

Fig. 5.161 Axial view of pelvis - acetabular fractures
Courtesy of the Trustees of the British Museum

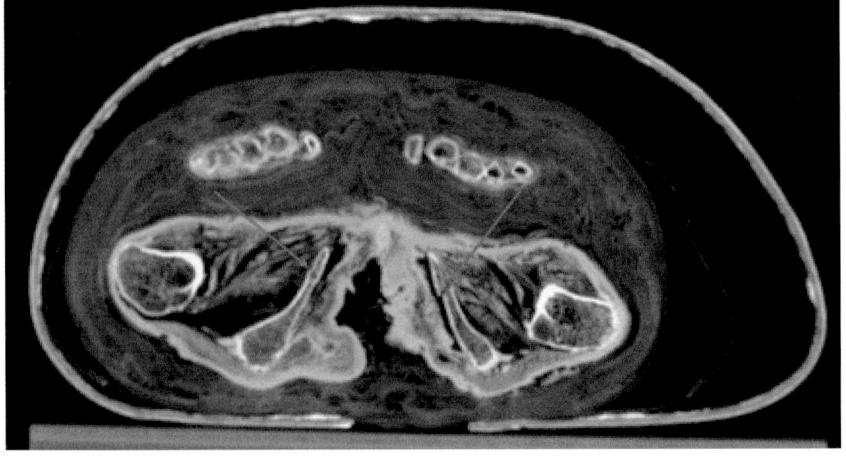

Fig. 5.162 Axial view of pelvis - fractured inferior pubic rami
Courtesy of the Trustees of the British Museum

XXXVI. Unnamed. - Bern (AE 9)

Thorax

The rib cage is a normal shape with no dislocations or fractures of the ribs. The mediastinum is detached from the sternum, but there is a structure in the mid-line which is almost certainly biological tissue (probably heart and great vessels) - Fig. 5.163 - arrow 2.

A layer of resin is seen in the posterior part of the thorax on both sides with two canopic packages in the right side of the chest - arrows 1 and one in the left side - arrow 3 (See Fig. 5.163).

Abdomen

A left sided flank incision is noted with linen protruding through it into the abdominal cavity (See Fig. 5.164). Evisceration has been complete with no evidence of returned loose viscera within the cavity.

Pelvis and Hips

Some disruption of the left SIJ and the pubic symphysis is seen but this is probably secondary to mummification (See Figs. 5.165 and 5.166 - circles). The pelvic organs are absent and the cavity filled with a linen pack. Evisceration has been complete with no evidence of returned loose viscera within the cavity. There is evidence of a phallus seen in cross section within circle in Fig. 5.167.

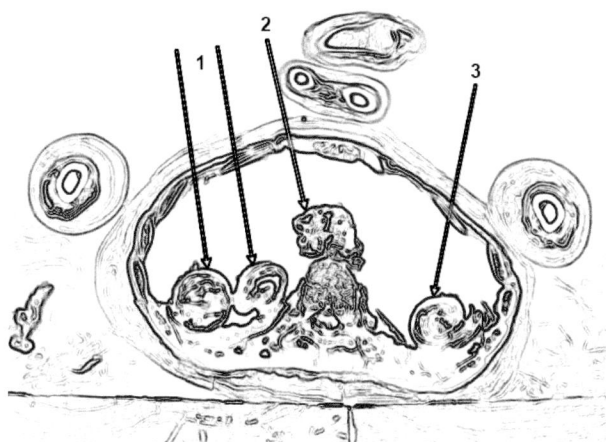

FIG. 5.163 Axial view of thorax - mediastinum and canopic packages. (After IEM image)

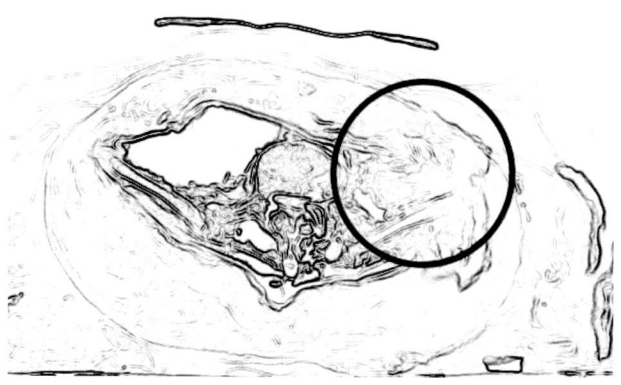

FIG. 5.164 Axial view showing abdominal incision (**After IEM** image)

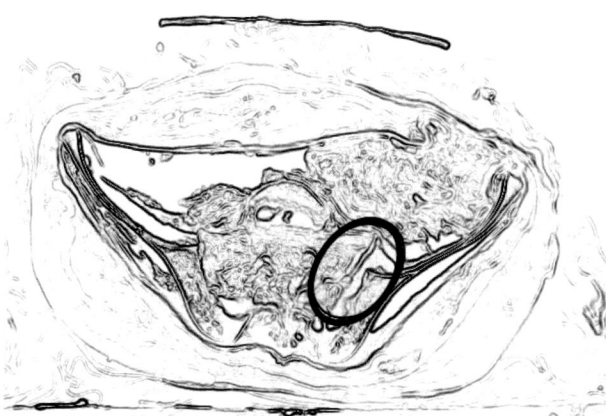

FIG. 5.165 Axial view of pelvis - disrupted left SIJ (After IEM image)

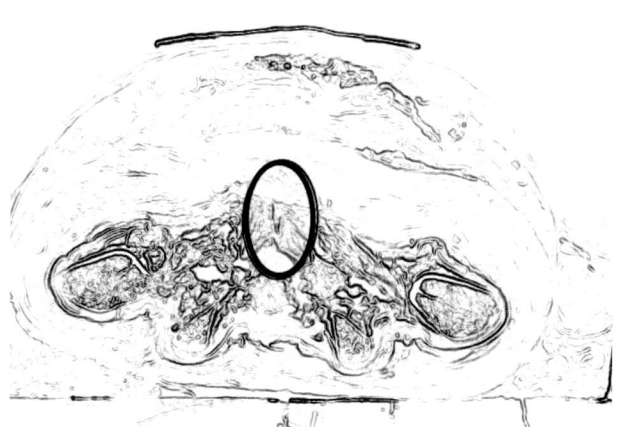

FIG. 5.166 Axial view of pelvis - disrupted pubic symphysis (After IEM image)

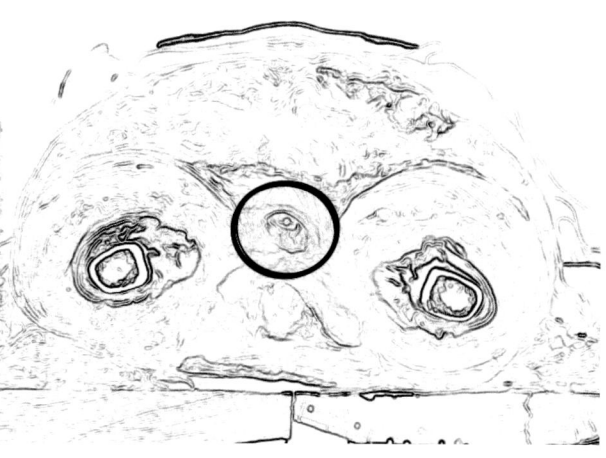

FIG. 5.167 Axial view inferior to pelvis - cross section of phallus (After IEM image)

XXXVIII. Shepenese - St. Gallen (no Number).

Thorax

The rib cage is intact and a normal shape having no fractures or posterior dislocations. The mediastinum is in situ and contains the heart (Fig. 5.168), great vessels (Fig. 5.169) remnants of lungs and both hemi-diaphragms (See Fig. 5.170).

The thoracic cavity is, largely, filled with low radio-dense granular material (possibly clay) and contains two canopic packages of granular radio-dense material in the upper thorax, lying on either side of the spine (See Fig. 5.171).

Superior to the left package, there is a regular, cuboid object with appearances similar to wood (See arrow 2). In the posterior aspect of the right 9th rib there is a small regular hole measuring 0.5 x 2.5 cms, probably a recent bone biopsy site (see Fig. 5.173).

Abdomen

The left flank incision, measures about 11.5 cms in length and is crossed by linen packing. Evisceration has been thorough and performed via both the abdominal incision and a perineal approach. The latter has been closed with a linen pack (Fig. 5.174 - circle). No organs remain.

Pelvis and Hips

The bony pelvis is intact, but contains no organs. There is a void where the bladder normally sits. The hip joints are intact and show a layer of articular cartilage indicating relative youth (See Fig. 5.175).

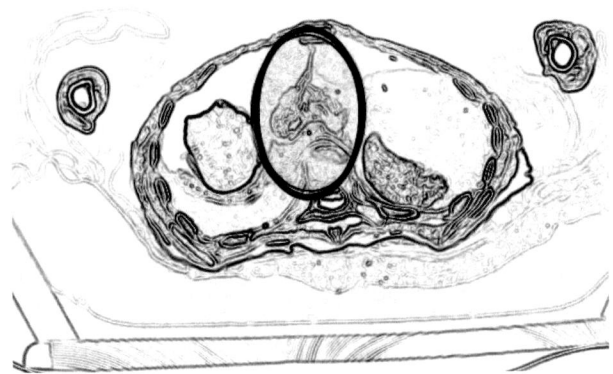

Fig. 5.168 Axial view of thorax - mediastinum (After IEM image)

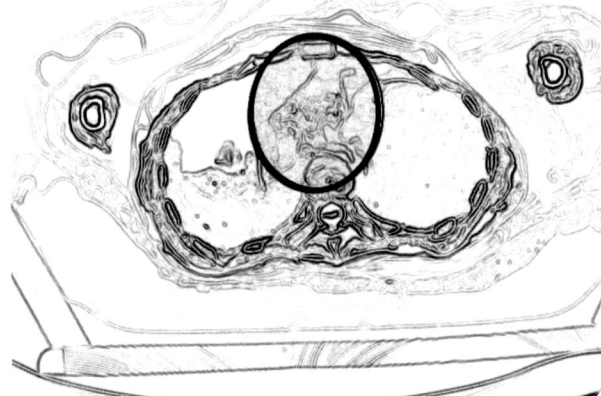

Fig. 5.169 Axial view of thorax - mediastinum and great vessels (After IEM image)

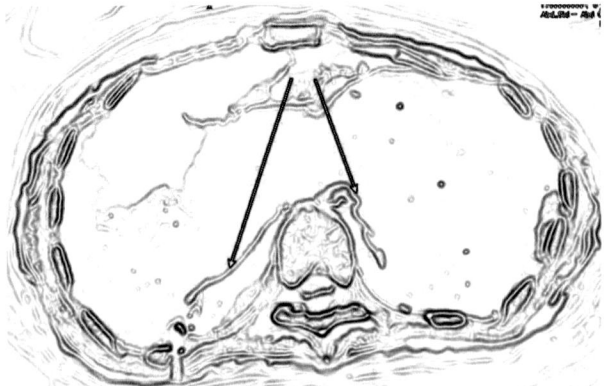

Fig. 5.170 Axial view of thorax demonstrating diaphragm (After IEM image)

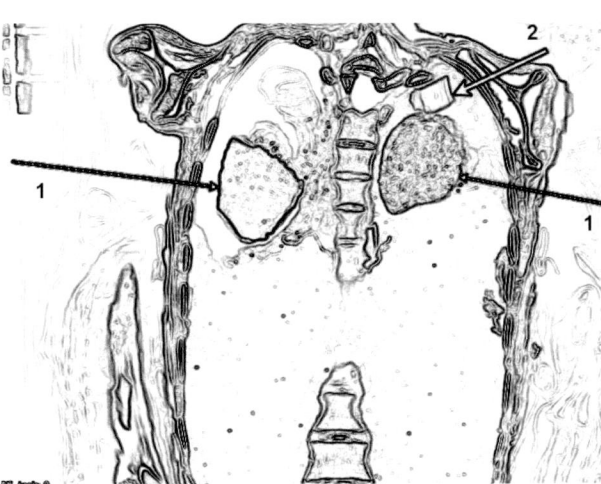

Fig. 5.171 Axial view of lower thorax - probable canopic packages (After IEM image)

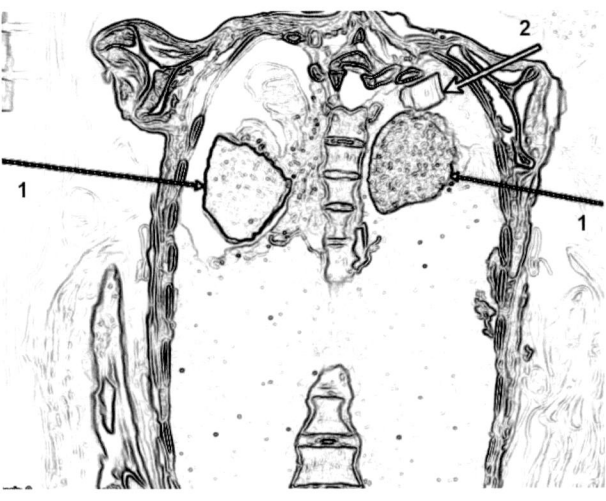

Fig. 5.172 Coronal view of thorax - canopic packages and 'cuboid' structure (After IEM image)

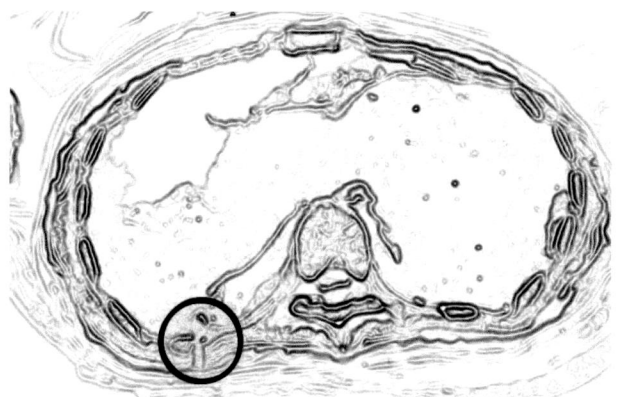

Fig. 5.173 Axial view of lower thorax - biopsy site in right rib posteriorly (After IEM image)

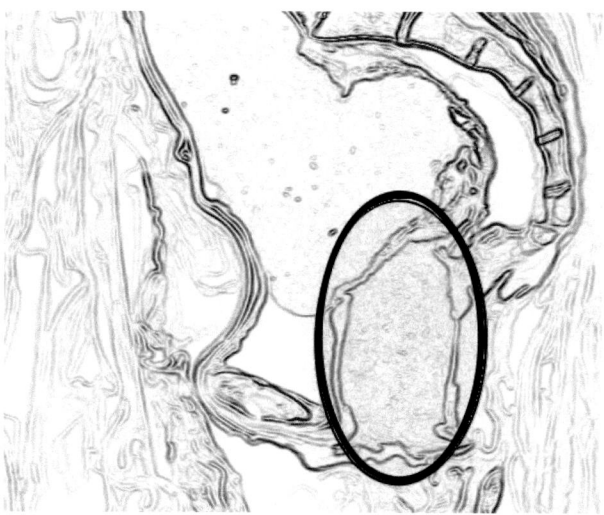

Fig. 5.174 Sagittal view of pelvis - linen pack in perineum (After IEM image)

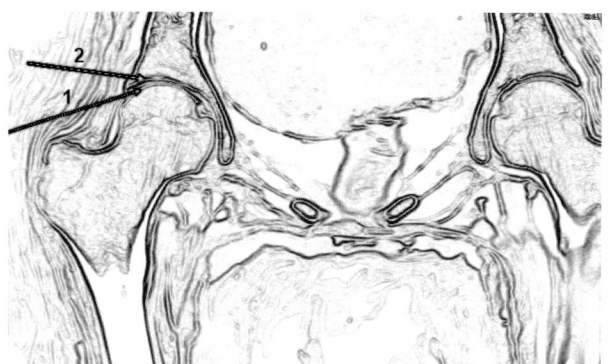

Fig. 5.175 Coronal view of pelvis showing hip joints (After IEM image)

XXXIX. Unnamed - St. Gallen (Cat. No.C3530)

Thorax

Whilst the spinal disruption ceases in the thoracic region, the upper ribs are disorganised anteriorly with the right 1st rib significantly displaced (See Fig. 5.176). The sternum lies posteriorly near the spine (See Fig. 5.177).

There are remnants of midline structures (not a true mediastinum) and some 'biological' tissue (See Fig.5.178 - arrows 1), lying on a layer of radio-dense granular material in the paraspinal gutters (Fig.5.178 - arrows 2). Whilst there are no canopic packages, the returned viscera lie between layers of the granular material. There is no evidence of the diaphragm.

Abdomen

There is a left flank incision measuring some 9.4 cms in length but no linen crosses this incision (See Fig. 5.179. - black lines). The abdomen is filled with a mixture of returned viscera (Fig. 5.179 - circle on the left), clay and resin (Fig. 5.179 - circle on the right).

Pelvis and Hips

The sacro-iliac joints are intact, with diastasis of the pubic symphysis (See Fig. 5.180 - circle). The hips are normal. There are no organs within the pelvis. The perineum has been disrupted to gain access to the pelvic cavity. Hence, there are no external genitalia.

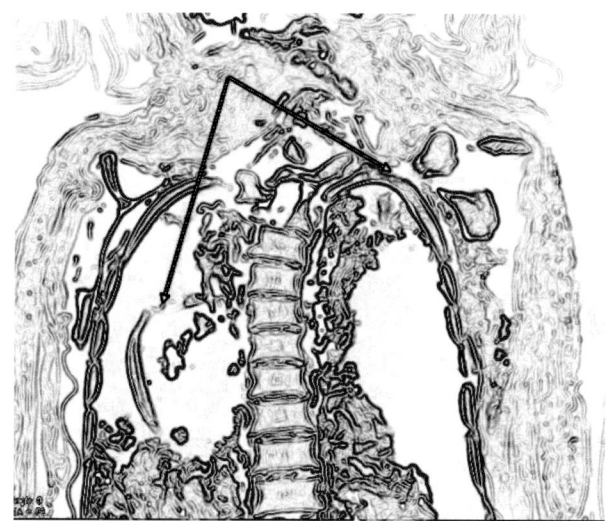

Fig. 5.176 Coronal view of thorax - comparison of 1st ribs (After IEM image)

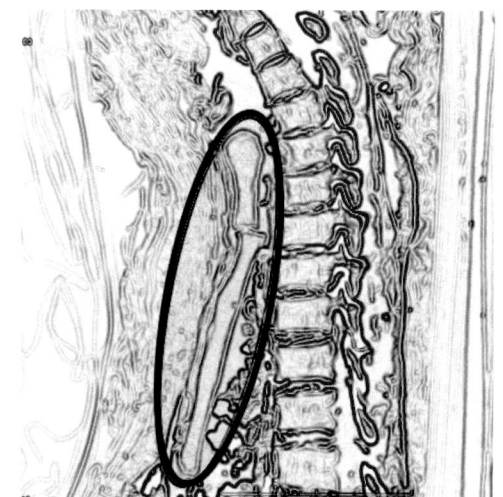

Fig. 5.177 Sagittal view of thorax - posterior position of sternum (After IEM image)

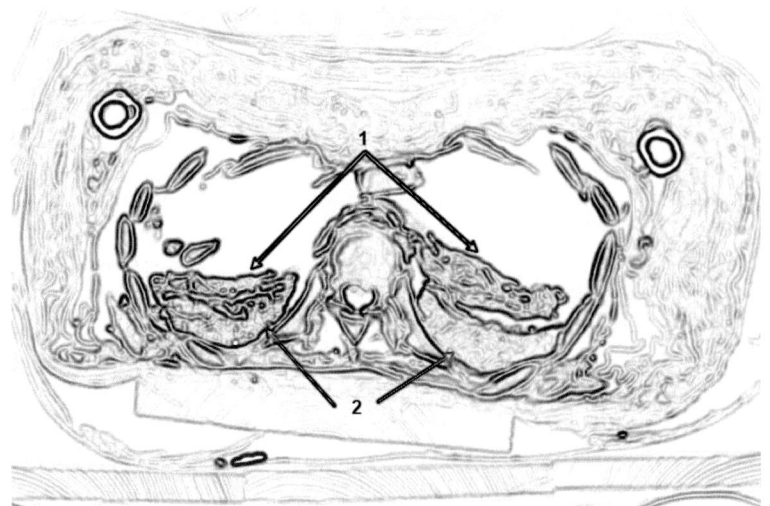

Fig. 5.178 Axial view of thorax - tissues and material on posterior wall (After IEM image)

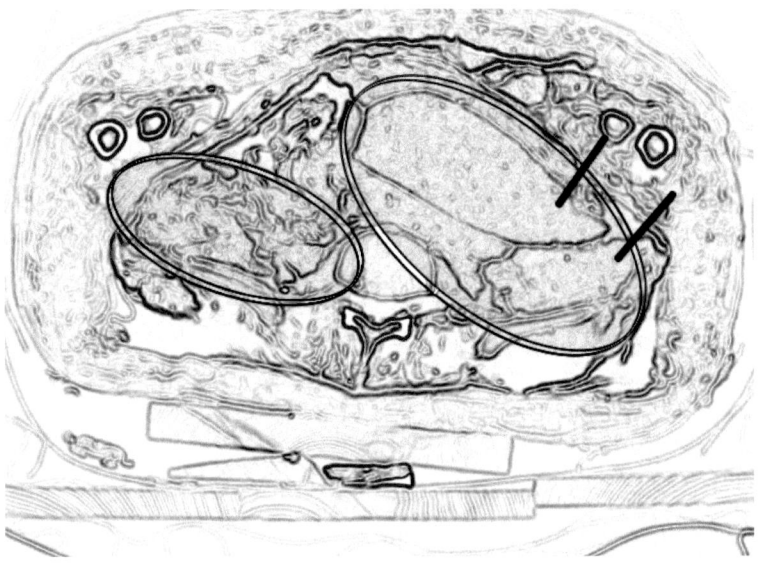

Fig. 5.179 Axial view - viscera and material in abdomen (After IEM image) (After IEM image)

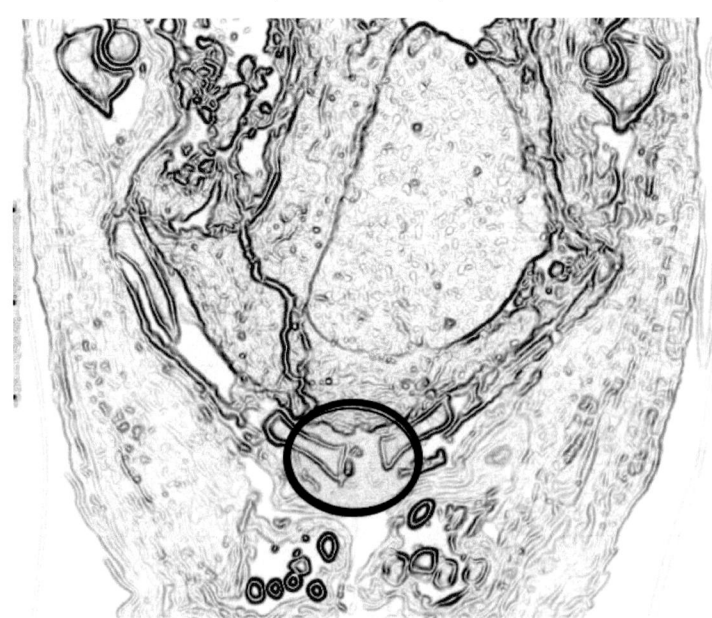

Fig. 5.180 Coronal view of pelvis - disruption of symphysis pubis (After IEM image)

XL. Unnamed - Lausanne (Cat. No.492)

Thorax

The rib cage is intact, with no evidence of compression. The mediastinum remains in situ with a large heart with a massive ventricle (See Fig. 5.181; arrow). Whether this is pathological or the result of desiccation is unknown, however, the more common feature of desiccation is to make the heart smaller and contracted. This would favour an interpretation of pathology.

The left hemi-thorax is empty, but on the right side, there is a series of fibrotic bands such as those seen in post inflammatory adhesions, although several of these structures could well represent the outlines of the lobes of the right lung (See circle in Fig.5.181). The hemi-diaphragms are seen below the heart with an intact right hemi-diaphragm and a small hole in the periphery of the left hemi-diaphragm (arrows in Fig. 5.182) measuring only 1.5 x1.0 cms. This would be too small to admit a hand, but would admit a hooked instrument, which could have been used to cut through the root of the left lung and hence allow its removal after collapse. This could explain how the other thoracic structures remained in place.

Abdomen

No evidence of a left flank incision is identified, but evisceration has been performed and the viscera returned to the abdominal cavity. These are seen within the circles in Fig. 5.183.

Although there is no flank incision, there are one or two defects in the supra-pubic region, which could represent incisions. These are seen in Figs. 5.184, 5.185 and 5.186 - arrows and in Fig. 5.187, arrows and circles.

Pelvis and Hips

The bony pelvis is intact. The hip joints are congruous and show no evidence of arthritis. There is a very small cyst in the sub-chondral region of the left acetabular superior rim, measuring 3x1 mms. It penetrates the articular cartilage in one region, measuring 1 mm. This is unlikely to be of significance in terms of degenerative change.

The pelvic organs remain in situ, with the perineal orifices visible (See Fig. 5.188 - Urethra=3, Vagina=2, Anus=1). It is of note that, although the viscera have been returned to the body cavity, the anterior body wall has been compressed against the spine.

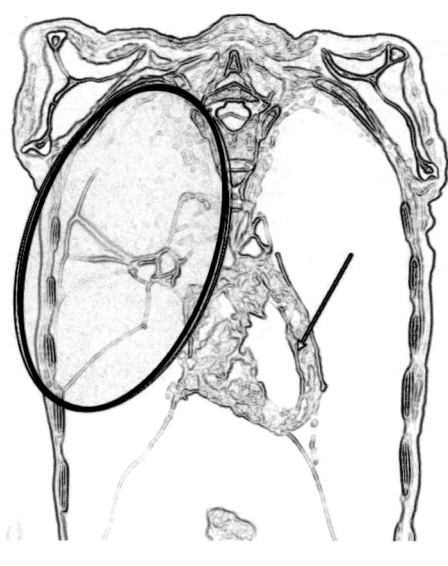

FIG. 5.181 CORONAL VIEW OF THORAX - OUTLINE OF RIGHT LUNG AND DILATED HEART (AFTER IEM IMAGE)

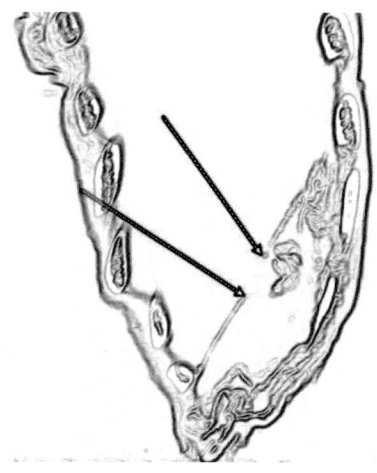

FIG. 5.182 SAGITTAL VIEW OF THORAX - DEFECT IN DIAPHRAGM (AFTER IEM IMAGE)

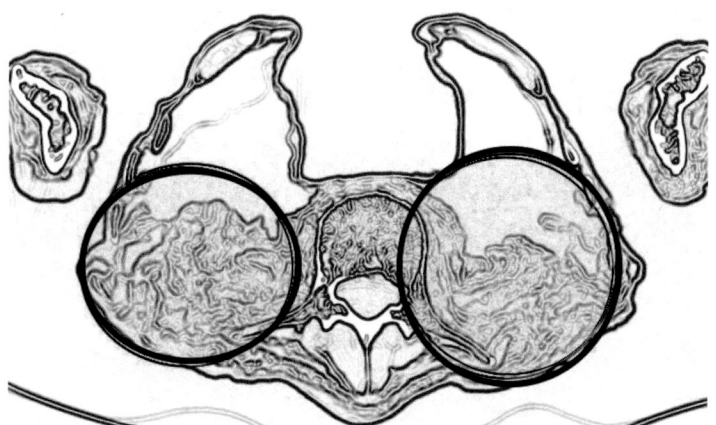

FIG. 5.183 AXIAL VIEW SHOWING VISCERA WITHIN THE ABDOMINAL CAVITY (AFTER IEM IMAGE)

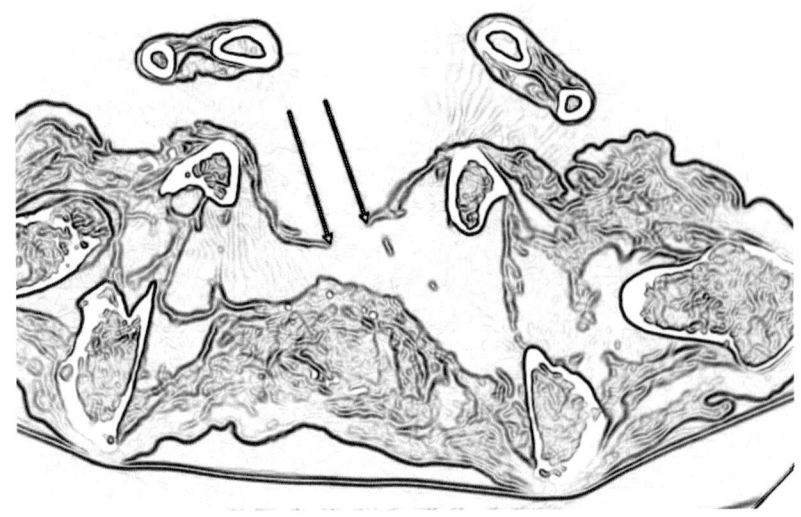

Fig. 5.184 Axial view of lower abdomen - lower abdominal wall defect (incision)

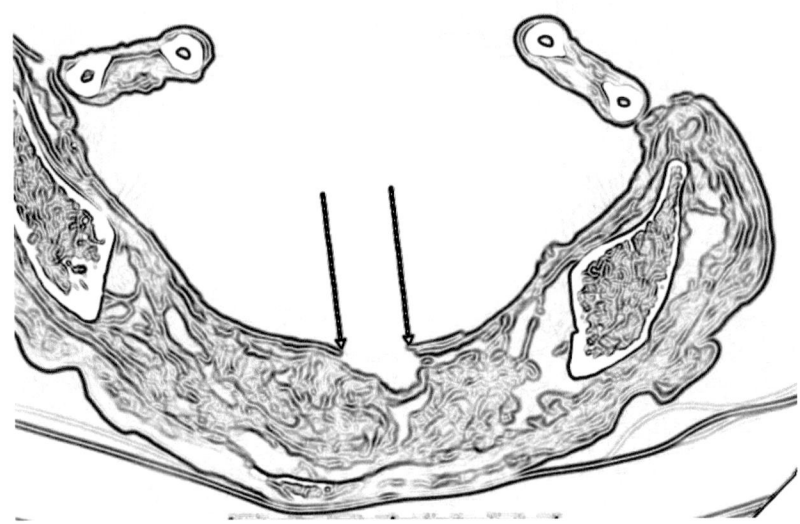

Fig. 5.185 Axial view of lower abdomen - lower abdominal wall defect (incision) (After IEM image)

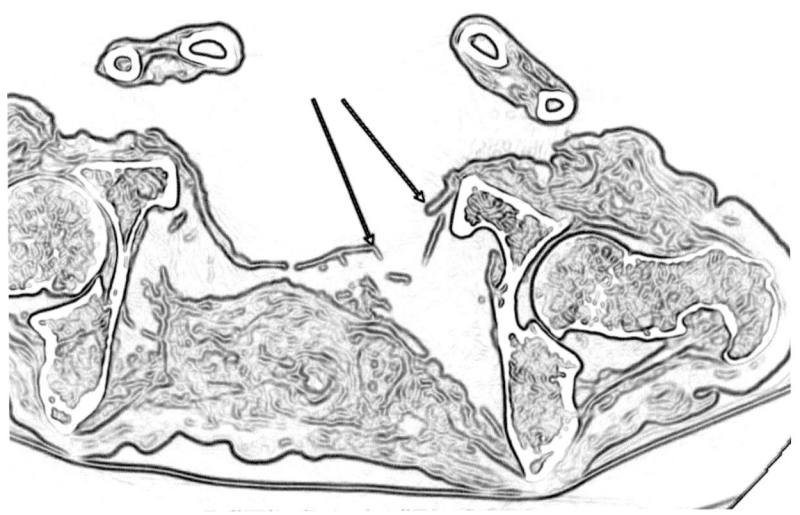

Fig. 5.186 Axial view of lower abdomen - lower abdominal wall defect (incision) (After IEM image)

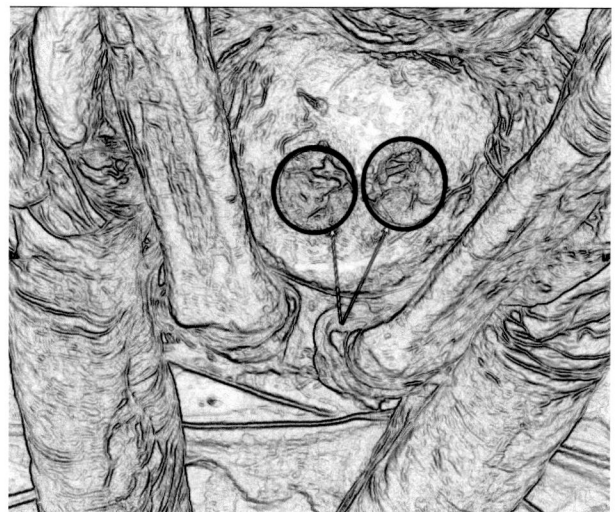

FIG. 5.187 3D RECONSTRUCTION - LOWER ABDOMINAL WALL DEFECTS

XLI. Unnamed child - Lenzburg (Cat. No.K-10351)

Thorax

The rib cage is a normal shape (See Fig. 5.189).

There has been complete evisceration of the thorax with no evidence of the mediastinum or its contents. The thorax is packed with linen (See Fig. 5.189).

There is no evidence of the diaphragm.

Abdomen

There is a left flank incision, which is more posterior than usual in its upper part. It measures some 7.5 cms. in length

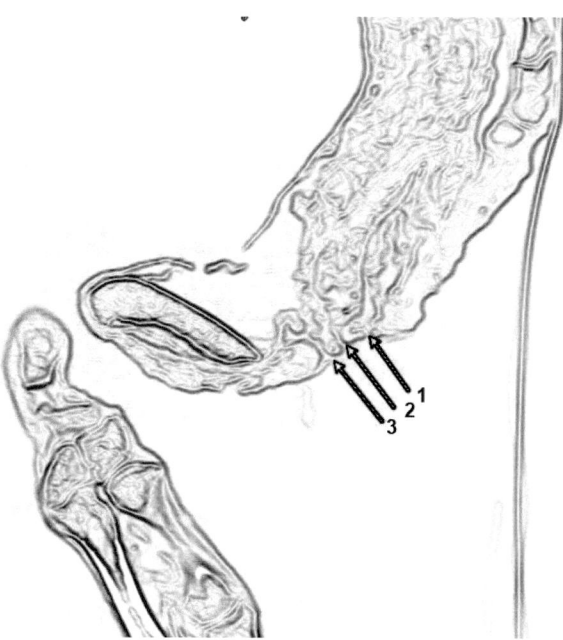

FIG. 5.188 SAGITTAL VIEW OF PELVIS - PERINEAL STRUCTURES

(See Fig. 5.190. - lines). Evisceration is complete with no viscera returned to the cavity, which is packed with linen.

Pelvis and Hips

The bony pelvis and hip joints are intact. The pelvic cavity is completely empty, the linen packing being restricted to the thorax. No external genitalia are visible. The tri-radiate cartilage (epiphysis) is still visible between the pubic and ischial bones in the acetabulum indicating that the child was aged less than seven years.

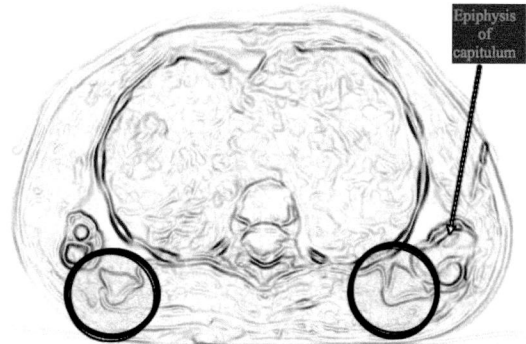

FIG. 5.189 AXIAL VIEW SHOWING THORACIC SHAPE AND PACKING (AFTER IEM IMAGE)

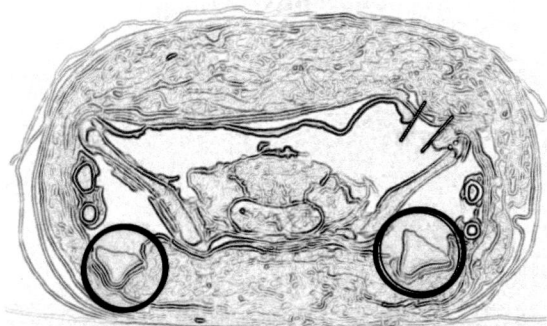

FIG. 5.190 AXIAL VIEW OF LOWER ABDOMEN SHOWING INCISION (AFTER IEM IMAGE)

XLIII. Unnamed from Tebtynis - Turin (Cat. No. Suppl.19691)

Thorax

The rib cage is intact and of a normal shape. The chest is not compressed.

The thoracic cavity is empty with no evidence of mediastinal contents, lungs or pleura. No packing is seen but some debris is noted.

Abdomen

Because of loss of the anterior abdominal wall by fragmentation, there is no evidence of a flank incision. However, there is the characteristically shaped linen pack indicating previous penetration through such an incision. No returned viscera or canopic packages are seen within the abdominal cavity.

Pelvis and Hips

There are no abnormalities in the bony pelvis.

The viscera have been removed from the pelvis and not returned. There are four packages, possibly containing viscera, within the pelvis. Inferior to them is a pack of linen. The pelvic floor is intact.

XLIV. Unnamed -Turin (Cat. No. Prov. 610)

Thorax

The rib cage is intact and of a normal shape. The mediastinum has been retained and contains the remnant of the heart and great vessels. Lung remnants are also present (See Fig. 5.191). Both hemi-diaphragms are present, but have been perforated medially.

A small package is observed within the right side of the chest (it may contain viscera) but there is no resin. Within the left side of the thorax there is a layered collection of resin containing a canopic package of rolled linen, the contents of which are difficult to interpret.

Abdomen

There is a left flank incision, with linen crossing it. Inferior to the linen, resin is seen crossing into the abdominal cavity and running into the pelvic cavity. Four canopic packages are seen lying longditudinally within the resin in the lower abdomen.

Pelvis and Hips

The bony pelvis is intact. The pelvic cavity contains no viscera and is filled with resin. The hips are congruous and show no signs of arthritis.

XLVIII. Unnamed - Manchester Museum (Cat. No. 3496)

Thorax

The upper part of the thorax has been lost in terms of recognizable structure and has, like the neck, been filled with linen.

There is no evidence of mediastinal contents, but there are remnants of the mediastinal wall, which has been infiltrated by resin. Both hemi-diaphragms are visible (See Fig. 5.192). The integrity of the rib cage is maintained to a large extent and the shape is normal (See Fig. 5.193). There are, however, posterior fractures of the left 7th, 8th and 9th ribs.

Abdomen

There is a left flank incision as shown in Fig. 5.194, between the lines. Compare this with the intact body wall in the figure on the left of Fig. 5.194. (arrow). A few structures on the posterior wall of the abdomen (and the pelvic cavity) represent retained or returned viscera (See Fig. 5.195).

Pelvis and Hips

The bony pelvis is intact. The hips joints are congruous and in joint. Ossification centres have not appeared in the upper femoral epiphyses, which again points towards the lower end of the age range of eighteen to twenty-four months (they have usually appeared by the age of one year).

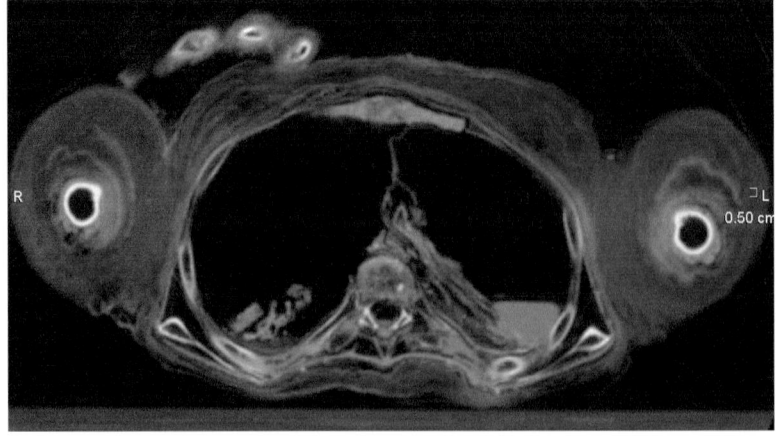

FIG. 5.191 AXIAL VIEW OF THORAX - MEDIASTINUM AND LUNGS

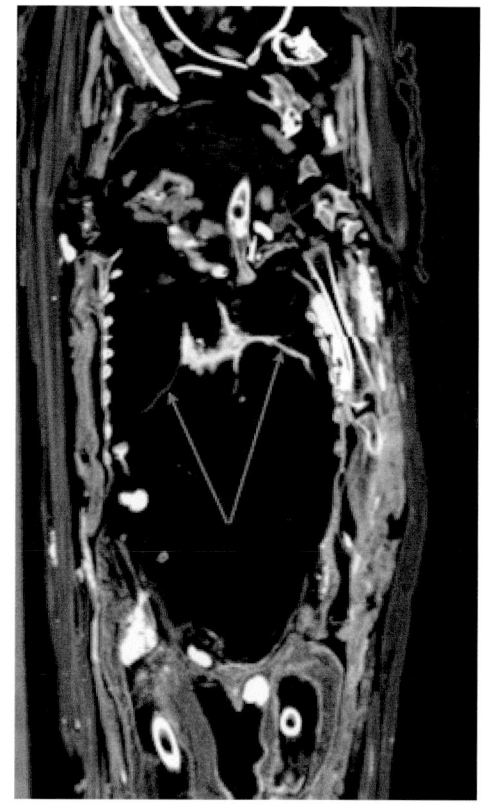

Fig. 5.192 Coronal view of trunk - remnants of diaphragm

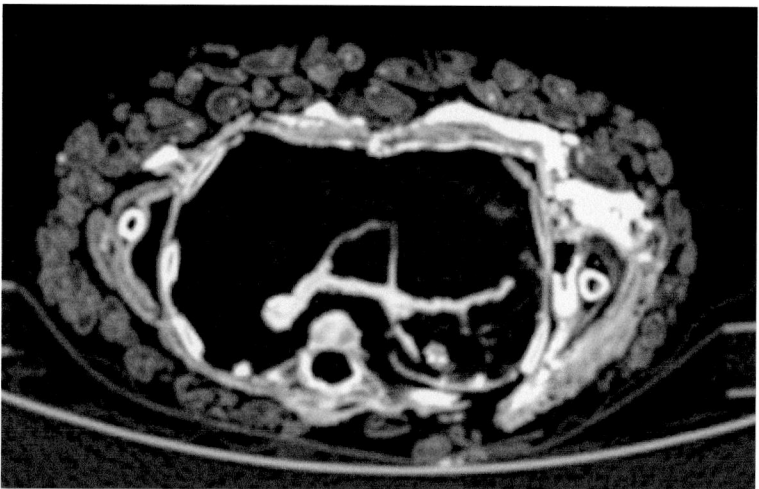

Fig. 5.193 Axial view of thorax demonstrating shape of rib cage

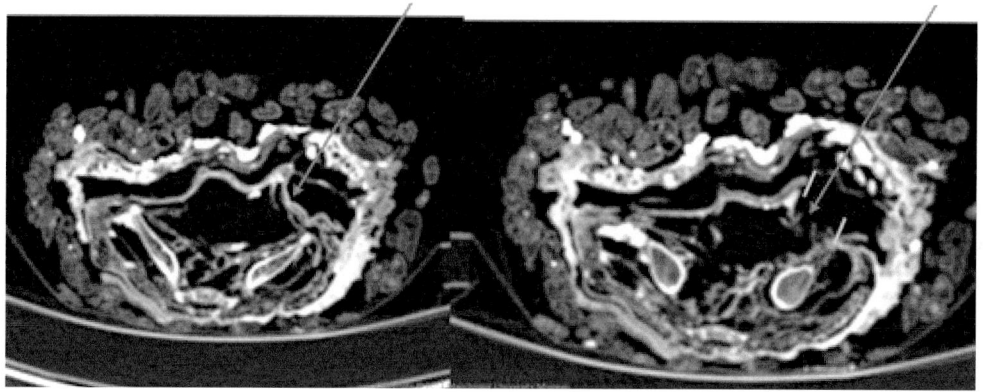

Fig. 5.194 Axial view showing abdominal wall incision

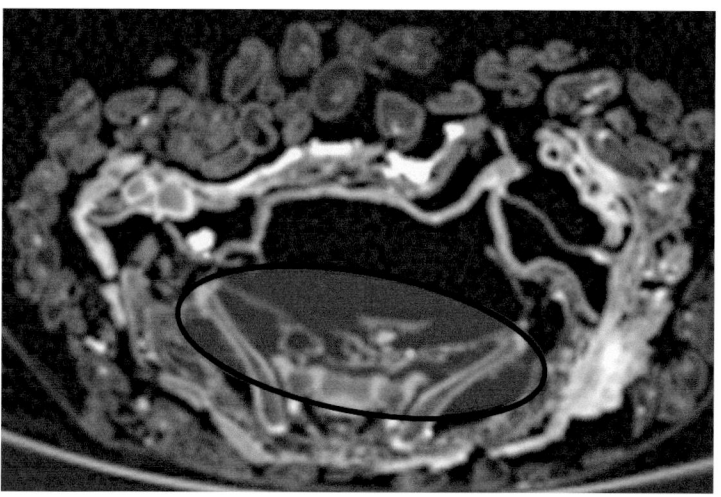

Fig. 5.195 Axial view - viscera on posterior pelvic wall

XLIX. Perenbast - Manchester University Museum (Accession No. MM5053.a)

Thorax

The thorax is symmetrical and a normal shape. Packing has pushed the mediastinum posteriorly. It does, however, contain structures including vessels and, probably, the heart lying over the posterior wall of the thorax (Fig. 5.196).

The thoracic cavity is filled with the granular material, which is a continuation of the neck packing (Fig. 5.197 - arrow 3). A more radio dense material on the right (Fig. 5.197 - arrow 1) may be a mixture of sawdust, resin and canopic packages (Fig. 5.197- arrows 2). These canopic packages extend into the abdominal cavity (See Fig. 5.198).

Abdomen

There is a left flank incision, through which a canopic package is seen protruding (See Fig. 5.199 - arrow 2). The incision is covered by a metal (probably gold) plate, which has a *Wadjet* eye upon it (See Fig. 5.199 - arrow 1 and Fig. 5.200).

Evisceration has been thorough. The viscera have been returned to the abdomen in four or five canopic packages, which have had resin added to them. The exact count is difficult as they are not in a defined plane. The lowest of these packages lies at the brim of the pelvis (See Fig. 5.201), a layer of granular material is seen on the posterior wall of the abdomen.

Pelvis and Hips

The bony pelvis is intact.

The pelvic cavity has some granular material of two radio densities lying over the posterior wall (See Fig. 5.202 - arrow 1). This Figure also shows the rectum - arrow 2, the vagina - arrow 3 and the possible remnant of the uterus - arrow 4. The perineum is intact.

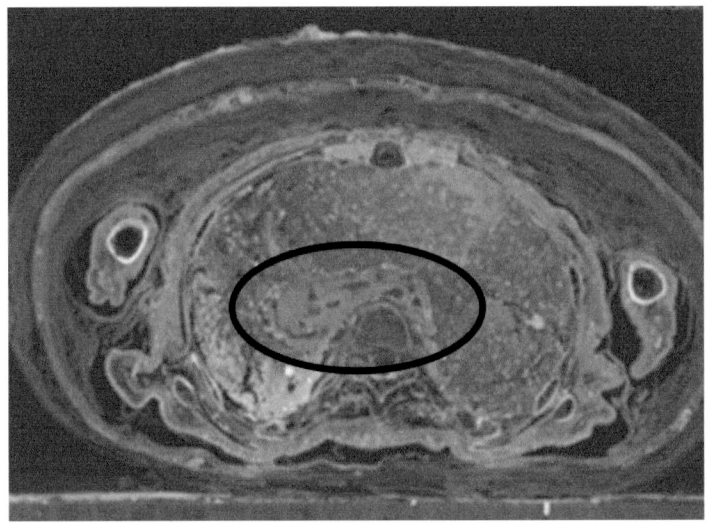

FIG. 5.196 AXIAL VIEW OF THORAX - MEDIASTINUM

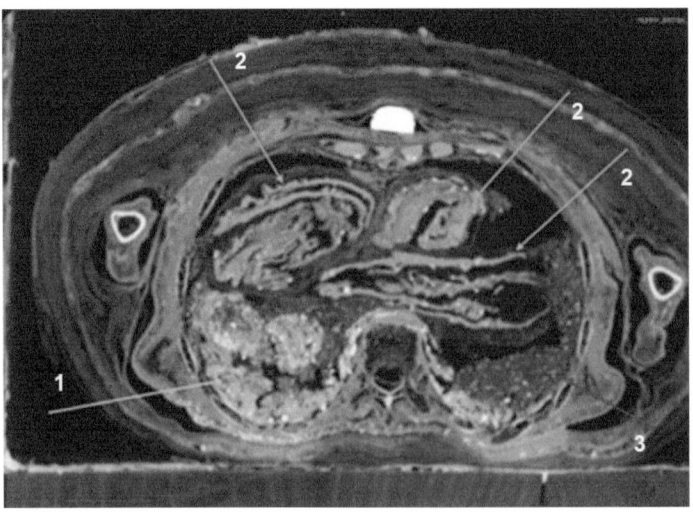

FIG. 5.197 AXIAL VIEW OF LOWER THORAX - CANOPIC PACKAGES

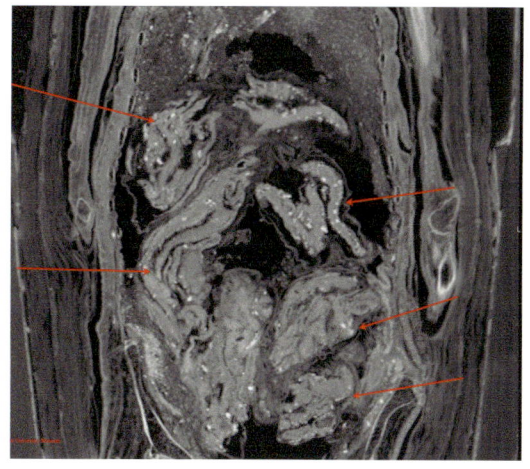

FIG. 5.198 CORONAL VIEW OF TRUNK - CANOPIC PACKAGES IN ABDOMEN

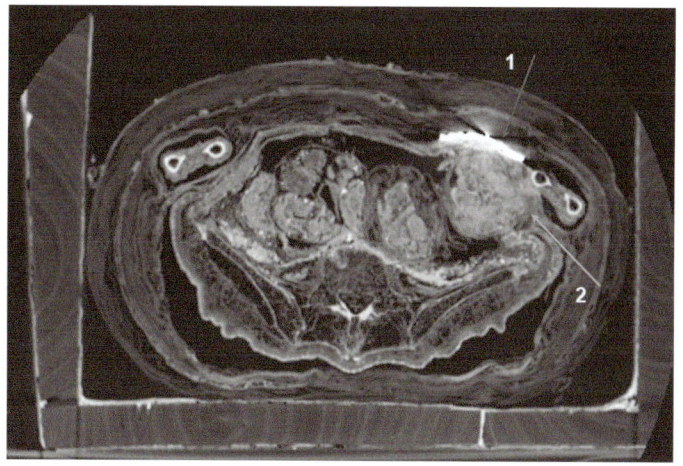

FIG. 5.199 AXIAL VIEW OF ABDOMEN - METAL PLATE COVERING INCISION

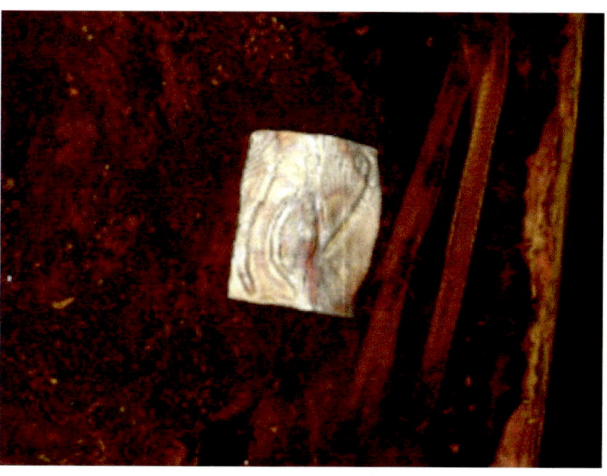

FIG. 5.200 3D RECONSTRUCTION OF INCISION PLATE

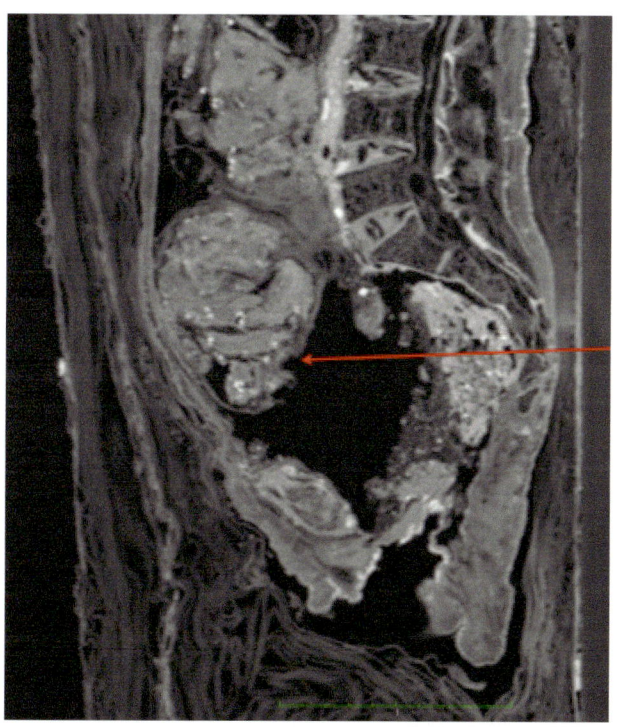

FIG. 5.201 SAGITTAL VIEW OF PELVIS - CANOPIC PACKAGE AT BRIM OF PELVIS

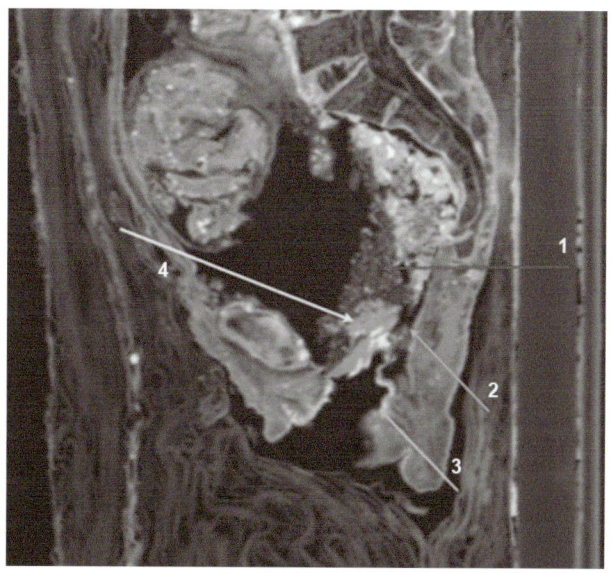

FIG. 5.202 SAGITTAL VIEW OF PELVIS - PERINEAL STRUCTURES AND MATERIAL IN PELVIS

LIII. Unnamed - Manchester Museum (Accession No. MM1976.51.a)

Thorax

The rib cage is a normal shape with the viscera completely removed and no evidence of the mediastinum or diaphragm. There is loosely packed linen within the thoracic cavity. See Fig. 5.203 (circles). Over the anterior surface of the vertebrae is a layer of (probably) resin most of which has been broken off (See Fig. 5.204) and may be represented by the fragments of material seen in the upper abdominal area (See Fig. 5.205 - circle).

Abdomen

A left flank incision is clearly seen (See Fig. 5.206 - between lines).

There are four separate packages in the abdomen that appear to be false canopic packages. Three of these packages are seen in Fig. 5.207. However, the two indicated by the arrows 1 are almost certainly two halves of one original package. The other two packages may well also be two halves of one original package, indicating a total of only two ORIGINAL packages. The packages are seen in the left side of the abdomen, the right side being completely empty.

Pelvis and Hips

The bony pelvis is intact but with complete clearance of the pelvic viscera. The posterior part of the pelvis contains a few fragments of (probable) resin (See Fig. 5.208). The perineal floor is seen, but no midline structures or orifices can be identified (See Fig. 5.209). This illustrates that the tissues are overlapped as if the rectum, vagina and urethra have been excised and skin flaps fashioned and fixed together.

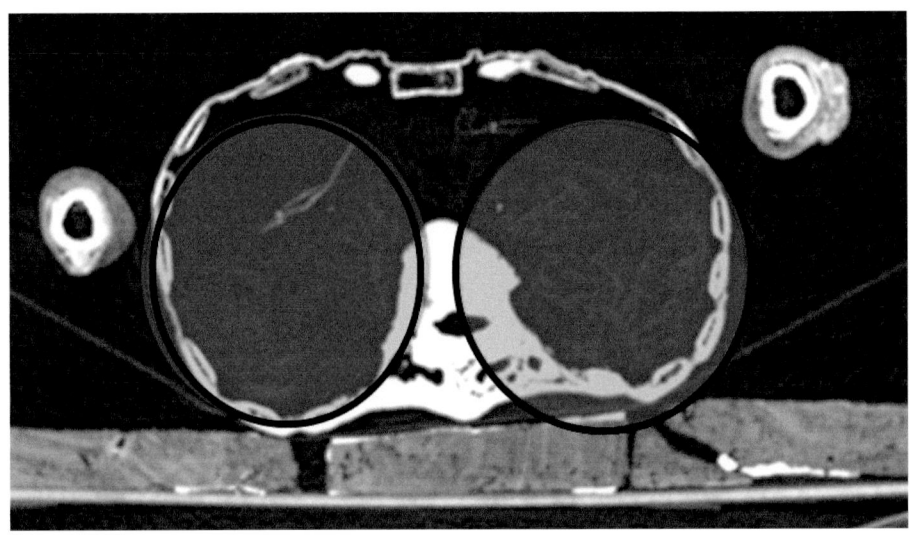

FIG. 5.203 AXIAL VIEW SHOWING LOOSE PACKING IN THORAX

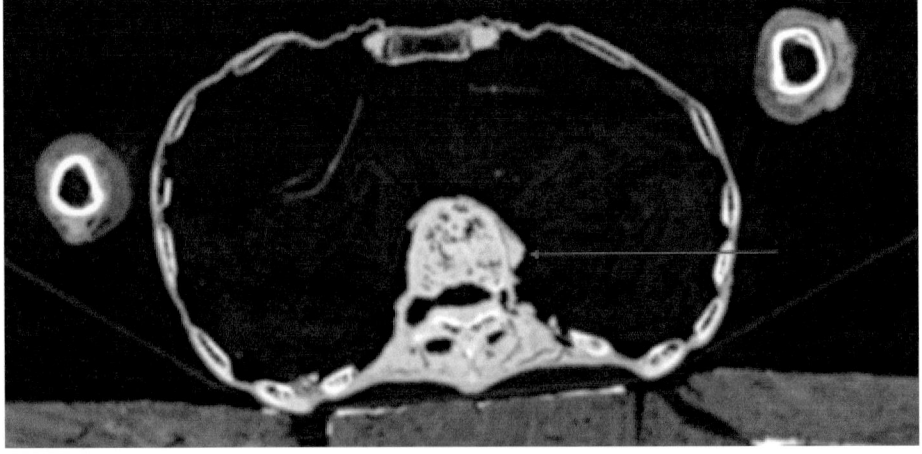

FIG. 5.204 AXIAL VIEW OF THORAX - RESIN OVER ANTERIOR SURFACE OF VERTEBRAE

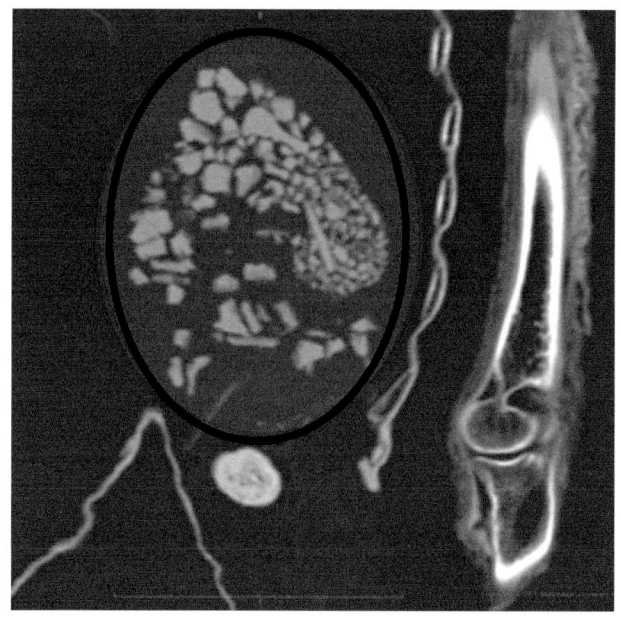

Fig. 5.205 Coronal view of trunk - fragmented resin

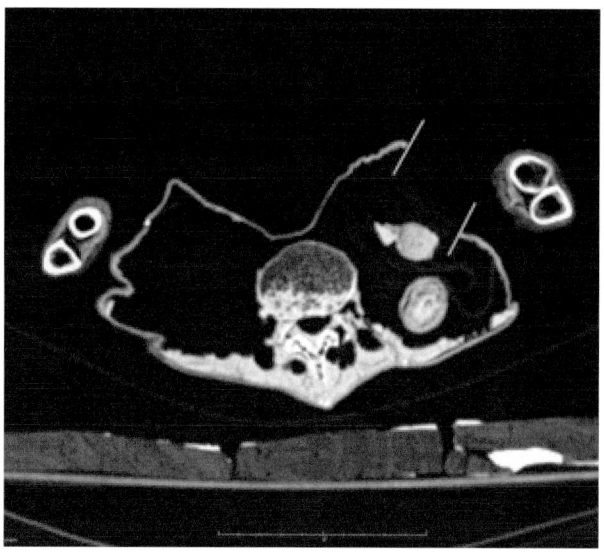

Fig. 5.206 Axial view showing abdominal incision

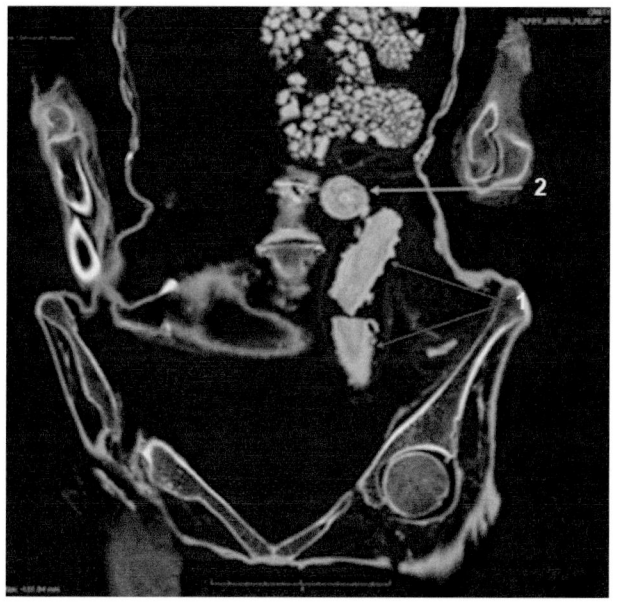

Fig. 5.207 Coronal view of abdomen - canopic packages

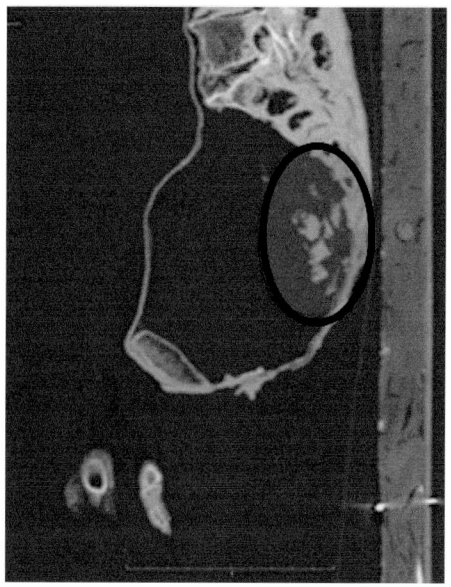

Fig. 5.208 Sagittal view of pelvis - fragments of resin in pelvis

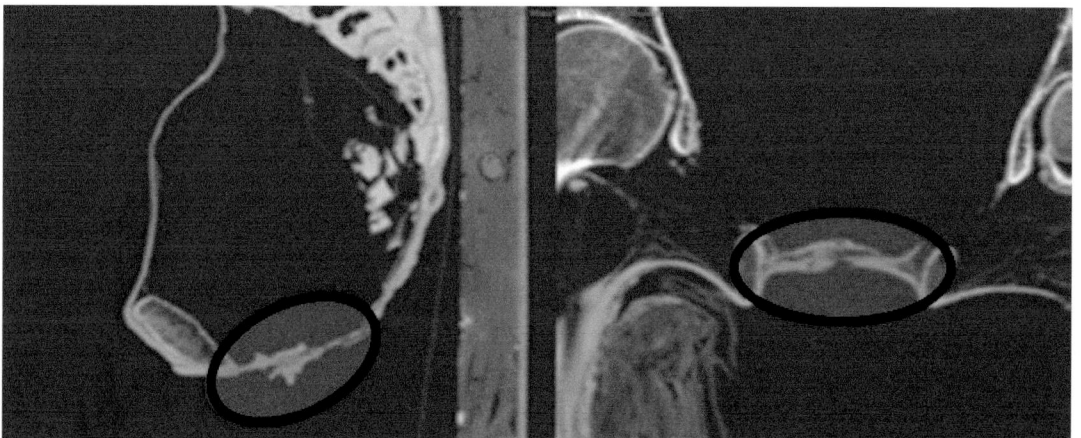

Fig. 5.209 Sagittal and coronal views of pelvis - perineal floor

LX. Unnamed - British Museum (Cat. No. EA 6704)

Thorax

The shape of the rib cage is normal (See Fig. 5.210).

The mediastinum and contained structures is absent but remnants of the diaphragm can be seen (See Fig. 5.210 - 2).

There are two layers of material (possibly resin and granular material) within the posterior part of the thoracic cavity (See Fig. 5.210 - 3 = resin and 4 = resin + granular material).

Abdomen

There is a left flank incision (See Fig. 5.211 - between lines) with linen passing through the incision. No viscera remain in the abdomen, but three canopic packages lie within the body cavity (See Fig. 5.212 - 1). Resin has been introduced into the abdominal cavity, in direct continuity with that in the thorax.

Pelvis and Hips

The bony pelvis is intact and the pelvic organs have been removed. There is a false canopic package within the pelvis (See Fig. 5.213 - 1). This Figure also shows resinous material within the pelvis - arrow 2. The pelvic organs such as rectum, bladder +/- vagina are not visulised but the pelvic floor (skin) is seen in Fig. 5.214 - circle. The tip of the coccyx is also identified in this figure - arrow.

Fig. 5.215 shows the pubic symphysis in the mid-line (arrow) and folded linen, but no convincing evidence of a true phallus (circle). There is, however, an object that could well be a false phallus (See Fig. 5.216 - circle). That this is a false phallus is indicated by its appearance in section, where layers of linen are shown (See Figs. 5.217 and 5.218- circles). An anatomical phallus would have a totally different sectional appearance.

Of the above thirty-eight mummies with an abdominal incision, six were not absolutely certain. Of these one was presumed although the abdominal wall was not well shown (V). Two were highly likely but not scientifically provable (VII and VIII). One was likely although the abdominal wall was so folded and convoluted that certainty could not be assured (XXVII) and one was assumed because of the presence of linen in the shape of that seen traversing an abdominal incision in other cases (XLIII).

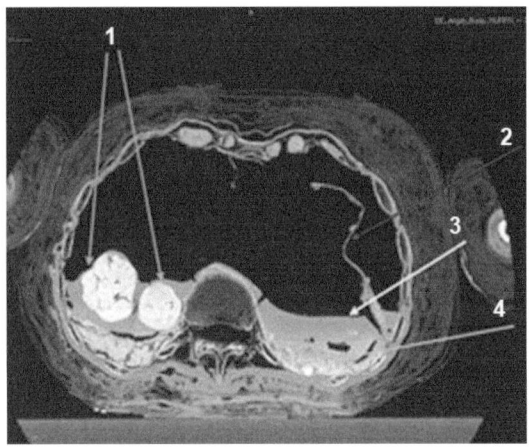

Fig. 5.210 Axial view of thorax demonstrating shape and contents
Courtesy of the Trustees of the British Museum

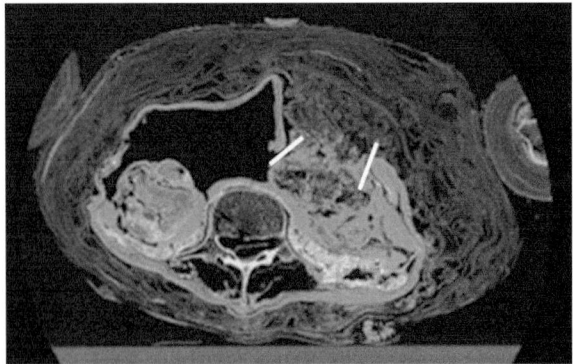

Fig. 5.211 Axial view showing abdominal incision
Courtesy of the Trustees of the British Museum

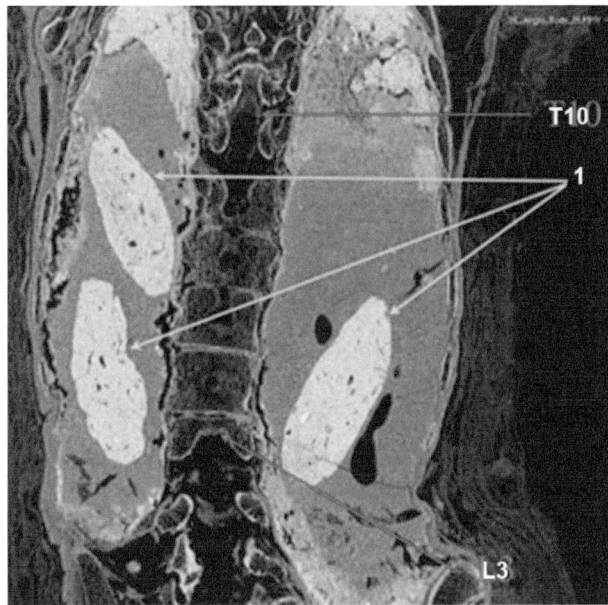

Fig. 5.212 Coronal view of abdomen - canopic packages
Courtesy of the Trustees of the British Museum

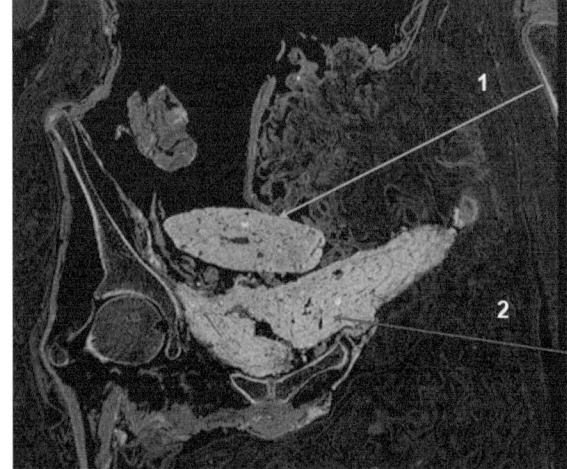

Fig. 5.213 Coronal view of pelvis - canopic package within the pelvis
Courtesy of the Trustees of the British Museum

RESULTS – THE TRUNK

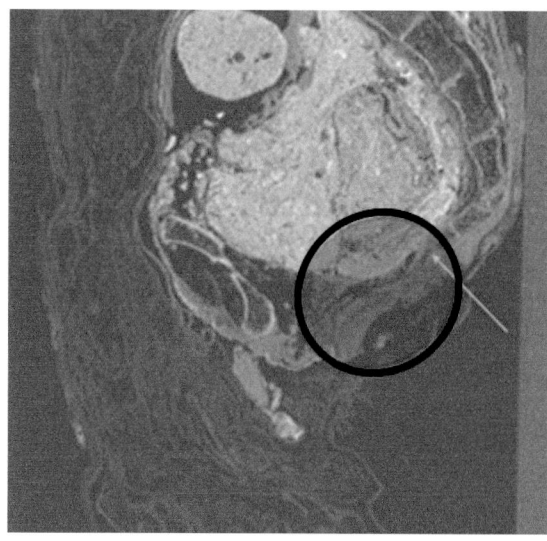

FIG. 5.214 SAGITTAL VIEW OF PELVIS - COCCYX AND PELVIC FLOOR
COURTESY OF THE TRUSTEES OF THE BRITISH MUSEUM

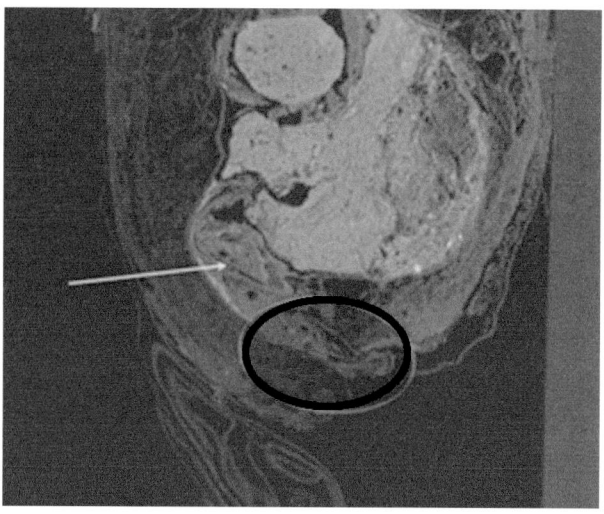

FIG. 5.215 SAGITTAL VIEW OF PELVIS - SYMPHYSIS PUBIS AND FALSE PHALLUS
COURTESY OF THE TRUSTEES OF THE BRITISH MUSEUM

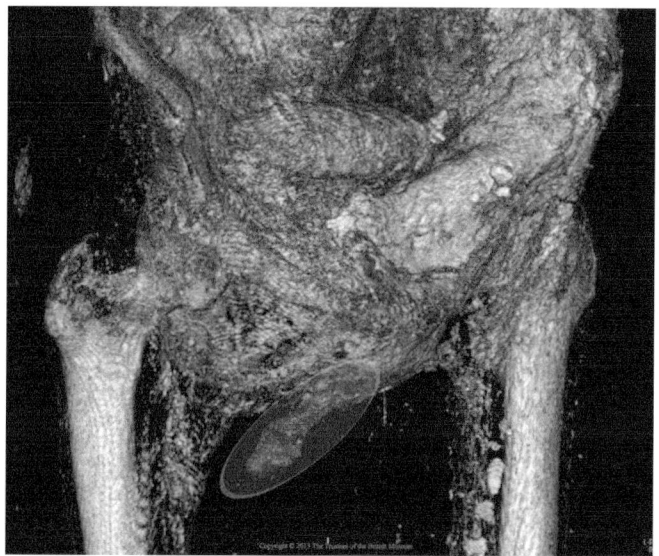

FIG. 5.216 3D RECONSTRUCTION DEMONSTRATING FALSE PHALLUS
COURTESY OF THE TRUSTEES OF THE BRITISH MUSEUM

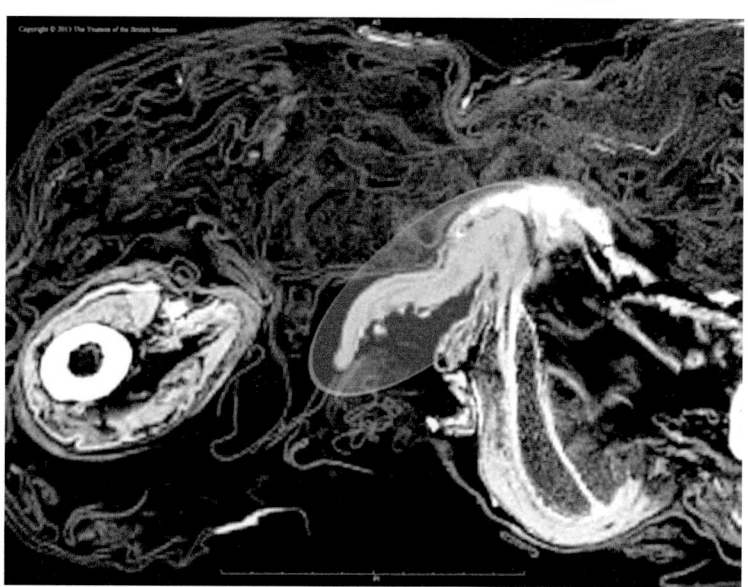

FIG. 5.217 OBLIQUE AXIAL VIEW OF PELVIS - FALSE PHALLUS
COURTESY OF THE TRUSTEES OF THE BRITISH MUSEUM

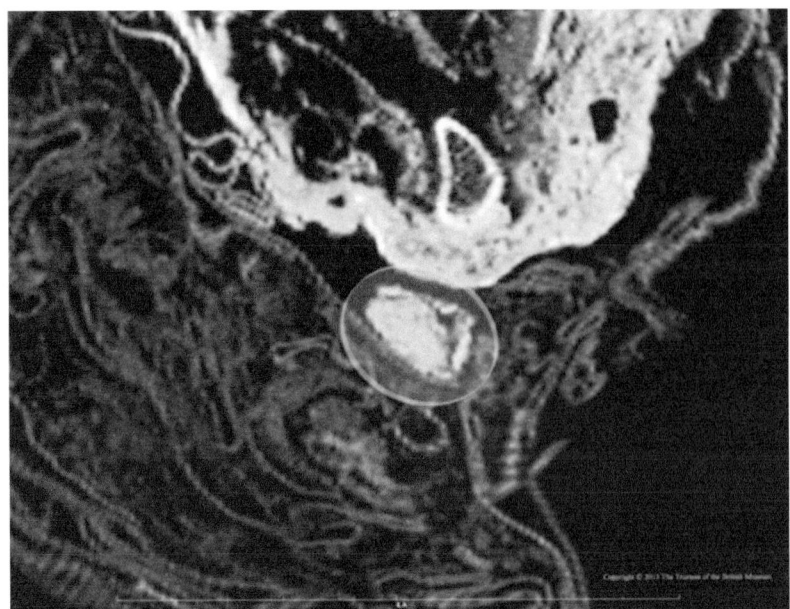

FIG. 5.218 OBLIQUE SAGITTAL VIEW OF PELVIS - FALSE PHALLUS
COURTESY OF THE TRUSTEES OF THE BRITISH MUSEUM

5.2.2 Perineal Approach

The perineal approach was found in combination with an abdominal incision in nine cases as described above. These were in mummies number: X, XVI, XVIII, XXII, XXIII, XXXVIII, XXXIX, LIII and LX. In a further four cases, a perineal approach alone was used. These are described below.

XXIV. Unnamed - Basel Museum (Cat. No.BSAE.1030)

Thorax

There are fractures (2) and posterior dislocations (1) of the upper ribs on both sides. On the left the 2nd, 3rd, 4th and 5th ribs are fractured just lateral to the costo-transverse ligaments. There are, also, fractures of the antero-lateral angles of the left 4th, 5th and 6th ribs. There are dislocations of the right 2nd, 3rd and 4th costo-vertebral joints and fractures of the right 3rd, 4th, 6th and 7th ribs laterally (See Fig. 5.219). The sternum is compressed backwards, flat against the spine.

The remnants of the mediastinum are visible but it is not positively certain that one can see the heart (2). However, biological tissue is seen on both sides, in the lower thorax (1) (See Fig. 5.220). Also arrows 1 in Fig. 5.221. This may well be the remnant of the lungs. There is no evidence of the left hemi-diaphragm. There are two granular packages within the left lower thorax, on the left (one shown - arrow 2 in Fig. 5.221).

Abdomen

No evidence of an abdominal incision is seen. There is an opening in the right side of the perineum indicating a trans-perineal evisceration, as there are no organs within the abdomen. There are some round fragments of granular material within the pelvis (See Fig. 5.222). The finding of most curiosity is the inclusion within the anterior wrappings of the abdomen, of two packages, one of rolled linen and the other containing a bird - an Ibis (See Fig. 5.220 - arrow 3 and Figs. 5.223 and 5.224 - circle).

Pelvis and Hips

Slight disruption of both sacro-iliac joints is seen, but this could well have occurred during mummification. The pubic symphysis is normal. There is a fracture of the floor of the right acetabulum and another of the right inferior pubic ramus (See Fig. 5.225).

As there is no associated haematoma or callus formation, it is presumed that these injuries may have occurred just before death or post-mortem. Due to the distortion of the perineum, there is no evidence of external genitalia.

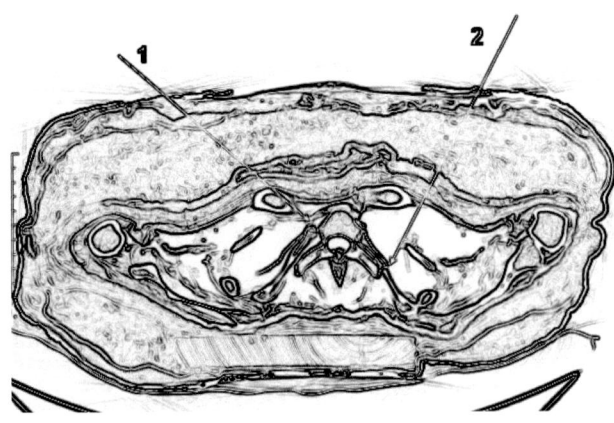

FIG. 5.219 AXIAL VIEW OF UPPER THORAX - COSTO-VERTEBRAL DISLOCATION AND RIB FRACTURE (AFTER IEM IMAGE)

RESULTS – THE TRUNK

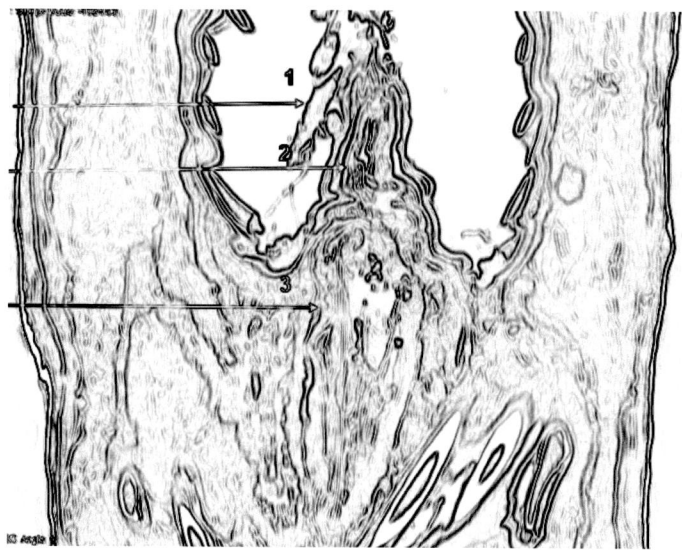

FIG. 5.220 CORONAL VIEW OF TRUNK - MEDIASTINAL STRUCTURES AND IBIS
(AFTER IEM IMAGE)

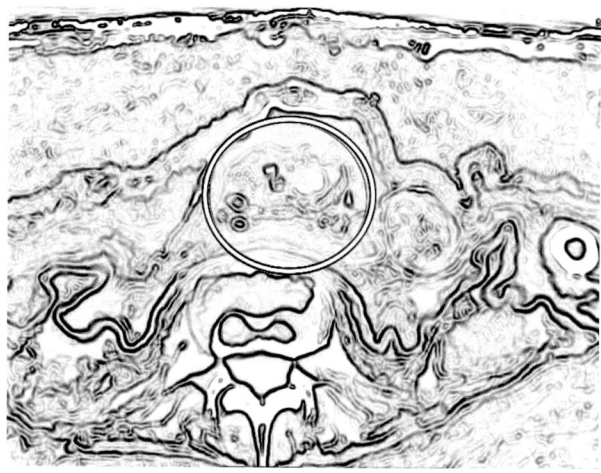

FIG. 5.223 AXIAL VIEW OF ABDOMEN - IBIS
(AFTER IEM IMAGE)

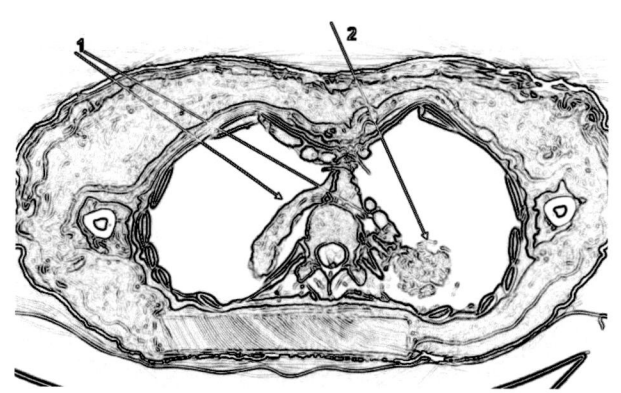

FIG. 5.221 AXIAL VIEW SHOWING STRUCTURES IN THORAX
(AFTER IEM IMAGE)

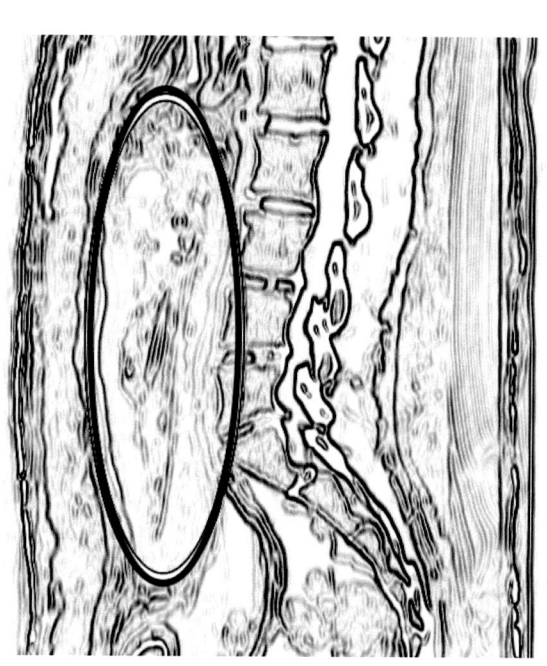

FIG. 5.224 SAGITTAL VIEW OF ABDOMEN - IBIS
(AFTER IEM IMAGE)

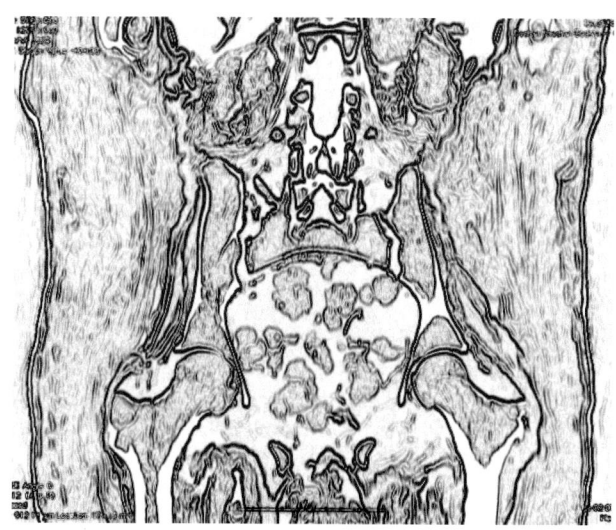

FIG. 5.222 CORONAL VIEW - GRANULAR MATERIAL WITHIN PELVIS.
(AFTER IEM IMAGE)

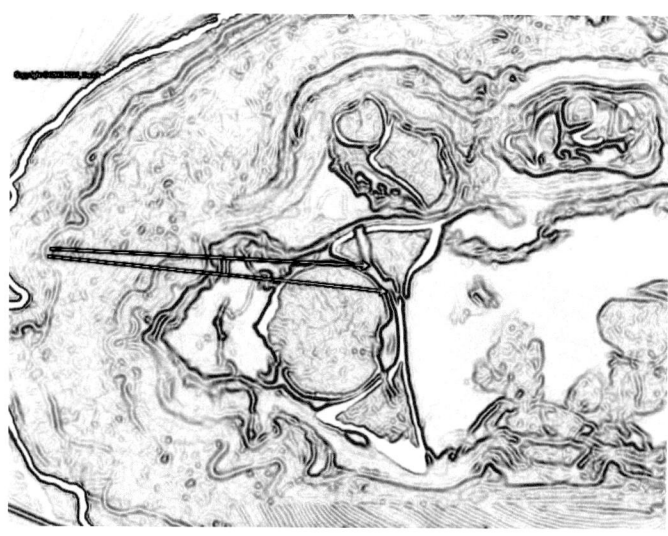

FIG. 5.225 AXIAL VIEW OF PELVIS - ACETABULAR FRACTURES
(AFTER IEM IMAGE)

XXXVII. Sherit-Min - Lenzburg (K10352).

Thorax

The rib cage is of a normal (or, if anything, narrow) shape with no compression of the ribs and no fractures or dislocations.

The mediastinum has been retained and contains the great vessels (Fig. 5.226). The heart is almost certainly present within the pericardium (Fig. 5.227 - smaller circle) and remnants of the diaphragm are retained (See Fig. 5.228). There is no extraneous tissue in the thoracic cavity, although the right lung outline remains, almost certainly indicating its retention (See Fig.5.227 - large circle).

Abdomen

The abdomen is empty and collapsed with a small amount of tissue in both paraspinal gutters (See Fig. 5.229). There is no evidence of an abdominal incision. No linen or canopic packages are seen within the abdomen.

Pelvis and Hips

The sacro-iliac joints and the symphysis pubis are intact. A healed fracture of the right inferior pubic ramus is noted (See Fig. 5.230). No organs are seen in the pelvic cavity and the perineum is entirely absent, with a linen pack placed at the site of the perineum (See Fig. 5.231 - Upper end of pack and Fig. 5.232 - Lower end of perineal pack).

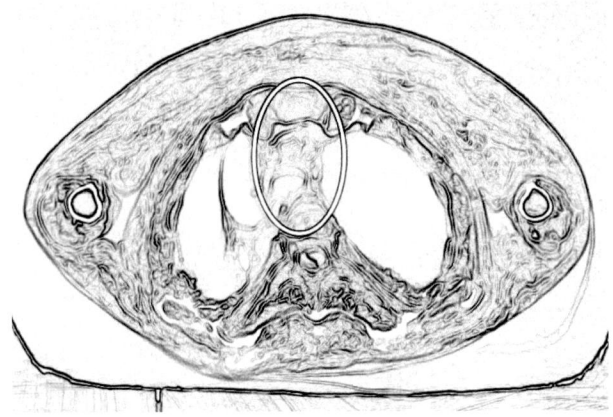

FIG. 5.226 AXIAL VIEW OF UPPER THORAX - GREAT VESSELS (**AFTER IEM** IMAGE)

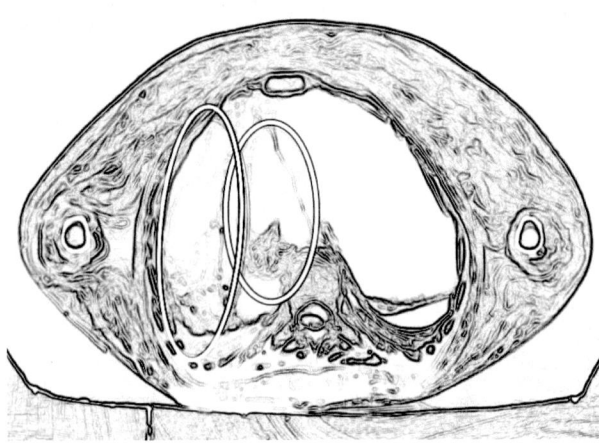

FIG. 5.227 AXIAL VIEW OF THORAX - HEART AND RIGHT LUNG (**AFTER IEM** IMAGE)

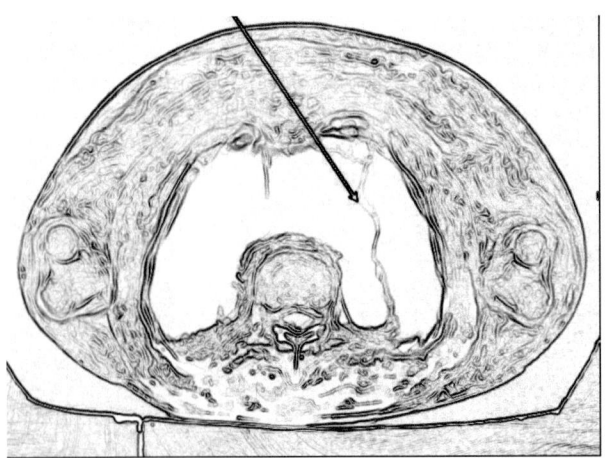

FIG. 5.228 AXIAL VIEW OF LOWER THORAX - REMAINS OF DIAPHRAGM (AFTER IEM IMAGE)

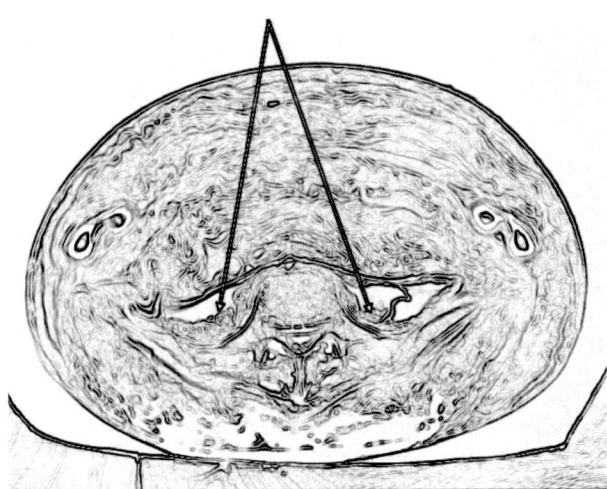

FIG. 5.229 AXIAL VIEW OF LOWER ABDOMEN - TISSUES IN PARASPINAL GUTTERS (AFTER IEM IMAGE)

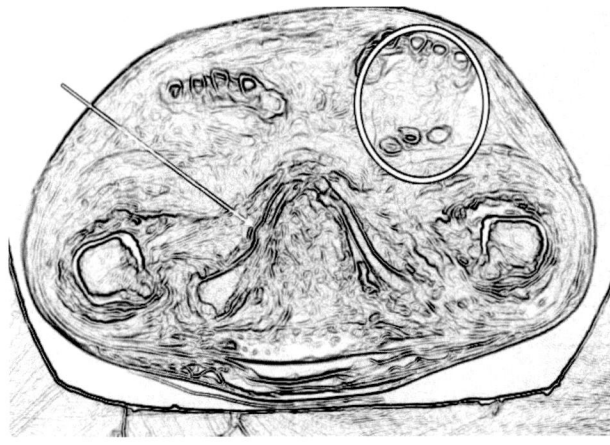

FIG. 5.230 AXIAL VIEW OF PELVIS - HEALED FRACTURE OF RIGHT PUBIC RAMUS (AFTER IEM IMAGE)

RESULTS – THE TRUNK

XLII. Ta-aset - Turin (Cat. No. Suppl. 9480)

Thorax

There is a kyphosis centred on T6 and with an angle of 50° and arthritic change throughout the thoracic spine.

The rib cage is intact with no evidence of fractures of the ribs or dislocation of the costo-vertebral joints. However, the sternum is depressed to be closer to the spine than normal and as a result, the ribs are overlapped and imbricated (See Fig. 5.233).

This same figure shows tissue lying over the spine with no definite evidence of a heart and therefore these tissues probably represent the lungs. The diaphragm is not seen. There is some granular (possibly clay) packing in the thorax, which has been introduced from below.

Abdomen

No observable abdominal incision can be confirmed, but the viscera have been removed.

The abdomen contains clay, which is in continuity with the lower thorax.

Pelvis and Hips

The bony pelvis is intact.

The perineum has been used as the portal of entry for evisceration and, subsequently, packed with linen and resin to seal the opening. There is a suggestion of female external genitalia.

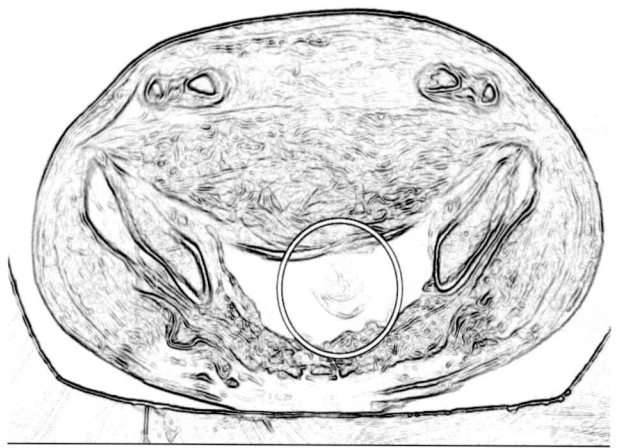

FIG. 5.231 AXIAL VIEW OF PELVIS - PACK IN UPPER PERINEUM (**AFTER IEM** IMAGE)

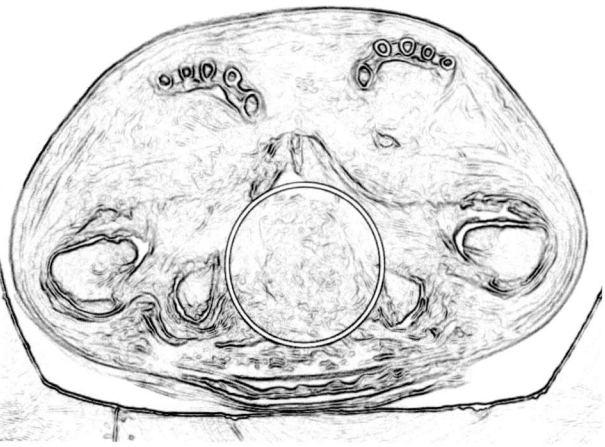

FIG. 5.232 AXIAL VIEW OF PELVIS - PACK IN LOWER PERINEUM (**AFTER IEM** IMAGE)

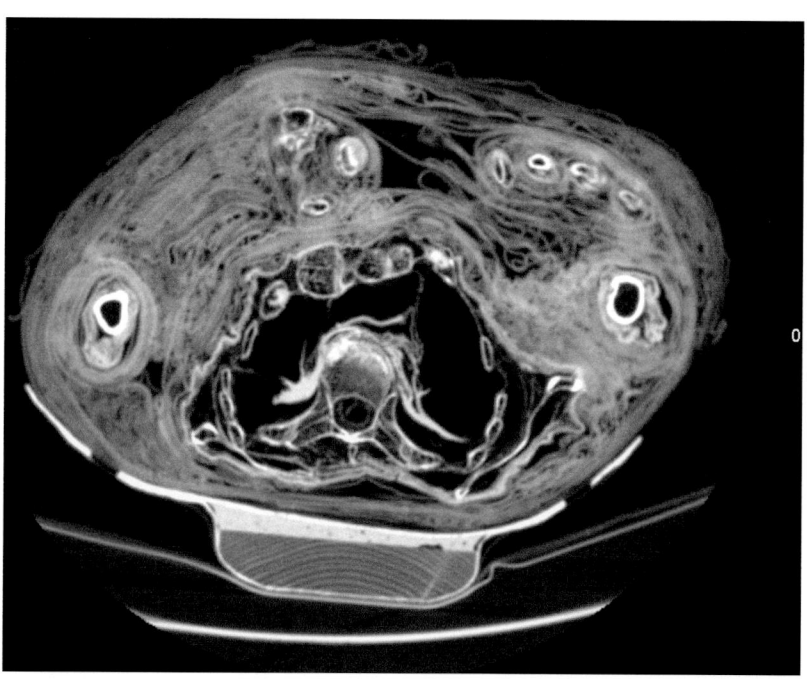

FIG. 5.233 AXIAL VIEW OF THORAX - IMBRICATED RIBS

XLV. Unnamed - Manchester Museum (Cat. No.MM1766)

Thorax

The rib cage/chest wall is asymmetrical, with the right side compressed. See Figs. 5.234 and 5.235.

The left ribs are more or less normal but the left 11th and 12th ribs are subluxed posteriorly. On the right side the ribs are disorganized, with costo-vertebral dislocations and subluxations. Some of the ribs are lying free. Although it is accepted that recent intervention might have damaged the rib cage, this has not altered the shape, as is seen by the conforming shape of the bandaging.

There is no evidence of the mediastinum or its contents. However, Fig. 5.236 does show some biological material over the right side of the body of the twelfth thoracic vertebra. There is, also, some granular material within the thoracic cavity - as well as debris, which may well be the result of the endoscopy. Fig. 5.236 also shows the asymmetry of the rib cage.

Abdomen

Evisceration is complete with no returned viscera or canopic packages. Furthermore, there is no evidence of an abdominal incision. The only portal for evisceration is the perineum. The abdominal cavity is empty apart from some debris within the pelvic cavity. A pad of resin impregnated linen lies on the front of the anterior abdominal wall.

Pelvis and Hips

There is significant disruption of the bony pelvis. Both sacro-iliac joints are subluxated (See Fig. 5.237 - arrows 1 and 2 and circle) with a fracture of the right ala of the sacrum (See Fig. 5.237 - arrow 1 and circle). The pubic symphysis is dislocated and overlapped (see Fig. 5.238). There are fractures of both the superior (Fig. 5.239) and inferior (Fig. 5.240) pubic rami and of the ischium (Fig. 5.241).

The perineum is largely absent and a resin impregnated linen pad has been placed over the perineal site (See Fig. 5.242).

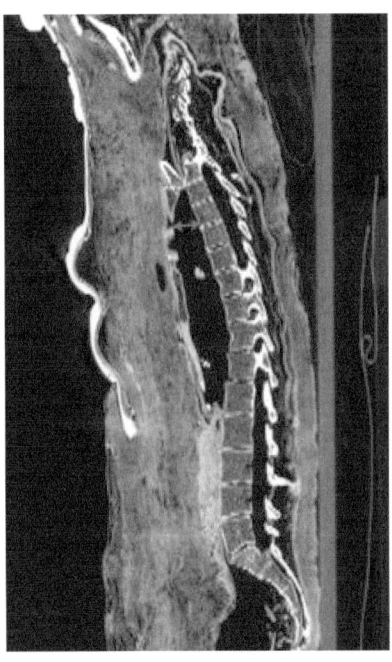

FIG. 5.234
SAGITTAL VIEW OF TRUNK - ANTEROPOSTERIORLY COMPRESSED THORAX

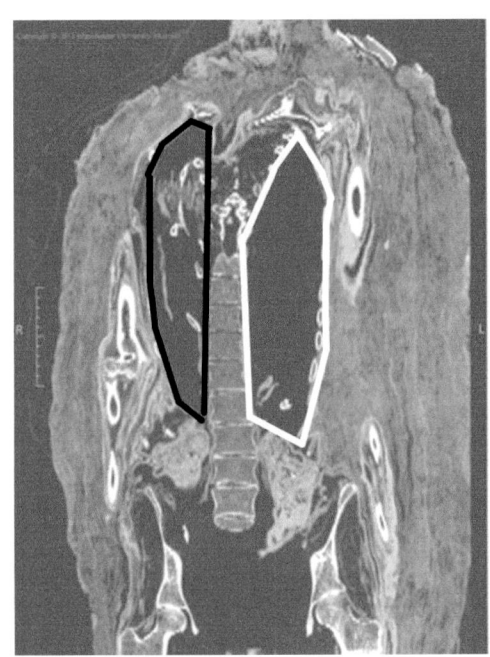

FIG. 5.235
CORONAL VIEW OF TRUNK - ASYMMETRY OF THORAX

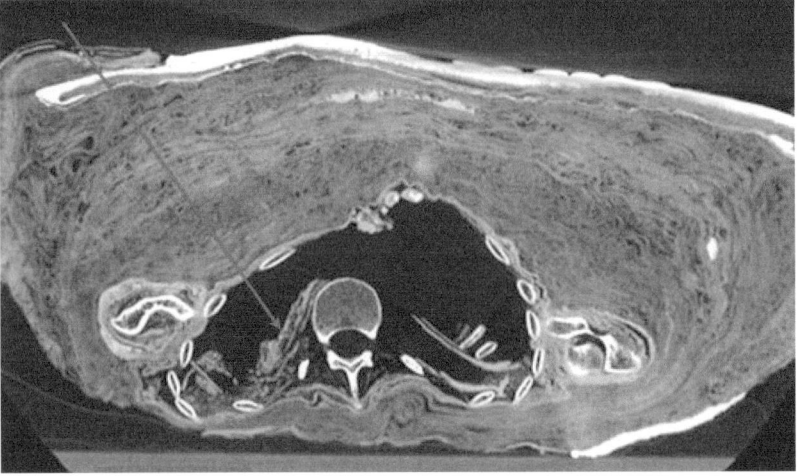

FIG. 5.236 AXIAL VIEW OF THORAX - TISSUE ON POSTERIOR WALL

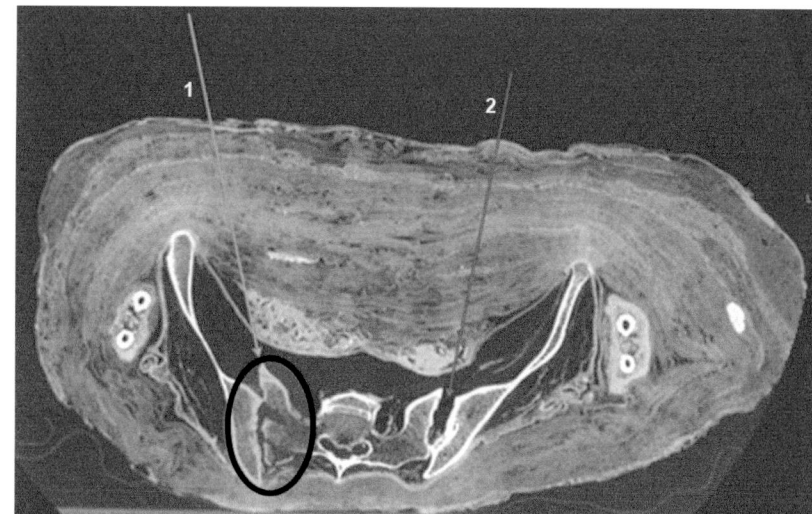

Fig. 5.237 Axial view of pelvis - sacro-iliac joint (SIJ) disruption

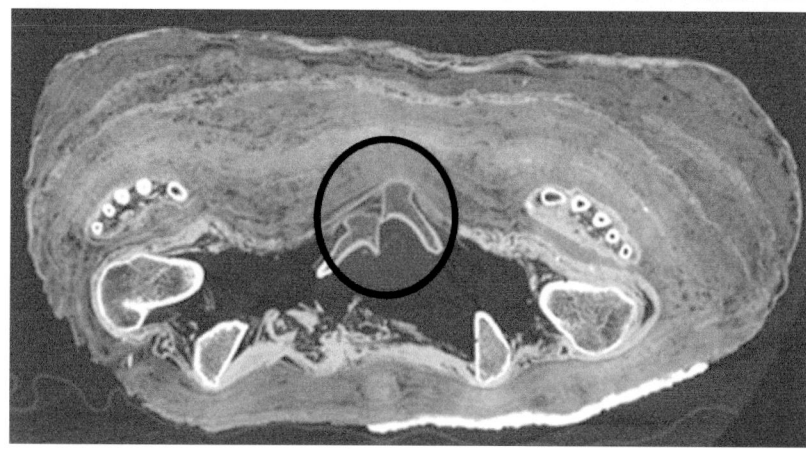

Fig. 5.238 Axial view of pelvis - dislocation of symphysis pubis

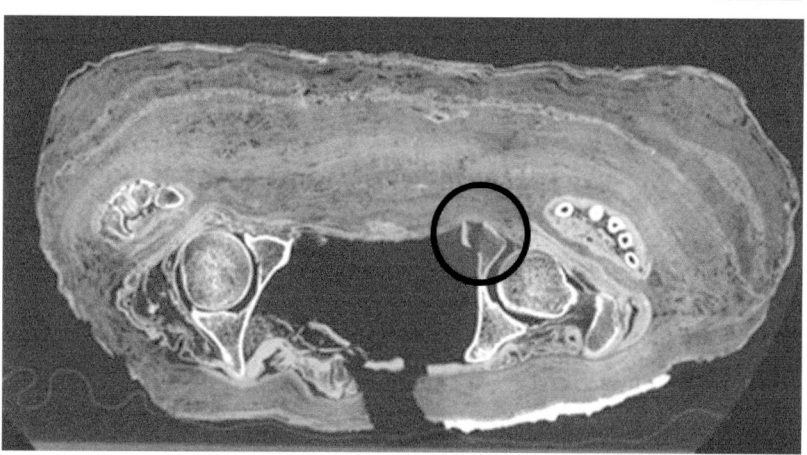

Fig. 5.239 Axial view of pelvis - superior pubic ramus fracture

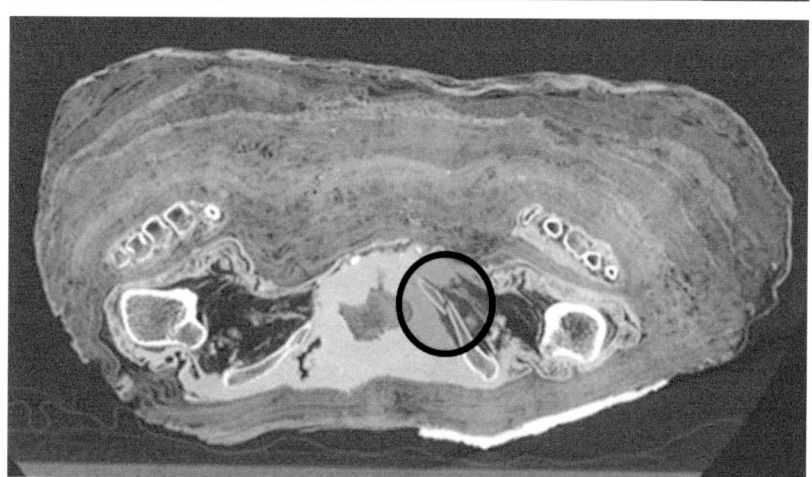

Fig. 5.240 Axial view of pelvis - inferior pubic ramus fracture

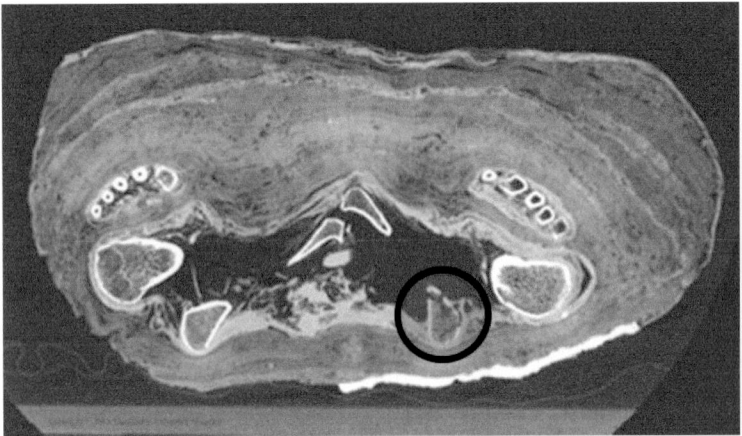

FIG. 5.241 AXIAL VIEW OF PELVIS - ISCHIAL FRACTURE

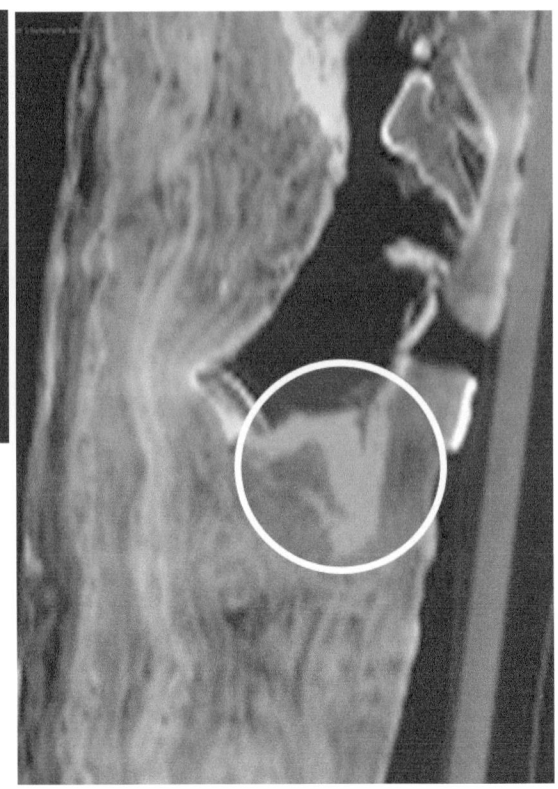

FIG. 5.242 SAGITTAL VIEW OF PELVIS - PERINEAL PAD

5.2.3 No evidence of incision or evisceration:

In eleven cases there was no visible evidence of an abdominal incision or of an approach via the perineum. In other words, there was no evidence of evisceration. There was, therefore, as expected, evidence of remaining viscera within the cavity of the torso. Table 5.2 shows these cases.

NUMBER	ORIGIN	ERA
XII	Manchester - MM1768	Roman
XIII	Manchester - MM1767	Roman
XV	Liverpool - 13.10.11.25	Roman
XLVII	Manchester - MM1769	Roman
LI	Manchester - MM9354a - Khary	D19/ Ptolemaic?
LII	Manchester - MM9319 - child	Roman
LIV	Manchester - Salford 2	3IP
LV	Manchester - MM13011	Ptolemaic
LVI	Manchester - MM2109	Roman
LVII	Manchester - MM1775 - Artemidorus	Roman
LIX	BM - EA 22108 Child	Roman

TABLE 5.2 MUMMIES WITH NO INCISION AND NO EVISCERATION

XII Unnamed - Manchester University Museum (Accession No. MM1768)

Thorax

Due to complete disruption of the normal bony anatomy it is difficult to interpret the contents of the thorax. However there is evidence of biological material (probably lung) bilaterally in the posterior parts of the thoracic cavity this being more obvious on the right (See Fig. 5.243 - arrow). Not only is the thoracic spine completely disrupted, but also the rib cage is compressed in an antero-posterior direction, with depression and distortion of the sternum (See Fig. 5.244 - circle). Due to the thoracic distortion, it is not possible to see any evidence of the mediastinum and its normal contents.

Abdomen

As with the thorax, there is major disruption to the spine in this region and compression of the abdomen in an antero-posterior direction. A significant amount of biological material remains within the abdominal cavity but it is not possible to visualize the abdominal wall sufficiently clearly to identify an abdominal incision (or, indeed, to exclude one); however, the presence of so much biological material makes the probability of such an incision unlikely. There is a breach in the posterior abdominal wall, through which several vertebrae have extruded (see arrow in Fig. 5.245).

Pelvis and Hips

There is complete disruption of both sacro-iliac joints. The pubic symphysis is intact and the hip joints congruent with no evidence of arthritis in the hips.

The bladder appears to be present (Fig. 5.246 Bladder - 1 and the rectum - 2).

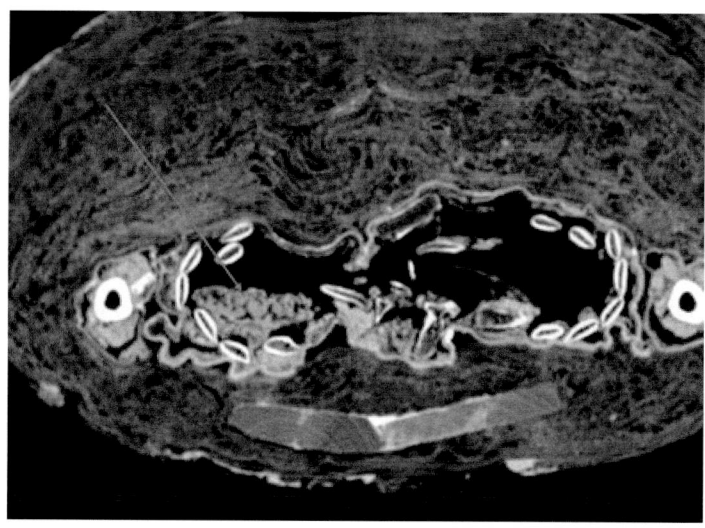

FIG. 5.243 AXIAL VIEW OF THORAX - VISCERA IN THORACIC CAVITY

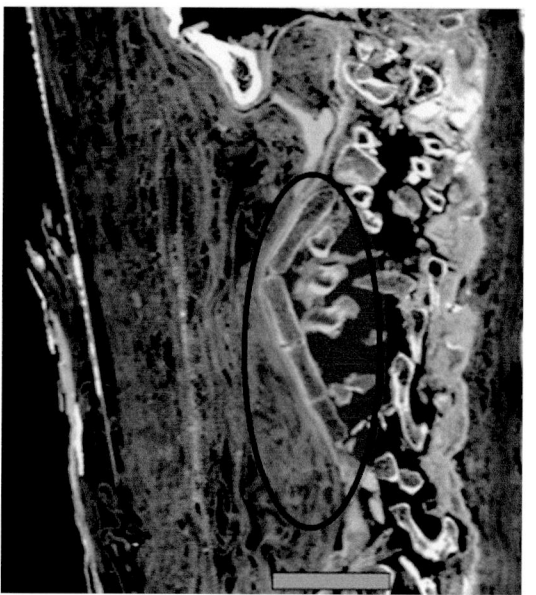

FIG. 5.244 SAGITTAL VIEW OF THORAX - DEPRESSED AND DISTORTED STERNUM

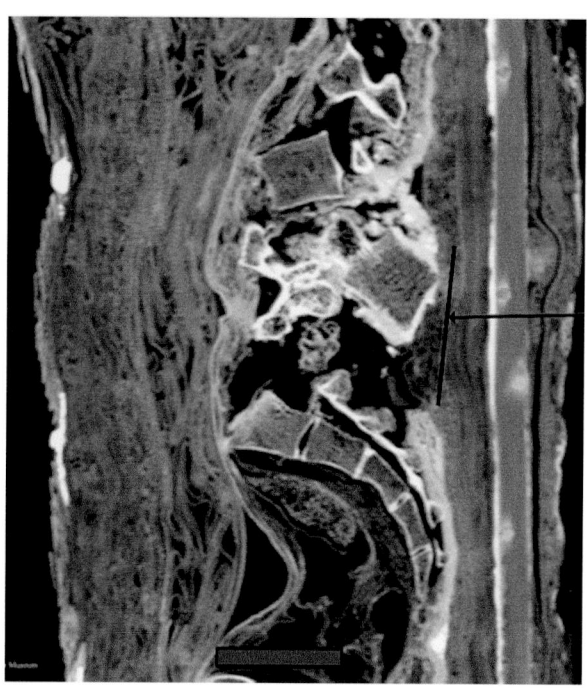

FIG. 5.245 SAGITTAL VIEW OF ABDOMEN - EXTRUDED LUMBAR VERTEBAE

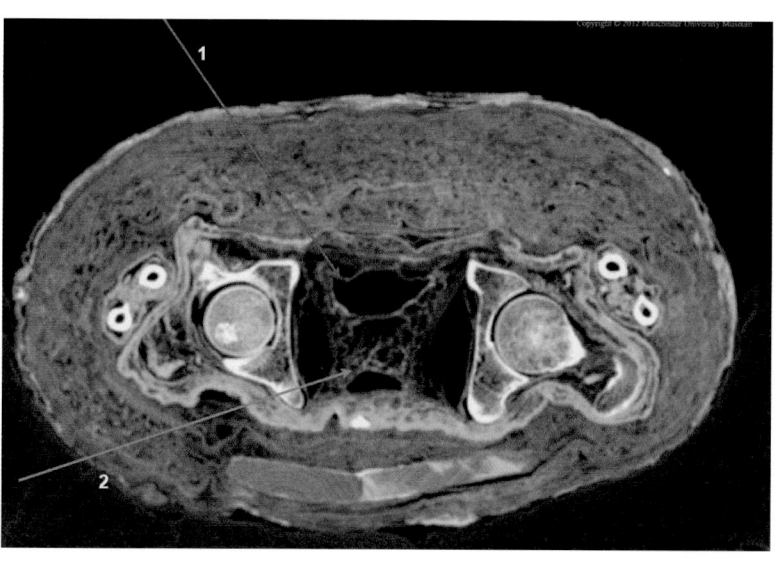

FIG. 5.246 AXIAL VIEW OF PELVIS - BLADDER AND RECTUM

XIII   Unnamed - Manchester University Museum (Accession No. MM1767)

Thorax

There is antero-posterior compression of the thoracic wall but no evidence of rib fractures (Fig. 5.247 - 2). This figure also shows some biological material in the posterior part of the thoracic cavity - presumably lung tissue - arrows 1. No mediastinal contents are visualized.

Abdomen

As with the thorax, there is antero-posterior compression of the abdomen. This is so profound that there is virtually no abdominal cavity remaining. No abdominal incision is identifiable. The only feature of note is the inclusion within the abdominal wrappings of a single vertebra, which is clearly the atlas, the first cervical vertebra (Fig. 5.248). Its inclusion within the wrappings indicates that it was recovered and included within those wrappings after bandaging had been commenced.

Pelvis and Hips

There is slight subluxation of both the sacro-iliac joints that may well be post-wrapping disruption. The pubic symphysis is intact and there are some soft tissue structures within the bony pelvis.

The hips are congruent with no evidence of arthritis.

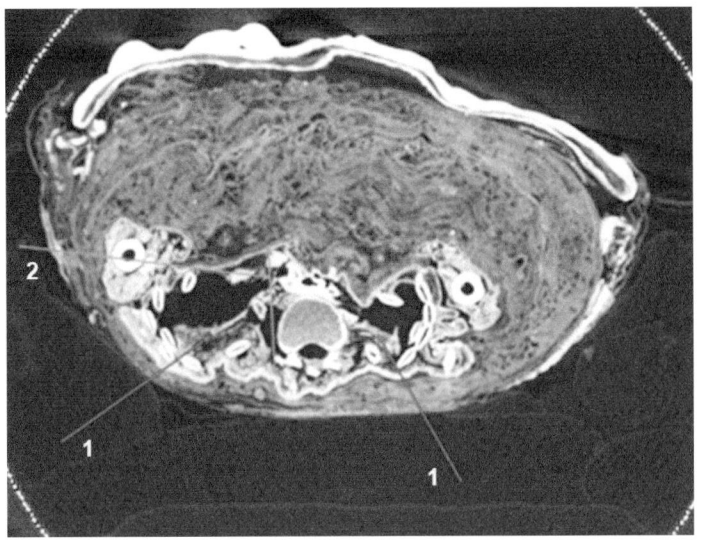

Fig. 5.247   Axial view - thoracic wall compression and thoracic visceral contents

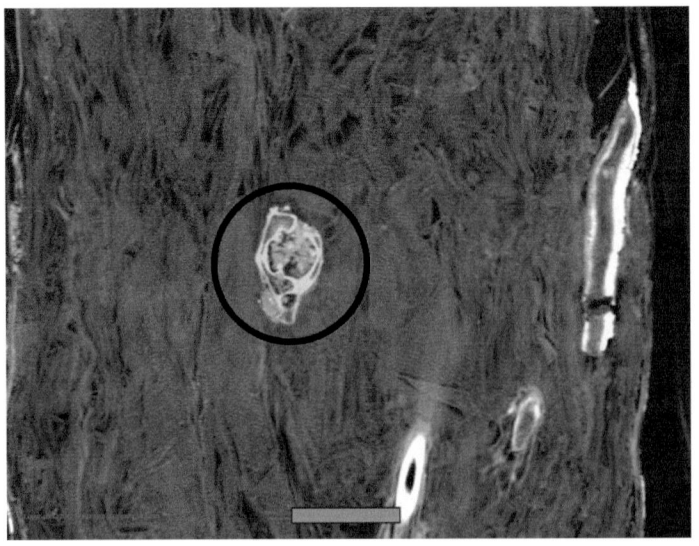

Fig. 5.248   Coronal view of abdomen - atlas within abdominal wrappings

XV. Unnamed - National Museums Liverpool (accession No. 13.10.11.25)

Thorax

There is disruption of the thoracic spine between the lower border of T2 and the upper border of T5. In other words there is loss of alignment of the T3 and 4 vertebrae (as mentioned above) and some curvature of the upper thoracic spine towards the left (See Fig. 5.249 - circle) but there is no rotation. It, therefore, does not indicate a true scoliosis, just a postural deformity - probably post-mortem.

There is no neural or meningeal tissue within the thoracic spinal canal.

The rib cage is compressed antero-posteriorly with rib disruption, but there is no evidence of rib fracture (See Fig. 5.250). Amorphous material is seen in both para-vertebral gutters, which is almost certainly biological tissue (Fig. 5.251 - arrow 1 and Fig. 5.251 - arrow 2). There is no evidence of a structured mediastinum or diaphragm.

Abdomen

The amorphous material in the thorax continues into the abdominal cavity on both sides, but is relatively sparse. This may represent organs in the abdomen. The abdominal cavity is, like the thorax, collapsed and flattened antero-posteriorly. As a result, the anterior abdominal wall is convoluted in axial section, which makes the recognition of an abdominal incision difficult. Whilst it is not possible to be dogmatic the evidence for a left flank (or other abdominal) incision is poor.

Pelvis and Hips

The bony pelvis is intact. The pelvis contains evidence of the lower colon, rectum and bladder. The external genitalia are covered anteriorly and to the left with a metal plate of apparently similar radio-density to the plate overlying the tongue. This could, therefore, also be gold (See Figs. 5.252 and 5.253). As stated above, in the General Description, the genitalia appear to be male.

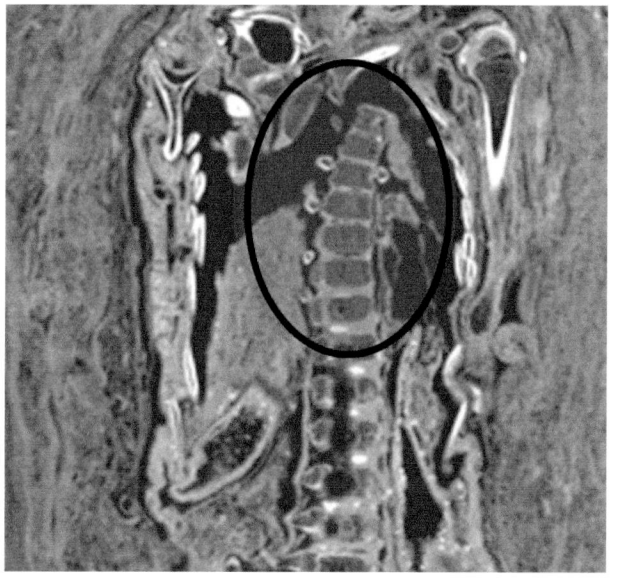

FIG. 5.249 CORONAL VIEW OF TRUNK - SPINAL CURVATURE - SCOLIOSIS

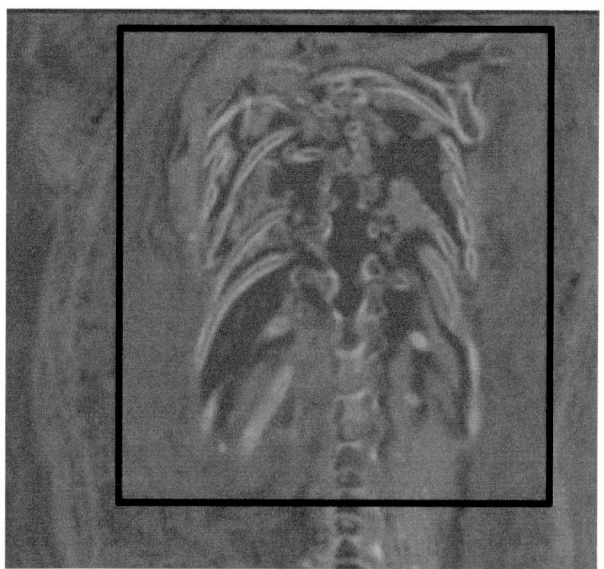

FIG. 5.250 CORONAL VIEW OF TRUNK - DISRUPTED RIBS

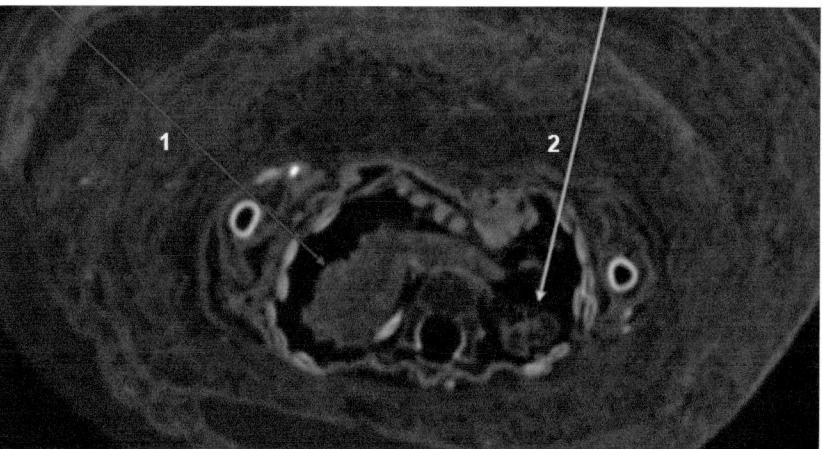

FIG. 5.251 AXIAL VIEW OF THORAX - VISCERA IN THORACIC CAVITY

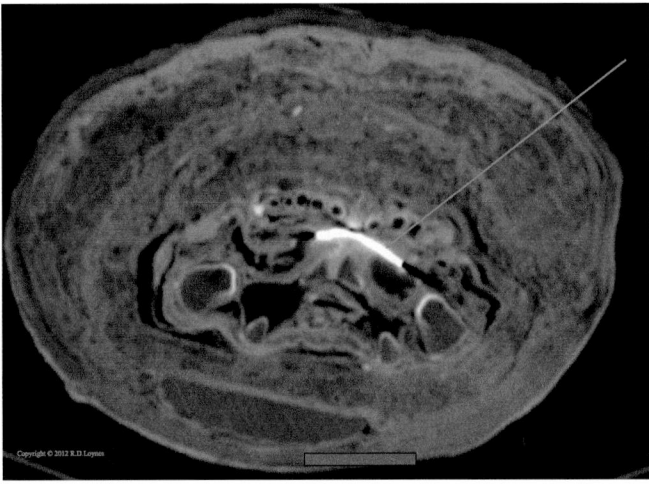

FIG. 5.252 AXIAL VIEW OF PELVIS - METAL PLATE OVER GENITALIA

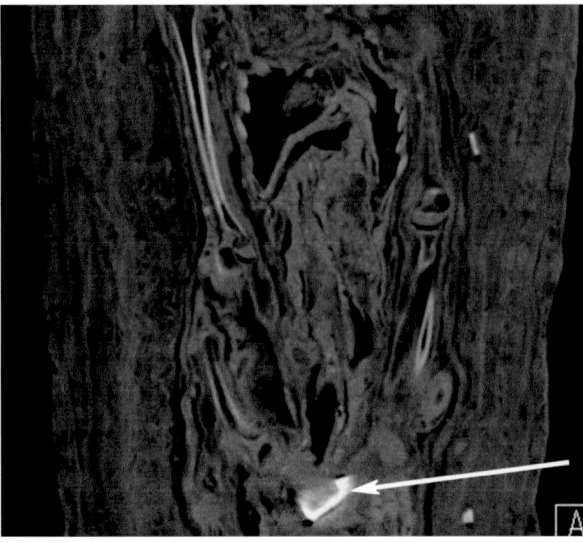

FIG. 5.253 CORONAL VIEW OF TRUNK - METAL PLATE OVER GENITALIA

XLVII. Unnamed - Manchester Museum (Cat. No.MM1769)

Thorax

Whilst the overall symmetry of the ribs is maintained, there is subluxation of the costo-vertebral joints affecting the right 4th, 5th, 6th, 7th, 8th and 9th ribs and the left 5th and 7th ribs. This is clearly seen in the right 8th costo-vertebral joint (See Fig. 5.254) - compare the black and white-circled arrows. Although there is no attachment of the mediastinum to the sternum, the intra-thoracic viscera appear to be in situ and are seen draped over the vertebrae in the axial views (See Fig. 5.255). No individual organs are visualised.

Abdomen

No abdominal incision is visible and the anterior abdominal wall is compressed against the spine. There is evidence of some viscera within the abdomen, but less than expected (See Fig. 5.256). Compression of the abdominal wall is seen well in Fig. 5.257.

Pelvis and Hips

There is subluxation of the left sacro-iliac joint, but no accompanying disruption of the right sacro-iliac joint or pubic symphysis.

The pelvic cavity contains viscera (See Fig. 5.258). As mentioned above, the external genitalia are not clearly visible. Although there is a suggestion of an external male urethra, the evidence is not conclusive.

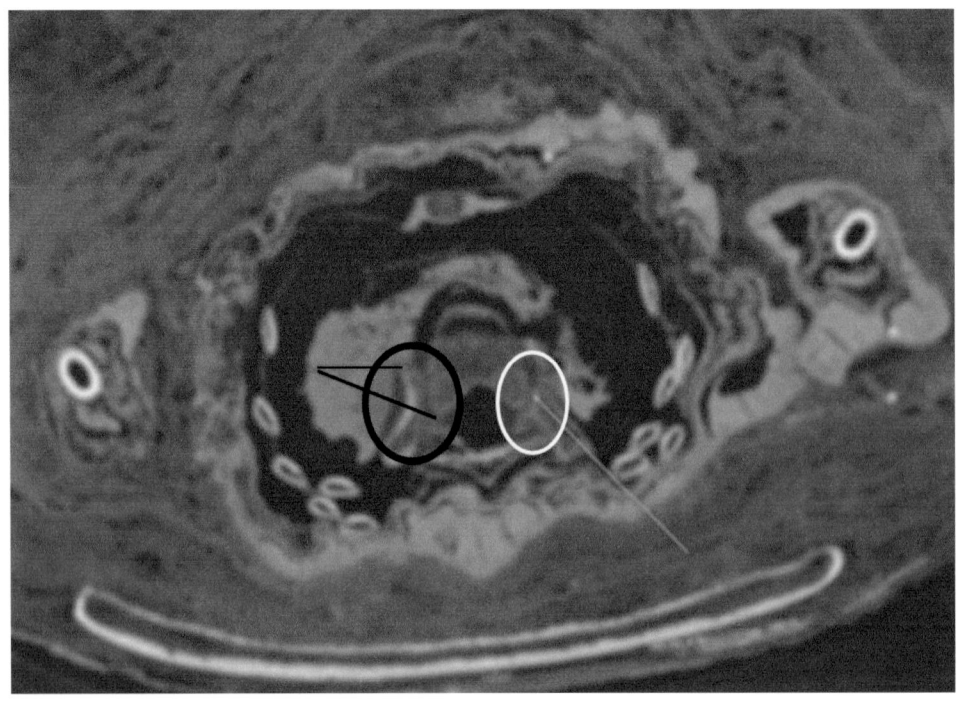

FIG. 5.254 AXIAL VIEW OF THORAX - COSTO-VERTEBRAL JOINTS

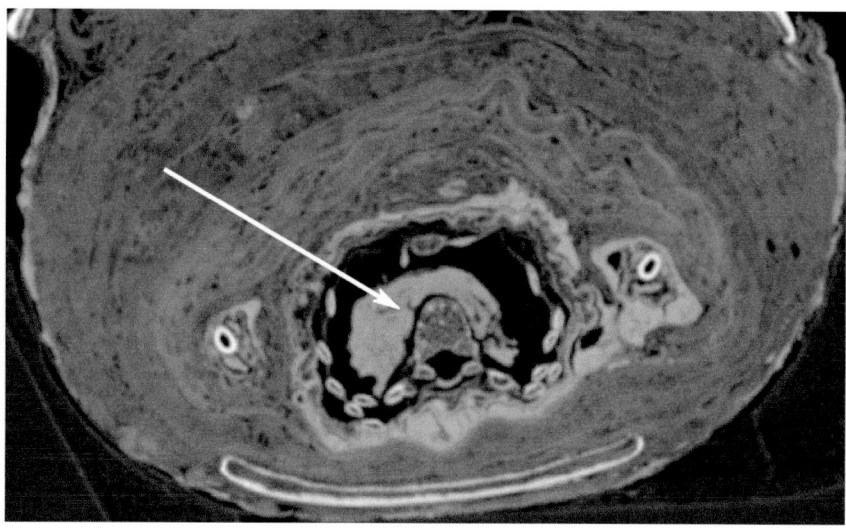

Fig. 5.255 Axial view of thorax - viscera overlying thoracic vertebral body

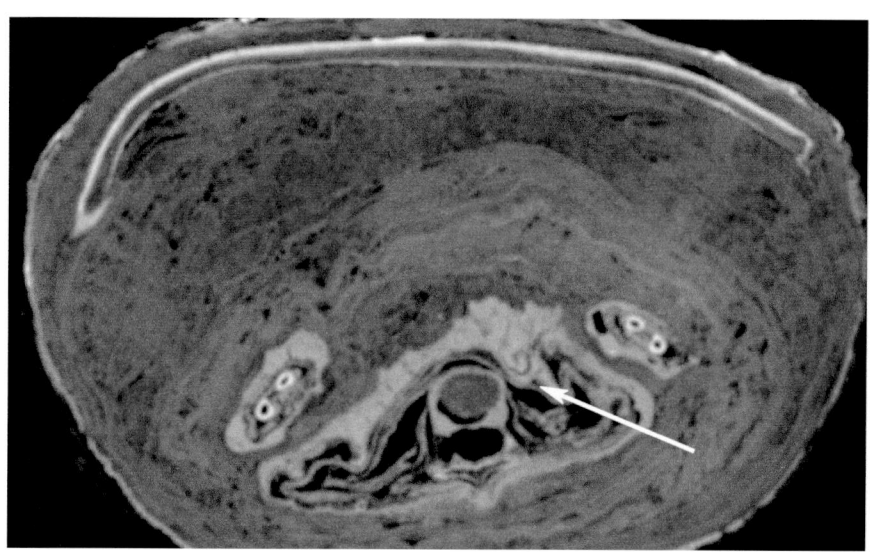

Fig. 5.256 Axial view of abdomen - viscera in abdomen

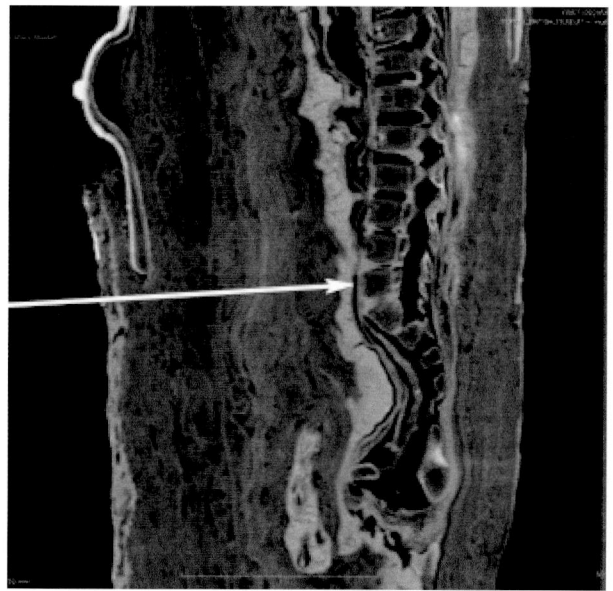

Fig. 5.257 Sagittal view of trunk - compression of abdominal wall against the spine

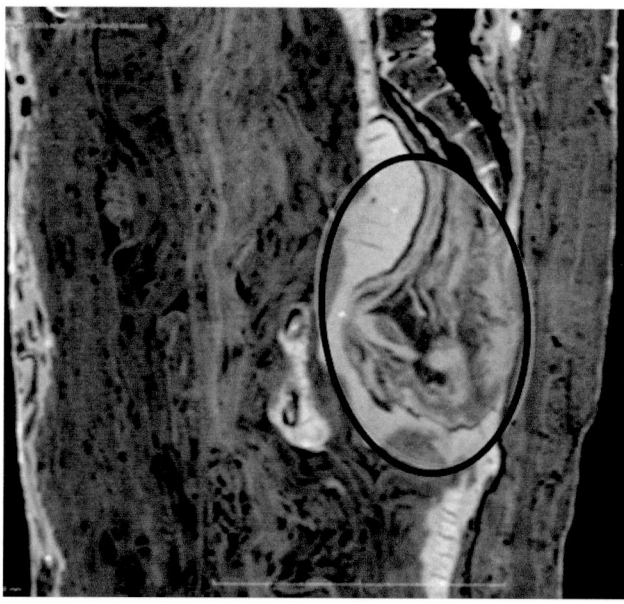

Fig. 5.258 Sagittal view showing viscera within pelvic cavity

Ll. Khary - Manchester Museum (Accession No. MM9354a)

Thorax

The thorax has not been eviscerated. The lungs can be seen desiccated and lying on the posterior wall. Although not seen separately, the heart is presumably within this tissue. Some calcification is noted at the root of both lungs that may indicate old healed TB (See Fig. 5.259 - 1). The left hemi-diaphragm is also clearly seen (See Fig. 5.259 - 2).

Abdomen

There is no evidence of an abdominal incision. Whilst the anterior abdominal wall has been compressed against the vertebral bodies, the remnants of the viscera can be seen displaced laterally within the abdominal cavity (See Fig. 5.260). Liver remnants can be seen on the right with calcified (and probably previously caseated) glands to the left of L1 (again secondary to healed TB) (See Fig. 5.261 - arrow 1 = liver; arrow 2 = calcified glands/lymph nodes).

Pelvis and Hips

The bony pelvis is intact and of a normal shape. The hip joints are congruous with visible evidence of articular cartilage (Fig. 5.262. - arrows). The pelvic viscera are in situ and the perineum is intact with normal external genitalia (See Fig. 5.263).

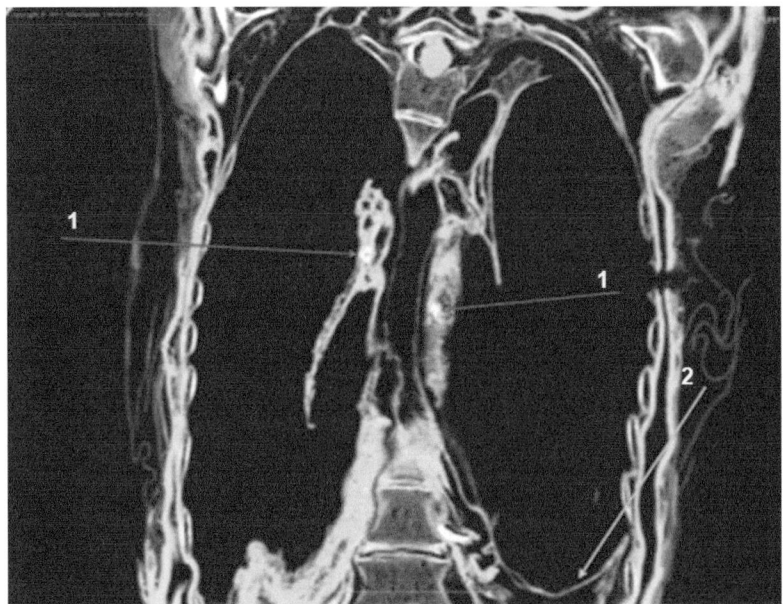

Fig. 5.259 Coronal view showing intra-thoracic structures

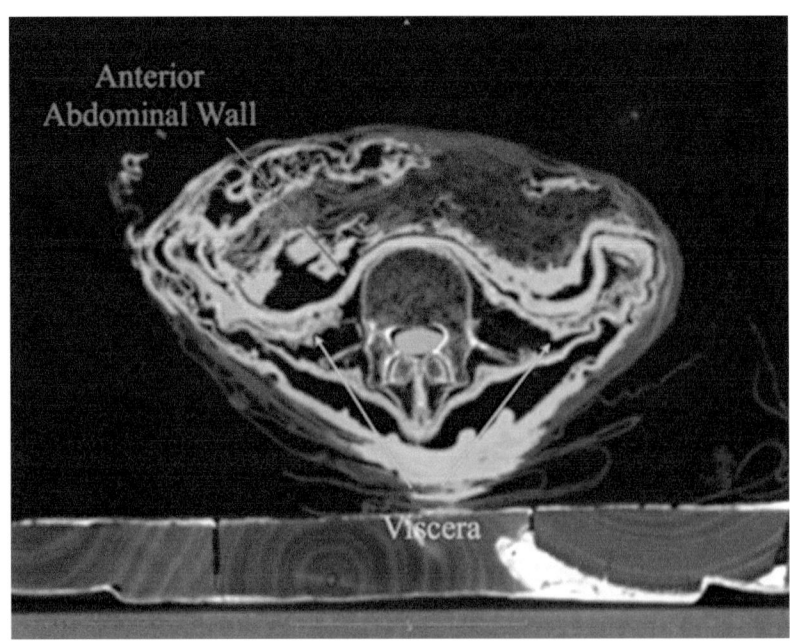

Fig. 5.260 Axial view of abdomen - compression of abdomen and contained structures

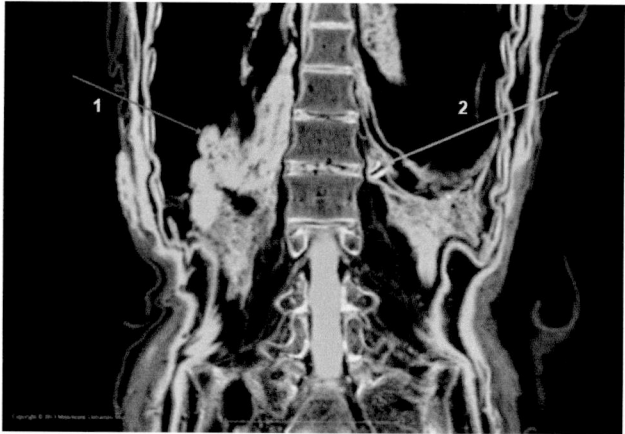

FIG. 5.261 CORONAL VIEW OF TRUNK - LIVER AND CALCIFIED NODE

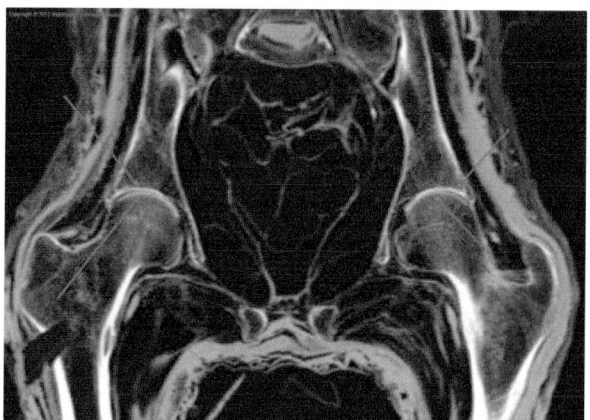

FIG. 5.262 CORONAL VIEW OF PELVIS - HIP JOINTS

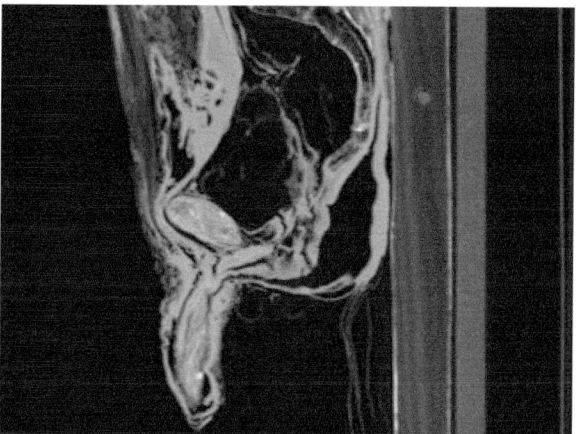

FIG. 5.263 SAGITTAL VIEW SHOWING PELVIC VISCERA

LII. Unnamed child - Manchester Museum (Accession No. MM9319)

Thorax

The normal thoracic kyphosis has been lost and the spine is straight. There are no other abnormalities in the thoracic spine, which contains the remnants of meningeal tissue but little else.

The rib cage is of a normal shape and the thoracic contents (lungs and mediastinum) are desiccated and lie in the posterior gutters of the thorax. Although remnants of both hemi-diaphragms are present they are not complete.

Abdomen

There is no abdominal wall incision and no evidence of evisceration. The abdominal contents lie, desiccated, on the posterior wall of the abdomen.

Pelvis and Hips

The bony pelvis is intact and the pelvic viscera are in situ. The perineum is intact and the phallus clearly seen. The hips are congruous and normal.

LIV. Unnamed - Manchester Museum (Accession. No. Salford2)

Thorax

The rib cage is a normal shape. There has been no attempt at evisceration. The heart and great vessels lie in the posterior mediastinum and the lungs in the paraspinal gutters (Fig. 5.264 (arrow 3 = mediastinal contents, arrows 1 and 2 = lungs and Fig. 5.265 shows a lateral view of the thorax).

Abdomen

There is no abdominal incision and there has been no attempt at evisceration. The viscera lie on the posterior abdominal wall (See Fig. 5.266).

Pelvis and Hips

Minimal disruption of the sacro-iliac joints and symphysis pubis is seen, but this could be post-mortem (See Fig. 5.267).

The hips are congruous and exhibit good articular cartilage cover (See Fig. 5.268 - 1. Fused epiphyses are still clearly visible, indicating early adulthood (See Fig. 5.268 - 2).

The perineum is intact, as has already been discussed. Remnants of the pelvic viscera are clearly seen (See Fig. 5.269).

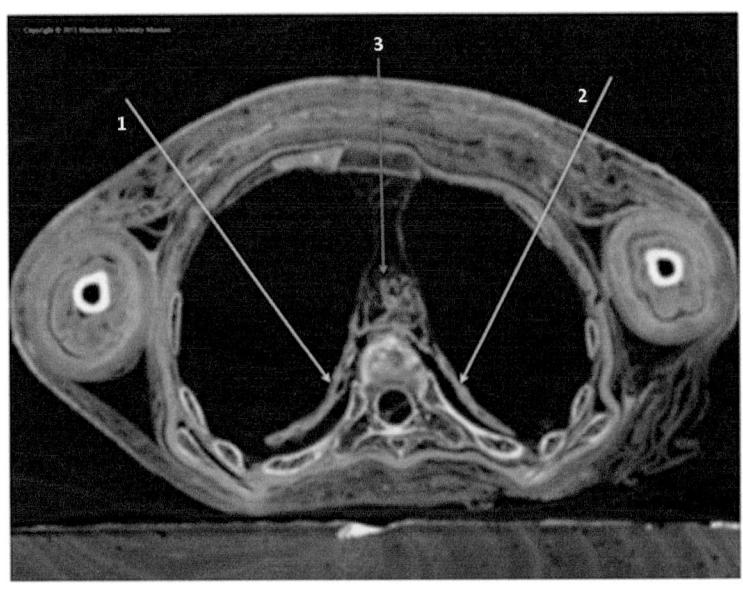

FIG. 5.264 AXIAL VIEW DEMONSTRATING INTRA-THORACIC CONTENTS

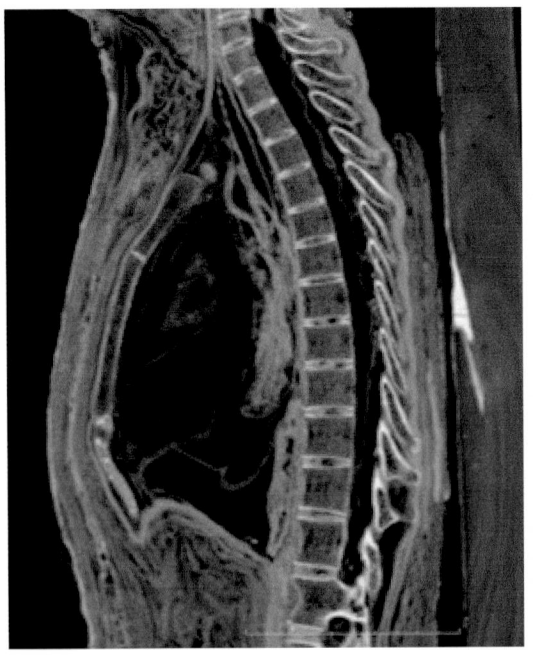

FIG. 4.265 SAGITTAL VIEW SHOWING INTRA-THORACIC CONTENTS

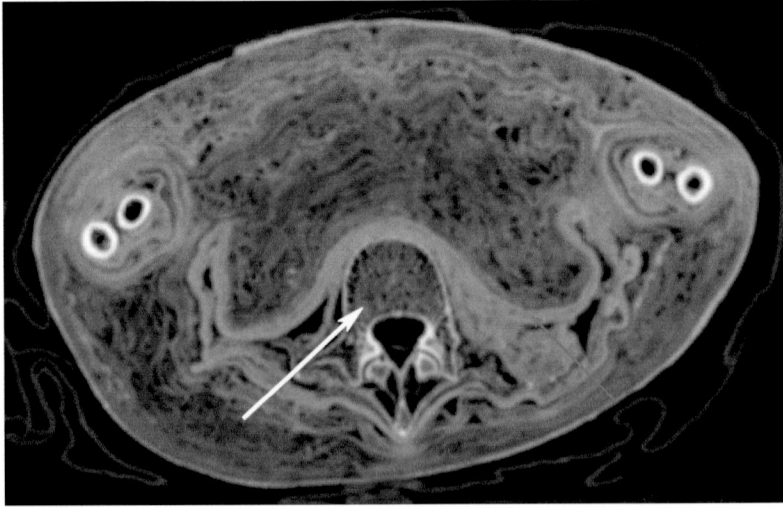

FIG. 5.266 AXIAL VIEW OF LOWER ABDOMEN - VISCERA ON POSTERIOR ABDOMINAL WALL

RESULTS – THE TRUNK

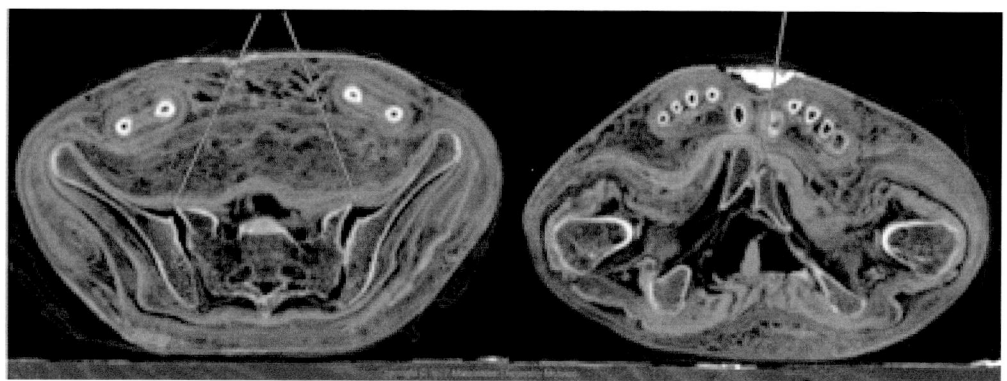

FIG. 5.267 AXIAL VIEW OF PELVIS - SLIGHT DISRUPTION OF THE BONY PELVIS

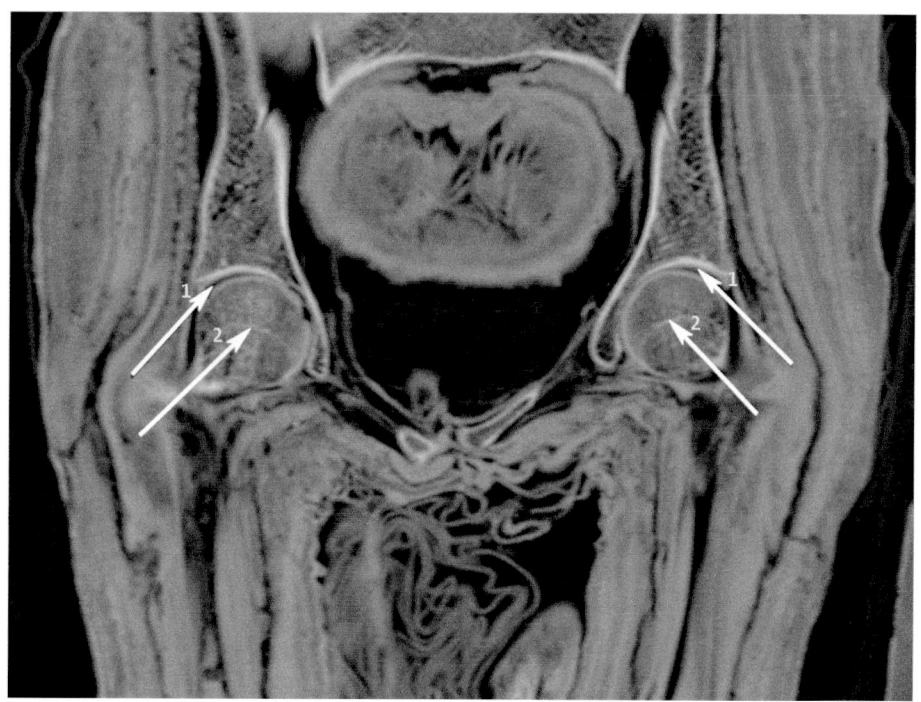

FIG. 5.268 CORONAL VIEW OF HIP JOINTS

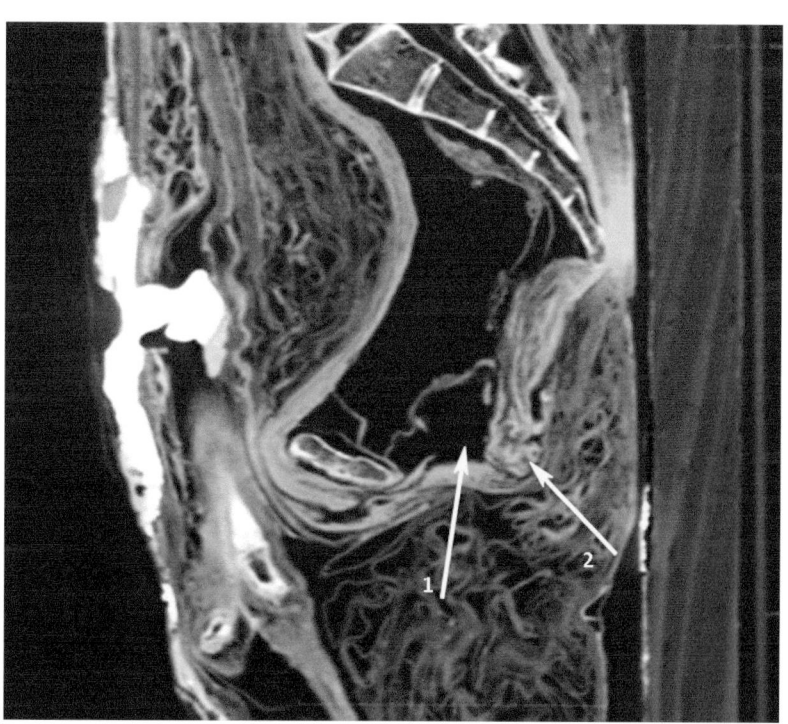

FIG. 5.269 SAGITTAL VIEW OF PELVIC CONTENTS

LV. Unnamed child - Manchester Museum (Accession No. MM 13011)

Thorax

The rib cage is almost symmetrical with only slight reduction in cross sectional area on the left, as seen in Fig. 5.270. This is, however, not a significant feature when viewed from posteriorly, anteriorly or laterally. Significantly, there is no evidence of fractures or dislocations of the ribs. The mediastinum remains intact and the heart and great vessels are seen to the left of the mid-line (See Fig. 5.271 - arrow). Remnants of the lungs lie on the posterior thoracic wall. Evisceration of the thorax has not been performed.

Abdomen

There is no abdominal incision or evisceration.

The anterior abdominal wall lies against the lumbar vertebrae (See Fig. 5.272 - arrow 2) with abdominal viscera on either side of the spine (See Fig. 5.272 - arrows 1).

Pelvis and Hips

Minimal right SI joint subluxation is seen but the left SI joint is intact (Fig. 5.273 - arrow 1 and arrow 2). The symphysis pubis and hip joints are normal.

The pelvic organs remain in situ and the perineum is undisturbed. The presence of the phallus has already been mentioned.

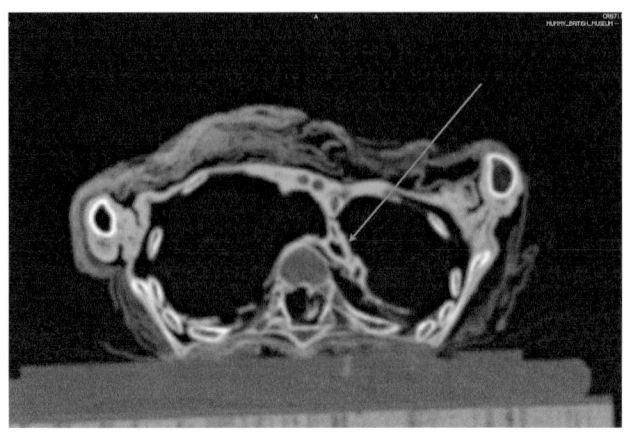

FIG. 5.271 Axial view of thorax - mediastinum

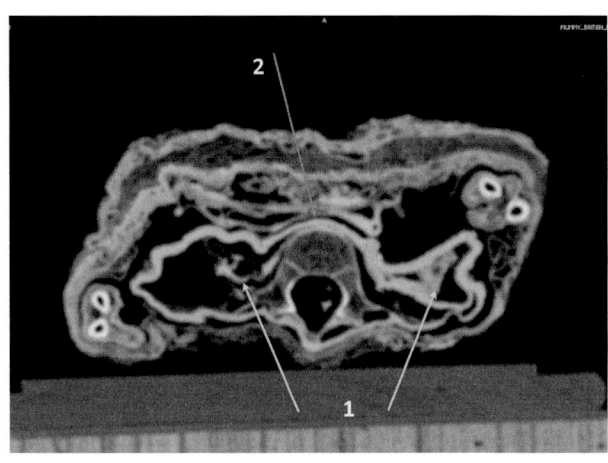

FIG. 5.272 Axial view showing abdominal compression and viscera

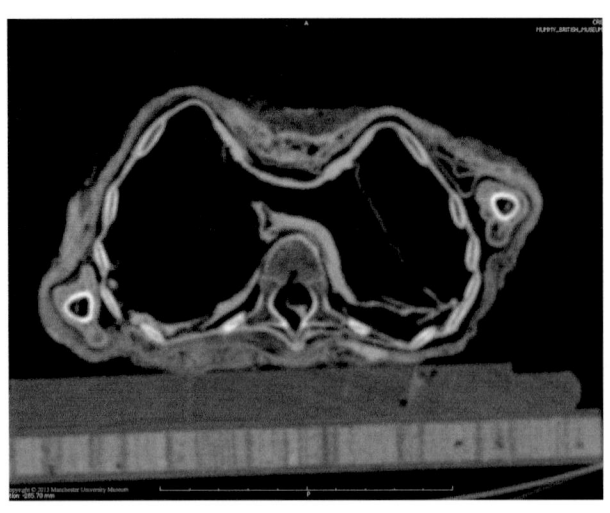

FIG. 5.270 Axial view of thorax - slight asymmetry of thoracic wall

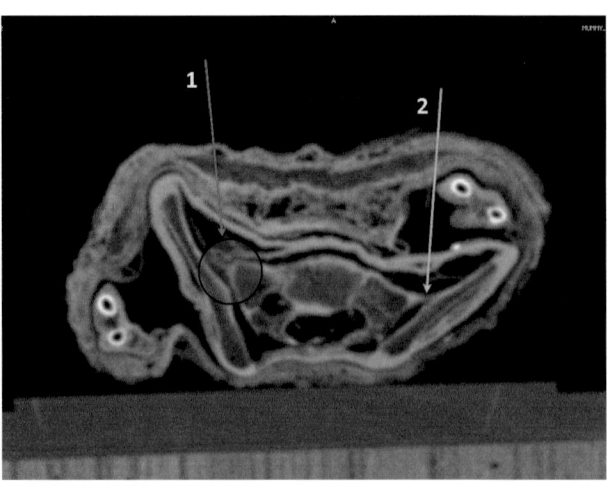

FIG. 5.273 Axial view of sacro-iliac joints

LVI. Unnamed child - Manchester Museum (Accession. No. MM 2109)

Thorax

There is compression of the thorax with the sternum (Fig. 5.274 - 1) lying against the thoracic vertebrae (Fig. 5.274 - 2). Many ribs are completely dislocated and displaced (Fig. 5.275). The desiccated thoracic organs are seen within the cavity (See Fig. 5.276 - larger circle). This figure also shows the sternum (2), the thoracic vertebral body (arrow 4) and the displaced ribs (smaller circle).

Abdomen

There is no abdominal incision and no abdominal evisceration, the viscera lying within the compressed abdominal cavity. Fig. 5.277 shows the viscera - arrow 2 and the anterior abdominal wall - arrow 1.

Pelvis and Hips

The bony pelvis is intact with normal, congruous hip joints. The pelvic viscera are present and there is a small pack of linen within the rectum (See Fig. 5.278 - circles). The sacrum is shown - arrow. The perineum is intact.

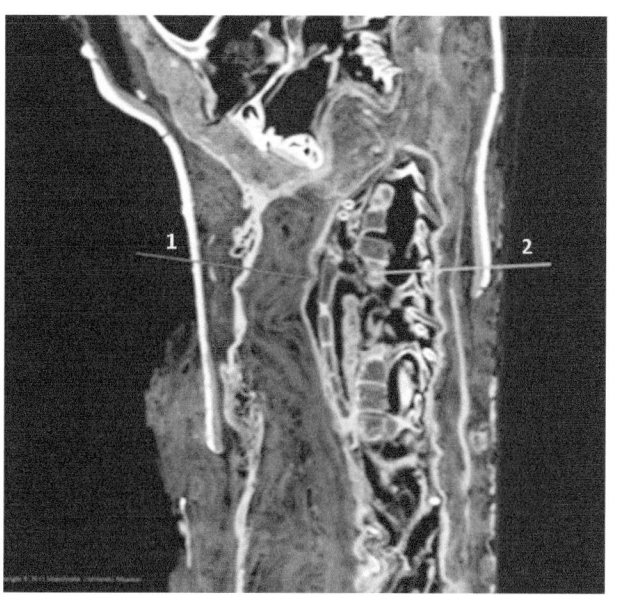

FIG. 5.274 SAGITTAL VIEW OF THORAX SHOWING COMPRESSION

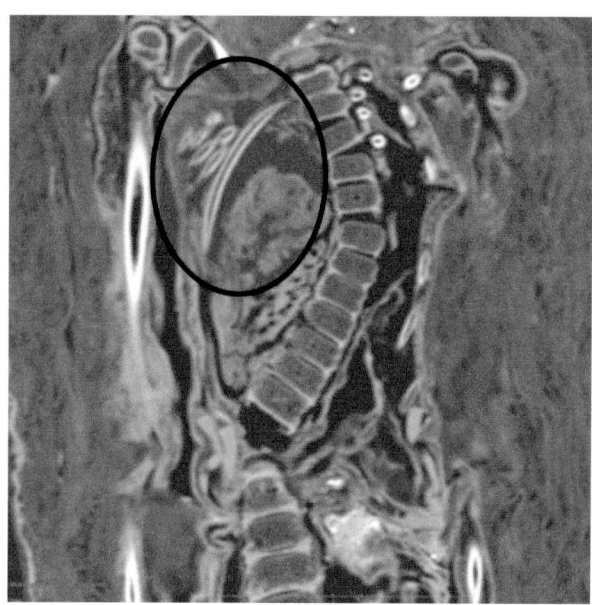

FIG. 5.275 CORONAL VIEW OF DISRUPTED RIBS AND SPINE

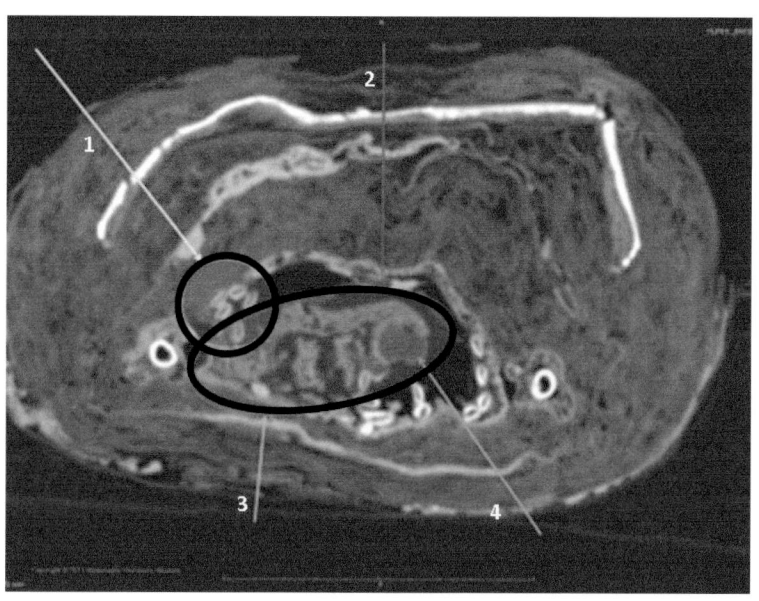

FIG. 5.276 AXIAL VIEW OF COMPRESSED THORAX AND CONTENTS

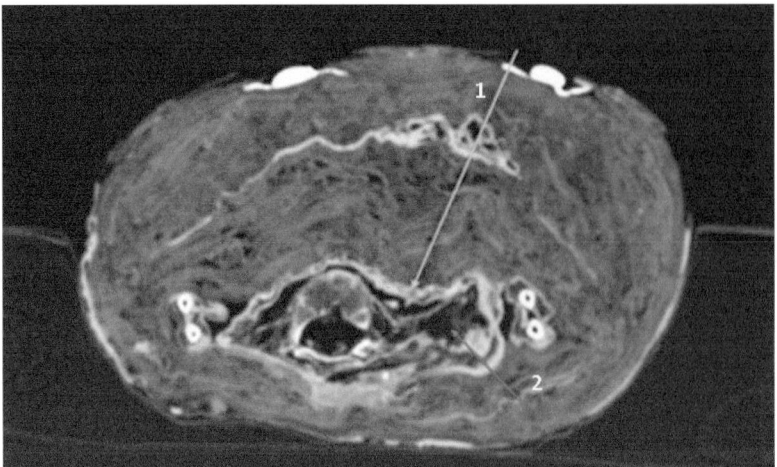

FIG. 5.277 AXIAL VIEW OF COMPRESSED ABDOMEN AND CONTAINED VISCERA

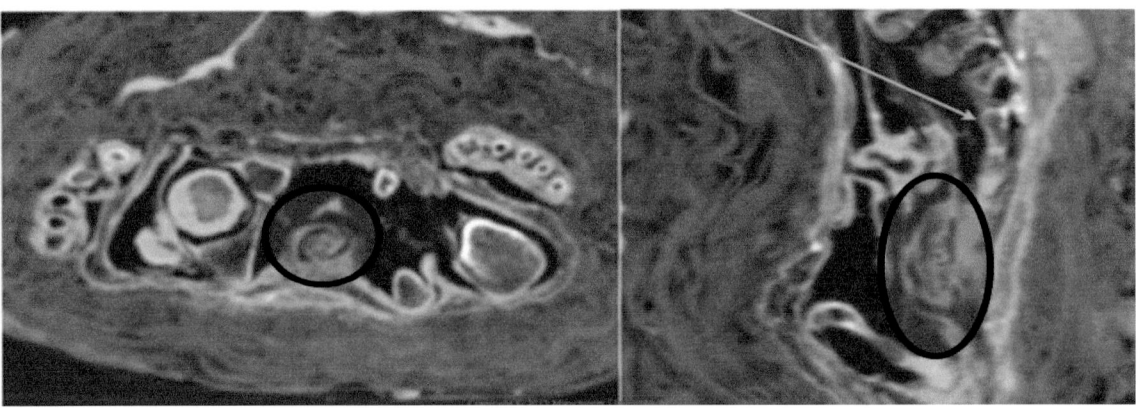

FIG. 5.278 AXIAL AND SAGITTAL VIEWS OF PACK IN RECTUM

LVII. Artemidorus - Manchester Museum (Cat. No. MM 1775)

Thorax

The rib cage is asymmetrical with compression of the left ribs and dislocation of some of the right costo-vertebral joints (1st, 5th, 6th, 7th, 8th). These are accompanied by fractures of the left 2nd, 3rd, 4th, 5th, 6th, 7th, 8th ribs. The asymmetry can be seen in Fig. 5.279 (cf black and white outlines). An example of right costo-vertebral dislocation is seen in Fig. 5.280 (cf the heads of the right and left ribs).

The mediastinal contents are visible with the great vessels shown in Fig. 5.281 and a structure, which may well be the heart shown in Figs. 5.282 and 5.283.

In the left thoracic cavity there is tissue, which could well be lung tissue. The diaphragm is seen in Fig. 5.284 - arrow. As can be seen in this figure, there is a radio-dense mass on the right side of the torso - circles. It is difficult to identify this tissue, it may be the desiccated liver but as there is no abdominal incision it is unlikely to be foreign material.

Abdomen

There is no evidence of a flank incision. Some desiccated viscera are seen on the posterior abdominal wall.

Pelvis and Hips

The bony pelvis is slightly disorganised in that there is disruption of the left sacro-iliac joint and pubic symphysis (Figs. 5.285 and 5.286 - circles) and a fracture of the right acetabulum (Fig. 5.286 - black circle). The hip joints are congruous (Fig. 5.287).

Whilst there are some disorganised structures in the pelvis, there is no evidence of definite organs. The perineum is intact.

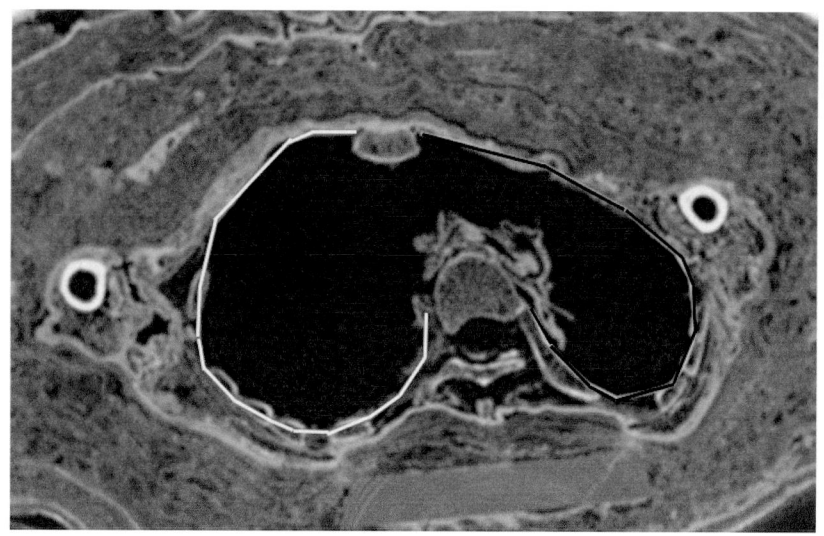

FIG. 5.279 AXIAL VIEW SHOWING ASYMMETRY OF RIB CAGE

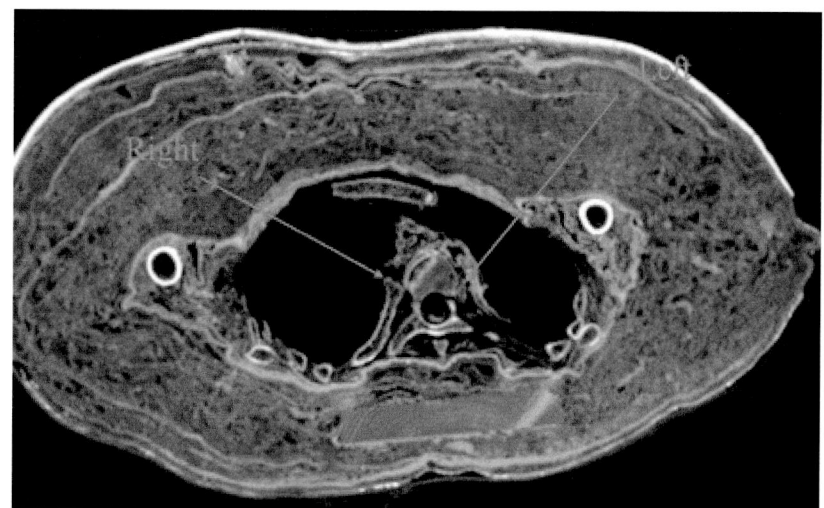

FIG. 5.280 AXIAL VIEW OF THORAX - COSTO-VERTEBRAL JOINTS

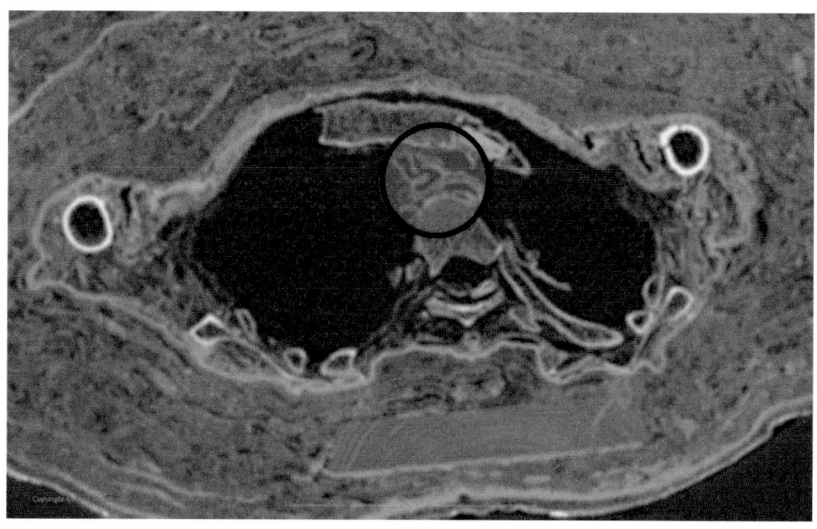

FIG. 5.281 AXIAL VIEW OF THORAX - MEDIASTINUM – GREAT VESSELS

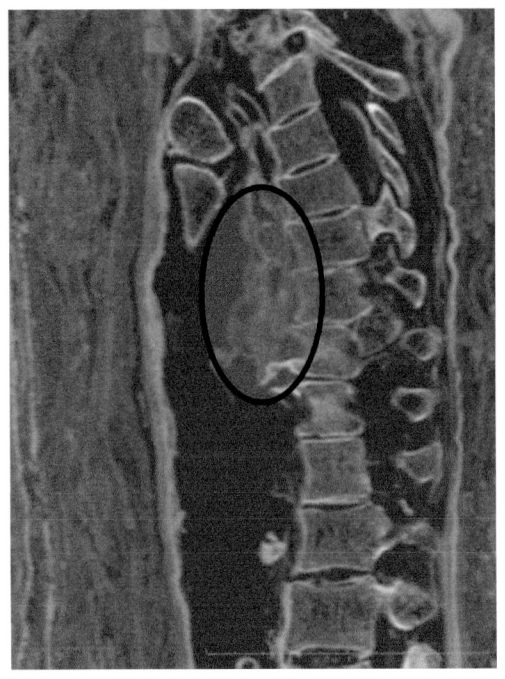

Fig. 5.282 Sagittal view of thorax - mediastinum - heart

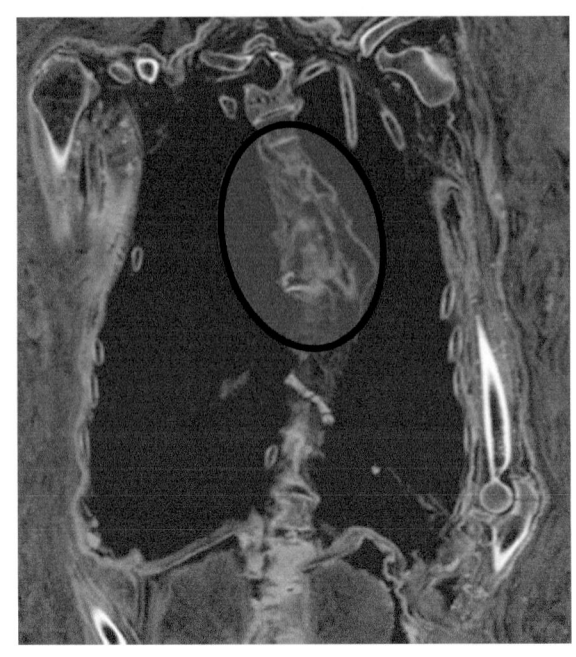

Fig. 5.283 Coronal view of thorax - mediastinum - heart

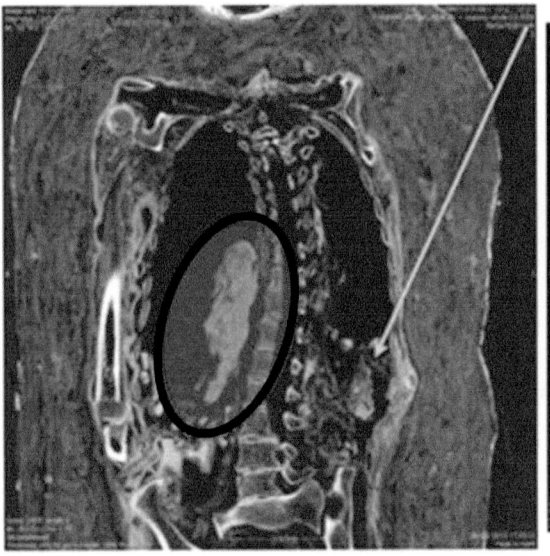
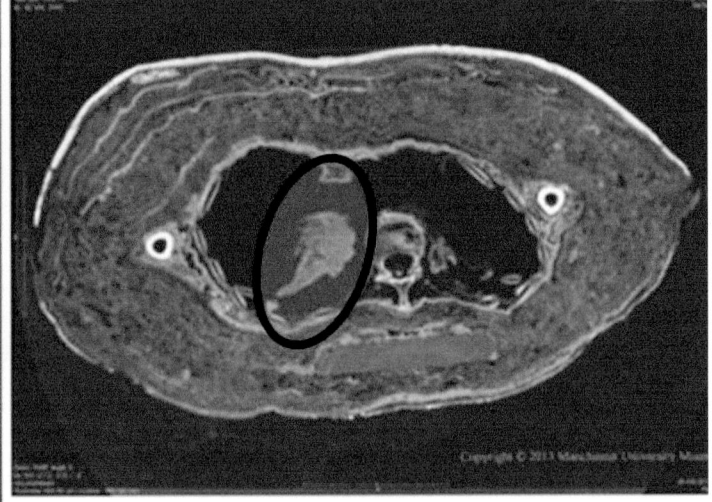

Fig. 5.284 Coronal view of trunk and axial view of thorax - diaphragm and liver

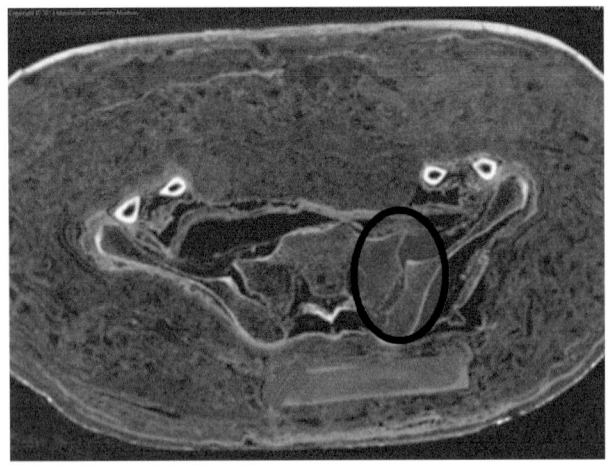

Fig. 5.285 Axial view of pelvis - disrupted SIJ

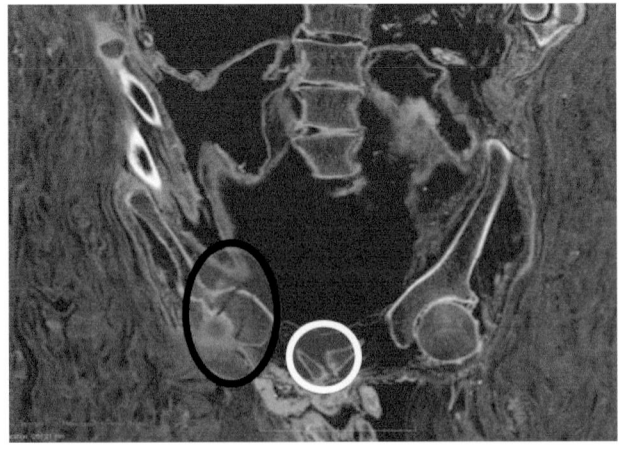

Fig. 5.286 Coronal view of pelvis - disrupted symphysis pubis and fractured acetabulum

RESULTS – THE TRUNK

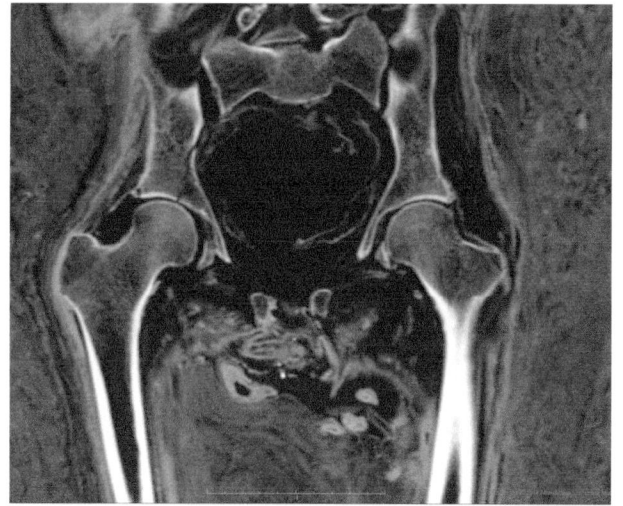

FIG. 5.287 CORONAL VIEW OF CONGRUOUS HIP JOINTS

Abdomen

The abdomen has no evidence of a flank incision, nor any evidence of evisceration.

Pelvis and Hips

There is slight disruption of the left sacro-iliac joint but no such damage on the right. The symphysis pubis and hips are intact. There has not been any disturbance of the perineum. As mentioned above, the phallus is almost certainly present.

LIX. Unnamed - British Museum (Cat. No.EA 22108)

Thorax

The rib cage is compressed antero-posteriorly with the sternum lying against the thoracic vertebral bodies (see Fig. 5.288 white circle = sternum; black circle = vertebral body). Evisceration has not been performed and remnants of the lungs can be seen lying over the vertebral bodies (See Fig. 5.289). The compression of the rib cage has resulted in the dislocation of some costo-vertebral joints, as shown in Fig. 5.290 - 1 = head of rib - 2 = corresponding point on vertebral body with which it should articulate (dislocation of CVJ 7th, 8th, 9th, 10th on right and 5th, 6th, 7th, 8th on left). There is, also, crowding of the left ribs (See Fig. 5.291 - 1= right ribs; 2 = left ribs).

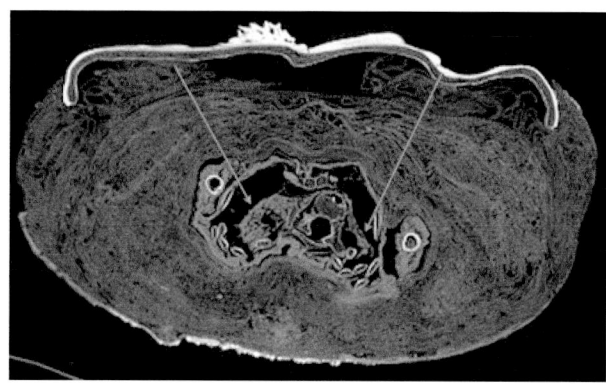

FIG. 5.289 AXIAL VIEW OF THORAX - VISCERA LYING OVER VERTEBRAL BODIES

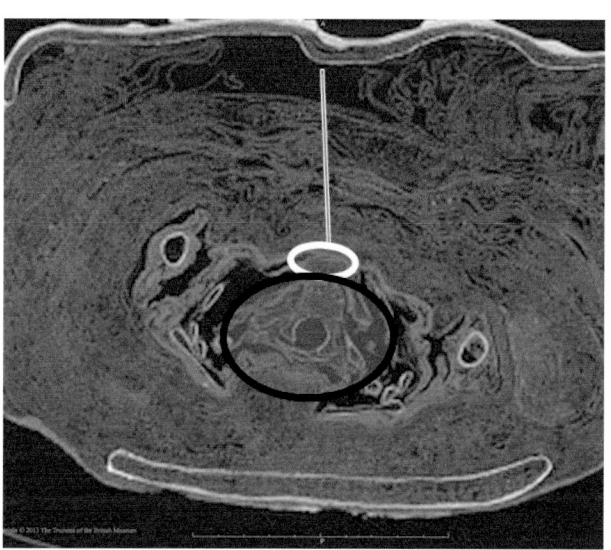

FIG. 5.288 AXIAL VIEW OF THORAX - STERNUM LYING AGAINST VERTEBRAL BODIES
COURTESY OF THE TRUSTEES OF THE BRITISH MUSEUM

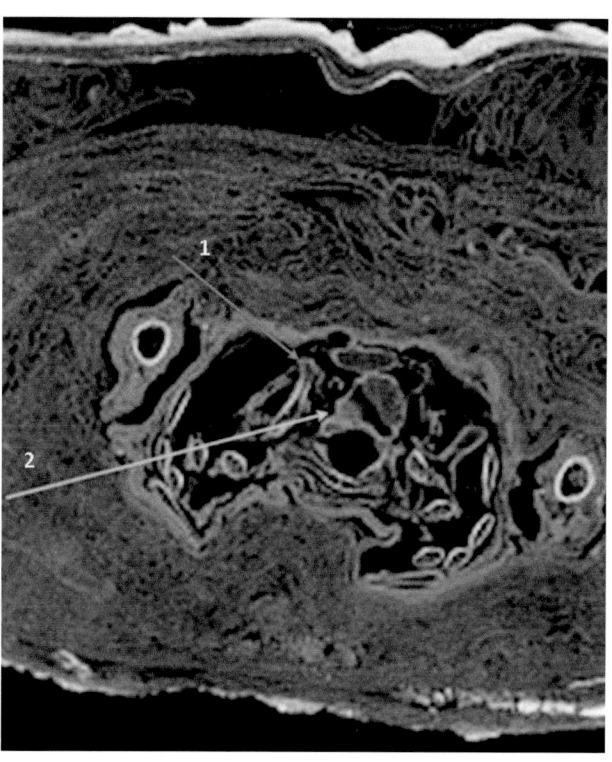

FIG. 5.290 AXIAL VIEW OF THORAX - COSTO-VERTEBRAL DISLOCATION
COURTESY OF THE TRUSTEES OF THE BRITISH MUSEUM

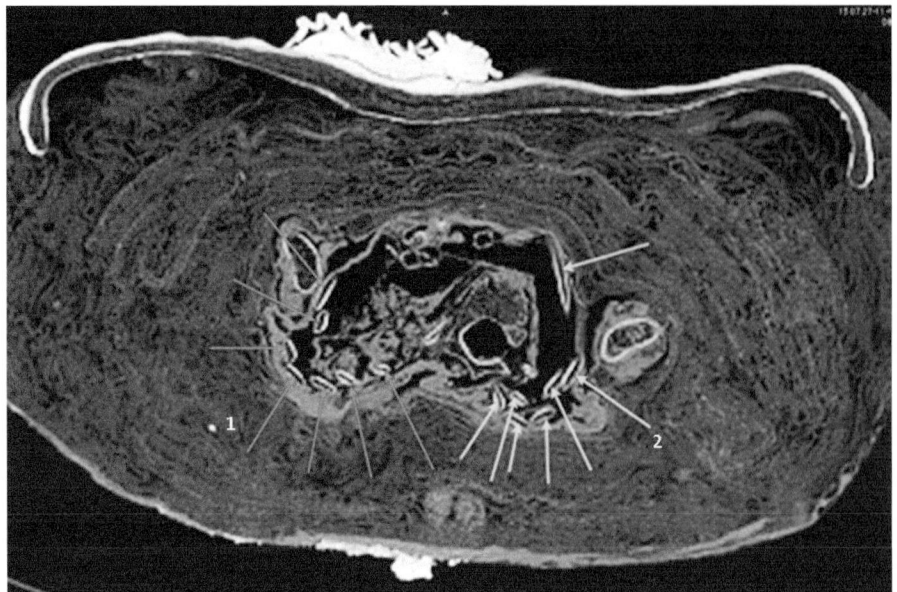

Fig. 5.291 Axial view of thorax - crowded ribs
Courtesy of the Trustees of the British Museum

5.2.4 Evisceration. The extent of visceral clearance:

Evisceration or visceral clearance affects three regions. These are the thoracic cavity, the abdominal cavity and the pelvic cavity. Whilst it might be initially assumed that clearance would be performed on all three regions, this is not necessarily the case. The appearance of these three regions of the body cavity in cases where there has been no apparent entry portal (covered in section 5.2.3) gives an indication of the appearance of tissues when they have been subjected to desiccation only.

5.2.4.1 Thorax

Of the eleven cases shown in Table 5.2 the rib cage is distorted in six cases and the structure of the mediastinum lost in these cases. However, in the other cases (Mummies LI, LII, LIV, LV and LVII) there is little or no distortion and the mediastinal structures are still recognizable. In the cases of rib cage distortion, the remains of the viscera (heart, lungs and great vessels) are visible lying on the posterior thoracic wall. A good example of mediastinal structure retention can be seen in Figure 5.264 – (P 164). The loss of mediastinal structure but with retention of tissues is shown in Figure 5.255 – (P 161). The loss of recognizable structure seems to be due more to external deformation than anything else. The interesting feature is that the cavity of the thorax sometimes appears empty as the internal structures desiccate and fall away to the posterior aspect of the cavity as seen in Figure 5.264 and 5.281. The conclusion that can be drawn is that the presence of viscera posteriorly may reflect either incomplete or absent attempts at evisceration of the thorax. The presence, absence or incomplete nature of the diaphragm is not a reflection of attempts at its removal but of its fragile and friable nature (when desiccated) secondary to its thinness.

5.2.4.2 Abdomen

In seven of the eleven cases of lack of evisceration, there is marked compression of the anterior abdominal wall against the posterior wall of the abdomen and against the spine. In mummies LV and LVII there is less compression and some remaining cavity seen in the abdomen and in Mummies LII and LIV there is no compression of the abdomen. As anticipated, there is obvious evidence of the remaining viscera on the posterior abdominal wall.

5.2.4.3 Pelvic cavity

In most of the non-evisceration cases there is clear evidence of pelvic organs remaining as seen in Figures 5.262, 5.263 and 5.269. In only one case above is there evidence of a linen pack in the rectum – Figure 5.278.

5.2.4.4 Evisceration of the thorax

Two of the forty mummies in this study that had evidence of evisceration were disrupted so that a true picture could not be analysed and one had evidence pointing to the fact that thoracic evisceration had, probably, not been attempted. Therefore there were thirty-seven mummies with evisceration of the thorax that could be analysed.

There is no evidence either in the literature or in this study of evisceration being performed by any route other than the abdominal one. Whether the abdominal route is via a left flank incision or via the perineum (or both) the approach to the thorax is from below. Therefore, to eviscerate the thorax it is necessary to penetrate the diaphragm. This will either destroy or deform this structure. However, as mentioned in section 5.2.4.1, the presence, absence or incomplete nature of the diaphragm reflects nothing more than the delicate nature of this structure. For the sake of completeness, the presence of the diaphragm is seen in the following mummies (See Table 5.3).

NUMBER	ORIGIN	ERA
II	Birmingham - Namenkhetamun	D26
III	Birmingham - Padimut	D20-21
IX	Liverpool - Padiamunnebnesuttauwy	D25
X	Liverpool - Nesmin	Ptolemaic
XIV	Manchester – MM1777 - Asru	D26
XVI	Liverpool - M13997a	Roman
XXV	Zurich - Geneva - TjesMoutPert - D0242	D22-25
XXVI	Zurich - Geneva - Infant	Unknown
XXXII	BM - EA20744	D22
XXXVIII	Zurich - St. Gallen - Shepenese	D26
XL	Zurich - Lausanne - 492	3IP
XLIV	Turin - Provv.610	Ptolemaic ??
XLVIII	Manchester - MM3496	D18
LX	BM - EA 6704	Roman

TABLE 5.3 EVIDENCE OF THE PRESENCE OF PART OF THE DIAPHRAGM

In the case of Mummy XXXII the diaphragm is possibly completely intact and the structures in the thorax may represent complete viscera. In other words, although the abdomen has been eviscerated, the thorax may not have been similarly treated (See Figs. 5.144 and 5.145 (P 129). The converse of this is Mummy XLIII where the thoracic cavity is completely empty and there is no packing. In other cases there is complete absence of thoracic viscera but packing of some description has been added (See Table 5.4). In Mummies XVI and LX remnants of the diaphragm are also seen – but not in the others.

NUMBER	ORIGIN	ERA
I	Birmingham - Graeco-Roman	Roman
V	Sheffield - Nesitanebetasheru	D25
VII	Ipswich - Tahathor	D25
VIII	Liverpool - Padiamun - 53.72a	D22
XV	Liverpool - 13.10.11.25	Roman
XVI	Liverpool - M13997a	Roman
XVII	Liverpool - Ankhesenaset - 14000	3IP
XVIII	Liverpool- M14048	Roman
XIX	Zurich - Altdorf Child	Roman
XXIII	Zurich - Yverdon - Nes-Shou - MY/3775	Ptolemaic
XXIX	BM - Hor - EA6659	D22
XXXIII	BM - EA22939	D22
XXXIV	BM - EA25258	D22
XLI	Zurich - Lenzburg - K10351	Roman
LIII	Manchester - MM1976.51a	D25
LX	BM - EA 6704	Roman

TABLE 5.4 THORACIC EVISCERATION COMPLETE, WITH THE ADDITION OF PACKING.

The contents of the thorax are, essentially, the lungs and the mediastinum. The mediastinum lies in the midline and contains the great vessels superiorly and the heart in the lower part. Also running through the mediastinum are the trachea and the oesophagus (See Fig. 5.292 - from Cardiac Vascular and Thoracic Surgery Associates).

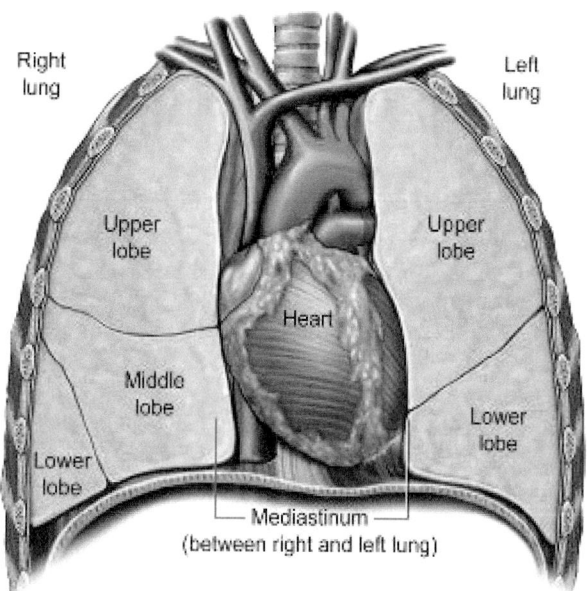

FIG. 5.292 THE ANATOMY OF THE THORAX AND MEDIASTINUM.
http://www.cvtsa.com

Evisceration of the thoracic cavity, if incomplete, will leave various organs behind. As mentioned in section 5.2.4.1 if left in situ, the lung tissue will fall to the posterior aspect of the thoracic cavity. There are two exceptions to this statement. These are mummies number XL and XXXVII, where the right lung and heart are both seen clearly. The right lung has not collapsed to the posterior wall. This may well indicate the presence of pleural adhesions secondary to previous pulmonary disease. In both cases the left lung is absent or only partially retained (See Figs. 5.181, 5.226 and 5.227). It is interesting to note that such adhesions are found in 90% of people dying of tuberculosis and in nearly as high a percentage of people with gross tuberculous lesions dying of other causes (Bogen and Pasternack, 1954: 170). To complete the picture, lung tissue is found in the following mummies where some degree of evisceration has been performed (see Table 5.5).

NUMBER	ORIGIN	Viscera Present	ERA
IX	Liverpool - Padiamunnebnesuttauwy	L,D,P	D25
XII	Manchester - MM1768	L	Roman
XIV	Manchester – MM1777 - Asru	GV,M,L,D	D26
XXVII	Manchester - Demetria - MM11630	L	Roman
XXXVIII	Zurich - St. Gallen - Shepenese	M,H,GV,L,D,P	D26
XXXIX	Zurich - St. Gallen - C3530	L,P	D21
XL	Zurich - Lausanne - 492	M,H,GV,L,D	3IP
XLIV	Turin - Provv.610	M,H,GV,L,D,P	Ptolemaic ??
XLIX	Manchester - MM5053.a - Perenbast	H,L,P	D22

L= Lung tissue present GV=Great Vessels present H=Heart present
M=Mediastinal outline present D=Diaphragm present P=Packing present in thorax

TABLE 5.5 PRESENCE OF LUNG AND OTHER TISSUES AND PACKING MATERIAL

Mediastinal structures are of particular interest as the heart lies within the mediastinum. The significance of the heart to ancient Egyptians is well known and described by Diodorus Siculus (P 2). Spell 27 in the Book of the Dead ('for not permitting a man's heart to be taken from him in the realm of the dead') relates to the need for the heart to be present for the Weighing of the Heart Ceremony (Taylor, 2010: 160). It is interesting to note that Wade and Nelson found little evidence to show that retention of the heart was commonplace. (Wade, Nelson, 2013: 29). Only nine of the thirty-seven mummies available for analysis of thoracic evisceration had evidence of a retained heart (See Table 5.6). In these nine there was evidence that in five cases the great vessels had been retained and in four cases lung tissue had been retained. All except one of the nine cases of heart retention had packing present in the thorax. The mummy with no packing was number XL from the Third Intermediate Period. A full discussion on the use of packing will follow later (P 180).

NUMBER	ORIGIN	VISCERA PRESENT	ERA
III	Birmingham - Padimut	H	D20-21
VI	Sheffield - Djedma'atiuesankh	H	D26
XXII	Zurich - Bern - 00/2	H	Unknown
XXV	Zurich - Geneva - TjesMoutPert - D0242	GV	D22-25
XXXVI	Zurich - Bern - AE9	GV	Ptolemaic
XXXVIII	Zurich - St. Gallen - Shepenese	GV,L	D26
XL	Zurich - Lausanne - 492	GV,L	3IP
XLIV	Turin - Provv.610	GV,L	Ptolemaic ??
XLIX	Manchester - MM5053.a - Perenbast	L	D22

H= Heart only GV= Heart and Great Vessels L= Heart and Lungs

TABLE 5.6 RETENTION OF THE HEART, GREAT VESSELS AND LUNGS

5.2.4.5 Evisceration of the abdomen

For the purposes of this research, the abdomen will be defined as the body cavity below the diaphragm and above the pelvic inlet. This definition has been chosen to reflect the practicality of manual clearance of the cavity by an embalmer. In view of the constriction of the pelvis at the pelvic inlet, this would make pelvic clearance from above more difficult. It will be seen below (P 176) that this is reflected in the findings of this study.

This section will cover the treatment of the abdominal cavity and exclude discussion of the treatment of the pelvic cavity, which will be addressed separately.

Of the mummies studied, thirty-eight had an abdominal incision. Five of these had only presumptive evidence of the incision– these are identified in Table 5.7 by the inclusion of '?'. Nine mummies had an additional perineal approach demonstrated by 'P'.

Whilst accepting that the process of evisceration may not, on all occasions, be total and that the finding of a few remnants of viscera is accepted as conforming to the concept of evisceration having taken place, the presence of significant amounts of viscera confirms one of two things. They are that evisceration has taken place and the loose viscera returned to the cavity or that evisceration has not been performed fully. To further complicate the issue it is difficult to distinguish the use of small linen strips treated with resin from cleaned and desiccated bowel similarly treated with resin.

Retroperitoneal organs such as the kidneys and pancreas, which have been subjected to significant desiccation are, on many occasions, difficult to identify. This leaves the liver to be accounted for. It is a large, solid organ (although containing some large blood vessels) and should be easy to identify even after desiccation. However, distortion of the liver's shape and displacement from its usual anatomical site can make identification problematic. If the remains of the bowels can be identified and are clearly in the wrong place anatomically, then it can be assumed that they were returned after evisceration.

Armed with these concepts it is possible on some occasions to comment on the evidence of evisceration of the abdomen with some confidence.

The subject of the use of canopic packages (real or false) will be discussed separately (P 179).

NUMBER	ORIGIN	CODE	ERA
I	Birmingham - Graeco-Roman	V	Roman
II	Birmingham - Namenkhetamun	V	D26
III	Birmingham - Padimut	V	D20-21
V	Sheffield - Nesitanebetasheru	?A?,V,C	D25
VI	Sheffield - Djedma'atiuesankh	C	D26
VII	Ipswich - Tahathor	?A?,V	D25
VIII	Liverpool - Padiamun - 53.72a	?A?,V	D22
IX	Liverpool - Padiamunnebnesuttauwy	V	D25
X	Liverpool - Nesmin	C,V, P	Ptolemaic
XI	Liverpool - Padiamun - M14003	C,V	D26
XIV	Manchester – MM1777 - Asru	V	D26
XVI	Liverpool - M13997a	V,C,P	Roman
XVII	Liverpool - Ankhesenaset - 14000	C,V	3IP
XVIII	Liverpool- M14048	C,V,P	Roman
XIX	Zurich - Altdorf Child	C,V	Roman
XXII	Zurich - Bern - 00/2	V,C,P	Unknown
XXIII	Zurich - Yverdon - Nes-Shou - MY/3775	C,P	Ptolemaic
XXV	Zurich - Geneva - TjesMoutPert - D0242	V,IM	D22-25
XXVI	Zurich - Geneva - Infant	V	Unknown
XXVII	Manchester - Demetria - MM11630	?A?,V	Roman

NUMBER	ORIGIN	CODE	ERA
XXVIII	Manchester – Ta-Sheri-Ankh – MM13783	A,?V?,C	Ptolemaic
XXIX	BM - Hor - EA6659	V	D22
XXX	BM - Ankh-Unen-Nefer - EA6681	C	D25
XXXI	BM - Padiamunet - EA6682	V	D25
XXXII	BM - EA20744	V,C	D22
XXXIII	BM - EA22939	V,C	D22
XXXIV	BM - EA25258	V	D22
XXXVI	Zurich - Bern - AE9	V,C	Ptolemaic
XXXVIII	Zurich - St. Gallen - Shepenese	V,C,P	D26
XXXIX	Zurich - St. Gallen - C3530	V,P	D21
XL	Zurich - Lausanne - 492	V	3IP
XLI	Zurich - Lenzburg - K10351		Roman
XLIII	Turin - (Tebtynis) - Suppl.19691	C	Ptolemaic ??
XLIV	Turin - Provv.610	C,V	Ptolemaic ??
XLVIII	Manchester - MM3496	V	D18
XLIX	Manchester - MM5053.a - Perenbast	V,C	D22
LIII	Manchester - MM1976.51a	C,P	D25
LX	BM - EA 6704	C,P	Roman

P=perineal approach C=canopic package V=visible viscera

TABLE 5.7 MUMMIES WITH AN ABDOMINAL INCISION AND SOME EVIDENCE OF EVISCERATION

Further analysis of the abdominal contents reveals the distribution of observable structures within the cavity. Only one case has reasonably convincing evidence of a liver being present. That is Mummy XVIII, Accession number 14048 from the National Museums, Liverpool (See Fig. 5.293, where the white circle indicates the liver and the black circles indicate the canopic packages).

NUMBER	ORIGIN	CODE	ERA
VII	Ipswich - Tahathor	R(few)	D25
VIII	Liverpool - Padiamun - 53.72a	R,L	D22
IX	Liverpool - Padiamunnebnesuttauwy	R	D25
XIV	Manchester – MM1777 - Asru	R(few)	D26
XXVII	Manchester - Demetria - MM11630	R	Roman
XXIX	BM - Hor - EA6659	R,L	D22
XXXI	BM - Padiamunet - EA6682	R(few)	D25
XXXII	BM - EA20744	R,L,?C	D22
XXXIV	BM - EA25258	R,L	D22
XXXVI	Zurich - Bern - AE9	R,C	Ptolemaic
XXXIX	Zurich - St. Gallen - C3530	R,L,P	D21
XL	Zurich - Lausanne - 492	R,L	3IP
XLVIII	Manchester - MM3496	R	D18
XLIX	Manchester - MM5053.a - Perenbast	R,C	D22
LX	BM - EA 6704	R,C,P	Roman

L=Loose viscera R=Retained viscera C=Canopic package
P=Perineal approach

TABLE 5.8 MUMMIES WITH RETAINED VISCERA DESPITE SOME EVISCERATION

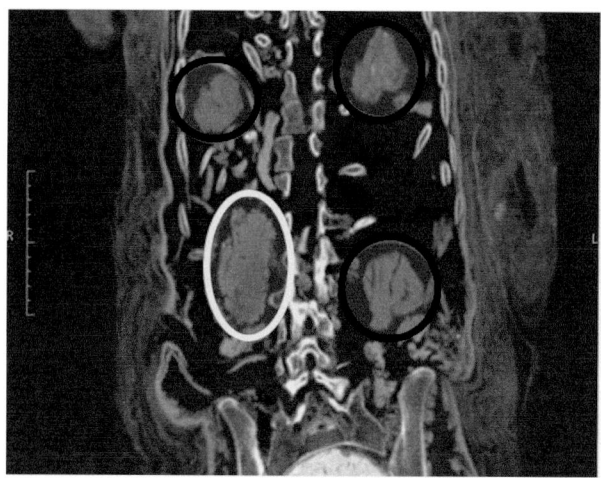

FIG. 5.293 CORONAL VIEW OF TRUNK - LIVER AND CANOPIC PACKAGES

Fifteen of the thirty-eight mummies with an abdominal incision were found to have some degree of visceral retention – that is, there was significant evidence of viscera found overlying the posterior wall of the abdomen. These are shown in Table 5.8. As can be seen there were three cases in which the retained viscera were only of modest volume (Mummies VII, XIV and XXXI).

An illustration of the appearance of residual (retained) visceral tissue is given in Fig. 5.294, which shows the appearance in Mummy IX (Padiamunnebnesuttauwy from Liverpool – Accession number 14050). Although there is a reasonably large amount of viscera seen in this case, smaller amounts are also found in other mummies – as in Fig 5.295 (Mummy VII – Tahathor from Ipswich Museum).

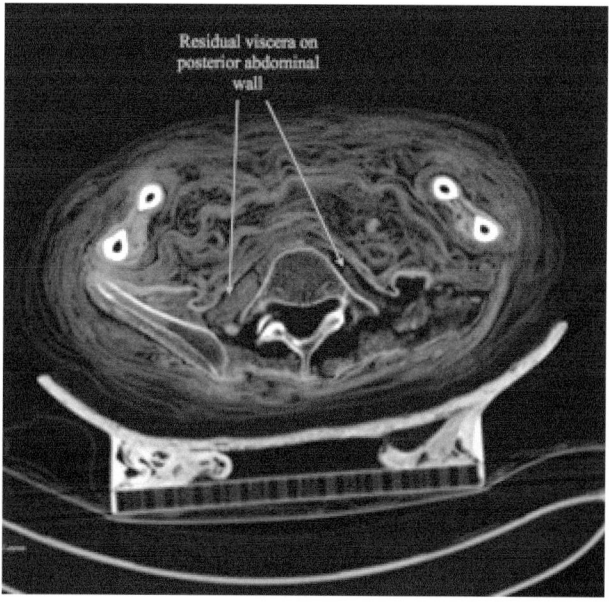

FIG. 5.294 AXIAL VIEW OF LOWER ABDOMEN - RESIDUAL VISCERAL TISSUE

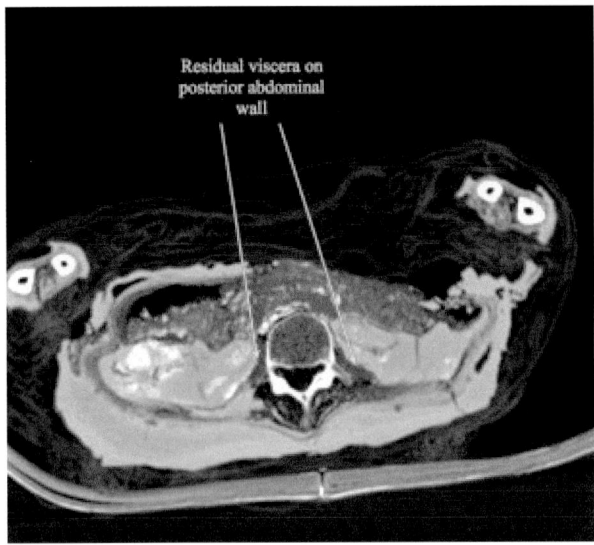

FIG. 5.295 AXIAL VIEW OF ABDOMEN - RESIDUAL VISCERAL TISSUE

On the other hand there is clear evidence when the viscera have been removed 'treated' (that is desiccated) and returned to the body cavity. In some cases the viscera are seen in the abdomen. In other cases the viscera are scattered throughout the whole body cavity. These cases are shown in Table 5.9.

NUMBER	ORIGIN	CODE	ERA
I	Birmingham - Graeco-Roman	L,C	Roman
II	Birmingham - Namenkhetamun	L,C	D26
III	Birmingham - Padimut	L	D20-21
V	Sheffield - Nesitanebetasheru	L,C	D25
VIII	Liverpool - Padiamun - 53.72a	L,R	D22
XVII	Liverpool - Ankhesenaset - 14000	L,C	3IP
XXII	Zurich - Bern - 00/2	L,C,P	Unknown
XXIX	BM - Hor - EA6659	L,R	D22
XXXII	BM - EA20744	L,R,?C	D22
XXXIII	BM - EA22939	L,?C	D22
XXXIV	BM - EA25258	L,R	D22
XXXIX	Zurich - St. Gallen - C3530	L,R,P	D21
XL	Zurich - Lausanne - 492	L,R	3IP

L=Loose viscera R=Retained viscera C=Canopic package P=Perineal approach

TABLE 5.9 VISCERA RETURNED TO THE BODY CAVITY AFTER INITIAL REMOVAL

A typical appearance of the 'random' nature of the distribution of the viscera in these cases is seen in the black circles in Figs. 5.296 and 5.297 (Mummy XXIX – EA6659 from the British Museum). This contrasts with the more 'formalized' nature of the viscera seen in a canopic package (See Fig. 5.297 – black circle). This latter example is from Mummy XXXII from the British Museum (EA20744). It can be seen from Table 5.9 that of the thirteen cases of mummies with returned viscera six also had evidence of some viscera being retained and, therefore, presumably not extracted at evisceration. There were seven cases of the use of canopic packages along with returned viscera. All three practices (retained and returned viscera and canopic packages) can be seen in Mummy XXXIII - British Museum EA22939 (see Figs. 5.298 and 5.299).

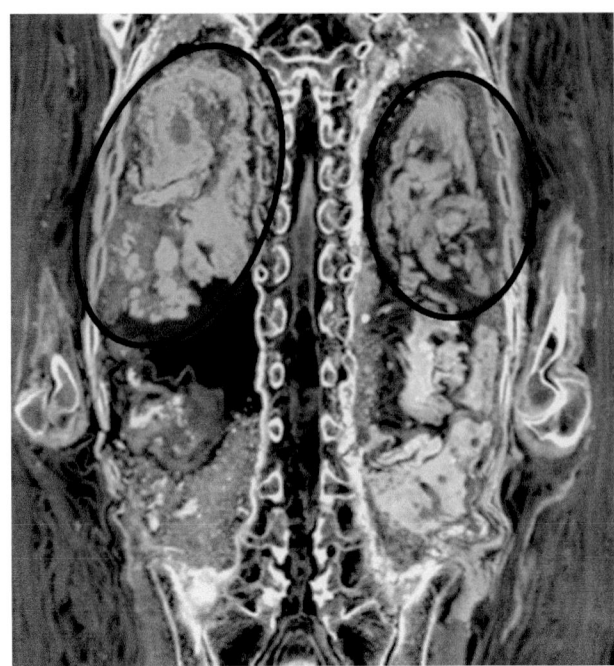

FIG. 5.296 CORONAL VIEW OF TRUNK - VISCERA RETURNED AFTER DESICCATION

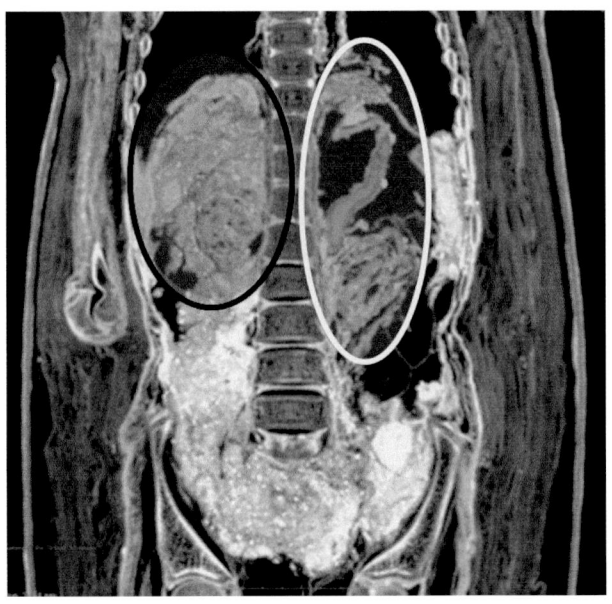

FIG. 5.297 CORONAL VIEW OF TRUNK - RETURNED VISCERA (WHITE CIRCLE) AND A CANOPIC PACKAGE (BLACK CIRCLE)
COURTESY OF THE TRUSTEES OF THE BRITISH MUSEUM

5.2.4.6 Evisceration of the pelvic cavity

The topic of evisceration of the pelvic cavity is approached separately because of the technical difficulties inherent in the process. It is accepted that the female pelvis has a larger inlet than the male (Johnston, Davies and Davies 1958: 406) and that the average measurements of the modern female pelvic inlet are in the region of 115 mms in diameter (Johnston, Davies and Davies v.s.: 405). This has to be compared with the transverse measurement of the average male hand at the level of the metacarpo-phalangeal joints of 95-100 mms (personal experience).

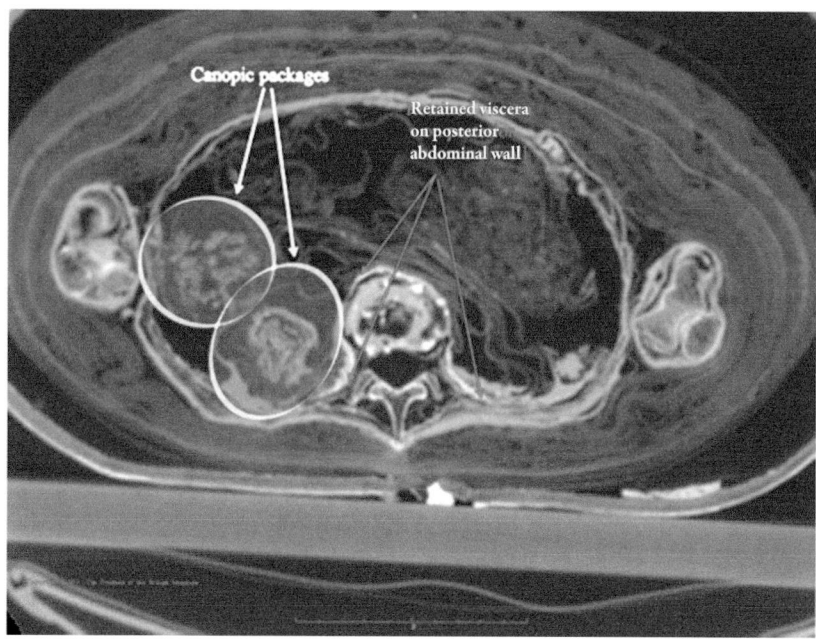

FIG. 5.298 AXIAL VIEW OF ABDOMEN - CANOPIC PACKAGES AND RETAINED VISCERA
COURTESY OF THE TRUSTEES OF THE BRITISH MUSEUM

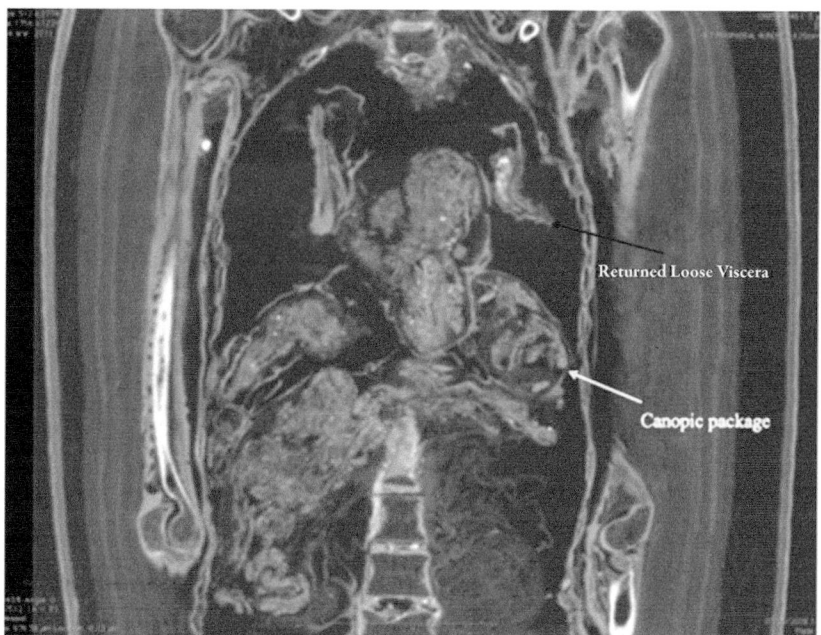

FIG. 5.299 CORONAL VIEW OF TRUNK - LOOSE VISCERA AND CANOPIC PACKAGE
COURTESY OF THE TRUSTEES OF THE BRITISH MUSEUM

It can be seen that, allowing for soft tissues, the space available for the 'surgical' manoeuvre of evisceration is very constrained. It is possible therefore, that clearance of this space may not be as thorough as in the main abdominal cavity. Reference to Table 5.10 shows that in the thirty-eight cases of evisceration via an abdominal incision, there was no data available in two cases (the CT scans were on analogue medium) and in a further two the pelvis was sufficiently disrupted to make analysis impossible. These cases are shown in bold for ease of identification. Therefore, the remaining thirty-four cases are available for analysis. These contain nine instances where the abdominal incision was augmented by a perineal approach. These are shown in italic. It can be seen that of these nine combined approaches to evisceration, there were three in which a false phallus had been attached – presumably after accidental removal secondary to the perineal destruction.

In one case the vagina and rectum were still visible as distinct entities. This was in Mummy number XVI from the National Museums, Liverpool. In this case closer examination shows that whilst the vagina is visible, there is no definite evidence of the uterus. There is no evidence of a bladder or of any bowel proximal to the rectum. There is an obvious pack in the perineum closing the aperture, presumably to prevent leakage of the resin, which has been introduced.

In all the other cases where a perineal approach has been used to augment the abdominal one there is either evidence of foreign material (in the form of linen, resin or granular material), debris or canopic package/s, but no evidence of organs.

In the twenty-five cases where there was no perineal approach, only an abdominal approach, there were four cases of males where the phallus alone was seen and no evidence of intra-pelvic organs. In another four cases the retention of the phallus was seen in combination with the presence of both the bladder and rectum. In other words, the pelvic organs appeared intact.

In females there were seven examples of retention of the vagina along with the rectum. In another two cases these organs were retained along with the bladder. That is, there were a total of thirteen cases where all or most of the pelvic organs were retained.

Whilst the numbers are too small to be statistically significant, it is interesting to note that in the cases where only an abdominal incision was used approximately half had retained organs in the pelvic cavity. This is in contrast with anticipated result of no organs being found in the pelvic cavity of the group of four with only a perineal approach (See section 5.2.2 - P 150).

NUMBER	ORIGIN	PELVIC CONTENTS	ERA
I	Birmingham - Graeco-Roman	M	Roman
II	Birmingham - Namenkhetamun	B,R,P	D26
III	Birmingham - Padimut	B,R,P,M	D20-21
V	Sheffield - Nesitanebetasheru	No data	D25
VI	Sheffield - Djedma'atiuesankh	No data	D26
VII	Ipswich - Tahathor	V,R,F	D25
VIII	Liverpool - Padiamun - 53.72a	F,M	D22
IX	Liverpool - Padiamunnebnesuttauwy	L,FF	D25
X	Liverpool - Nesmin	FF,M	Ptolemaic
XI	Liverpool - Padiamun - M14003	B,R,P,F	D26
XIV	Manchester – MM1777 - Asru	B,V,R,F	D26
XVI	Liverpool - M13997a	V,R,M	Roman
XVII	Liverpool - Ankhesenaset - 14000	M	3IP
XVIII	Liverpool- M14048	L,M	Roman
XIX	Zurich - Altdorf Child	L,R	Roman
XXII	Zurich - Bern - 00/2	Empty	Unknown
XXIII	Zurich - Yverdon - Nes-Shou - MY/3775	L,FF,M,C	Ptolemaic
XXV	Zurich - Geneva - TjesMoutPert - D0242	V,R	D22-25
XXVI	Zurich - Geneva - Infant	L,P,F	Unknown
XXVII	Manchester - Demetria - MM11630	V,R	Roman
XXVIII	Manchester – Ta-Sheri-Ankh – MM13783	D,M	Ptolemaic
XXIX	BM - Hor - EA6659	B,R,P,M	D22
XXX	BM - Ankh-Unen-Nefer - EA6681	Disrupted, P,M	D25
XXXI	BM - Padiamunet - EA6682	D,P,M	D25
XXXII	BM - EA20744	F,V	D22
XXXIII	BM - EA22939	L,D	D22
XXXIV	BM - EA25258	M	D22
XXXVI	Zurich - Bern - AE9	L,P,F	Ptolemaic
XXXVIII	Zurich - St. Gallen - Shepenese	Empty,M	D26
XXXIX	Zurich - St. Gallen - C3530	M	D21
XL	Zurich - Lausanne - 492	B,V,R	3IP
XLI	Zurich - Lenzburg - K10351	Empty	Roman
XLIII	Turin - (Tebtynis) - Suppl.19691	Empty,C	Ptolemaic ??
XLIV	Turin - Provv.610	M,C	Ptolemaic ??
XLVIII	Manchester - MM3496	Disrupted	D18
XLIX	Manchester - MM5053.a - Perenbast	V,R,M	D22
LIII	Manchester - MM1976.51a	Empty	D25
LX	BM - EA 6704	FF,C	Roman

L=Linen D=Debris B=Bladder V=Vagina or Uterus R=Rectum P=Phallus FF=False Phallus F=Fascia M='Mummification Material' C=Canopic Package

TABLE 5.10 PELVIC CONTENTS AFTER EVISCERATION.

5.2.5 The use of canopic packages

Following evisceration, the viscera may be returned 'loose' into the body cavity, returned in the form of canopic packages (or 'packets' – a term used by Dunand and Lichtenberg, 2006: 61) or not returned at all. In the latter case the possibilities include discarding the viscera or placing them in canopic jars, canopic chests or coffinettes.

To further complicate the picture the possible use of false canopic packages also has to be considered. This would be a parallel to the use of false canopic jars.

Of the thirty-eight cases where an abdominal incision was used, twenty-two mummies revealed the presence of canopic packages (See Table 5.11).

NUMBER	ORIGIN	CODE	ERA
I	Birmingham - Graeco-Roman	L,C	Roman
II	Birmingham - Namenkhetamun	L,C	D26
V	Sheffield - Nesitanebetasheru	L,C	D25
VI	Sheffield - Djedma'atiuesankh	C	D26
X	Liverpool - Nesmin	C,P	Ptolemaic
XI	Liverpool - Padiamun - M14003	C	D26
XVI	Liverpool - M13997a	C,P	Roman
XVII	Liverpool - Ankhesenaset - 14000	L,C	3IP
XVIII	Liverpool- M14048	Li,C,P	Roman
XIX	Zurich - Altdorf Child	C	Roman
XXII	Zurich - Bern - 00/2	L,C,P	Unknown
XXIII	Zurich - Yverdon - Nes-Shou - MY/3775	C,P	Ptolemaic
XXVI	Zurich - Geneva - Infant	C	Unknown
XXVIII	Manchester – Ta-Sheri-Ankh – MM13783	Disrupted,C	Ptolemaic
XXXII	BM - EA20744	L,R,C	D22
XXXIII	BM - EA22939	L,C	D22
XXXVI	Zurich - Bern - AE9	R,C	Ptolemaic
XLIII	Turin - (Tebtynis) - Suppl.19691	C	Ptolemaic ??
XLIV	Turin - Provv.610	C	Ptolemaic ??
XLIX	Manchester - MM5053.a - Perenbast	R,C	D22
LIII	Manchester - MM1976.51a	C,P	D25
LX	BM - EA 6704	R,C,P	Roman

Li=Liver L=Loose viscera R=Retained viscera C=Canopic package
P=Perineal approach

TABLE 5.11 PRESENCE OF CANOPIC PACKAGES

It can be seen that of these twenty-two cases, seven of the mummies also had returned 'loose' viscera – that is, not packaged. Unsurprisingly of the four cases where a perineal incision alone had been used three did not contain any packages. In the case of the fourth mummy there were two packages that appear to contain tightly packaged viscera (See Fig. 5.300).

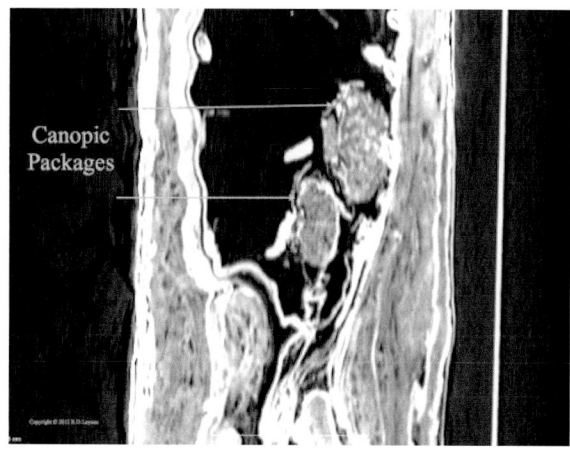

FIG. 5.300 SAGITTAL VIEW OF TRUNK - CANOPIC PACKAGES IN A MUMMY WITH ONLY A PERINEAL APPROACH

The question of the false canopic package is complicated by the fact that the appearance of a package is made difficult to interpret if a large amount of resin has been used, as this tends to obscure the contents. However on close examination of the available images, it appears that in only one case where modern images are available, is there any doubt as to whether the packages contain viscera; Nesmin, Mummy X from the National Museums, Liverpool. Comparing the images in Figs. 5.301 and 5.302 it is possible to see the dilemma. They both represent the same package with the only difference being the contrast alteration. Fig. 5.302 would tend towards the interpretation of this being a true package containing viscera. In the remaining twenty mummies there is no doubt that the packages do, in fact, contain viscera.

In the case of Mummy XLIV from Turin, it is currently impossible to reach a conclusion because of the absence of image availability for re-examination

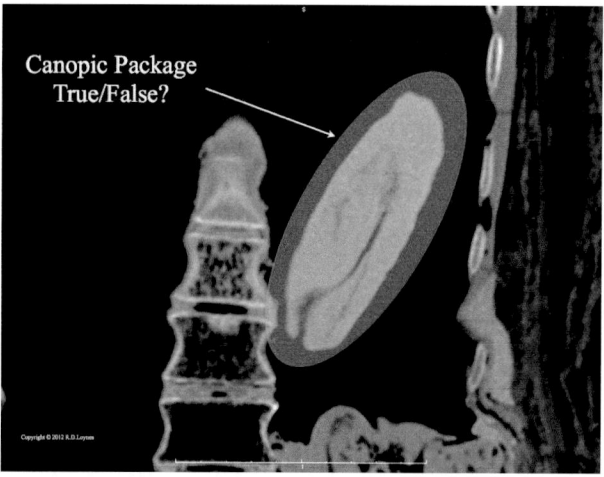

FIG. 5.301 CORONAL VIEW OF TRUNK - CANOPIC PACKAGE – TRUE OR FALSE?

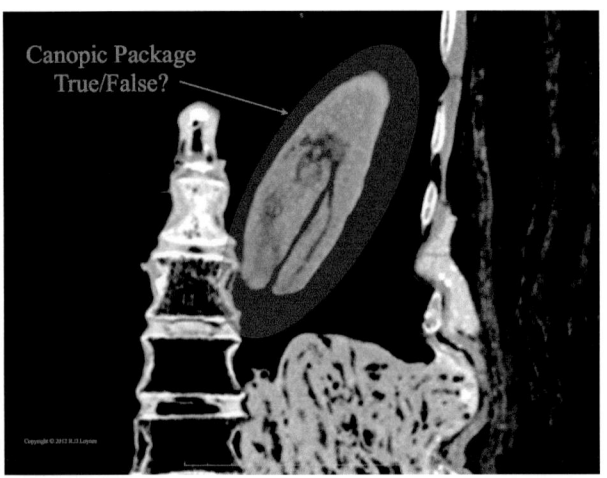

FIG. 5.302 CORONAL VIEW OF TRUNK - CANOPIC PACKAGE – TRUE OR FALSE?

5.2.6 Materials inserted into the body cavity after evisceration

Table 5.12 shows those mummies where there was definite insertion of foreign material after evisceration via an abdominal incision. To these should be added Mummy XXIV from Basel, where there is granular material in the thorax; Mummy XLII from Turin where there is also granular material in the thorax; and Mummy XLV from Manchester where there is granular material in the pelvis (these three mummies all have perineal approaches but no abdominal incision). Mummies where no incision or evisceration was performed or where it was impossible to judge the situation because of disruption of the mummy have been omitted from the Table.

It is difficult to be dogmatic about the true identity of inserted material as there is no accurate specific value to attribute to the radio density of substances used which can be relied upon as applying to all CT machines. Each substance has a range of Hounsfield Unit values and different machines tend to give slightly different estimations of this value. Further more, there can be a difference in value between two apparently similar substances.

Hounsfield introduced the concept of these units in his Nobel Lecture on 8th. December 1979 (Hounsfield G.N., 1980: 459-68). The Hounsfield Unit (HU) scale is a linear transformation of the attenuation coefficient of radiodensity. The value of water (at standard temperature and pressure) is defined as 0, the value of air as - 1000 and the value of dense bone as +1000. As the attenuation can vary according to radiological parameters and the density of other substances in the X-ray beam it is necessary to 'calibrate' the machine at each examination. Values within the ranges of hundreds are less susceptible to variations in radiographic parameters which affect the X-ray energy. Therefore readings of HU are more useful and reliable for soft tissues than more radio-dense objects such as might be used during mummification. The analysis of HU values in such substances (those found in mummies) was performed by Gostner et al. (Gostner et al., 2013: 1003-1011).

An attempt was made to obtain numerical values of the radio density of various objects but failed to be useful because of the overlap of some values and the differences in material values just mentioned. An example was the value of two samples of 'mud' provided by the National Museums, Liverpool. They were both from ancient Egypt, with one from the Archaic Period and the other from the New Kingdom (from Amarna). The values ranged from 800 to 1100 in one case (dependent upon where in the specimen the reading was taken) and from 1400 to 1600 in the other sample. Whilst these figures do not represent accurate Hounsfield Unit measurements they do illustrate the variations in the values attributable to objects of allegedly similar composition. There is also the problem of the variability of the chemical nature of substances such as resin. Amongst others, Buckley and Evershed have undertaken investigation of this subject (Buckley and

NUMBER	ORIGIN	CODE	ERA
I	Birmingham - Graeco-Roman	A,V,IM	Roman
III	Birmingham - Padimut	A,V,IM	D20-21
V	Sheffield - Nesitanebetasheru	?A?,V,C,IM	D25
VI	Sheffield - Djedma'atiuesankh_	A,C,IM	D26
VIII	Liverpool - Padiamun - 53.72a	?A?,V,IM	D22
IX	Liverpool - Padiamunnebnesuttauwy	A,V,IM	D25
X	Liverpool - Nesmin	A,P,C,V,IM	Ptolemaic
XI	Liverpool - Padiamun - M14003	A,C,V,IM	D26
XVI	Liverpool - M13997a	A,V,C,IM,P	Roman
XVII	Liverpool - Ankhesenaset - 14000	A,C,IM,V	3IP
XVIII	Liverpool- M14048	A,C,V,IM,P	Roman
XIX	Zurich - Altdorf Child	A,C,V,IM	Roman
XXII	Zurich - Bern - 00/2	A,V,IM,C,P	Unknown
XXIII	Zurich - Yverdon - Nes-Shou - MY/3775	A,P,C,IM	Ptolemaic
XXV	Zurich - Geneva - TjesMoutPert - D0242	A,V,IM	D22-25
XXVI	Zurich - Geneva - Infant	A,V,IM	Unknown
XXVIII	Manchester – Ta-Sheri-Ankh – MM13783	A,?V?,C,IM	Ptolemaic
XXIX	BM - Hor - EA6659	A,V,IM	D22
XXX	BM - Ankh-Unen-Nefer - EA6681	A,C,IM	D25
XXXI	BM - Padiamunet - EA6682	A,V,IM	D25
XXXII	BM - EA20744	A,V,C,IM	D22
XXXIII	BM - EA22939	A,V,IM,C	D22
XXXIV	BM - EA25258	A,V,IM	D22
XXXVI	Zurich - Bern - AE9	A,V,C,IM	Ptolemaic
XXXVIII	Zurich - St. Gallen - Shepenese	A,V,C,IM,P	D26
XXXIX	Zurich - St. Gallen - C3530	A,V,IM,P	D21
XLI	Zurich - Lenzburg - K10351	A,IM	Roman
XLII	Turin - Taaset - Suppl.9480	V,IM,P	Ptolemaic
XLIII	Turin - (Tebtynis) - Suppl.19691	A,C,IM	Ptolemaic ??
XLIV	Turin - Provv.610	A,C,V,IM	Ptolemaic ??
XLV	Manchester - MM1766	V,P,IM	Roman
XLIX	Manchester - MM5053.a - Perenbast	A,V,IM,C	D22
LIII	Manchester - MM1976.51a	A,IM,C,P	D25
LX	BM - EA 6704	A,IM,C,P	Roman

A=abdo inc P=perineal C=canopic package IM=inserted material V=visible viscera

TABLE 5.12 MUMMIES WITH FOREIGN MATERIAL INSERTED INTO THE BODY CAVITY

Evershed 2001: 837-841). Reference to resin in this work indicates a substance with a high radio density that exhibits a 'fluid level' indicating that it was fluid when introduced and subsequently hardened. A fine granular substance will be referred to as 'clay' or 'mud', although it is recognized that it could equally well be a mixture of something else like sawdust mixed with another material. In the context of this research, it is more the fact that material was introduced rather than its exact chemical nature, which is of importance.

For the sake of brevity the amount of material used will be classified as absent, small, medium, large or complete (the latter indicating complete or almost complete filling of the body cavity as illustrated in Fig. 5.303).

Mummies with X-rays or analogue records of the CT scans are eliminated from this analysis, as is the 'false' mummy – XXI from Lausanne (490). British Museum Mummy XXXV – EA29577 was also eliminated from consideration because of its advanced state of disintegration. The same decision was applied to Mummy XLVI from Manchester (MM10881). While not as badly affected, the mummy from Perth (23/1936) is sufficiently disrupted to make assessment of the volume of material used impossible. It is clear, however, that granular material has been used in the body cavity. The results are shown in Table 5.13.

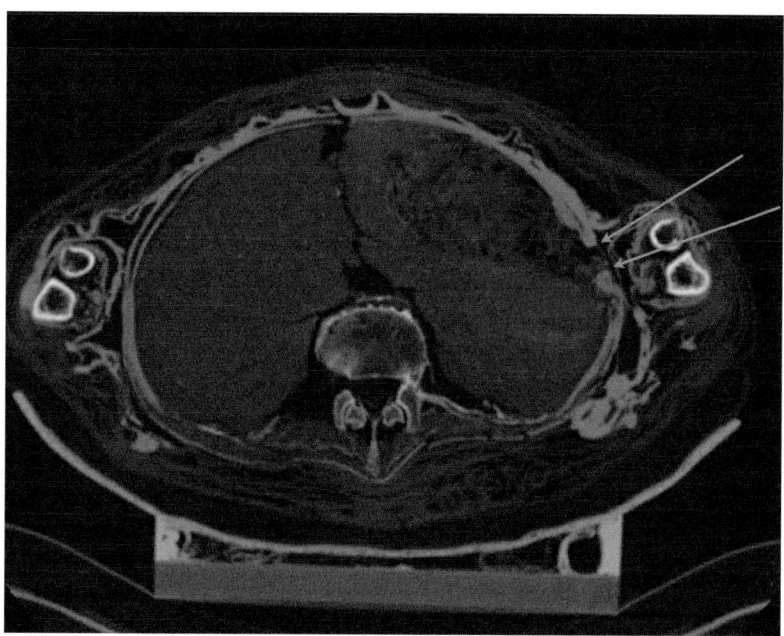

FIG. 5.303 AXIAL VIEW OF ABDOMEN - AN EXAMPLE OF TOTAL FILLING OF THE BODY CAVITY WITH 'MATERIAL' ('CLAY/MUD')

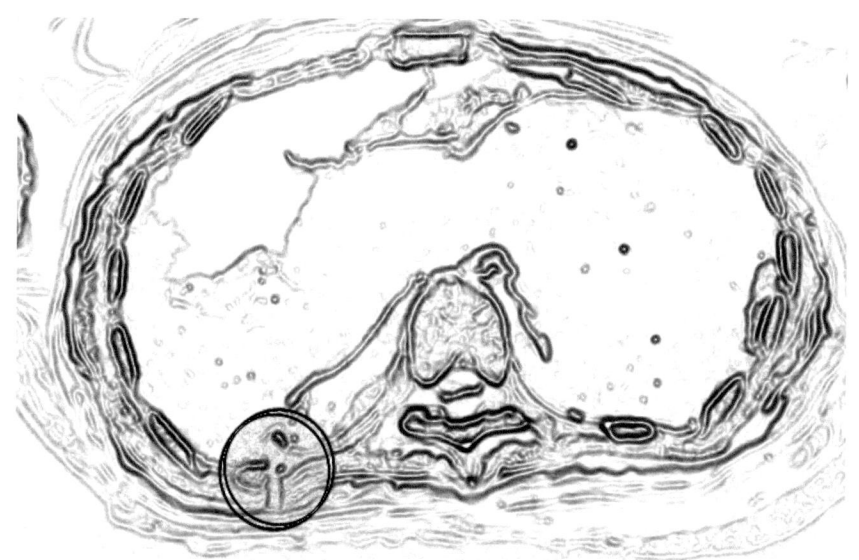

FIG. 5.304 AXIAL VIEW OF ABDOMEN - AN EXAMPLE OF A LARGE AMOUNT OF FILLING MATERIAL (AFTER IEM IMAGE)

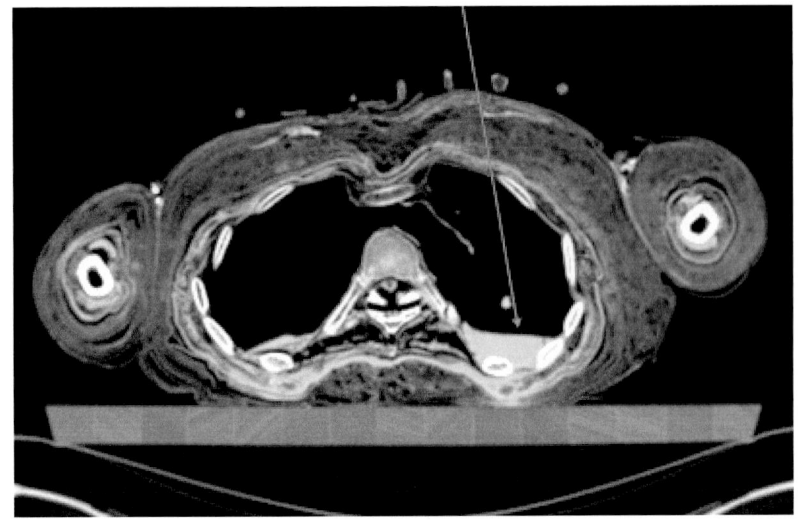

FIG. 5.305 AXIAL VIEW OF THORAX - AN EXAMPLE OF A SMALL AMOUNT OF 'MATERIAL' ('RESIN')

NUMBER	ORIGIN	FILLING	ERA
I	Birmingham - Graeco-Roman	M,R,G	Roman
II	Birmingham - Namenkhetamun	S,G	D26
III	Birmingham - Padimut	M,R,G	D20-21
VII	Ipswich - Tahathor	S/M,G	D25
VIII	Liverpool - Padiamun - 53.72a	M/L,R,G	D22
IX	Liverpool - Padiamunnebnesuttauwy	S,G	D25
X	Liverpool - Nesmin	M,R	Ptolemaic
XI	Liverpool - Padiamun - M14003	T,G	D26
XII	Manchester - MM1768	S,R,G	Roman
XVI	Liverpool - M13997a	S,R	Roman
XVII	Liverpool - Ankhesenaset	S/M,R,G	3IP
XVIII	Liverpool- M14048	PELVIS,R,G,Li	Roman
XIX	Zurich - Altdorf Child	S,Li	Roman
XX	Zurich - TaDjIsis - K1205	T,G	D26
XXII	Zurich - Bern - 00/2	M,R	Unknown
XXIII	Zurich - Yverdon - Nes-Shou - MY/3775	M,R	Ptolemaic
XXIV	Zurich - Basel - BSAE.1030	Pelvis,S,R	Roman
XXV	Zurich - Geneva - TjesMoutPert - D0242	S,G	D22-25
XXVI	Zurich - Geneva - Infant	M,R	Unknown
XXVII	Manchester - Demetria - MM11630	A	Roman
XXVIII	Manchester – Ta-Sheri-Ankh – MM13783	M,R	Ptolemaic
XXIX	BM - Hor - EA6659	L,R,G	D22
XXX	BM - Ankh-Unen-Nefer - EA6681	L,R,G	D25
XXXI	BM - Padiamunet - EA6682	M,G	D25
XXXII	BM - EA20744	M,G	D22
XXXIII	BM - EA22939	S,G+L,Li	D22
XXXIV	BM - EA25258	S,G	D22
XXXVI	Zurich - Bern - AE9	S,R	Ptolemaic
XXXVII	Zurich - Lenzburg - Sherit-Min	A	Ptolemaic
XXXVIII	Zurich - St. Gallen - Shepenese	L,G	D26
XXXIX	Zurich - St. Gallen - C3530	L,G	D21
XL	Zurich - Lausanne - 492	A	3IP
XLI	Zurich - Lenzburg - K10351	A	Roman
XLII	Turin - Taaset - Suppl.9480	S,G	Ptolemaic
XLIII	Turin - (Tebtynis) - Suppl.19691	A	Ptolemaic ??
XLIV	Turin - Provv.610	S,G	Ptolemaic ??
XLV	Manchester - MM1766	Thorax,S,G	Roman
XLVIII	Manchester - MM3496	S,R	D18
XLIX	Manchester - MM5053.a - Perenbast	L,G	D22
L	Perth - 23/1936	G	D26
LIII	Manchester - MM1976.51a	S,G	D25
LVIII	Manchester - MM13784	A	Middle Kingdom
LX	BM - EA 6704	M,R	Roman

A=ABSENT S=SMALL M=MEDIUM L=LARGE T=TOTAL R=RESIN G=GRANULAR Li=LINEN

TABLE 5.13 FOREIGN MATERIALS IN THE BODY CAVITY

Evaluation of these results shows that a granular substance was used in twenty-six cases of the forty-three mummies available for study. Resin was used in eighteen cases and linen in only two cases. The amount of packing used was judged to be total in two cases, large in six cases, medium in eleven cases and small in fourteen cases. Packing material was restricted to the pelvis in two cases and to the thorax in one case. It was entirely absent in six cases. These results are illustrated in Tables 5.14 and 5.15.

Granular	Resin	Linen
26	18	2

TABLE 5.14 MATERIAL USED IN PACKING THE BODY CAVITY

Total	Large	Medium	Small	Absent	Regional
2	6	11	14	6	Th=1/P=2

TABLE 5.15 DISTRIBUTION OF AMOUNTS OF MATERIAL

Chapter Six

Results - Treatment of the skin, subcutaneous tissues and position of the arms

6.1 The use of resin externally

Ikram and Dodson state, '…most mummies were covered in resin…' (Ikram and Dodson 1998: 117). However this is not always the case. In comparison to the use of resin as a material for introduction into the body cavity after evisceration, the use of resin poured over the skin as an unguent is restricted to just six mummies in this series. There is a seventh mummy where resin is seen outside the body, but this appears to have been introduced into the body cavity and suffused through the tissues to the outside - Mummy XXIII from Yverdon Museum (See Table 6.1). Reference to this table shows that there is no obvious pattern of technique with examples from three different locations and five different eras.

NUMBER	ERA	LOCATION	RESIN ON SKIN	RESIN IN BODY CAVITY
VIII	D22	Thebes	Y	Y
X	Ptol.	Akhmim	Y	Y
XXIII	Ptol.	Akhmim	Posterior -In>Out	Y
XXV	D22	Thebes	Y-Ant.2/3	Y
XXVIII	D21	Akhmim	Y	Y
XXX	D25	Thebes	Y but fragmented	Y
XLVII	Roman	Hawara	Y	N

TABLE 6.1 MUMMIES WHERE RESIN IS USED TO 'ANOINT' THE SKIN.

6.2 Subcutaneous packing

The practice of subcutaneous stuffing/packing is associated with Dynasty 21 (Ikram and Dodson, 1998: 124). In this cohort subcutaneous packing was found in eight of the sixty cases (See Table 6.2), but only in the cervical region.

NUMBER	ORIGIN	PACKING	ERA
III	Birmingham - Padimut	L	D20-21
VIII	Liverpool - Padiamun - 53.72a	L	D22
XVII	Liverpool - Ankhesenaset	L	3IP
XXIX	BM - Hor - EA6659	L	D22
XXX	BM - Ankh-wenen-nefer - EA6681	L	D25
XXXIII	BM - EA22939	G	D22
XXXIV	BM - EA25258	L	D22
XLIX	Manchester - MM5053.a - Perenbast	G	D22

L = LINEN PACKING   G = GRANULAR PACKING

TABLE 6.2 THE USE OF SUBCUTANEOUS PACKING

It can be seen that six of these mummies were from Dynasties 20 to 22, which would accord well with the perceived knowledge. One other is from the 'Third Intermediate Period' which includes Dynasty 21. The only outlier is from Dynasty 25. This is shown below as well as examples of granular and linen packing (See Figs. 6.2 and 6.3).

XXX. Ankh-wenen-nefer - British Museum - (Accession No. EA 6681)

Neck

The soft tissues have been destroyed. However, there is a linen pack, lying free in the cervical region. This may well have been a subcutaneous pack in the front of the neck (See Fig. 6.1). It is the correct size, shape and in the correct location for such a pack.

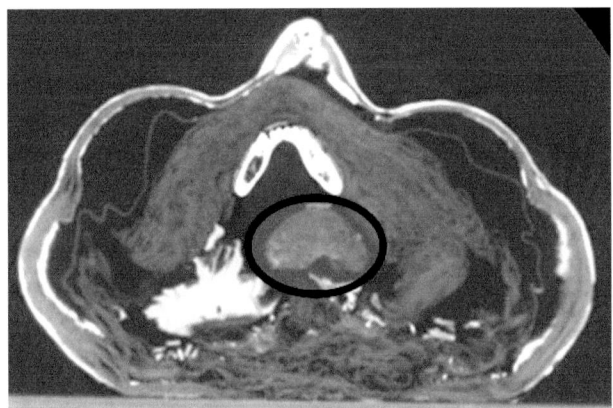

FIG. 6.1 AXIAL VIEW OF CERVICAL REGION - SUBCUTANEOUS PACKING
COURTESY OF THE TRUSTEES OF THE BRITISH MUSEUM

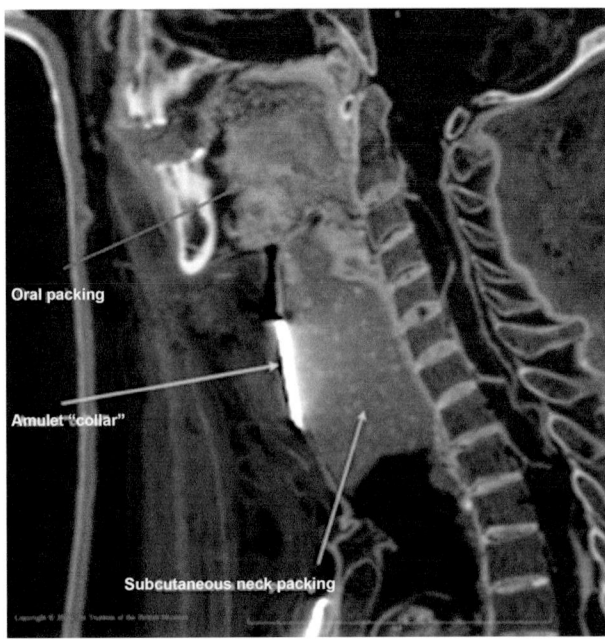

FIG. 6.2 SAGITTAL VIEW OF CERVICAL REGION - GRANULAR PACKING (MUMMY XXXIII)
COURTESY OF THE TRUSTEES OF THE BRITISH MUSEUM

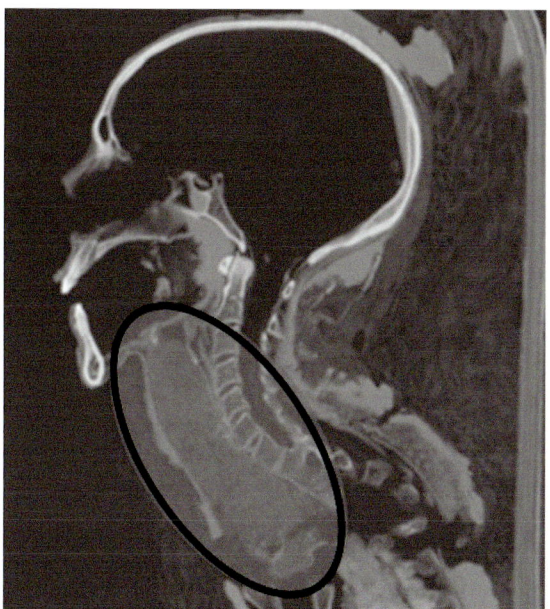

FIG. 6.3 SAGITTAL VIEW OF CERVICAL REGION - LINEN PACKING (MUMMY VIII)

6.3 Amulets

Although the presence of amulets within the bandaging and, occasionally, within the body cavity has been noted, it is difficult to assess the significance of their presence or absence in the light of the history of the wholesale removal of such objects in the past (Ikram and Dodson 1998:137). The statistics are, therefore, distorted to the point of being meaningless.

6.4 Position of the arms

The position of the arms has been noted. In fact, it is this feature that has prompted a discussion about the true date of Mummy LI – Khary from Manchester Museum. The original museum records date the mummy to Dynasty 19, but the arm position resulted in a re-assignment to the Ptolemaic Period. This opinion is based on a comment by Raven and Taconis (Raven and Taconis 2005: 133) that in turn refers to the conclusion reached by Gray (Gray 1972: 200-204). He expressed the opinion that 'A change in the position of the arms takes place: the favoured position shows them crossed upon the breast.' (that is in Ptolemaic mummies). This statement was made with reference to a comparison with 'Dynastic Mummies'. It is important to note that the term 'Dynastic Mummies' refers to some of the mummies he X-rayed between 1963 and 1972 that he defined as 'mummies dating from Dynasty 21 to the start of the Ptolemaic Period.' In other words his cohort does not include mummies prior to Dynasty 21. Therefore, re-assignment to the Ptolemaic Period may not be as sound as at first thought. However, this will be discussed separately (P 208).

Returning to the arm position in this series. This is demonstrated in Table 6.3.

F = arms flexed at the elbow, across each other and over the chest (See Fig. 6.4).

EL = arms extended at the elbow and lateral to the thighs (See Fig. 6.5). EA = arms extended at the elbow and lying anteriorly over the hips or upper thighs - the difference reflects the length of the arms rather than a positional change (See Fig. 6.6).

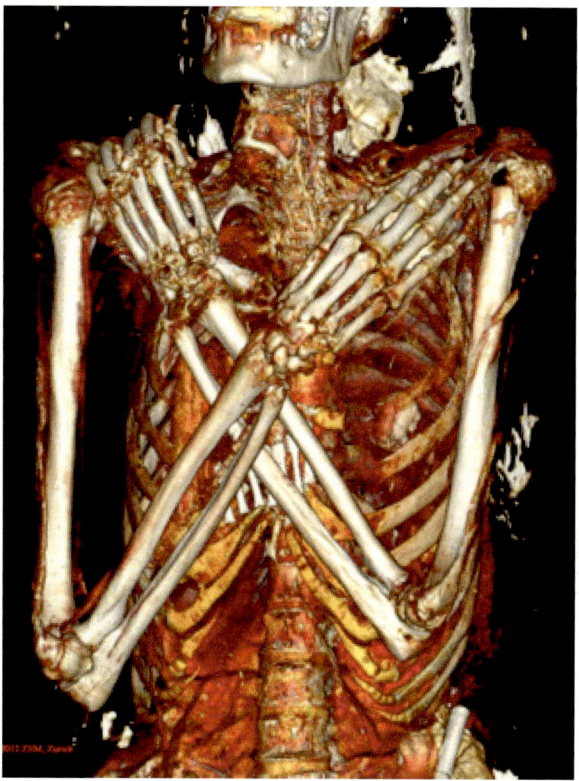

FIG. 6.4 3D RECONSTRUCTION SHOWING ARMS FLEXED AND ACROSS CHEST

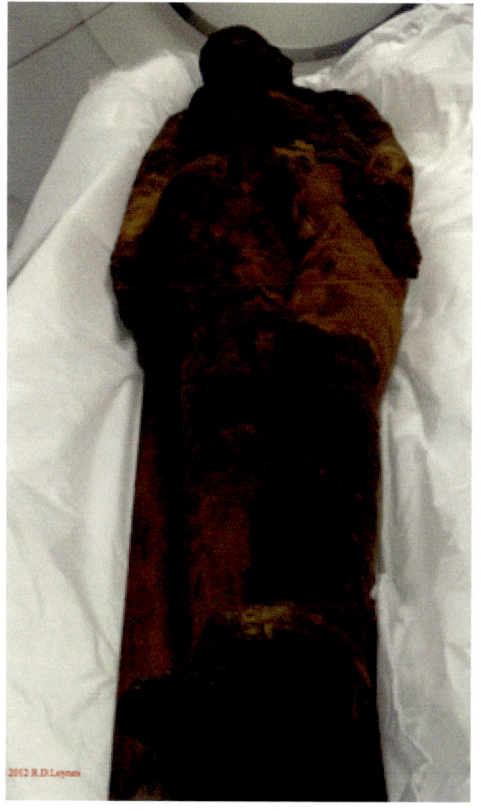

FIG. 6.5 ARMS EXTENDED AND LATERAL TO THE THIGHS

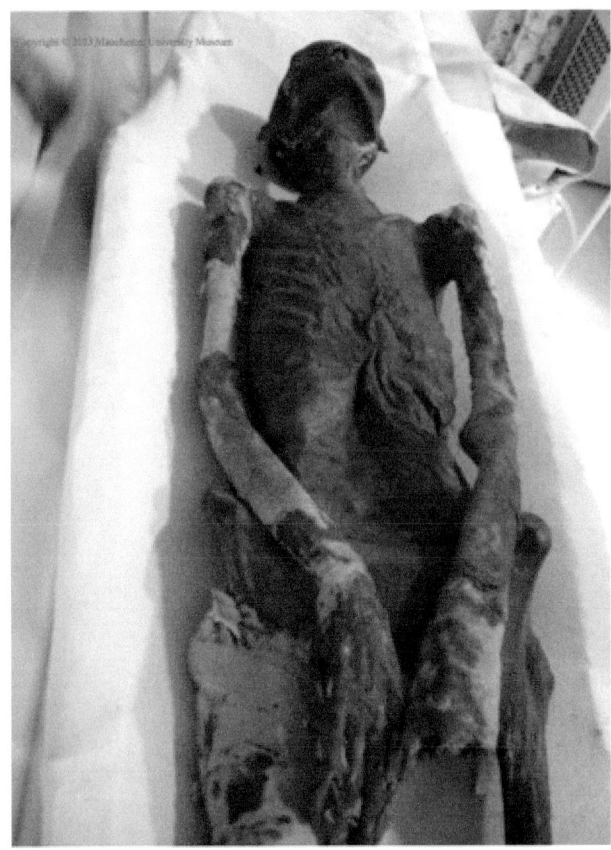

FIG. 6.6 ARMS EXTENDED AND OVER UPPER THIGHS/HIPS

As can be seen, there are three mummies where there is disorganization of the mummy or a false mummy. In a further mummy the analogue images do not give sufficient information to determine arm position. The remaining fifty-six mummies are divided into thirty-five with arms extended at the elbow and the hands over the front of the thighs/hips, ten where the extended arms are lateral to the hips and eight where the arms are flexed at the elbow and lie crossed over the chest. Of the mummies with flexed arms seven are from the Ptolemaic Period and one from Dynasty 26. Further discussion of these findings will be pursued in Chapter Eight. However three of the eight mummies with flexed arms had extended fingers in both hands. In contrast, five mummies had the fingers extended (open palm) in the right hand with flexed fingers (a closed fist as if grasping an object) in the left hand. In the remaining mummy the left hand had been destroyed and was therefore not available for analysis (See Table 6.4). Of these eight mummies seven had the right forearm superficial to the left. Only in the case of Mummy L – from Perth Museum and Art Gallery – was the left forearm superficial to the right. The mummy Khary has not been included in the above results as it will be discussed separately (P 208).

NUMBER	ORIGIN	POSITION	ERA
I	Birmingham - Graeco-Roman	EA	Roman
II	Birmingham - Namenkhetamun	EA	D26
III	Birmingham - Padimut	EA	D20-21
IV	Exeter - Shepenmut	EA	D22
V	Sheffield - Nesitanebetasheru	?	D25
VI	Sheffield - Djedma'atiuesankh	EA	D26
VII	Ipswich - Tahathor	EA	D25
VIII	Liverpool - Padiamun - 53.72a	EA	D22
IX	Liverpool - Padiamunnebnesuttauwy	EA	D25
X	Liverpool - Nesmin	F	Ptolemaic
XI	Liverpool - Padiamun - M14003	EA	D26
XII	Manchester - MM1768	EL	Roman

NUMBER	ORIGIN	POSITION	ERA
XIII	Manchester - MM1767	EA-C	Roman
XIV	Manchester – M1777 - Asru	EA	D26
XV	Liverpool - 13.10.11.25	EA	Roman
XVI	Liverpool - M13997a	EL	Roman
XVII	Liverpool - Ankhesenaset	EA	3IP
XVIII	Liverpool- M14048	EL	Roman
XIX	Zurich - Altdorf Child	EL	Roman
XX	Zurich - TaDjIsis - K1205	Disorganised	D26
XXI	Zurich - Lausanne - 490	FALSE	3IP
XXII	Zurich - Bern - 00/2	EL	Unknown
XXIII	Zurich - Yverdon - Nes-Shou - MY/3775	F	Ptolemaic
XXIV	Zurich - Basel - BSAE.1030	EA-C	Roman
XXV	Zurich - Geneva - TjesMoutPert - D0242	EA	D22-25
XXVI	Zurich - Geneva - Infant	EL	Unknown
XXVII	Manchester - Demetria - MM11630	EL	Roman
XXVIII	Manchester – Ta-Sheri-Ankh – MM13783	F	Ptolemaic
XXIX	BM - Hor - EA6659	EA	D22
XXX	BM - Ankh-Unen-Nefer - EA6681	EA	D25
XXXI	BM - Padiamunet - EA6682	EA	D25
XXXII	BM - EA20744	EA	D22
XXXIII	BM - EA22939	EA	D22
XXXIV	BM - EA25258	EA	D22
XXXV	BM - EA29577	EA	D22
XXXVI	Zurich - Bern - AE9	F	Ptolemaic
XXXVII	Zurich - Lenzburg - Sherit-Min	EA-Fist	Ptolemaic
XXXVIII	Zurich - St. Gallen - Shepenese	EA	D26
XXXIX	Zurich - St. Gallen - C3530	EA	D21
XL	Zurich - Lausanne - 492	EA	3IP
XLI	Zurich - Lenzburg - K10351	EL	Roman
XLII	Turin - Taaset - Suppl.9480	F	Ptolemaic
XLIII	Turin - (Tebtynis) - Suppl.19691	F	Ptolemaic ??
XLIV	Turin - Provv.610	F	Ptolemaic ??
XLV	Manchester - MM1766	EA	Roman
XLVI	Manchester - MM10881	Disorganised	D26
XLVII	Manchester - MM1769	EA	Roman
XLVIII	Manchester - MM3496	EA	D18
XLIX	Manchester - MM5053.a - Perenbast	EA	D22
L	Perth - 23/1936	F	D26
LI	Manchester - MM9354a - Khary	F	D19/ Ptolemaic?
LII	Manchester - MM9319 - child	EL	Roman
LIII	Manchester - MM1976.51a	EA	D25
LIV	Manchester - Salford 2	EA	3IP
LV	Manchester - MM13011	EA	Ptolemaic
LVI	Manchester - MM2109	EA(L)/EL(R)	Roman
LVII	Manchester - MM1775 - Artemidorus	EA	Roman
LVIII	Manchester - MM13784	EA	Middle Kingdom
LIX	BM - EA 22108 Child	EA	Roman
LX	BM - EA 6704	EL	Roman

F= FLEXED ACROSS CHEST   EL= EXTENDED LATERAL   EA= EXTENDED ANTERIOR

TABLE 6.3 POSITION OF ARMS

NUMBER	ORIGIN	POSITION	ERA
X	Liverpool - Nesmin	R and L =E	Ptolemaic
XXIII	Zurich - Yverdon - Nes-Shou - MY/3775	R=E, L=F	Ptolemaic
XXVIII	Manchester – Ta-Sheri-Ankh – MM13783	R=E, L=F	Ptolemaic
XXXVI	Zurich - Bern - AE9	R=E, L=F	Ptolemaic
XLII	Turin - Taaset - Suppl.9480	R=E, L=F	Ptolemaic
XLIII	Turin - (Tebtynis) - Suppl.19691	R and L =E	Ptolemaic ??
XLIV	Turin - Provv.610	R and L =E	Ptolemaic ??
L	Perth - 23/1936	R=E, L=?	D26

R=Right hand L=Left hand F=Fingers flexed E=Fingers extended

Table 6.4 Hand posture in mummies with flexed arms

Chapter Seven

Results related to Demographics and Palaeopathology

7.1 Age at Death

This was briefly discussed in Chapter Two 2.3 (P 13). In the context of this research project exact age at death is not required (as it would be in a forensic arena). In children (C) the age was estimated as accurately as dental and epiphyseal signs allowed. In adults the age grouping was given as 'young adult' (YA), 'middle aged' (MA) and 'elderly' (E). This grouping was assigned taking note of dental wear and pathology and skeletal wear (joints and spine). The transition from Child to Young Adult is taken as eighteen years. Transition from Young Adult to Middle Age is taken as thirty years. The transition from Middle Age to Elderly is taken as sixty years. However it is realized that these designations are arbitrary and inexact.

7.1.1 Results

Of the sixty mummies available for study, two were disorganized and two lacked sufficient detail in the images to determine age. After removing the false mummy the remaining fifty-five were analysed. The results are summarized in Table 7.1

NUMBER	ORIGIN	AGE	ERA
I	Birmingham – Graeco-Roman	YA	Roman
II	Birmingham – Namenkhetamun	MA	D26
III	Birmingham – Padimut	MA	D20-21
IV	Exeter – Shepenmut	?	D22
V	Sheffield – Nesitanebetasheru	?	D25
VI	Sheffield – Djedma'atiuesankh	C – 13-16	D26
VII	Ipswich – Tahathor	YA	D25
VIII	Liverpool – Padiamun – 53.72a	YA	D22
IX	Liverpool – Padiamunnebnesuttauwy	MA	D25
X	Liverpool – Nesmin	MA	Ptolemaic
XI	Liverpool – Padiamun – M14003	E	D26
XII	Manchester – MM1768	YA	Roman
XIII	Manchester – MM1767	MA	Roman
XIV	Manchester – MM1777 – Asru	MA	D26
XV	Liverpool – 13.10.11.25	C – 5	Roman
XVI	Liverpool – M13997a	YA	Roman
XVII	Liverpool – Ankhesenaset	MA	3IP
XVIII	Liverpool- M14048	YA	Roman
XIX	Zurich – Altdorf Child	C – 3-4	Roman
XX	Zurich – TaDjIsis – K1205	I	D26
XXI	Zurich – Lausanne – 490	FALSE	3IP
XXII	Zurich – Bern – 00/2	MA	Unknown
XXIII	Zurich – Yverdon – Nes-Shou – MY/3775	E	Ptolemaic
XXIV	Zurich – Basel – BSAE.1030	MA	Roman
XXV	Zurich – Geneva – TjesMoutPert – D0242	E	D22-25
XXVI	Zurich – Geneva – Infant	C – 6	Unknown
XXVII	Manchester – Demetria – MM11630	YA	Roman
XXVIII	Manchester – Ta-Sheri-Ankh – MM13783	YA	Ptolemaic
XXIX	BM – Hor – EA6659	MA	D22
XXX	BM – Ankh-Unen-Nefer – EA6681	MA	D25
XXXI	BM – Padiamunet – EA6682	MA	D25
XXXII	BM – EA20744	C – 15-19	D22
XXXIII	BM – EA22939	MA	D22
XXXIV	BM – EA25258	MA	D22
XXXV	BM – EA29577	?YA	D22
XXXVI	Zurich – Bern – AE9	YA	Ptolemaic
XXXVII	Zurich – Lenzburg – Sherit-Min	MA	Ptolemaic

NUMBER	ORIGIN	AGE	ERA
XXXVIII	Zurich – St. Gallen – Shepenese	MA	D26
XXXIX	Zurich – St. Gallen – C3530	MA	D21
XL	Zurich – Lausanne – 492	MA	3IP
XLI	Zurich – Lenzburg – K10351	C – 3-6 ?	Roman
XLII	Turin – Taaset – Suppl.9480	E	Ptolemaic
XLIII	Turin – (Tebtynis) – Suppl.19691	YA	Ptolemaic ??
XLIV	Turin – Provv.610	YA	Ptolemaic ??
XLV	Manchester – MM1766	YA	Roman
XLVI	Manchester – MM10881	I	D26
XLVII	Manchester – MM1769	C – 6	Roman
XLVIII	Manchester – MM3496	C – 1-2	D18
XLIX	Manchester – MM5053.a – Perenbast	E	D22
L	Perth – 23/1936	E	D26
LI	Manchester – MM9354a – Khary	MA	D19/ Ptolemaic?
LII	Manchester – MM9319 – child	C – 2	Roman
LIII	Manchester – MM1976.51a	MA	D25
LIV	Manchester – Salford 2	YA	3IP
LV	Manchester – MM13011	C – 2-3	Ptolemaic
LVI	Manchester – MM2109	C – 2-3	Roman
LVII	Manchester – MM1775 – Artemidorus	MA	Roman
LVIII	Manchester – MM13784	C – 16-17	Middle Kingdom
LIX	BM – EA 22108 Child	C – 2-3	Roman
LX	BM – EA 6704	MA	Roman

TABLE 7.1 Age at Death

AGE	CHILD	YOUNG ADULT	MIDDLE AGE	ELDERLY
Nos.	13	14	22	6

TABLE 7.2 Age distribution

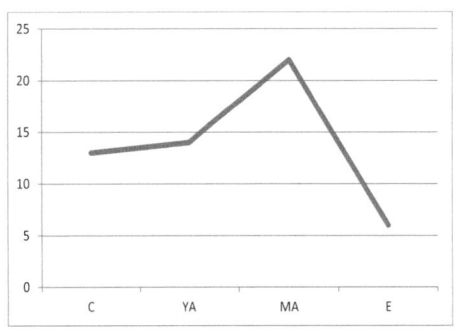

TABLE 7.3 Age distribution of this cohort

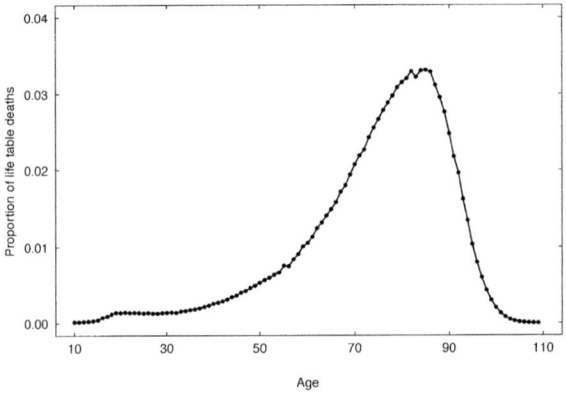

TABLE 7.4 Age at death distribution of US males 2002 (Ouellette and Bourbeau, 011: 598)

The distribution of deaths related to the arbitrary age groups previously described is shown in Table 7.2 in tabular form and in Table 7.3 in graphic form. Table 7.4 shows the distribution of deaths of US males in 2002 for comparison. But of more relevance may be a model of expected age at death distribution from the Roman Period (Pers. Comm. Chamberlain A. after Bagnall and Frier). See Table 7.5. It can be seen from this table that the 'modelled' expected pattern from the Roman Period is not followed. This may be due to cohort size or to the fact that the mummies in this study come from a wide time range (that is from the Middle Kingdom to the Roman Period – a period covering over two thousand years).

7.2 Sex

This topic is discussed in Chapter Two 2.4 (P 13). Although it is not possible to credibly assert the sex of an individual in all cases, those cases where it is possible are shown in Table 7.6. Where a '?' is shown this indicates that the sex was probably that indicated but there was no certainty.

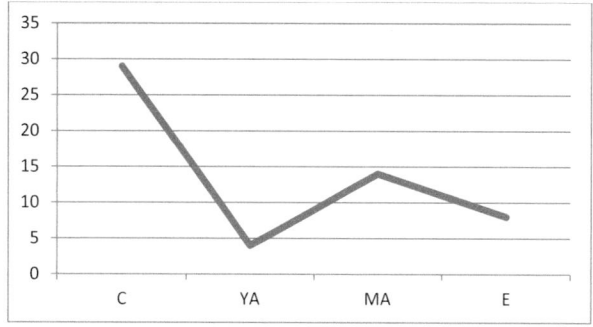

TABLE 7.5 AGE AT DEATH MODEL FOR THE ROMAN PERIOD

NUMBER	ORIGIN	SEX	ERA
I	Birmingham – Graeco-Roman	M	Roman
II	Birmingham – Namenkhetamun	M	D26
III	Birmingham – Padimut	M	D20-21
IV	Exeter – Shepenmut	?F	D22
V	Sheffield – Nesitanebetasheru	F	D25
VI	Sheffield – Djedma'atiuesankh	?F	D26
VII	Ipswich – Tahathor	F	D25
VIII	Liverpool – Padiamun – 53.72a	M	D22
IX	Liverpool – Padiamunnebnesuttauwy	M	D25
X	Liverpool – Nesmin	M	Ptolemaic
XI	Liverpool – Padiamun – M14003	M	D26
XII	Manchester – MM1768	M	Roman
XIII	Manchester – MM1767	M	Roman
XIV	Manchester – MM1777 – Asru	F	D26
XV	Liverpool – 13.10.11.25	M	Roman
XVI	Liverpool – M13997a	F	Roman
XVII	Liverpool – Ankhesenaset	F	3IP
XVIII	Liverpool- M14048	F	Roman
XIX	Zurich – Altdorf Child	M	Roman
XX	Zurich – TaDjIsis – K1205	I	D26
XXI	Zurich – Lausanne – 490	FALSE	3IP
XXII	Zurich – Bern – 00/2	?F	Unknown
XXIII	Zurich – Yverdon – Nes-Shou – MY/3775	M	Ptolemaic
XXIV	Zurich – Basel – BSAE.1030	M	Roman
XXV	Zurich – Geneva – TjesMoutPert – D0242	F	D22-25
XXVI	Zurich – Geneva – Infant	M	Unknown
XXVII	Manchester – Demetria – MM11630	F	Roman
XXVIII	Manchester – Ta-Sheri-Ankh – MM13783	F	Ptolemaic
XXIX	BM – Hor – EA6659	M	D22
XXX	BM – Ankh-Unen-Nefer – EA6681	M	D25
XXXI	BM – Padiamunet – EA6682	M	D25
XXXII	BM – EA20744	F	D22
XXXIII	BM – EA22939	F	D22
XXXIV	BM – EA25258	F	D22
XXXV	BM – EA29577	?M	D22
XXXVI	Zurich – Bern – AE9	M	Ptolemaic

NUMBER	ORIGIN	SEX	ERA
XXXVII	Zurich – Lenzburg – Sherit-Min	?M	Ptolemaic
XXXVIII	Zurich – St. Gallen – Shepenese	F	D26
XXXIX	Zurich – St. Gallen – C3530	M	D21
XL	Zurich – Lausanne – 492	F	3IP
XLI	Zurich – Lenzburg – K10351	?	Roman
XLII	Turin – Taaset – Suppl.9480	?F	Ptolemaic
XLIII	Turin – (Tebtynis) – Suppl.19691	F	Ptolemaic ??
XLIV	Turin – Provv.610	M	Ptolemaic ??
XLV	Manchester – MM1766	F	Roman
XLVI	Manchester – MM10881	I	D26
XLVII	Manchester – MM1769	?F	Roman
XLVIII	Manchester – MM3496	F	D18
XLIX	Manchester – MM5053.a – Perenbast	F	D22
L	Perth – 23/1936	?F	D26
LI	Manchester – MM9354a – Khary	M	D19/ Ptolemaic?
LII	Manchester – MM9319 – child	M	Roman
LIII	Manchester – MM1976.51a	F	D25
LIV	Manchester – Salford 2	F	3IP
LV	Manchester – MM13011	M	Ptolemaic
LVI	Manchester – MM2109	M	Roman
LVII	Manchester – MM1775 – Artemidorus	M	Roman
LVIII	Manchester – MM13784	?F	Middle Kingdom
LIX	BM – EA 22108 Child	M	Roman
LX	BM – EA 6704	M	Roman

TABLE 7.6 SEX DISTRIBUTION IN COHORT ANALYSED (AFTER BAGNALL AND FRIER)

7.2.1 Results

Table 7.6 shows that there were twenty-seven definite and two probable males. There were twenty definite and seven probable females. The remaining four were disorganized, false or impossible to define from the images. This represents a broadly 50/50 split, as one might expect.

7.3 Palaeopathology

This subject was discussed briefly in Chapter Two 2.5 (P 13). The majority of observable causes of death would be expected to be bony, but a few soft tissue diagnoses may be possible despite the distortion of the tissues by desiccation.

It should be noted that contemporary statistics (from the ONS) show that the majority of the causes of death relate to soft tissues with only cancers having the potential to show their presence as bony metastases. Primary bone cancers are very rare causing something in the region of 0.00045 % of deaths per annum (ONS) (See Tables 7.7 – 7.10).

Leading cause of death	No. of men	Percentage of men
Heart disease	37423	15.60%
Lung cancer	16698	7%
Emphysema/bronchitis	14378	6%
Stroke	14116	5.90%
Dementia and Alzheimer's	13984	5.80%
Flu/pneumonia	11063	4.60%
Prostate cancer	9698	4%
Bowel cancer	7841	3.30%
Lymphoid cancer	6301	2.60%
Throat cancer	4603	1.90%

TABLE 7.7 CAUSES OF DEATH IN 2011 IN UK – MEN – PRIMARY SOFT TISSUE CANCERS IN GREY

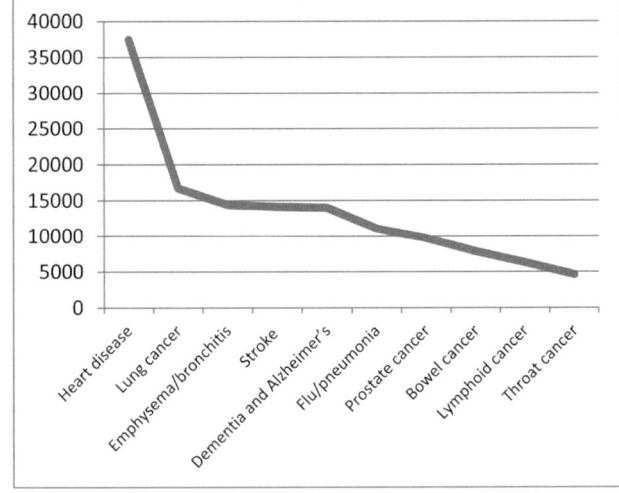

TABLE 7.8 CAUSES OF DEATH IN 2011 IN UK – MEN

Leading cause of death	No. of women	Percentage of women
Dementia and Alzheimer's	29873	11.50%
Heart disease	26741	10.30%
Stroke	21730	8.40%
Flu/pneumonia	15075	5.80%
Emphysema/bronchitis	14155	5.50%
Lung cancer	13575	5.20%
Breast cancer	10311	4%
Bowel cancer	6600	2.50%
Urinary disease	5570	2.10%
Heart failure	5065	2%

TABLE 7.9 CAUSES OF DEATH IN 2011 IN UK –WOMEN – PRIMARY SOFT TISSUE CANCERS IN GREY

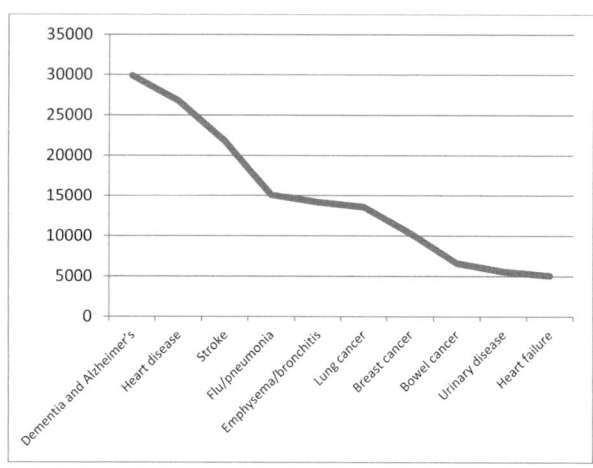

TABLE 7.10 CAUSES OF DEATH IN 2011 IN UK – WOMEN

One further cause of death in the past would have been severe bone infection, which could manifest itself in the CT scans. The cause of death in these cases would, probably, have been septicaemia. Other unusual causes of death are described below.

7.3.1 Results – Causes of death

The following are reports from those mummies exhibiting evidence of probable causes of death.

VII Tahathor – Ipswich Museum (Cat. No. COLEM 1871.3.7)

Cause of death

The fractures to both scapulae and the subluxation of the left sterno-clavicular joint could have been caused by a blow to, or a fall onto, the back with the body slightly rotated to the right. Whether this occurred just before death or by clumsy handling during the mummification process is not possible to determine.

Other abnormalities lie within the pelvis. There is widening of both sacro-iliac joints and the symphysis pubis in a young mature woman. This is a picture seen around the time of childbirth and it cannot be excluded that this woman died during or soon after childbirth.

X. Nesmin- National Museums Liverpool (Accession No. 56.22.79a)

Cause of death

Whilst there is no certainty, there is a good chance that the cause of death was a fall, causing a badly displaced fracture of the left wrist. Whilst such fractures are often seen in the elderly, they are also seen as the result of a 'high energy' impact in the young and middle-aged population. The comminution and displacement seen in this case would fit well with this latter scenario. At the same time it has to be acknowledged that the fracture occurred shortly before death. There is no evidence of healing callus but there is significant swelling of the soft tissues.

There are three fractured ribs on the left, again with no evidence of healing. It is distinctly possible that this man died of a complication of the fractured ribs. That is either pneumonia or pneumothorax (where air gains access to the pleural space between the rib cage and the lung and compresses the lung, so preventing proper breathing).

XVIII. Unnamed – National Museums Liverpool – (Accession No. M14048)

Cause of death

The extensive skeletal damage is at least in part post-mortem. This comment applies to the rib cage and the spine. The fractures of the left side of the pelvis and of the distal forearms conform to the patterns seen in life. They are injuries that occurred close to the time of death, there being no evidence of callus.

XXIV. Unnamed – Basel Museum (Cat. No.BSAE.1030)

Pelvis and Hips

There is slight disruption of both sacro-iliac joints, but this could well have occurred during mummification. The pubic symphysis is normal. There is a fracture of the floor of the right acetabulum and another of the right inferior pubic ramus.

XXXIII. Tjenmutengebtiu – British Museum - (Accession No. EA 22939)

Cause of death

Whilst there is no definite cause of death shown, the fractured left os calcis with the fracture of the fourth lumbar vertebral body and unhealed fractured ribs are highly suggestive of significant trauma (for example a fall from a height, landing on the feet) shortly before death.

XXXVI. Unnamed – Bern (AE 9)

Cause of death

Whilst the disruption at the C4/5 level is almost certainly postmortem, the abnormalities in the lumbar spine are pathological and premortem. There appears to be collapse of the first lumbar vertebral body with a resulting gibbus (See Fig. 7.1).

Also, some disease process has replaced the body of the fourth lumbar vertebra. The diagnosis lies between infection and tumour, but the presence of several affected vertebral bodies in continuity and the collapse of one of them favors infection. One of the lower inter-vertebral discs is intact but the others may be reduced in height. This would indicate an infection such as TB. Whilst the presence of a para-spinal abscess would be helpful in the diagnosis, its absence may have resulted from the mummification process (See Fig. 7.2, 7.3 and 7.4 – circles).

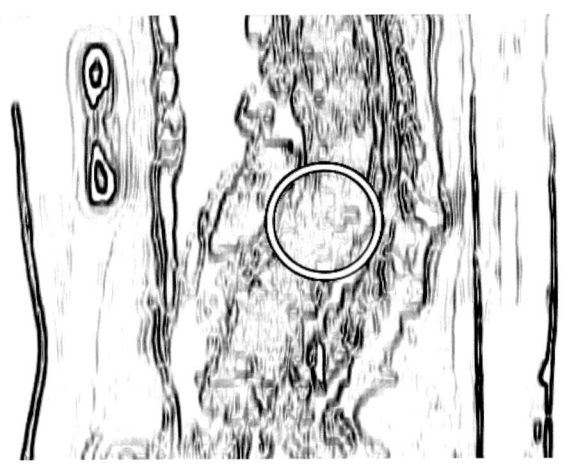

FIG. 7.1 SAGITTAL VIEW OF TRUNK - COLLAPSE OF THE FIRST LUMBAR VERTEBRA (AFTER IEM IMAGE)

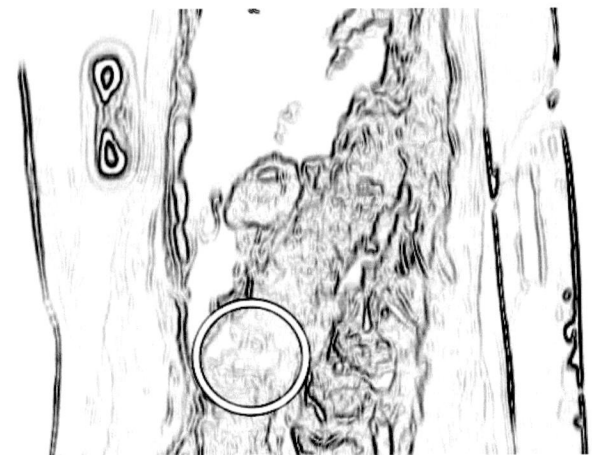

FIG. 7.2 SAGITTAL VIEW OF ABDOMEN - FOURTH LUMBAR VERTEBRA PATHOLOGY (AFTER IEM IMAGE)

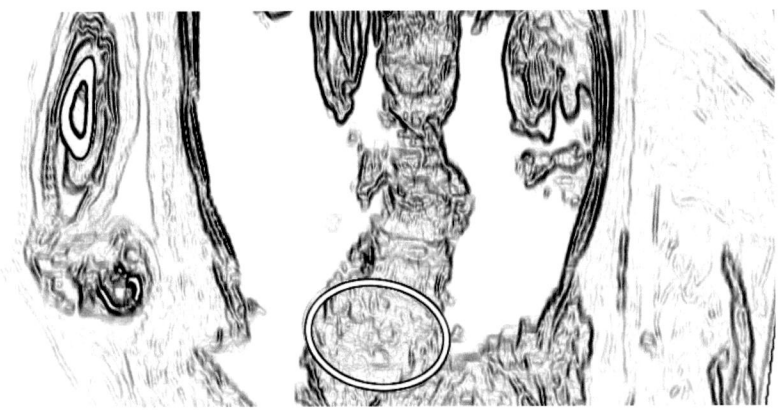

FIG. 7.3 CORONAL VIEW OF FOURTH LUMBAR VERTEBRA PATHOLOGY (AFTER IEM IMAGE)

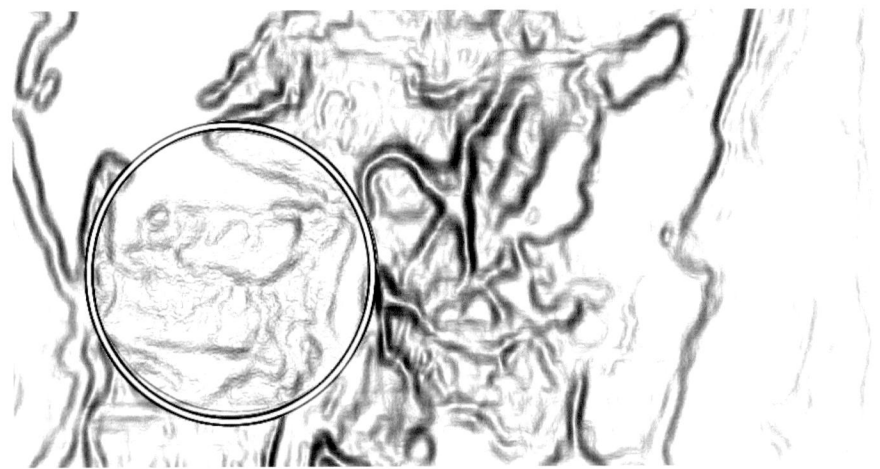

FIG. 7.4 SAGITTAL VIEW OF FOURTH LUMBAR VERTEBRA PATHOLOGY (AFTER IEM IMAGE)

This finding may indicate a severe infection with abscess formation or, less likely, tumours in the lumbar vertebrae leading to severe deformity and possible paralysis. This, in turn, could lead to urinary tract infection, septicaemia and subsequent death.

XL. Unnamed – Lausanne (Cat. No.492)

Cause of death

There is no definite cause of death shown, but the apparently grossly enlarged heart may be an indication of a cardiac problem such as chronic failure (See Fig. 5.181).

XLIX. Perenbast – Manchester University Museum (Accession No. MM5053.a)

Cause of death

Depending on the interpretation of the spinal pathology, this may be due to carcinoma of unknown primary origin (See Fig. 7.5).

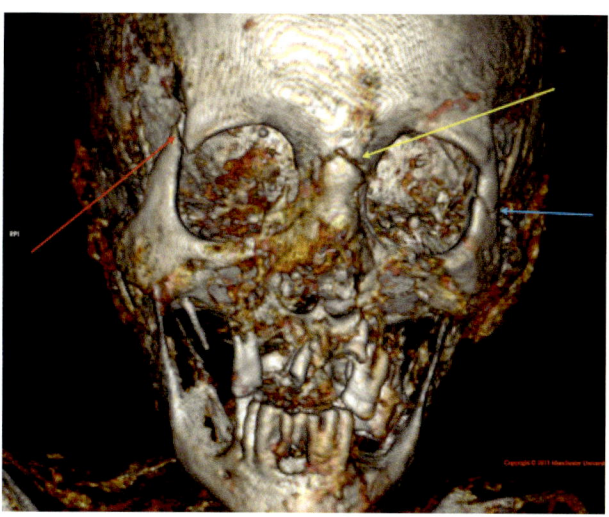

FIG. 7.6 3D RECONSTRUCTION OF FACIAL FRACTURES

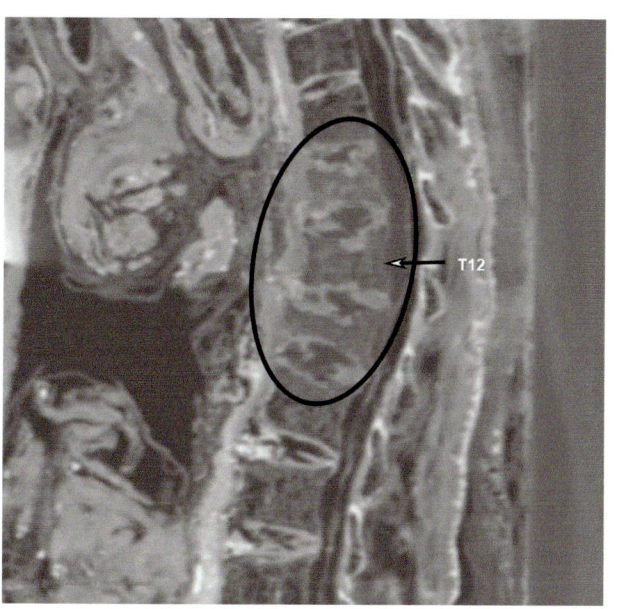

FIG. 7.5 SAGITTAL VIEW OF THORACO-LUMBAR JUNCTION - COLLAPSED VERTEBRAE

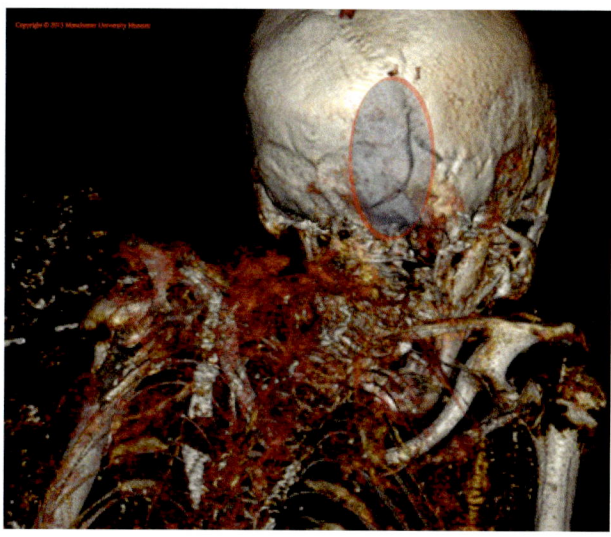

FIG. 7.7 3D RECONSTRUCTION OF FRACTURED RIGHT OCCIPUT

LVII. Artemidorus – Manchester Museum (Cat. No. MM 1775)

Cause of death

In view of the fractures of the occiput and facial bones, it is highly likely that death was due to violent trauma to the head and face and that the fractures of the left humeral neck and olecranon were caused as a result of the subsequent fall to the ground, a twisting injury to the left upper arm or defence injuries. The fractures of the eleventh thoracic vertebrae and the right side of the pelvis could all have been caused at this time but could equally well have been post-mortem (See Figs. 7.6, 7.7 and 7.8).

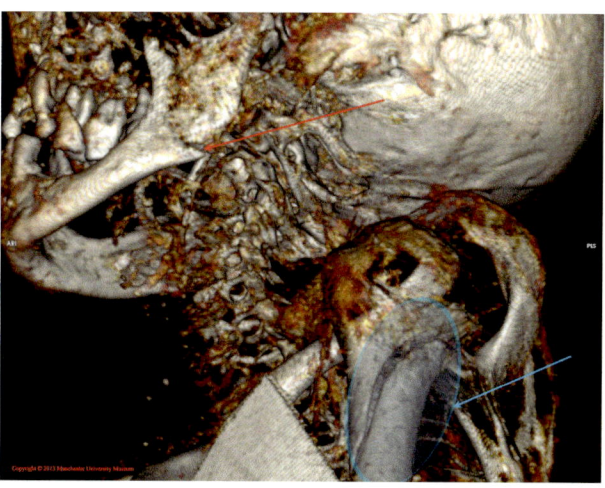

FIG. 7.8 3D RECONSTRUCTION OF FRACTURED LEFT ANGLE OF MANDIBLE AND LEFT HUMERAL NECK

LX. Unnamed – British Museum (Cat. No. EA 6704)

Cause of death

There is evidence of a spinal infection in the cervical region (namely marked intervertebral disc space reduction, vertebral body endplate irregularity, osteophyte formation and thickening of the anterior longitudinal ligament). There is a possibility that this was associated with the cause of death. No other cause of death is demonstrated (see Fig. 7.9).

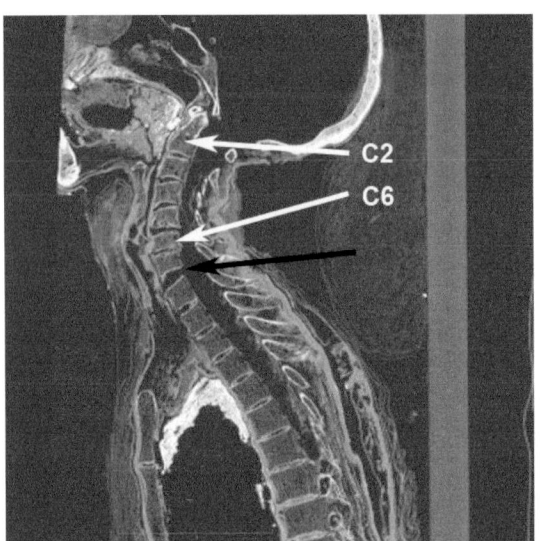

FIG. 7.9 SAGITTAL VIEW OF INFECTED CERVICAL SPINE. COURTESY OF THE TRUSTEES OF THE BRITISH MUSEUM

Of these ten cases (15% of the total), the distribution of causes is shown in Table 7.11.

7.3.2 Results – Non-Fatal Pathologies

Of passing interest is the finding of non-fatal pathology such as healed fractures, possible vitamin deficiencies and a possible haemoglobinopathy (See Table 7.12).

TRAUMA	INFECTION	HEART FAILURE	POST-PARTUM	METASTASES
5	2	1	1	1

TABLE 7.11 DISTRIBUTION OF OBSERVED PROBABLE CAUSES OF DEATH

NUMBER	ORIGIN	COMPLETE	ERA
VII	Ipswich – Tahathor	Scurvy	D25
XIV	Manchester – MM1777 – Asru	Cervical OA	D26
XVI	Liverpool – M13997a	Spondylolisthesis	Roman
XXVI	Zurich – Geneva – Infant	? Sickle Cell Dis.	Unknown
XXXIII	BM – EA 220744	Gall stones+Fract. Os calcis+L4	D22
XXXIX	Zurich – St. Gallen – C3530	IOVNS + Healed Fracture Radius	D21
XLII	Turin – Taaset – Suppl.9480	OA Spine + Healed Fracture Tibia	Ptolemaic
XLVIII	Manchester – MM3496	CTEV	D18
LI	Manchester – MM9354a – Khary	TB	D19/ Ptolemaic?
LII	Manchester – MM9319 – child	Dense Metaphyses	Roman
LVI	Manchester – MM2109	Scoliosis	Roman
LX	BM – EA 6704	Synovioma	Roman

OA = OSTEO-ARTHRITIS IOVNS = INTRA-OSSEOUS VILLONODULAR SYNOVITIS CTEV = CONGENITAL TALIPES EQUINOVARUS

TABLE 7.12 NON-FATAL PATHOLOGIES

Chapter Eight

Discussion of mummification techniques related to era, geographic location and age at death

8.1 Introduction

The above results have been presented in an order related to anatomical regions. The decision to do this emanated from the fact that analysis of the CT scans was akin to performing a 'virtual autopsy'. Many authors have described the concept of performing a 'virtual autopsy' by CT scan – examples are Donchin et al. in 1994 (Donchin et al., 1994: 552-555) and Dirnhofer et al in 2006 (Dirnhofer et al., 2006: 1305-1333). The use of a CT scan as a 'Virtual autopsy' was also used by Taylor in the Egyptology arena (Taylor, 2004). There are many other examples of the use of this term in the radiological and forensic medicine literature. The value of this technique is that there is no damage to the mummy and therefore the process is repeatable if thought desirable. The only risk to the mummy is a physical one during the period of transport. There is no evidence to support the concept of damage to the ancient DNA when using medical diagnostic equipment (Wanek, Speller, Rühli, 2013: 397-410). Furthermore, the resultant Dicom image files can easily be transmitted to researchers and can be analysed with whichever software packages are considered appropriate at that point in time.

The topic of Dicom Reader software has been mentioned before (Chapter Two - P 11) but it should be mentioned here that the choice of Reader software can make fundamental differences to the outcome of the analysis. Initial reports in this project were composed using the Dicom reader software from the hospital where the examination was performed. This either linked to the installed CT machine or to the PACS software used to handle images at the hospital. The limitation of such an approach is that all manipulation and reconstruction of images has to be performed in the hospital prior to downloading the files to the researcher/museum. Subsequently in the project, images were analysed using stand-alone software. This was, initially, the Osirix 32 bit programme. In April 2013, Osirix 64 bit software was obtained. This resulted in a significant increase in the detail of the images, so leading to the need to revise some details of several of the reports. An example of this relates to the course of the skin around the region of the lower jaw. In earlier analyses this appeared to be superficial to 'packing' in some cases. However, with the newer software it became apparent that the skin was, in fact, deep to that packing. Clearly, this resulted in the diagnosis of subcutaneous packing being revised. As a result, all available image files were re-examined.

The foregoing suggests that CT scans of mummies need to be reviewed from time to time and a decision made as to whether further examinations should be undertaken on more modern machines and re-analysed using current software (Loynes et al, 2013)

Other concepts that require discussion are 'burden of proof' and 'Occam's Razor'. There are two different 'burden of proof' requirements set in English Law. The first is in the field of criminal justice where the burden is that of 'beyond reasonable doubt'. This is difficult to define mathematically but is supposed to be close to 100%. However, in civil law, the burden is 'on the balance of probabilities'. This is much easier to define and is 51% and above. Where opinions are given in this document they are 'on the balance of probabilities'.

Occam's Razor is a principle attributed to a Franciscan friar in the fourteenth century from the village of Ockham in Surrey (William of Ockham). In simple terms it states that entities should not be multiplied unnecessarily and that where two competing theories make the same predictions, the simpler one is better (this used to be taught in the medical curriculum as 'commonest things are commonest!' and 'sparrows are far more plentiful than canaries'). This principle will be followed in this document.

The initial aim of this research was to find patterns of embalming technique related to historical era and to locations in ancient Egypt. There is insufficient reliable information in the available provenance of mummies to detect patterns of embalming/mummification related to status (which had been another of the initial aims).

Within this cohort of cases there are several which have been damaged somewhere along the 'journey' from the death of the individual to their current location in museums. These continue to provide useful but not complete information. All available information will be used where possible.

8.2 Patterns of mummification related to era

A list of the mummies studied, grouped in similar eras is shown in Table 8.1 and the numbers in each era are shown in Tables 8.2 and 8.3.

NUMBER	ORIGIN	ERA
LVIII	Manchester – MM13784	Middle Kingdom
XLVIII	Manchester – MM3496	D18
LI	Manchester – MM9354a – Khary	D19/ Ptolemaic?
III	Birmingham – Padimut	D20
XXXIX	Zurich – St. Gallen – C3530	D21
IV	Exeter – Shepenmut	D22
VIII	Liverpool – Padiamun – 53.72a	D22
XXIX	BM – Hor – EA6659	D22
XXXII	BM – EA20744	D22
XXXIII	BM – EA22939	D22
XXXIV	BM – EA25258	D22
XXXV	BM – EA29577	D22
XLIX	Manchester – MM5053.a – Perenbast	D22
XXV	Zurich – Geneva – TjesMoutPert – D0242	D22-25
V	Sheffield – Nesitanebetasheru	D25
VII	Ipswich – Tahathor	D25
IX	Liverpool – Padiamunnebnesuttauwy	D25
XXX	BM – Ankh-Unen-Nefer – EA6681	D25
XXXI	BM – Padiamunet – EA6682	D25
LIII	Manchester – MM1976.51a	D25
XVII	Liverpool – Ankhesenaset	3IP
XXI	Zurich – Lausanne – 490	3IP
XL	Zurich – Lausanne – 492	3IP
LIV	Manchester – Salford 2	3IP
II	Birmingham – Namenkhetamun	D26
VI	Sheffield – Djedma'atiuesankh	D26
XI	Liverpool – Padiamun – M14003	D26
XIV	Manchester – MM1777 – Asru	D26
XX	Zurich – TaDjIsis – K1205	D26
XXXVIII	Zurich – St. Gallen – Shepenese	D26
XLVI	Manchester – MM10881	D26
L	Perth – 23/1936	D26
X	Liverpool – Nesmin	Ptolemaic
XXIII	Zurich – Yverdon – Nes-Shou – MY/3775	Ptolemaic
XXVIII	Manchester – Ta-Sheri-Ankh – MM13783	Ptolemaic
XXXVI	Zurich – Bern – AE9	Ptolemaic
XXXVII	Zurich – Lenzburg – Sherit-Min	Ptolemaic
XLII	Turin – Taaset – Suppl.9480	Ptolemaic
LV	Manchester – MM13011	Ptolemaic
XLIII	Turin – (Tebtynis) – Suppl.19691	Ptolemaic ??
XLIV	Turin – Provv.610	Ptolemaic ??
I	Birmingham – Graeco-Roman	Roman
XII	Manchester – MM1768	Roman
XIII	Manchester – MM1767	Roman
XV	Liverpool – 13.10.11.25	Roman
XVI	Liverpool – M13997a	Roman
XVIII	Liverpool- M14048	Roman
XIX	Zurich – Altdorf Child	Roman
XXIV	Zurich – Basel – BSAE.1030	Roman
XXVII	Manchester – Demetria – 11630	Roman
XLI	Zurich – Lenzburg – K10351	Roman
XLV	Manchester – MM1766	Roman
XLVII	Manchester – MM1769	Roman
LII	Manchester – MM9319 – child	Roman
LVI	Manchester – MM2109	Roman
LVII	Manchester – MM1775 – Artemidorus	Roman
LIX	BM – EA 22108 Child	Roman
LX	BM – EA 6704	Roman
XXII	Zurich – Bern – 00/2	Unknown
XXVI	Zurich – Geneva – Infant	Unknown

TABLE 8.1 DISTRIBUTION OF MUMMIES BY ERA

Discussion of mummification techniques related to era, geographic location and age at death

M K	D18	D19	D20/21	D22	D25	3IP	D26	Ptol	Rom
1	1	1	2	8	7	4	8	9	17

TABLE 8.2 NUMBERS IN EACH ERA

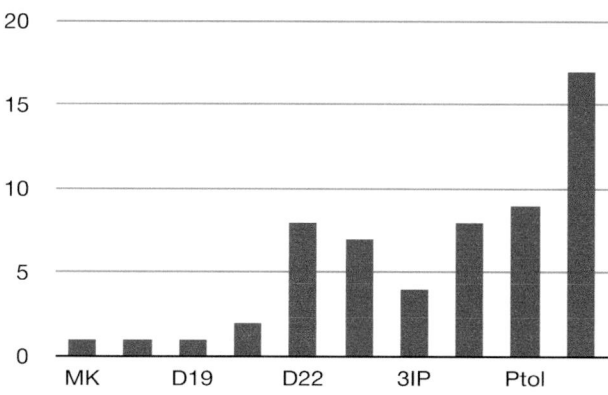

TABLE 8.3 NUMBERS IN EACH ERA

Although the small numbers associated with the Middle Kingdom and Dynasties 18, 19 and 20 make assertions impossible, they may be used to indicate concordance (or otherwise) with the perceived knowledge concerning mummification techniques in those eras. On the other hand, from Dynasty 22 onwards the cohort numbers increase and more reliable conclusions can be formed.

8.2.1 Middle Kingdom

The example of a Middle Kingdom mummy (Mummy LVIII) reveals evidence of excerebration, probably via the trans-foraminal route. Evisceration has been through a left flank incision with retention of some of the mediastinal tissues. Otherwise the evisceration has been thorough. Although there has been significant posterior disruption, the body is grossly intact and the arms can be seen lying over the front of the thighs. The reported mummification practices of this era are varied (Ikram and Dodson, 1998: 113-116) and the data relating to Mummy LVIII correlates well with the descriptions given.

8.2.2 Dynasty 18

The Dynasty 18 mummy (Mummy XLVIII) is of a child aged one to two years. The body is wrapped in a reed mat and has been considerably distorted – possibly due to the constriction caused by the mat and the rope bindings at either end (See Fig. 8.1). Although a left flank incision is seen, there is evidence of incomplete evisceration. This conforms to the concept that Dynasty 18 saw the appearance of the 'classic' method of mummification referred to by Ikram and Dodson (Ikram and Dodson, vs: 118), the zenith of mummification technique only being reached in Dynasty 21 (Ikram and Dodson, vs: 124). The fact that the skull bones are completely disarticulated from one another bears testimony to the fact that the child was young and cranial fusion had not taken place. Lack of fusion of the individual cranial bones would accord well with the proposed age of one to two years (Johnston, Davies and Davies, 1958: 353).

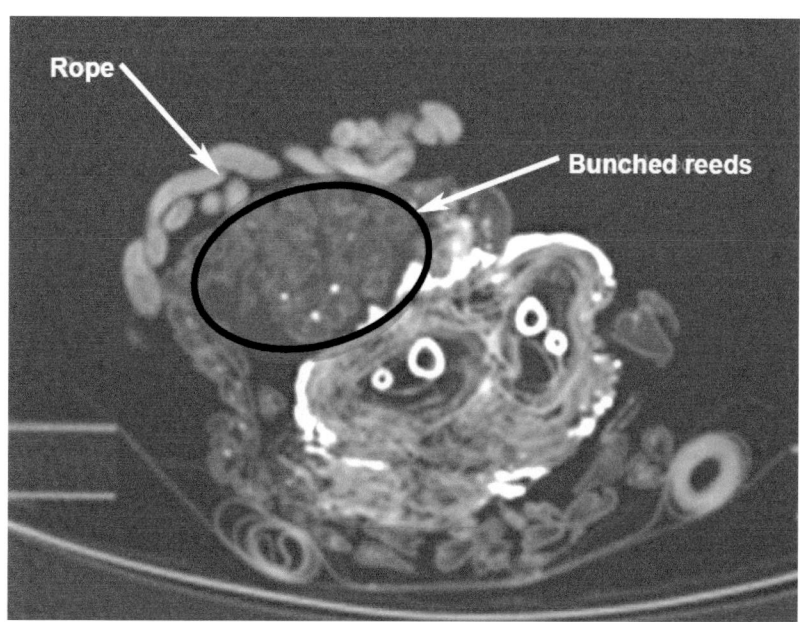

FIG. 8.1 AXIAL VIEW OF ROPE AND REEDS AT ONE END OF THE MAT 'COFFIN'

8.2.3 Dynasty 19

Dynasty 19 is represented by the mummy of Khary (Mummy LI from Manchester Museum). However, there is some uncertainty about the era of origin of this mummy as records show it to be from Dynasty 19 but there are characteristics, such as the arm position, which might place it in a much later era. For this reason it will be discussed separately after all eras have been considered.

8.2.4 Dynasty 20

The mummy of Padimut (Mummy III) from Birmingham Museum and Art Gallery was the subject of three separate reports in 1973. One of these was prepared by a John Ruffle of that institution and dated the coffins and mummy to the late Ramesside Period, that is Dynasty 20. The mummy was originally encased in a cartonnage coffin and then in two further wooden anthropoid coffins. It was removed and publically unwrapped in Warwick in 1850. Excerebration has been through a limited perforation of the ethmoid sinuses and the cribriform plate, with preservation of the sphenoid sinuses and some of the structures of the nasal cavity. This would imply a certain degree of care in this process. Despite the limited access the brain has been completely removed, but no foreign material subsequently introduced. The eyes have been retained and are covered with 'eye plates' ('false eyes'). The mouth contains packing and the neck subcutaneous packing. The mediastinum including the heart had been retained in situ but other viscera removed, desiccated and then returned to the body cavity after the introduction of two layers of resin. Evisceration has been performed via a left flank incision with layers of linen crossing through the incision into the abdomen. The arms lie beside the body with the hands over the front of the hips.

Overall the appearance is one of a well-performed complex procedure of mummification, in this case with some subcutaneous packing.

The picture is one that complies with the expected level and detail of mummification in this era. The specific treatment of the eyes has been only briefly discussed in the past (Aufderheide, 2010: 318 and 343; Cockburn, Cockburn and Reyman, 1998: 76, 79, 108 and 114) and will be the subject of a more detailed discussion below.

8.2.5 Dynasty 21

This era is represented by one mummy, namely Mummy XXXIX from St. Gallen Museum. This mummy is damaged, which slightly limits its value. However, there is much information to be gleaned. The head of Mummy XXXIX has been detached from the body and unwrapped, with the mandible being disarticulated from the skull. There is also trauma to the left maxilla. As a result, analysis of the skull, the brain, the eyes and the mouth are difficult. There is no evidence of subcutaneous packing in the neck. There is a left flank incision but no evidence of the use of linen or resin within the body cavity – only granular material along with returned loose viscera.

8.2.6 Dynasty 22

There are eight mummies from Dynasty 22. These are shown in Table 8.4.

NUMBER	ORIGIN	ERA
IV	Exeter – Shepenmut	D22
VIII	Liverpool – Padiamun – 53.72a	D22
XXIX	BM – Hor – EA6659	D22
XXXII	BM – EA20744	D22
XXXIII	BM – EA22939	D22
XXXIV	BM – EA25258	D22
XXXV	BM – EA29577	D22
XLIX	Manchester – MM5053.a – Perenbast	D22
XXV	Zurich – Geneva – TjesMoutPert – D0242	D22-25

TABLE 8.4 MUMMIES FROM DYNASTY 22

The mummy of TjesMoutPert (Mummy XXV) has been given a provenance of Dynasty 22-25 and will be considered separately (P 208). Therefore, for the sake of uniformity there are eight mummies assigned to this particular cohort. Unfortunately, the mummy from Exeter has only been X-rayed and therefore analysis is very basic. As other cases have been the subject of far more sophisticated investigation, this case will not be included in the evaluation. Of the seven remaining mummies the treatment of the head and the body/torso will be considered separately.

Mummy	Exc. Route	Cranial Packing	Eyes	Mouth	Neck	Location
VIII	E+Sp	Res	L+Gr	L+Res	L	Thebes
XXIX	E+FM	Gr	Rem+L/Res+Pl	Gr(Sm)	L+Gr	Thebes
XXXII	Bas	-----	Des	L+Gr	-----	D-E-B
XXXIII	E	L	Des+Res+Pl	Gr	Gr	Thebes
XXXIV	E+Sp	----	L+Pl	Res+Gr	Gr	Thebes
XXXV	E+Sp	Gr	Disrupted	Disrupted	Disrupted	Thebes
IL	Sp	L	L	Gr	Gr	Thebes

E=ETHMOID SP=SPHENOID FM=FORAMEN MAGNUM RES=RESIN GR=GRANULAR MATERIAL L=LINEN REM=REMOVAL PL=PLATES DES=DESICCATED D-E-B=DEIR EL BAHARI

TABLE 8.5 MUMMIFICATION TECHNIQUES USED IN THE HEAD

8.2.6.1 Treatment of the Head and Neck

Five points will be considered. These are the route used for excerebration, the filling/packing used in the cranial cavity, the treatment of the eyes, the treatment of the mouth and the treatment of the neck. These are summarized in Table 8.5.

The first point to note is that the route used for excerebration is almost always more horizontal than used in previous eras, resulting in the more common perforation of the sphenoid air sinus as well as (or alternative to) the ethmoid sinuses. The extreme example of this horizontal approach is seen in Mummy XXXII, where the perforation involves the base of the skull (in a teenager where the base of the skull may well be somewhat softer than in the adult) (See Figures 4.106 and 4.107 – P 62 and 63). The second point of note is that cranial cavity packing has been performed in all cases except Mummy XXXII that has the basal perforation. This has been combined in all cases with packing of the subcutaneous tissues of the neck (except Mummy XXXII). The curious detail is that where linen has been used to pack the neck, a different material has been used in the cranial cavity (granular material being used – or vice versa) except for Mummy XXIX where granular material is used in both locations with the addition of linen in the neck. Mummy XXXV has had the head and neck severely disrupted so preventing comment on these areas. In most other cases the eyes have been retained.

In the six cases available for comment on eye treatment, one has retention with desiccation alone. The other five have retention of the globe of the eye with packing of the eye with linen or resin or both. Eye plates (or 'false eyes') have been used in three cases.

Wherever granular material has been used to pack the neck it has also been used alone or with other material (resin) in the mouth. Where linen has been used for subcutaneous packing in the neck it has also been used to pack the mouth and eyes (Mummy VIII). The only mummy without either neck or cranial cavity packing came from Deir el Bahari, all others originating in Thebes. It is interesting to note that mummies shown in Table 6.2 (P 184) where subcutaneous neck packing has been performed are all from Thebes. This would indicate strongly that such packing might well have been a Theban custom.

8.2.6.2 Treatment of the Trunk

The factors to be considered here are the route of evisceration, the completeness or otherwise of that evisceration, whether the viscera were returned to the body – either in canopic packages or loose - and what, if any, foreign material was used for packing. Table 8.6 summarises the findings. For the sake of clarity it can be stated that there was no evidence of the use of a perineal approach in this era.

With the exception of Mummy XXXV where disruption prevented comment on the treatment of the trunk it can be seen that a left flank incision has been used on all occasions. In the six remaining cases there are two examples of incomplete evisceration. In these cases the abdomen was eviscerated, but the thorax evisceration was incomplete in that the mediastinum was retained. It is possible that this was in an attempt to retain the heart in situ. This goal appears to have been achieved in both cases. However, Mummy XXXII was from Deir el Bahari and Mummy IL from Thebes. Therefore the theme of varying practices in Thebes and Deir el Bahari seen in the treatment of the head and neck is not repeated when it comes to the treatment of the body. The use of canopic packages does not appear to have a distinct pattern in this group. Although granular material is used throughout the group, the addition of resin, linen or both does not conform to a pattern in this era.

8.2.7 Dynasty 25

There are only six mummies in this cohort as shown in Table 8.7. They were all obtained in Thebes.

A similar technique to that used in sections 8.2.6.1 and 8.2.6.2 will be used for the analysis of this cohort.

NUMBER	ORIGIN	ERA	LOCATION
V	Sheffield – Nesitanebetasheru	D25	Thebes
VII	Ipswich – Tahathor	D25	Thebes
IX	Liverpool – Padiamunnebnesuttauwy	D25	Thebes
XXX	BM – Ankh-Unen-Nefer – EA6681	D25	Thebes
XXXI	BM – Padiamunet – EA6682	D25	Thebes
LIII	Manchester – MM1976.51a	D25	Thebes

TABLE 8.7 MUMMIES FROM DYNASTY 25

Mummy	Evisceration Route	Complete Evisceration?	Returned Viscera	Packing Material
VIII	L. Flank	Complete	Loose	Res+Gr
XXIX	L. Flank	Complete	Loose	Res+Gr+L
XXXII	L. Flank	Med. Ret.	Loose+CP	Gr
XXXIII	L. Flank	Complete	CP	L+Gr
XXXIV	L. Flank	Complete	Loose	Gr
XXXV	Disrupted	Disrupted	Disrupted	Gr
IL	L. Flank	Med. Ret.	CP	Gr

RES=RESIN GR=GRANULAR MATERIAL L=LINEN CP=CANOPIC PACKAGES

TABLE 8.6 MUMMIFICATION TECHNIQUES USED IN THE TRUNK

Mummy	Exc. Route	Cranial Packing	Eyes	Mouth	Neck	Location
V	E+Sp	Res	L+Pl	L+Res	----	Thebes
VII	FM	Gr	Rem+L	L	-----	Thebes
IX	E	Res	Des+Res	Res	-----	Thebes
XXX	E	Gr	L+Pl	-----	L	Thebes
XXXI	E	----	L	L	L+Stick	Thebes
LIII	E	Res	Des	L	-----	Thebes

E=Ethmoid Sp=Sphenoid FM=Foramen Magnum Res=Resin Gr=Granular material L=Linen Rem=Removal Pl=Plates Des=Desiccated

TABLE 8.8 Mummification techniques used in the head

Mummy	Evisceration Route	Complete Evisceration?	Returned Viscera	Packing Material
V	?	Complete	Loose+CP	Res+Gr
VII	? L. Flank	Complete	Loose	Gr
IX	Supra-pubic	Incomplete	Loose	Gr
XXX	L. Flank	Complete	CP	Res+Gr
XXXI	L. Flank	Incomplete	Loose	Gr
LIII	L. Flank+Per.	Complete	CP	Res+L

Res=Resin Gr=Granular material L=Linen CP=Canopic Packages

TABLE 8.9 Mummification techniques used in the trunk

NUMBER	ORIGIN	ERA	LOCATION
XVII	Liverpool – Ankhesenaset	3IP	Thebes
XXI	Zurich – Lausanne – 490	3IP	Unknown
XL	Zurich – Lausanne – 492	3IP	Unknown
LIV	Manchester – Salford 2	3IP	Unknown

TABLE 8.10 Mummies from the Third Intermediate Period

Mummy	Exc. Route	Cranial Packing	Eyes	Mouth	Neck	Location
XVII	E	L	L+Pl	Gr	L+Gr	Thebes
XL	E+Sp	Res	Des	-----	-----	Unknown
LIV	E	Res	Des	-----	-----	Unknown

E=Ethmoid Sp=Sphenoid FM=Foramen Magnum Res=Resin Gr=Granular material L=Linen Rem=Removal Pl=Plates Des=Desiccated

TABLE 8.11 Mummification techniques used in the head in Third Intermediate Period

8.2.7.1 Treatment of the Head and Neck

As with Dynasty 22 mummies there is a case of excerebration via the foramen magnum. This route is only found in four of the cases analysed in this series. In all other cases from Dynasty 25 excerebration has been performed via the trans-nasal route – and in particular via the ethmoid sinus. In one of these cases there is evidence of additional damage to the sphenoid sinus but unfortunately the CT scans are in analogue format and this phenomenon is only seen in the axial view. It is not possible to reconstruct a sagittal view that could have given more information as to how horizontal the perforation was. In the other cases the perforation was more vertical than in Dynasty 22 mummies seen above (P 200). Excerebration has been thorough in all cases and some form of cranial packing used in all except one case - that is in the case of Mummy XXXI where the absence of cranial cavity packing is accompanied by packing of the mouth and cheeks to better restore the facial contours.

With regard to the eyes these have been removed in one case (Mummy VII – where excerebration was via the trans-foraminal route), left in situ and desiccated in two cases (with resin packs inserted superficial to the remains of the globes in one case) and retained with linen packing to restore the shape of the eye in three cases two of which had eye plates added.

Packing of the mouth has been mentioned already in one of the cases and is seen in four other cases (but without the addition of cheek packing).

Subcutaneous packing of the neck is less used than in Dynasty 22 examples. It is seen in only two cases. In one of these cases there is the addition of a rod in the neck and mouth, presumably to add stability to these areas.

8.2.7.2 Treatment of the Trunk

In these Dynasty 25 mummies an abdominal incision has been used in five out of six cases (the sixth being disrupted in the region of the abdomen). A perineal approach has been added to the abdominal incision in Mummy LIII. The viscera have always been returned to the body cavity, sometimes in canopic packages and sometimes unpackaged. Packing material has always been introduced into the cavity. Granular material is the more common material, sometimes with resin as a second component. Linen is only used for packing in one case. Complete body cavity packing has not been used in any mummy in this dynasty cohort.

8.2.8 Mummies assigned to the 'Third Intermediate Period' (Dynasty 21-25)

It is uncertain to which dynasty these mummies belong. This coincides well with the fact that their origin is also unknown and this reflects the sparse information about the provenance. There are only four such mummies in this series (of which one is a 'false' mummy – Mummy XXI) and they are shown in Table 8.10.

For the sake of completeness they will be considered in a similar fashion to those mummies who have been assigned to a particular dynasty.

8.2.8.1 Treatment of the Head and Neck

There is no exact match for any of the above mummies but similarities would point to Mummy XVII being closer to a Dynasty 22 example. Similarly Mummies XL and LIV do not match exactly but are closer to Dynasty 25 examples than those from Dynasty 22.

8.2.8.2 Treatment of the Trunk

Unlike the treatment of the head and neck, there is no convincing match or similarity to either Dynasties 22 or 25 in the treatment of the trunk. Therefore, it could be that these mummies are from Dynasties 23 or 24 or that the mummification techniques in the Third Intermediate Period were wide-ranging and varied. The other possibility is that these mummies have been attributed to the wrong period in history.

8.2.9 Dynasty 26

There are eight mummies in this group. Six are from Thebes, one from Akhmim and for a further one the museum records show an origin of Thebes although recent examination of the anthropoid coffin indicates that Akhmim is a distinct possibility as provenance. This is currently under investigation and the final outcome is awaited. Of further note is Mummy II. The anthropoid coffin is of Namenkhetamun, a Chantress in the temple of Amun at Thebes. Examination of the CT scans reveals that this mummy is male. The provenance is therefore in doubt. The mummies in this cohort are shown in Table 8.13.

In the first instance all mummies will be included in the analysis of this cohort and consideration of the characteristics of the treatment of the head will be followed by a similar analysis of the treatment of the trunk.

Mummy	Evisceration Route	Complete Evisceration?	Returned Viscera	Packing Material
XVII	L. Flank	Complete	Loose+CP	Gr
XL	Supra-pubic	Incomplete	Loose	-----
LIV	None	None	-----	-----

RES=RESIN GR=GRANULAR MATERIAL L=LINEN CP=CANOPIC PACKAGES
TABLE 8.12 MUMMIFICATION TECHNIQUES USED IN THE TRUNK IN THIRD INTERMEDIATE PERIOD

NUMBER	ORIGIN	ERA	LOCATION
II	Birmingham – Namenkhetamun	D26	Thebes
VI	Sheffield – Djedma'atiuesankh	D26	Thebes
XI	Liverpool – Padiamun – M14003	D26	Thebes
XIV	Manchester – MM1777 – Asru	D26	Thebes
XX	Zurich – TaDjIsis – K1205	D26	Thebes
XXXVIII	Zurich – St. Gallen – Shepenese	D26	Akhmim
XLVI	Manchester – MM10881	D26	Thebes
L	Perth – 23/1936	D26	Thebes/Akhmim

TABLE 8.13 MUMMIES FROM DYNASTY 26

8.2.9.1 Treatment of the Head and Neck

It can be seen that of the eight mummies, five had excerebration performed via the trans-nasal route and one via the trans-orbital route (this route will be discussed in further detail below P 228). One mummy had no excerebration and the last was too disrupted to analyse. Of the four cases of excerebration via the ethmoid all failed to show evidence of the introduction of foreign material into the cranial cavity. However, where the excerebration route was through the sphenoid or the orbit resin was introduced.

All six cases suitable for analysis had retained eyes. Of these six cases the eye globe was packed with linen in five, the sixth being only retained and desiccated. In only one case were eye plates used.

It was possible to see the contents of the mouth in five cases. In these cases the mouth was packed with resin, granular material or linen in four of the cases and left empty in only one.

Where it was possible to analyse the cervical region it was found that no packing had been used in any of the cases.

8.2.9.2 Treatment of the Trunk

With the disruption of the body of three of this cohort only five remain for analysis. All of these had a left flank incision used for evisceration. In the case of Mummy XXXVIII a further, perineal, route was used. This mummy was from Akhmim.

In all these five cases a part or whole of the mediastinum was retained.

It is interesting to note that in Table 8.16 showing the mediastinal contents there is retention of all components of the mediastinum in only two cases. These include Mummy VI where the analogue CT scan images make interpretation difficult, but there is a pack in the perineal area. Although not certain, this may indicate a perineal route for evisceration as well as an abdominal one. In the second case, Mummy XXXVIII, a perineal route has definitely been used in conjunction with an abdominal route. This mummy is from Akhmim.

8.2.10 Ptolemaic Period

There are no mummies in this series from Dynasty 27 to Dynasty 31. Nine mummies represent the Ptolemaic Period. Of these Mummies XLIII and XLIV are only 'probably' from this period. The records accompanying the CT scans were vague in that these mummies were referred to as 'Graeco-Roman' but personal communication with museum staff in Turin indicated that the mummies were regarded as almost certainly from the Ptolemaic Period. The mummies are shown in Table 8.17

These mummies will be analysed in a similar way as those from previous eras.

8.2.10.1 Treatment of the Head and Neck

Excerebration has been performed in all mummies except Mummy LV. It is interesting to note that this is the mummy of a child aged between two and three years. Following excerebration in the other cases the cranial cavity has been packed to an extent with resin. The exceptions to this statement are the two mummies from Turin where the

Mummy	Exc. Route	Cranial Packing	Eyes	Mouth	Neck	Location
II	None	-----	L	L	-----	Thebes
VI	E	-----	L	?	?	Thebes
XI	E	-----	L+Pl	L	-----	Thebes
XIV	TO	Res	Des	Gr	-----	Thebes
XX						Thebes
XXXVIII	E	-----	L	Res	-----	Akhmim
XLVI	Sp	Res	-----			Thebes
L	E	-----	L	-----	-----	Thebes/Akhmim

E=Ethmoid Sp=Sphenoid FM=Foramen Magnum TO=Trans-orbital Res=Resin Gr=Granular material L=Linen
Res=Resin Gr=Granular material L=Linen REM=Removal Pl=Plates Des=Desiccated Blue shading = Disrupted

Table 8.14 Mummification techniques used in the head in Dynasty 26

Mummy	Evisceration Route	Complete Evisceration?	Returned Viscera	Packing Material
II	L. Flank	Med. Ret.	Loose	Gr
VI	L. Flank	Med. Ret.	-----	Res
XI	L. Flank	Sup.Med. Ret.	CP	Gr
XIV	L. Flank	Med. Ret.	Loose	-----
XX				
XXXVIII	L. Flank+Peri.	Med. Ret.	CP	Gr
XLVI				
L				

Res=Resin Gr=Granular material L=Linen CP=Canopic Packages Per.=Perineal Blue shading = Disrupted

Table 8.15 Mummification techniques used in the trunk in Dynasty 26

Mummy	Heart	Great Vessels	Pleura	Evisceration Route
II	NO	YES	YES	L. Flank
VI	YES	YES	YES	L. Flank
XI	NO	YES	NO	L. Flank
XIV	NO	YES	YES	L. Flank
XXXVIII	YES	YES	YES	L. Flank+Peri.

TABLE 8.16 CONTENTS OF MEDIASTINUM

NUMBER	ORIGIN	ERA	LOCATION
X	Liverpool – Nesmin	Ptolemaic	Akhmim
XXIII	Zurich – Yverdon – Nes-Shou – MY/3775	Ptolemaic	Akhmim
XXVIII	Manchester –Ta- Sheri –Ankh – MM13783	Ptolemaic	Akhmim
XXXVI	Zurich – Bern – AE9	Ptolemaic	Akhmim
XXXVII	Zurich – Lenzburg – Sherit-Min	Ptolemaic	Akhmim
XLII	Turin – Taaset – Suppl.9480	Ptolemaic	Assiut
LV	Manchester – MM13011	Ptolemaic	Unknown
XLIII	Turin – (Tebtynis) – Suppl.19691	Ptolemaic ??	Fayum
XLIV	Turin – Provv.610	Ptolemaic ??	Unknown

TABLE 8.17 MUMMIES FROM THE PTOLEMAIC PERIOD

Mummy	Exc. Route	Cranial Packing	Eyes	Mouth	Neck	Location
X	E+Sp	Res	Des	Res	-----	Akhmim
XXIII	E	Res	REM	Res	-----	Akhmim
XXVIII	E	Res	Des	-----	-----	Akhmim
XXXVI	E	Res	Des	L	-----	Akhmim
XXXVII	E	Res	Des	-----	-----	Akhmim
XLII	E	Res	L	L+Res	-----	Assiut
LV	None	Brain	Des	-----	-----	Unknown
XLIII	E	-----	Des	L	-----	Fayum
XLIV	E	-----	Des	-----	-----	Unknown

E=ETHMOID SP=SPHENOID FM=FORAMEN MAGNUM TO=TRANS-ORBITAL RES=RESIN GR=GRANULAR MATERIAL L=LINEN
REM=REMOVAL PL=PLATES DES=DESICCATED

TABLE 8.18 MUMMIFICATION TECHNIQUES USED IN THE HEAD IN THE PTOLEMAIC PERIOD

Mummy	Evisceration Route	Complete Evisceration?	Returned Viscera	Packing Material
X	L. Flank+Per	Med. Ret.	CP	Res
XXIII	L. Flank+Per	Complete	CP	Res
XXVIII	L. Flank	Complete	CP	Res
XXXVI	L. Flank+Per	Med. Ret.	CP	Res
XXXVII	Per	Med. Ret.	Loose	-----
XLII	Per	Incomplete	-----	Gr
LV	None	None	-----	-----
XLIII	L. Flank	Complete	CP	-----
XLIV	L. Flank	Med. Ret.	CP	Res

RES=RESIN GR=GRANULAR MATERIAL L=LINEN CP=CANOPIC PACKAGES PER.=PERINEAL

TABLE 8.19 MUMMIFICATION TECHNIQUES USED IN THE TRUNK IN THE PTOLEMAIC PERIOD

provenance was uncertain with regard to the era of origin. In one case the eyes were removed, but in all others they were retained. Packing of the eye globe was performed in only one case (from the Fayum). The treatment of the mouth varied from no filling in four cases to the use of small amounts of linen or resin in five cases. As anticipated the subcutaneous tissues of the neck have not been packed.

8.2.10.2 Treatment of the Trunk

The results of the treatment of the trunk in these cases are shown in Table 8.19. As there are four cases of mediastinal retention the extent of this is shown in Table 8.20. The great vessels have been retained in all cases and the heart in three cases. Whether this is related to the route used for evisceration is difficult to say, as the perineal route would make access to the mediastinum difficult. However, an abdominal route was also used in conjunction with the perineal route in two of these cases. The whole subject of the practicalities of access will be discussed later (P 238).

Mummy	Heart	Great Vessels	Pleura	Evisceration Route
X	NO	YES	NO	L. Flank+Per
XXXVI	YES	YES	NO	L. Flank+Per
XXXVII	YES	YES	YES	Per
XLIV	YES	YES	YES	L. Flank

TABLE 8.20 CONTENTS OF MEDIASTINUM

NUMBER	ORIGIN	ERA	LOCATION
I	Birmingham – Graeco-Roman	Roman	Unknown
XII	Manchester – MM1768	Roman	Fayum
XIII	Manchester – MM1767	Roman	Fayum
XV	Liverpool – 13.10.11.25	Roman	Hawara
XVI	Liverpool – M13997a	Roman	Thebes
XVIII	Liverpool- M14048	Roman	Thebes
XIX	Zurich – Altdorf Child	Roman	Unknown
XXIV	Zurich – Basel – BSAE.1030	Roman	El-Hibe
XXVII	Manchester – Demetria – 11630	Roman	Hawara
XLI	Zurich – Lenzburg – K10351	Roman	Unknown
XLV	Manchester – MM1766	Roman	Hawara
XLVII	Manchester – MM1769	Roman	Hawara
LII	Manchester – MM9319 – child	Roman	?Hawara
LVI	Manchester – MM2109	Roman	Hawara
LVII	Manchester – MM1775 – Artemidorus	Roman	Hawara
LIX	BM – EA 22108 Child	Roman	Hawara
LX	BM – EA 6704	Roman	Thebes

TABLE 8.21 MUMMIES FROM THE ROMAN PERIOD

NUMBER	ORIGIN	ERA	LOCATION
XII	Manchester – MM1768	Roman	Faiyum
XIII	Manchester – MM1767	Roman	Faiyum
XV	Liverpool – 13.10.11.25	Roman	Hawara
XXVII	Manchester – Demetria – MM11630	Roman	Hawara
XLV	Manchester – MM1766	Roman	Hawara
XLVII	Manchester – MM1769	Roman	Hawara
LII	Manchester – MM9319 – child	Roman	?Hawara
LVI	Manchester – MM2109	Roman	Hawara
LVII	Manchester – MM1775 – Artemidorus	Roman	Hawara
LIX	BM – EA 22108 Child	Roman	Hawara
XXIV	Zurich – Basel – BSAE.1030	Roman	El-Hibe
XVI	Liverpool – M13997a	Roman	Thebes
XVIII	Liverpool- M14048	Roman	Thebes
LX	BM – EA 6704	Roman	Thebes
I	Birmingham – Graeco-Roman	Roman	Unknown
XIX	Zurich – Altdorf Child	Roman	Unknown
XLI	Zurich – Lenzburg – K10351	Roman	Unknown

TABLE 8.22 MUMMIES FROM THE ROMAN PERIOD GROUPED BY LOCATION OF ORIGIN

8.2.11 Roman Period

The largest cohort of mummies was from the Roman Period. There are seventeen such mummies in this group. Table 8.21 shows their identity and place of origin.

As can be seen there are three mummies of un-known origin, three from Thebes, one from El-Hibe and the remaining ten from Hawara or the Fayum. If it is accepted that Hawara is a location within the Fayum then these mummies can be taken as a distinct cohort. For the sake of clarity these mummies will be re-arranged in order of location as seen in Table 8.22

As with previous groups the methods of treating the head and the trunk will be considered separately.

8.2.11.1 Treatment of the Head and Neck

Table 8.23 shows significant variety in the approach to excerebration. In the Theban group, all three cases had trans-nasal excerebration via the ethmoid. This was

Mummy	Exc. Route	Cranial Packing	Eyes	Mouth	Neck	Location
XII	None	None	Des	Res	-----	Faiyum
XIII	None	None	REM	Res	Disrupt	Faiyum
XV	FM	Gr	Des	Plate	-----	Hawara
XXVII	E	Res	Des	L	-----	Hawara
XLV	E	Res	Des	L	-----	Hawara
XLVII	TN+TO	Res	Des	L	-----	Hawara
LII	None	None	Des	-----	-----	?Hawara
LVI	E	-----	Des	-----	-----	Hawara
LVII	E	-----	Des	-----	-----	Hawara
LIX	Sp	Res	Des	-----	-----	Hawara
XXIV	None	None	Des	-----	-----	El-Hibe
XVI	E	Res	L	Res	-----	Thebes
XVIII	E	Res	Des	-----	-----	Thebes
LX	E	Res	Res/L	L+Res+Gr	-----	Thebes
I	E	-----	Des	-----	-----	Unknown
XIX	E	-----	L	-----	-----	Unknown
XLI	E	-----	Des	Res	-----	Unknown

E=Ethmoid Sp=Sphenoid FM=Foramen Magnum TO=Trans-orbital Res=Resin Gr=Granular material L=Linen
REM=Removal Pl=Plates Des=Desiccated

Table 8.23 Mummification techniques used in the head in the Roman Period

followed by the introduction of varying amounts of resin. The treatment of the eyes and the packing of the mouth are also variable.

In contrast the cases from the Fayum (ten in number) received a variety of approaches from a lack of excerebration (three cases) through use of the trans-nasal route in five cases to the use of less common routes such as the trans-foraminal route and the trans-orbital route. As the trans-orbital route had commenced in the nose and deviated through the medial wall of the orbit, the superior orbital fissure may have been more an arbitrary choice than a deliberate point of skull entry. One of the trans-nasal routes was very horizontal (Mummy LIX) as previously noted in mummies from Dynasty 22.

The mummy from El-Hibe did not undergo excerebration and the eyes were left in situ and desiccated.

The three mummies with an unknown place of origin all had excerebration via the trans-nasal route (ethmoid) but without the introduction of any intracranial material. This would fit less well with an origin from Thebes rather than from Hawara or some other place.

The eyes were treated most often by retention and desiccation alone.

8.2.11.2 Treatment of the Trunk

If the disrupted mummy is excluded, the remaining sixteen mummies fall into two groups. There are eight mummies where there has been no attempt at evisceration and therefore no incision.

In the case of Mummy XXVII the anterior abdominal wall has been convoluted so much in the desiccation process that an incision cannot be confirmed or excluded. In the remaining eight there is evidence of an abdominal incision,

Mummy	Evisceration Route	Complete Evisceration?	Returned Viscera	Packing Material
XII	Disrupted	Incomplete	Disrupted	Disrupted
XIII	None	None	-----	-----
XV	None	None	-----	-----
XXVII	?None	Incomplete	-----	-----
XLV	Per	Incomplete	-----	-----
XLVII	None	None	-----	-----
LII	None	None	-----	-----
LVI	None	None	-----	-----
LVII	None	None	-----	-----
LIX	None	None	-----	-----
XXIV	Per	Incomplete	-----	Gr
XVI	L. Flank+Per	Complete	CP	Res
XVIII	L. Flank+Per	Complete	CP	Res
LX	L. Flank+Per.	Complete	CP	Res
I	L. Flank	Complete	Loose+CP	Gr
XIX	L. Flank	Complete	CP	L
XLI	L. Flank	Complete	-----	L

Res=Resin Gr=Granular material L=Linen CP=Canopic Packages Per.=Perineal

Table 8.24 Mummification techniques used in the trunk in the Roman Period

a perineal approach or both. Unsurprisingly, where a perineal approach alone has been used the evisceration is incomplete. Where a left flank incision has been used, then complete evisceration has been effected.

The viscera have not been returned to the body as either canopic packages or loose in any of the ten mummies from the Fayum region, nor has any intra-corporeal packing been used in these mummies.

One feature of mummies from the Roman era is the distortion of the chest wall seen in many of them. This will be discussed as a separate issue later.

8.3 Analysis of Specific Mummies

8.3.1 Mummy XXV – TjesMoutPert

This mummy is from Geneva Museum. The rationale for considering it separately is that the provenance places it vaguely in ' Dynasty 22 to 25'. Given that this covers almost three hundred years and most of the Third Intermediate Period, an attempt to associate it within a shorter timescale was thought to be appropriate.

Analysis will follow that previously used.

Excerebration has been performed via the ethmoid and most of the brain removed. There are remnants of the brain within the cranial cavity. There is some debris and a little resin in the posterior cranial fossa.

The eyes have been retained and packed with resin soaked linen. The amount of resin used to 'soak' the linen is much greater in the left globe packing than in the right.

A small amount of linen has been introduced into the back of the mouth.

There is no subcutaneous packing in the neck.

The abdomen has been thoroughly eviscerated through a left flank incision and granular material introduced into the cavity compressing the remains of the pelvic organs from above. It is possible to see the remains of the pelvic viscera and the usual orifices in the perineum.

Although the abdomen has been eviscerated and the diaphragm perforated, only the lungs have been removed from the thoracic cavity. The mediastinum and its contents (heart and great vessels) can be seen clearly.

Comparing these findings with those of Dynasties 22 and 25, they show a greater affinity with Dynasty 25 than 22. The support for this statement is that the excerebration route was more horizontal in Dynasty 22 and granular packing material is used more frequently in the abdomen in that dynasty. However, retention of the mediastinal structures occurs more frequently in Dynasty 22 (in fact, not at all in Dynasty 25 – in this series). With the intervening dynasties being unrepresented it is difficult to be dogmatic, but the findings may indicate a dynasty between the twenty-third and the twenty-fourth with a greater likelihood of the latter.

8.3.2 Mummy LI – Khary

The mummy of Khary in Manchester Museum was originally thought to be from Dynasty 19 and until recently the museum records reflected this. The original designation of Dynasty 19 was acquired from the coffin in which the mummy was contained on arrival at the museum (David, 1979:1). The mummy's provenance was challenged because the arm position – crossed over the chest with the left hand flexed – was thought by Raven (Raven and Taconis, 2005: 133) to be far more characteristic of the Ptolemaic Period. However, the Leiden mummy with which it was compared did not have the left hand flexed and, uncharacteristically, had the left arm superficial to the right. Furthermore, the reference used by them is that of Gray (Gray, 1972: 200-204). This is discussed on page 185.

Further confusion arises from the fact that in the series under consideration, there is one mummy – Mummy L – that is not from the Ptolemaic period. Although not in this series, the mummy described by Dr. Granville that has been discussed by several authors including Donoghue et al (Donoghue et al, 2010: 51-56) is illustrated with crossed arms with the right superficial to the left and with the fingers of the left hand flexed. This mummy is from Dynasty 26. Therefore the case for all non-royal mummies with flexed arms being from the Ptolemaic Period is far from proven.

Under these circumstances the provenance in the case of Mummy LI should be regarded as 'open'.

The manner in which other mummies have been analysed will be followed in this case.

Excerebration has been performed via a relatively small perforation in the cribriform plate (through the ethmoid) and the brain completely removed. This is despite the fact that the meninges have, in large part, been retained. A copious amount of resin has then been introduced into the cranial cavity (sufficient to run into the spinal canal in the upper cervical region). The nose has then been sealed with two linen tampons.

The eyes have been retained and the globes packed with resin-soaked linen.

Although there is a small amount of resin within the posterior part of the naso- and oro-pharynx, there has been no attempt to pack the mouth.

There is no subcutaneous packing in the neck.

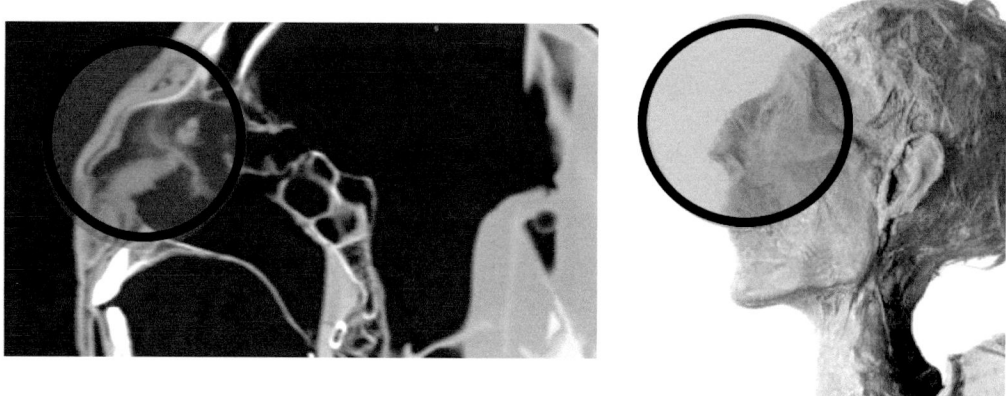

FIG. 8.2 THE NASAL PROFILE OF MUMMY LI – KHARY COMPARED WITH RAMESSES II

No attempt has been made to eviscerate the thorax, abdomen or pelvic cavity, there being no abdominal or perineal portal for evisceration. The phallus has been retained and is wrapped separately.

Although the place of origin is not known for certain it is thought likely that it originated from Western Thebes.

The arm position is of flexed arms with the right forearm superficial to the left and the fingers of the left hand flexed.

Wrappings are difficult to interpret, as the mummy was partly unwrapped prior to entering the museum collection.

All of the above facts indicate a mummy from the Ptolemaic Period rather than Dynasty 19. The only feature (apart from original provenance) to link it with Dynasty 19 is the rather unusual profile of the nose, which is reminiscent of the Ramesside period (See Fig. 8.2)

8.4 Patterns of mummification related to location

A brief analysis of the locations from which the mummies were said to originate reveals the following information as shown in Fig 8.3 and Table 8.25.

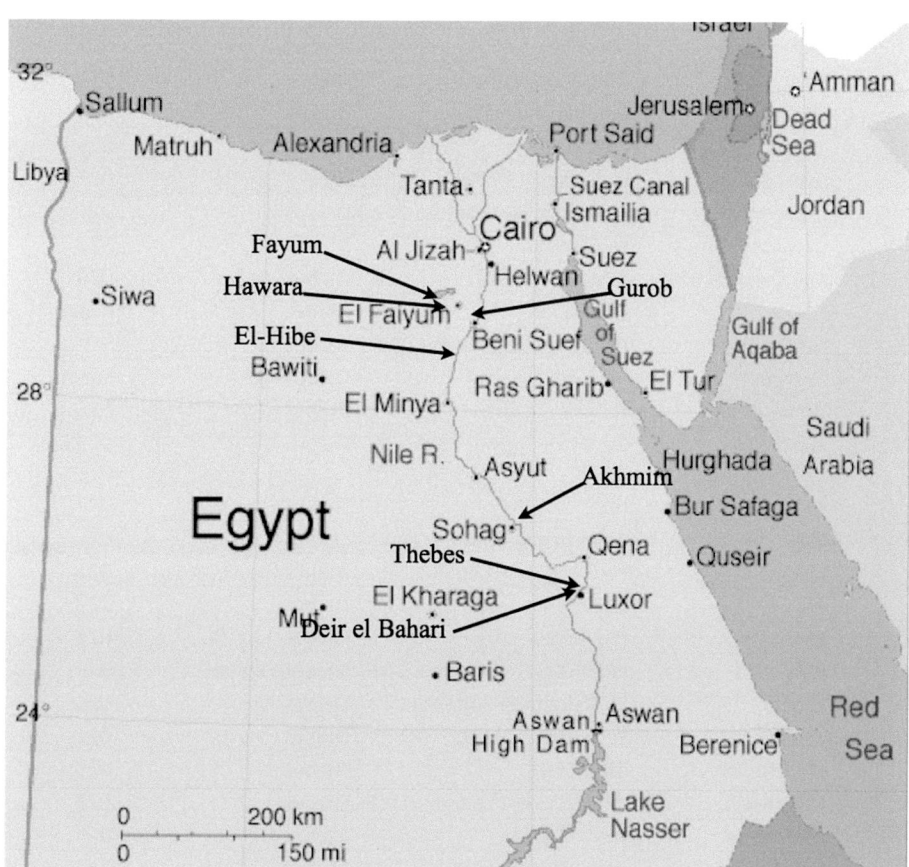

FIG. 8.3 LOCATION OF PLACES OF ORIGIN OF MUMMIES
(AFTER MAGELLAN GEOGRAPHIC)

The argument that the resilience of the provenance of stated locations may be questioned by suggesting that mummies could have been transported to Thebes (for example) to increase value in the 'tourist' market, may have some merit but the <u>evidence</u> for this is slight. Under the circumstances of more robust information being unavailable, the stated locations have been used. The distribution of mummies by location can be found in Table 3.3.

NUMBER	MUSEUM	MUMMY NAME	ORIGIN	PERIOD
XII	Manchester	MM1768	Fayum	Roman
XIII	Manchester	MM1767	Fayum	Roman
XLIII	Turin	(Tebtynis) – Suppl.19691	Fayum	Ptolemaic ??
XV	Liverpool	13.10.11.25	Hawara	Roman
XXVII	Manchester	Demetria – MM11630	Hawara	Roman
XLV	Manchester	MM1766	Hawara	Roman
XLVII	Manchester	MM1769	Hawara	Roman
LII	Manchester	MM9319 – child	?Hawara	Roman
LVI	Manchester	MM2109	Hawara	Roman
LVII	Manchester	MM1775 – Artemidorus	Hawara	Roman
LIX	BM	EA 22108 Child	Hawara	Roman
XLVIII	Manchester	MM3496	Gurob	D18
XXIV	Zurich	Basel – BSAE.1030	El-Hibe	Roman
XLII	Turin	Taaset – Suppl.9480	Assiut	Ptolemaic
X	Liverpool	Nesmin	Akhmim	Ptolemaic
XXIII	Zurich	Yverdon – Nes-Shou – MY/3775	Akhmim	Ptolemaic
XXVIII	Manchester	Ta-Sheri-Ankh – MM13783	Akhmim	Ptolemaic
XXXVI	Zurich	Bern – AE9	Akhmim	Ptolemaic
XXXVII	Zurich	Lenzburg – Sherit-Min	Akhmim	Ptolemaic
L	Perth	23/1936	Akhmim/Thebes	D26
II	Birmingham	Namenkhetamun	Thebes	D26
III	Birmingham	Padimut	Thebes	D20-21
IV	Exeter	Shepenmut	Thebes	D22
V	Sheffield	Nesitanebetasheru	Thebes	D25
VI	Sheffield	Djedma'atiuesankh	Thebes	D26
VII	Ipswich	Tahathor	Thebes	D25
VIII	Liverpool	Padiamun – 53.72a	Thebes	D22
IX	Liverpool	Padiamunnebnesuttauwy	Thebes	D25
XI	Liverpool	Padiamun – M14003	Thebes	D26
XIV	Manchester	MM1777 – Asru	Thebes	D26
XVI	Liverpool	M13997a	Thebes	Roman
XVII	Liverpool	Ankhesenaset – M 14000	Thebes	3IP
XVIII	Liverpool	M14048	Thebes	Roman
XX	Zurich	TaDjIsis – K1205	Thebes	D26
XXV	Zurich	Geneva – TjesMoutPert – D0242	Thebes	D22-25
XXIX	BM	Hor – EA6659	Thebes	D22
XXX	BM	Ankh-Unen-Nefer – EA6681	Thebes	D25
XXXI	BM	Padiamunet – EA6682	Thebes	D25
XXXIII	BM	EA22939	Thebes	D22
XXXIV	BM	EA25258	Thebes	D22
XXXV	BM	EA29577	Thebes/Faiyum	D22
XXXVIII	Zurich	St. Gallen – Shepenese	Thebes	D26
XXXIX	Zurich	St. Gallen – C3530	Thebes	D21
XLVI	Manchester	MM10881	Thebes	D26
XLIX	Manchester	MM5053.a – Perenbast	Thebes	D22
LIII	Manchester	MM1976.51a	Thebes	D25
LX	BM	EA 6704	Thebes	Roman
XXXII	BM	EA20744	Deir El Bahari	D22

NUMBER	MUSEUM	MUMMY NAME	ORIGIN	PERIOD
I	Birmingham	Graeco-Roman	Unknown	Roman
XIX	Zurich	Altdorf Child	Unknown	Roman
XXI	Zurich	Lausanne – 490	Unknown	3IP
XXII	Zurich	Bern – 00/2	Unknown	Unknown
XXVI	Zurich	Geneva – Infant	Unknown	Unknown
XL	Zurich	Lausanne – 492	Unknown	3IP
XLI	Zurich	Lenzburg – K10351	Unknown	Roman
XLIV	Turin	Provv.610	Unknown	Ptolemaic ??
LI	Manchester	MM9354a – Khary	Unknown	D19/ Ptolemaic?
LIV	Manchester	Salford 2	Unknown	3IP
LV	Manchester	MM13011	Unknown	Ptolemaic
LVIII	Manchester	MM13784	Unknown	Middle Kingdom

TABLE 8.25 MUMMIES ARRANGED BY LOCATION OF ORIGIN

Evaluating the results by location and era will follow and be observed in locations from North to South.

8.4.1 The Fayum and Hawara

The mummies from the Fayum, including those from Hawara, are seen in Table 8.26. As can be seen and as expected only Ptolemaic and Roman era mummies originated from this area. Referring to Tables 8.17 – 8.24 it can be seen that excerebration was performed via the ethmoid in the Ptolemaic mummy and in four of the ten Roman mummies. In the latter era this was followed in 50% of cases with the introduction of resin and in the other 50% by the use of no foreign material.

NUMBER	MUMMY NAME	ORIGIN	PERIOD
XLIII	(Tebtynis) – Suppl.19691	Fayum	Ptolemaic ??
XII	M1768	Fayum	Roman
XIII	M1767	Fayum	Roman
XV	13.10.11.25	Hawara	Roman
XXVII	Demetria – 11630	Hawara	Roman
XLV	M1766	Hawara	Roman
XLVII	M1769	Hawara	Roman
LII	M9319 – child	?Hawara	Roman
LVI	MM2109	Hawara	Roman
LVII	MM1775 – Artemidorus	Hawara	Roman
LIX	EA 22108 Child	Hawara	Roman

TABLE 8.26 MUMMIES FROM FAYUM AND HAWARA

In the Roman Period there seems to have been experimentation with other routes of excerebration. These included the trans-foraminal, the basal and a trans-nasal route deviating into the orbit and into the cranial cavity via the superior orbital fissure. In this group there are three cases where there has been no attempt at excerebration. These are Mummies XII, XIII and LII. In this whole series of mummies there are only six cases where there has been no attempt at excerebration. The other three are Mummies II, XXIV and LV. The provenance of Mummy II is under question as the mummy is definitely male but the coffin refers to a 'Chantress' – in other words a female. Therefore the era (Dynasty 26) may also need to be called into question. The provenance of Mummy LV is from an 'unknown' origin but it is Ptolemaic (although reference to the museum records would allow for the possibility that it is from the Roman Period) and Mummy XXIV is from El-Hibe and said to be from the Roman Period. Although Hawara and El-Hibe are eighty-five kilometers apart on modern roads there may be an indication of a common influence on their funerary practices.

8.4.2 Gurob

Since Gurob is close to Hawara and the Fayum it might be expected that there would be similar practices to those in Hawara and the Fayum. The only mummy from this location is that of a child from Dynasty 18 interred in a reed mat (Mummy XLVIII). Therefore it may well stand alone with regard to mummification technique. Unfortunately the skull has been completely disorganized due to the fact that the mummy is that of a child between one and two years of age and the individual skull bones have not yet fused together. Subsequently, the skull has completely collapsed due to pressure during mummification and the weight of the wrappings.

Evisceration has been performed via a left flank incision and the mediastinum spared to an extent from full evisceration. Remnants of the pleura remain, as do some of the viscera within the abdomen. There is damage to the spine in the cervical and upper and lower thoracic regions further disrupting the mummy. The most that can be said about this mummy is that evisceration is incomplete and performed via an abdominal incision. There is insufficient evidence to allow further comment.

8.4.3 El-Hibe

Fifty miles South-east of Fayum, this is the location of origin of Mummy XXIV. It is the mummy of a male in early middle age and said to be from the Roman Period. Excerebration has not been performed. The eyes have been retained but are not packed. The mouth may well be empty and there is no subcutaneous packing in the neck.

Evisceration has been via a perineal route and has removed the abdominal but not thoracic organs. Granular material has been introduced into the abdomen.

The unusual feature of this case is the inclusion within the wrappings of two Ibises – one over the abdomen and one between the thighs. The inclusion of an Ibis within mummy wrappings has been described before by Corcoran and Svoboda (Corcoran and Svoboda, 2010: 66-71). In this book they deal with Roman portrait mummies including the Red Shroud mummies of which Herakleides and Mummy XXIV (from Basel). The significance of the contained ibis is not resolved but the association with writing and scribes may be important.

8.4.4 Assiut

There is only one mummy from Assiut, north of Akhmim - Mummy XLII, Ta-aset, from the Ptolemaic Period. In this case complete excerebration has been performed via the ethmoid route. The eyes have been opened and packed with linen and the mouth loosely packed with linen. Complete evisceration has been performed via the perineal route without recourse to a left flank incision. There is granular material within the body cavity.

8.4.5 Akhmim

Recognised as the cult centre of Min, the ithyphallic fertility god, Akhmim was the provenance of at least five mummies in this series. A sixth mummy will be discussed in this section as the names of the parents of the mummy from Perth Museum (shown on the coffin lid) include the name Min and the currently available provenance material points to this location, although Thebes is also a possible location. The mummies to be considered are shown in Table 8.27.

NUMBER	MUMMY NAME	ORIGIN	PERIOD
X	Nesmin	Akhmim	Ptolemaic
XXIII	Yverdon – Nes-Shou – MY/3775	Akhmim	Ptolemaic
XXVIII	Sheri-Ankh – MM13783	Akhmim	Ptolemaic
XXXVI	Bern – AE9	Akhmim	Ptolemaic
XXXVII	Lenzburg – Sherit-Min	Akhmim	Ptolemaic
L	Perth 23/1936	Akhmim/Thebes	D26

TABLE 8.27 MUMMIES FROM AKHMIM

The common features of the mummies from Akhmim are the ethmoid route for excerebration (with sphenoid perforation added in one case) followed by the introduction of resin into the cranial cavity in all cases. The eyes are retained and desiccated but not packed in all cases except one where they are removed. The introduction of material into the mouth is variable with nothing in the mouth in two cases, resin used in two cases and linen in one case.

In four cases a perineal route is used for evisceration, enhanced in three cases by a left flank incision. In one

NUMBER	MUMMY NAME	ORIGIN	PERIOD
III	Padimut	Thebes	D20-21
XXXIX	St. Gallen – C3530	Thebes	D21
IV	Shepenmut	Thebes	D22
VIII	Padiamun – 53.72a	Thebes	D22
XXIX	Hor – EA6659	Thebes	D22
XXXIII	EA22939	Thebes	D22
XXXIV	EA25258	Thebes	D22
XXXV	EA29577	Thebes/Fayum	D22
XLIX	MM5053.a – Perenbast	Thebes	D22
XXV	Geneva – TjesMoutPert – D0242	Thebes	D22-25
V	Nesitanebetasheru	Thebes	D25
VII	Tahathor	Thebes	D25
IX	Padiamunnebnesuttauwy	Thebes	D25
XXX	Ankh-Unen-Nefer – EA6681	Thebes	D25
XXXI	Padiamunet – EA6682	Thebes	D25
LIII	MM1976.51a	Thebes	D25
XVII	Ankhesenaset – M 14000	Thebes	3IP
II	Namenkhetamun	Thebes	D26
VI	Djedma'atiuesankh	Thebes	D26
XI	Padiamun – M14003	Thebes	D26
XIV	MM1777 – Asru	Thebes	D26
XX	TaDjIsis – K1205	Thebes	D26
XXXVIII	St. Gallen – Shepenese	Thebes	D26
XLVI	MM10881	Thebes	D26
XVI	M13997a	Thebes	Roman
XVIII	M14048	Thebes	Roman
LX	EA 6704	Thebes	Roman

TABLE 8.28 MUMMIES FROM THEBES

case the perineal route alone is used and in one case the abdominal route alone used. In three of the cases with a perineal route the mediastinum is retained, complete evisceration taking place in the other two cases. In the four cases where an abdominal incision is used the viscera have been returned in canopic packages and resin introduced into the body cavity. In the fifth case a perineal route has been used in exclusion for evisceration and the viscera have been returned in loose form. No further packing material had been used in this case.

Unlike previous groups of mummies there is a fairly consistent picture of technique seen in Akhmim.

The concentration on the use of the perineal route for evisceration and the association of Akhmim with an ithyphallic fertility god are interesting coincident facts.

All of the above remarks exclude consideration of Mummy L. In this case an ethmoid route is used for excerebration but no resin inserted into the cranial cavity. The eyes are retained and packed with linen. The mouth is empty. Unfortunately the thorax and abdomen have been destroyed and do not reveal any detail. Under these circumstances the case for inclusion in the Akhmim group relies entirely on the coffin hieroglyphs and comparison with the group from Thebes should also be performed.

8.4.6 Thebes

There are twenty-seven mummies from Thebes

8.4.6.1 Thebes in Dynasties 21-24 – the delta capitals

Rulers from the south of Egypt conquered and took control of the country in Dynasty 25. Previously the country had been governed from cities in the Nile Delta (Tanis, Bubastis, Leontopolis and Sais). Mummies from Dynasty 21 to 24 will be considered separately from those of Dynasty 25.

Although Egypt was ruled from the cities mentioned above the following mummies were all from Thebes (see Table 8.29).

NUMBER	MUMMY NAME	ORIGIN	DYNASTY
III	Padimut	Thebes	D20-21
XXXIX	St. Gallen – C3530	Thebes	D21
IV	Shepenmut	Thebes	D22
VIII	Padiamun – 53.72a	Thebes	D22
XXIX	Hor – EA6659	Thebes	D22
XXXIII	EA22939	Thebes	D22
XXXIV	EA25258	Thebes	D22
XXXV	EA29577	Thebes/Faiyum	D22
XLIX	MM5053.a – Perenbast	Thebes	D22

TABLE 8.29 THEBAN MUMMIES FROM DYNASTY 20 TO 24

The characteristics of the mummies will be analysed as previously by exploring the techniques used in the head and then in the body.

8.4.6.1.1 Treatment of the Head and Neck

It can be seen in Table 8.30 that there are no results for Mummy IV. This is because this mummy was only X-rayed and the images provide very little information. The remainder of the cohort has been excerebrated, some with subsequent packing of linen, resin or granular material and some (37.5%) without any packing. In only six cases was it possible to assess the eyes. In all these cases the eyes had been retained and in five of the six cases the globes were opened and packed. Four cases had the addition of plates in front of the globes. In all cases where assessment was possible the mouth was packed and subcutaneous packing used in the neck.

8.4.6.1.2 Treatment of the Trunk

It can be seen from Table 8.31 that in the seven cases where analysis could be made all had a left flank incision (one with the addition of a perineal approach) and complete evisceration was performed in four of the seven cases. In the remaining three cases two had incomplete evisceration with retention of the mediastinum and the other one had incomplete evisceration without retention of the mediastinum. In all these cases the viscera were returned to the body. The viscera were loose in five cases and in canopic packages in the other two.

Mummy	Exc. Route	Cranial Packing	Eyes	Mouth	Neck
III	E	-----	Des+Pl	RGr	L
XXXIX	FM	-----	Dis	Dis	Dis
IV					
VIII	E+Sp	Res	L+Gr	L+Res	L
XXIX	E+FM	Gr	Rem+L/Res+Pl	Gr(Sm)	L+Gr
XXXIII	E	L	Des+Res+Pl	Gr	Gr
XXXIV	E+Sp	----	L+Pl	Res+Gr	Gr
XXXV	E+Sp	Gr	Dis	Dis	Dis
XLIX	Sp	L	L	Gr	Gr

E=Ethmoid Sp=Sphenoid FM=Foramen Magnum Res=Resin
Gr=Granular material L=Linen Rem=Removal Pl=Plates Des=Desiccated Dis=Disrupted

TABLE 8.30 MUMMIFICATION TECHNIQUES USED IN THE HEAD IN DYNASTY 20 TO 24

Mummy	Evisceration Route	Complete Evisceration?	Returned Viscera	Packing Material
III	L. Flank	Med. Ret.	Loose	Res+Gr
XXXIX	L. Flank+Per	Incomplete	Loose	Gr
IV				
VIII	L. Flank	Complete	Loose	Res+Gr
XXIX	L. Flank	Complete	Loose	Res+Gr+L
XXXIII	L. Flank	Complete	CP	L+Gr
XXXIV	L. Flank	Complete	Loose	Gr
XXXV	Disrupted	Disrupted	Disrupted	Gr
XLIX	L. Flank	Med. Ret.	CP	Gr

RES=RESIN GR=GRANULAR MATERIAL L=LINEN CP=CANOPIC PACKAGES PER.=PERINEAL MED. RET.=MEDIASTINUM RETAINED

TABLE 8.31 MUMMIFICATION TECHNIQUES USED IN THE TRUNK IN DYNASTY 20 TO 24

NUMBER	MUMMY NAME	ORIGIN	PERIOD
XXV	Geneva – TjesMoutPert – D0242	Thebes	D22-25
V	Nesitanebetasheru	Thebes	D25
VII	Tahathor	Thebes	D25
IX	Padiamunnebnesuttauwy	Thebes	D25
XXX	Ankh-Unen-Nefer – EA6681	Thebes	D25
XXXI	Padiamunet – EA6682	Thebes	D25
LIII	MM1976.51a	Thebes	D25

TABLE 8.32 THEBAN MUMMIES FROM DYNASTY 25

Mummy	Exc. Route	Cranial Packing	Eyes	Mouth	Neck
XXV	E	Res	Res+L	L	-----
V	E+Sp	Res	L+Pl	L	-----
VII	FM	Gr	REM+L	L	-----
IX	E	Res+Gr	Res	-----	-----
XXX	E	------	L+Pl	-----	-----
XXXI	E	------	Des	L	-----
LIII	E	Res	Des	L	-----

E=ETHMOID SP=SPHENOID FM=FORAMEN MAGNUM RES=RESIN
GR=GRANULAR MATERIAL L=LINEN PL=PLATES DES=DESICCATED REM=REMOVED

TABLE 8.33 MUMMIFICATION TECHNIQUES USED IN THE HEAD IN DYNASTY 25

Mummy	Evisceration Route	Complete Evisceration?	Returned Viscera	Packing Material
XXV	L. Flank	Med. Ret.	Loose	Gr
V	L. Flank	Incomplete	Loose+CP	Res
VII	L. Flank	Incomplete	Loose	Gr
IX	L. Flank	Incomplete	Loose	Gr
XXX	L. Flank	Complete	CP	Res+Gr
XXXI	L. Flank	Incomplete	Loose	Gr
LIII	L. Flank+Per.	Complete	CP	Res+L

RES=RESIN GR=GRANULAR MATERIAL L=LINEN
CP=CANOPIC PACKAGES PER.=PERINEAL

TABLE 8.34 MUMMIFICATION TECHNIQUES USED IN THE TRUNK IN DYNASTY 25

In all cases foreign material was introduced into the body cavity after evisceration. Some granular material was used in all cases with the addition of resin in three cases and linen in two cases.

8.4.6.2 Thebes in Dynasty 25 – Kushite rule

With the conquest of Egypt by Piankhy from Napata, the kingdom was reunited and a southern influence imposed on the land. Although the capital was now situated further south at Napata, the cult of Amun, having been previously adopted by the Kushites, flourished in both lands and was especially prominent in Thebes (Shaw, 2000: 354).

The mummies in this series from Dynasty 25 Thebes are shown in Table 8.32.

These include Mummy XXV that has been discussed earlier (P 208), as it is closer to Dynasty 25 than 22.

Mummy	Exc. Route	Cranial Packing	Eyes	Mouth	Neck
XVII	E	L	L+Pl	Gr	L+Gr

TABLE 8.35 MUMMIFICATION TECHNIQUES USED IN THE HEAD OF MUMMY XVII

Mummy	Evisceration Route	Complete Evisceration?	Returned Viscera	Packing Material
XVII	L. Flank	Complete	CP	Gr

TABLE 8.36 MUMMIFICATION TECHNIQUES USED IN THE TRUNK OF MUMMY XVII

The first point to stand out here is that all cases have been excerebrated via the ethmoid, with the exception of one via the foramen magnum. Five of the seven have had foreign material introduced into the skull following excerebration. In this respect it is interesting to note that of five cases of trans-foraminal excerebration three are from Thebes in Dynasties 21, 22 and 25. The fourth is from an unknown origin and the fifth from Hawara (in the Roman era).

Six of the seven cases have had the eyes preserved with the addition of packing in the globes in four cases with the addition of eye plates in two of them. The seventh case has had the eyes removed but linen has been subsequently inserted into the orbits.

All cases have had evisceration performed via a left flank incision (enhanced with a perineal approach in the case of Mummy LIII) and some form of foreign material inserted afterwards. Evisceration has been incomplete in five of the seven cases with return of the viscera in all cases – sometimes as loose viscera and sometimes in the form of canopic packages.

Mummy XVII has not been included in Table 8.32 as it is assigned only to 'the Third Intermediate Period'.

However, as mentioned on page 203, the characteristics of this mummy are closer to those of Dynasty 22 than to other dynasties (See Tables 8.35 and 8.36).

8.4.6.3 Thebes in Dynasty 26

Egypt was conquered by Assyria in Dynasty 26 but then became independent for a period prior to the arrival of the Persian influence in Dynasty 27. There are seven mummies from Dynasty 26 Thebes. These are shown in Table 8.37.

As can be seen from Tables 8.38 and 8.39, Mummies XX and XLVI have disruption of the head and trunk making analysis difficult. The only exception to this statement is that it is possible to determine that excerebration has been via the sphenoid with the subsequent introduction of resin in the case of Mummy XLVI.

Excerebration has been performed in five of the six cases available for scrutiny, three via the ethmoid, one via the sphenoid and one via the orbit. Resin has been introduced into the cranial cavity of those excerebrated via the sphenoid and trans-orbital routes.

NUMBER	MUMMY NAME	ORIGIN	PERIOD
II	Namenkhetamun	Thebes	D26
VI	Djedma'atiuesankh	Thebes	D26
XI	Padiamun – M14003	Thebes	D26
XIV	MM1777 – Asru	Thebes	D26
XX	TaDjIsis – K1205	Thebes	D26
XXXVIII	St. Gallen – Shepenese	Thebes	D26
XLVI	MM10881	Thebes	D26

TABLE 8.37 THEBAN MUMMIES FROM DYNASTY 26

Mummy	Exc. Route	Cranial Packing	Eyes	Mouth	Neck
II	None	-----	L	L	-----
VI	E	-----	L	?	?
XI	E	-----	L+Pl	L	-----
XIV	TO	Res	Des	Gr	-----
XX					
XXXVIII	E	-----	L	Res	-----
XLVI	Sp	Res	-----		

E=ETHMOID SP=SPHENOID TO=TRANS-ORBITAL RES=RESIN GR=GRANULAR MATERIAL L=LINEN PL=PLATES DES=DESICCATED
SHADING = DISRUPTED

TABLE 8.38 MUMMIFICATION TECHNIQUES USED IN THE HEAD IN THEBAN DYNASTY 26

Mummy	Evisceration Route	Complete Evisceration?	Returned Viscera	Packing Material
II	L. Flank	Med. Ret.	Loose	Gr
VI	L. Flank	Med. Ret.	-----	Res
XI	L. Flank	Sup.Med. Ret.	CP	Gr
XIV	L. Flank	Med. Ret.	Loose	-----
XX				
XXXVIII	L. Flank+Peri.	Med. Ret.	CP	Gr
XLVI				

Res=Resin Gr=Granular material L=Linen
CP=Canopic Packages Per.=Perineal Shading = Disrupted

Table 8.39 Mummification techniques used in the trunk in Theban Dynasty 26

It is interesting to note that the eyes have been retained in five of the six available for study. In Mummy VI the analogue CT images do not allow assessment of the mouth, but in the remaining four, packing has been used, varying from linen to resin or granular material.

In the body a left flank incision can be seen in all cases available for assessment. This is combined with only partial evisceration, the whole or part of the mediastinum being retained in all these cases.

The viscera have been returned to the body cavity, either as loose viscera or canopic packages, in all cases (the images of Mummy VI are inadequate to allow an assessment). The use of packing material is also widely seen.

8.4.6.4 Thebes in the Roman Period

There are only three mummies from Thebes relating to this period. These are shown in Table 8.40 and analysed in Tables 8.41 and 8.42.

Reference to Tables 8.41 and 8.42 shows that in all three cases excerebration was performed via the ethmoid and that resin was then introduced into the cranial cavity. The eyes were retained and packed in two of the three cases. The mouth was also packed in the same two cases.

A left flank incision enhanced by a perineal approach was used in all cases with complete evisceration and return of the viscera in canopic packages. Resin was also introduced into the body cavity in all cases.

Whilst the numbers are small a consistent picture emerges.

8.4.7 Deir El Bahari

There is only one mummy from this particular site. Mummy XXXII is from the British Museum and from Dynasty 22. The age of the female is in dispute since the dental evidence suggests an age of about nine years while the bone age indicates sixteen or seventeen years. The causes of such a disparity are both rare and difficult to detect except in cases of pituitary tumours (where the pituitary fossa would be expanded). Most conditions that cause accelerated bone age also accelerate dental development. If the causes of delayed dental eruption are considered, then most of those that cause abnormalities of skeletal morphology can be eliminated if their signs are not present. The subject of delayed tooth eruption

NUMBER	MUMMY NAME	ORIGIN	PERIOD
XVI	M13997a	Thebes	Roman
XVIII	M14048	Thebes	Roman
LX	EA 6704	Thebes	Roman

Table 8.40 Theban mummies from the Roman Period

Mummy	Exc. Route	Cranial Packing	Eyes	Mouth	Neck
XVI	E	Res	L	Res	-----
XVIII	E	Res	Des	-----	-----
LX	E	Res	Res/L	L+Res+Gr	-----

E=Ethmoid Res=Resin Gr=Granular material L=Linen Des=Desiccated

Table 8.41 Mummification techniques used in the head in Roman Period Thebes

Mummy	Evisceration Route	Complete Evisceration?	Returned Viscera	Packing Material
XVI	L. Flank+Per	Complete	CP	Res
XVIII	L. Flank+Per	Complete	CP	Res
LX	L. Flank+Per.	Complete	CP	Res

Res=Resin CP=Canopic Packages

Table 8.42 Mummification techniques used in the trunk in Roman Period Thebes

Mummy	Exc. Route	Cranial Packing	Eyes	Mouth	Neck
XXXII	Bas	-----	Des	L+Gr	-----

BAS=BASAL GR=GRANULAR MATERIAL L=LINEN DES=DESICCATED

TABLE 8.43 MUMMIFICATION TECHNIQUES USED IN THE HEAD

Mummy	Evisceration Route	Complete Evisceration?	Returned Viscera	Packing Material
XXXII	L. Flank	Med. Ret.	Loose+CP	Gr

MED=MEDIASTINUM RETAINED CP=CANOPIC PACKAGES GR=GRANULAR MATERIAL

TABLE 8.44 MUMMIFICATION TECHNIQUES USED IN THE TRUNK

is well documented by Peedikayil (Peedikayil, 2011: 81-86). Advanced bone age is usually linked with increased hormone production.

From the Egyptological point of view the mummification techniques used are summarized in Tables 8.43 and 8.44.

It can be seen that the excerebration route is novel in that it is through the base of the skull. Excerebration has been complete without any material added subsequently. The eyes have been retained and desiccated and the mouth filled with layers of linen and radio dense material that may be a mixture of resin and some other material such as sawdust. The neck is not packed.

Partial evisceration has been performed via a left flank incision with the return of the viscera in canopic packages plus granular material. In this case the mediastinum has been retained with clear evidence of the heart, lungs, great vessels and pleura.

The common features of mummification with those in Thebes in Dynasty 22 are the novel route for excerbration, retention of the eyes, packing of the mouth and the use of a left flank incision with return of the viscera in both loose form and in canopic packages along with packing of the abdomen with foreign material.

8.5 Techniques related to age at death

If comparison is made of the mummification techniques used in adults and children (below the age of eighteen) the whole series can be shown in Table 8.45. In this table mummies are excluded if the age is not known (where the images provide too little information), they are disrupted or if it is a false mummy.

The children are shown in Table 8.46 arranged by age and in Table 8.47 arranged by era.

NUMBER	AGE	MUMMY NAME	ORIGIN	PERIOD
XLVIII	C – 1-2	MM3496	Gurob	D18
LII	C – 2	MM9319 – child	?Hawara	Roman
LV	C – 2-3	MM13011	Unknown	Ptolemaic
LVI	C – 2-3	MM2109	Hawara	Roman
LIX	C – 2-3	EA 22108 Child	Hawara	Roman
XIX	C – 3-4	Altdorf Child	Unknown	Roman
XV	C – 5	13.10.11.25	Hawara	Roman
XLI	C – 3-6 ?	Lenzburg – K10351	Unknown	Roman
XXVI	C – 6	Geneva – Infant	Unknown	Unknown
XLVII	C – 6	MM1769	Hawara	Roman
VI	C – 13-16	Djedma'atiuesankh	Thebes	D26
XXXII	C – 15-19	EA20744	Deir El Bahari	D22
LVIII	C – 16-17	MM13784	Unknown	Middle Kingdom
I	YA	Graeco-Roman	Unknown	Roman
VII	YA	Tahathor	Thebes	D25
VIII	YA	Padiamun – 53.72a	Thebes	D22
XII	YA	MM1768	Fayum	Roman
XVI	YA	M13997a	Thebes	Roman
XVIII	YA	M14048	Thebes	Roman
XXVII	YA	Demetria – 11630	Hawara	Roman
XXVIII	YA	Ta-Sheri-Ankh – MM13783	Akhmim	D21
XXXV	?YA	EA29577	Thebes/ Fayum	D22

NUMBER	AGE	MUMMY NAME	ORIGIN	PERIOD
XXXVI	YA	Bern – AE9	Akhmim	Ptolemaic
XLIII	YA	(Tebtynis) – Suppl.19691	Fayum	Ptolemaic ??
XLIV	YA	Provv.610	Unknown	Ptolemaic ??
XLV	YA	MM1766	Hawara	Roman
LIV	YA	Salford 2	Unknown	3IP
II	MA	Namenkhetamun	Thebes	D26
III	MA	Padimut	Thebes	D20-21
IX	MA	Padiamunnebnesuttauwy	Thebes	D25
X	MA	Nesmin	Akhmim	Ptolemaic
XIII	MA	MM1767	Fayum	Roman
XIV	MA	MM1777 – Asru	Thebes	D26
XVII	MA	Ankhesenaset – M 14000	Thebes	3IP
XXII	MA	Bern – 00/2	Unknown	Unknown
XXIV	MA	Basel – BSAE.1030	El-Hibe	Roman
XI	E	Padiamun – M14003	Thebes	D26
XXIII	E	Yverdon – Nes-Shou – MY/3775	Akhmim	Ptolemaic
XXV	E	Geneva – TjesMoutPert – D0242	Thebes	D22-25
XXIX	MA	Hor – EA6659	Thebes	D22
XXX	MA	Ankh-Unen-Nefer – EA6681	Thebes	D25
XXXI	MA	Padiamunet – EA6682	Thebes	D25
XXXIII	MA	EA22939	Thebes	D22
XXXIV	MA	EA25258	Thebes	D22
XXXVII	MA	Lenzburg – Sherit-Min	Akhmim	Ptolemaic
XXXVIII	MA	St. Gallen – Shepenese	Thebes	D26
XXXIX	MA	St. Gallen – C3530	Thebes	D21
XL	MA	Lausanne – 492	Unknown	3IP
LI	MA	MM9354a – Khary	?Thebes	D19/ Ptolemaic?
LIII	MA	MM1976.51a	Thebes	D25
LVII	MA	MM1775 – Artemidorus	Hawara	Roman
LX	MA	EA 6704	Thebes	Roman
XI	E	Padiamun – M14003	Thebes	D26
XXIII	E	Yverdon – Nes-Shou – MY/3775	Akhmim	Ptolemaic
XXV	E	Geneva – TjesMoutPert – D0242	Thebes	D22-25
XLII	E	Taaset – Suppl.9480	Fayum	Ptolemaic
XLIX	E	MM5053.a – Perenbast	Thebes	D22
L	E	23/1936	Akhmim/ Thebes	D26

TABLE 8.45 MUMMIES SORTED BY AGE AT DEATH

NUMBER	AGE	MUMMY NAME	ORIGIN	PERIOD
XLVIII	C – 1-2	MM3496	Gurob	D18
LII	C – 2	MM9319 – child	?Hawara	Roman
LV	C – 2-3	MM13011	Unknown	Ptolemaic
LVI	C – 2-3	MM2109	Hawara	Roman
LIX	C – 2-3	EA 22108 Child	Hawara	Roman
XIX	C – 3-4	Altdorf Child	Unknown	Roman
XV	C – 5	13.10.11.25	Hawara	Roman
XLI	C – 3-6 ?	Lenzburg – K10351	Unknown	Roman
XXVI	C – 6	Geneva – Infant	Unknown	Unknown
XLVII	C – 6	M1769	Hawara	Roman
VI	C – 13-16	Djedma'atiuesankh	Thebes	D26
XXXII	C – 15-19	EA20744	Deir El Bahari	D22
LVIII	C – 16-17	MM13784	Unknown	Middle Kingdom

TABLE 8.46 CHILDREN IN ORDER OF AGE

NUMBER	AGE	MUMMY NAME	ORIGIN	PERIOD
LVIII	C – 16-17	MM13784	Unknown	Middle Kingdom
XLVIII	C – 1-2	MM3496	Gurob	D18
XXXII	C – 15-19	EA20744	Deir El Bahari	D22
VI	C – 13-16	Djedma'atiuesankh	Thebes	D26
LV	C – 2-3	MM13011	Unknown	Ptolemaic
LII	C – 2	M9319 – child	?Hawara	Roman
LVI	C – 2-3	MM2109	Hawara	Roman
LIX	C – 2-3	EA 22108 Child	Hawara	Roman
XIX	C – 3-4	Altdorf Child	Unknown	Roman
XV	C – 5	13.10.11.25	Hawara	Roman
XLI	C – 3-6 ?	Lenzburg – K10351	Unknown	Roman
XLVII	C – 6	M1769	Hawara	Roman
XXVI	C – 6	Geneva – Infant	Unknown	Unknown

TABLE 8.47 CHILDREN IN ORDER OF ERA

Mummy	Exc. Route	Cranial Packing	Eyes	Mouth	Neck
XLVIII					
LII	None	None	Des	-----	-----
LV	None	None	Des	-----	-----
LVI	E	None	Des	-----	-----
LIX	Basal	Res	Des	-----	-----
XIX	E	None	L	-----	-----
XV	FM	Gr	Des	Plate	-----
XLI	E	None	Des	Res	-----
XXVI	E	None	Des	-----	-----
XLVII	TN+TO	Res	Des	L	-----
VI	E	None	L	?	?
XXXII	Bas	None	Des	L+Gr	-----
LVIII	TF	Res	Des	-----	-----

TABLE 8.48 TREATMENT OF THE HEAD IN CHILDREN IN ORDER OF AGE.
WHITE = 1-4 YRS. MEDIUM GREY = 5-6 YRS. DARK GREY = TEENAGE PALE GREY = DISORGANIZED.

Little can be learned from Mummy XLVIII as the head has been crushed and there is no discernable detail. Of the other mummies it can be said that there appears to be a disproportionate number of novel methods of excerebration used in the total group. The eyes have been retained in all cases. The numbers are too small to allow a firm conclusion, but there does not appear to be any significant difference between the way the head is treated in the groups of young children (1-4 years), the five and six year olds and the teenagers.

Analysis of the treatment of the head in children grouped into era adds nothing in terms of identifying a pattern.

A similar assessment of the abdomen reveals information as shown in Tables 8.50 and 8.51.

Mummy	Exc. Route	Cranial Packing	Eyes	Mouth	Neck
LVIII	TF	Res	Des	-----	-----
XLVIII	I	Dis	Dis	Dis	Dis
XXXII	Bas	None	Des	L+Gr	-----
VI	E	None	L	?	?
LV	None	None	Des	-----	-----
LII	None	None	Des	-----	-----
LVI	E	None	Des	-----	-----
LIX	Basal	Res	Des	-----	-----
XIX	E	None	L	-----	-----
XV	FM	Gr	Des	Plate	-----
XLI	E	None	Des	Res	-----
XLVII	TN+TO	Res	Des	L	-----
XXVI	E	None	Des	-----	-----

TABLE 8.49 TREATMENT OF THE HEAD IN CHILDREN GROUPED BY ERA. MEDIUM GREY=PTOLEMAIC; DARK GREY=ROMAN

Mummy	Evisceration Route	Complete Evisceration?	Returned Viscera	Packing Material
XLVIII	Disruption	Disruption	Disruption	Disruption
LII	None	None	-----	-----
LV	None	None	-----	-----
LVI	None	None	-----	-----
LIX	None	None	-----	-----
XIX	L. Flank	Complete	CP	L
XV	None	None	-----	-----
XLI	L. Flank	Complete	-----	L
XXVI	L. Flank	Med. Ret.	CP	Res
XLVII	None	None	-----	-----
VI	L. Flank	Med. Ret.	-----	Res
XXXII	L. Flank	Med. Ret.	Loose+CP	Gr
LVIII	L. Flank	Disruption	Disruption	-----

TABLE 8.50 TREATMENT OF THE TRUNK IN CHILDREN IN ORDER OF AGE.
WHITE = 1-4 YRS. MEDIUM GREY = 5-6 YRS. DARK GREY = TEENAGE

Mummy	Evisceration Route	Complete Evisceration?	Returned Viscera	Packing Material
LVIII	L. Flank	Disruption	Disruption	-----
XLVIII	Disruption	Disruption	Disruption	Disruption
XXXII	L. Flank	Med. Ret.	Loose+CP	Gr
VI	L. Flank	Med. Ret.	-----	Res
LV	None	None	-----	-----
LII	None	None	-----	-----
LVI	None	None	-----	-----
LIX	None	None	-----	-----
XIX	L. Flank	Complete	CP	L
XV	None	None	-----	-----
XLI	L. Flank	Complete	-----	L
XLVII	None	None	-----	-----
XXVI	L. Flank	Med. Ret.	CP	Res

TABLE 8.51 TREATMENT OF THE TRUNK IN CHILDREN GROUPED BY ERA.
MEDIUM GREY=PTOLEMAIC; DARK GREY=ROMAN

Of the twelve mummies available for analysis, six have been eviscerated via an abdominal incision and six left without evisceration. Canopic packages have been used in only three cases. Of those without evisceration all are at or below the age of six years. The three cases below the age of six that have undergone evisceration have had the viscera returned in canopic packages in two cases and not returned in the other case.

The one to four year olds have a higher rate of non-evisceration. However, the numbers are small and observations have to be viewed with caution.

If a similar approach is taken to the adult population in this series they can then be compared with the child population. To ensure that adults are all 'processed' in a similar manner during the evaluation process, they will initially be considered in groups – namely Young Adults, Middle Aged and Elderly, as defined in section 7.1. The lists of mummies in each age group are shown in Tables 8.52, 8.53 and 8.54. These groups will then be compared to show any similarities. The comparison relating to treatment of the head can be seen by referring to Tables 8.55, 8.56 and 8.57. From these tables it can be seen that the large majority of mummies were excerebrated via the ethmoid in all groups but the frequency of novel routes (trans-foraminal, basal and trans-orbital) was greater in the Middle Aged group. Some degree of cranial packing with resin in particular was used in 57% of the young adults, 36% in the middle-aged group and 50% in the elderly. Treatment of the eyes by packing the globe was seen in 21% of the young adults, 50% of the middle aged and 83% in the elderly. The mouth was packed in 57% of young adults, 64% of the middle-aged group and 83% of the elderly.

A fuller discussion of the treatment of eyes can be seen below (P 228).

Using the crude percentages that can be derived from Table 8.49 (children) it can be seen that the trans-nasal route was used in only 50% of cases of children. Cranial packing was used in 8% of cases and packing of the globe of the eye was performed in 16%. Introducing material into the oral cavity was seen in 33%.

With the caveat that the numbers in each group are small and, therefore caution needs to be applied, it can be deduced that the use of novel routes for excerebration is more prevalent in children and that cranial packing is much less frequently used in children. Packing of retained eyes is less frequently used in children (16% as opposed to an increasing use of packing as the age increases – from 21% to 83%). The introduction of material into the mouth (including a metal plate in one case) was seen in 33% of children as opposed to 57%, 64% and 83% respectively in the adult groups.

A review of treatment of the trunk in adults is presented in Tables 8.58, 8.59 and 8.60.

NUMBER	MUMMY NAME	ORIGIN	PERIOD
XXVIII	Ta-Sheri-Ankh – MM13783	Akhmim	D21
VIII	Padiamun – 53.72a	Thebes	D22
XXXV	EA29577	Thebes/Fayum	D22
VII	Tahathor	Thebes	D25
LIV	Salford 2	Unknown	3IP
XXXVI	Bern – AE9	Akhmim	Ptolemaic
XLIII	(Tebtynis) – Suppl.19691	Faiyum	Ptolemaic ??
XLIV	Provv.610	Unknown	Ptolemaic ??
I	Graeco-Roman	Unknown	Roman
XII	MM1768	Fayum	Roman
XVI	M13997a	Thebes	Roman
XVIII	M14048	Thebes	Roman
XXVII	Demetria – MM11630	Hawara	Roman
XLV	MM1766	Hawara	Roman

TABLE 8.52 Mummies within the Young Adult group – aged 18 to 29 years.

NUMBER	MUMMY NAME	ORIGIN	PERIOD
III	Padimut	Thebes	D20-21
XXXIX	St. Gallen – C3530	Thebes	D21
XXIX	Hor – EA6659	Thebes	D22
XXXIII	EA22939	Thebes	D22
XXXIV	EA25258	Thebes	D22
IX	Padiamunnebnesuttauwy	Thebes	D25
XXX	Ankh-Unen-Nefer – EA6681	Thebes	D25
XXXI	Padiamunet – EA6682	Thebes	D25
LIII	MM1976.51a	Thebes	D25
XVII	Ankhesenaset – M 14000	Thebes	3IP
XL	Lausanne – 492	Unknown	3IP
II	Namenkhetamun	Thebes	D26
XIV	MM1777 – Asru	Thebes	D26
XXXVIII	St. Gallen – Shepenese	Thebes	D26
X	Nesmin	Akhmim	Ptolemaic
XXXVII	Lenzburg – Sherit-Min	Akhmim	Ptolemaic
LI	MM9354a – Khary	?Thebes	D19/ Ptolemaic?
XIII	MM1767	Faiyum	Roman
XXIV	Basel – BSAE.1030	El-Hibe	Roman
LVII	MM1775 – Artemidorus	Hawara	Roman
LX	EA 6704	Thebes	Roman
XXII	Bern – 00/2	Unknown	Unknown

TABLE 8.53 Mummies within the Middle Age group – 30 to 60 years

NUMBER	MUMMY NAME	ORIGIN	PERIOD
XLIX	M5053.a – Perenbast	Thebes	D22
XXV	Geneva – TjesMoutPert – D0242	Thebes	D22-25
XI	Padiamun – M14003	Thebes	D26
L	23/1936	Akhmim/Thebes	D26
XXIII	Yverdon – Nes-Shou – MY/3775	Akhmim	Ptolemaic
XLII	Taaset – Suppl.9480	Fayum	Ptolemaic

TABLE 8.54 Mummies within the Elderly group - 60 years plus.

Mummy	Exc. Route	Cranial Packing	Eyes	Mouth	Neck
XXVIII	E	Res	Des	-----	-----
VIII	E+Sp	Res	L+Gr	L+Res	L
XXXV	E+Sp	Gr	Dis	Dis	Dis
VII	FM	Gr	REM+L	L	-----
LIV	E	Res	Des	-----	-----
XXXVI	E	Res	Des	L	-----
XLIII	E	-----	Des	L	-----
XLIV	E	-----	Des	-----	-----
I	E	-----	Des	-----	-----
XII	None	None	Des	Res	-----
XVI	E	Res	L	Res	-----
XVIII	E	Res	Des	-----	-----
XXVII	E	Res	Des	L	-----
XLV	E	Res	Des	L	-----

TABLE 8.55 TREATMENT OF THE HEAD IN YOUNG ADULTS.

Mummy	Exc. Route	Cranial Packing	Eyes	Mouth	Neck
III	E	-----	Des+Pl	RGr	L
XXXIX	FM	-----	Dis	Dis	Dis
XXIX	E+FM	Gr	Rem+L/ Res+Pl	Gr(Sm)	L+Gr
XXXIII	E	L	Des+Res+Pl	Gr	Gr
XXXIV	E+Sp	----	L+Pl	Res+Gr	Gr
IX	E	Res+Gr	Res	-----	-----
XXX	E	------	L+Pl	-----	-----
XXXI	E	------	Des	L	-----
LIII	E	Res	Des	L	-----
XVII	E	L	L+Pl	Gr	L+Gr
XL	E+Sp	Res	Des	-----	-----
II	None	-----	L	L	-----
XIV	TO	Res	Des	Gr	-----
XXXVIII	E	-----	L	Res	-----
X	E+Sp	Res	Des	Res	-----
XXXVII	E	Res	Des	-----	-----
LI	E	Res	Des+L+Res	-----	-----
XIII	None	None	REM	Res	Disrupt
XXIV	None	None	Des	-----	-----
LVII	E	-----	Des	-----	-----
LX	E	Res	Res/L	L+Res+Gr	E
XXII	E+Sp	-----	Des	L	-----

TABLE 8.56 TREATMENT OF THE HEAD IN MIDDLE AGE.

Mummy	Exc. Route	Cranial Packing	Eyes	Mouth	Neck
XLIX	Sp	L	L	Gr	Gr
XXV	E	Res	L+Res	L	-----
XI	E	-----	L+Pl	L	-----
L	E	-----	L	-----	-----
XXIII	E	Res	REM	Res	-----
XLII	E	Res	L	L+Res	-----

TABLE 8.57 TREATMENT OF THE HEAD IN THE ELDERLY

Mummy	Evisceration Route	Complete Evisceration?	Returned Viscera	Packing Material
XXVIII	L. Flank	Complete	CP	Res
VIII	L. Flank	Complete	Loose	Res+Gr
XXXV	Disrupted	Disrupted	Disrupted	Gr
VII	L. Flank	Incomplete	Loose	Gr
LIV	None	None	-----	-----
XXXVI	L. Flank+Per	Med. Ret.	CP	Res
XLIII	L. Flank	Complete	CP	-----
XLIV	L. Flank	Med. Ret.	CP	Res
I	L. Flank	Complete	Loose+CP	Gr
XII	Disrupted	Incomplete	Disrupted	Disrupted
XVI	L. Flank+Per	Complete	CP	Res
XVIII	L. Flank+Per	Complete	CP	Res
XXVII	?	Incomplete	------	-----
XLV	Per	Incomplete	-----	-----

TABLE 8.58 TREATMENT OF THE TRUNK IN YOUNG ADULTS.

Mummy	Evisceration Route	Complete Evisceration?	Returned Viscera	Packing Material
III	L. Flank	Med. Ret.	Loose	Res+Gr
XXXIX	L. Flank+Per	Incomplete	Loose	Gr
XXIX	L. Flank	Complete	Loose	Res+Gr+L
XXXIII	L. Flank	Complete	CP	L+Gr
XXXIV	L. Flank	Complete	Loose	Gr
IX	L. Flank	Incomplete	Loose	Gr
XXX	L. Flank	Complete	CP	Res+Gr
XXXI	L. Flank	Incomplete	Loose	Gr
LIII	L. Flank+Per.	Complete	CP	Res+L
XVII	L. Flank	Complete	CP	Gr
XL	Supra-pubic	Incomplete	Loose	-----
II	L. Flank	Med. Ret.	Loose	Gr
XIV	L. Flank	Med. Ret.	Loose	-----
XXXVIII	L. Flank+Per.	Med. Ret.	CP	Gr
X	L. Flank+Per	Med. Ret.	CP	Res
XXXVII	Per	Med. Ret.	Loose	-----
LI	None	None	-----	-----
XIII	None	None	-----	-----
XXIV	Per	Incomplete	-----	Gr
LVII	None	None	-----	-----
LX	L. Flank+Per.	Complete	CP	Res
XXII	L. Flank+Per	Med. Ret.	Loose+CP	Res

TABLE 8.59 TREATMENT OF THE TRUNK IN MIDDLE AGE.

Mummy	Evisceration Route	Complete Evisceration?	Returned Viscera	Packing Material
XLIX	L. Flank	Med. Ret.	CP	Gr
XXV	L. Flank	Med. Ret.	Loose	Gr
XI	L. Flank	Sup.Med. Ret.	CP	Gr
L	Disrupted	rupted	Disrupted	rupted
XXIII	L. Flank+Per	Complete	CP	Res
XLII	Per	Incomplete	-----	Gr

TABLE 8.60 TREATMENT OF THE TRUNK IN THE ELDERLY.

Comparing the treatment of the trunk in the three groups of adults shows that if the two disorganized mummies in the young adult group are discounted there are twelve in this group, twenty-two in the middle age group and five in the elderly group. Of these a left flank incision was used in 75 to 80% of all three groups. A perineal approach was used in 30% to 40% of all groups with a slight bias towards the elderly. The mediastinum was retained in increasing frequency with age, occurring in 60% of the elderly. Conversely complete evisceration was performed with decreasing frequency as age advanced. Canopic package use changed from 60% in the young adult to 35% in middle age and back to 60% in the elderly. Resin was used to pack the trunk cavity in 50% of cases in the young adult group, 32% in middle age and 20% in the elderly, with granular material used in 25% in the young adult, 55% in middle age and 80% of the elderly group. Whilst these figures may indicate significant differences between the groups the varying cohort sizes and small numbers involved do make comparison risky. This risk is compounded by the fact that different locations and eras are involved.

However, for the sake of completeness they will be used to compare the children's results with those of the adults.

If all the children are taken as one group a left flank incision was used in 50% of cases and no incision in 50%. The mediastinum was retained in 25% of cases and complete evisceration performed in 16%. Canopic packages were used in 25% of cases and the viscera returned loose in 8%. Granular material was inserted into the body cavity in 8% and resin used in 16% with linen also used in 16%.

The most obvious difference between child and adult mummification was the high percentage in which evisceration was omitted in the children. However, this finding must be tempered by the fact that numbers are relatively small and time-scale (era) may have played a part. Seven of the thirteen child mummies came from the Roman Period.

To complete the comparison it can be said that the use of novel routes for excerebration followed by less cranial packing is a feature of child mummification as are the less frequent use of eye globe packing and packing of the mouth. Evisceration is used less frequently in children. With the caveat regarding small cohort numbers this points to a more casual approach used in child mummification.

Chapter Nine

Discussion of specific mummification techniques

9.1 Introduction

In the past the most popular routes used for excerebration have been well described by many authors although variations in the trans-nasal route do require further discussion. Other techniques discussed below are alternative routes for excerebration, the treatment of the eyes, the use of the perineal route for evisceration, techniques used in the Roman Period and the use of devices to 'stiffen' the mummy. The influence exerted on Egyptian mummification practices by the arrival of immigrant populations will be discussed as will the subject of surgical practicality when considering mummification techniques.

9.2 Variations in the trans-nasal route of excerebration

Although the Trans-nasal route for excerebration was first described by Herodotus in the fifth century BC (Herodotus v.s.) a detailed analysis of the procedure is needed. In this research project the trans-nasal route has been considered under four headings related to the exact site of perforation in the floor of anterior cranial fossa. These are:

1. Through the ethmoid sinus only
2. Through both the ethmoid and sphenoid sinuses
3. Through the sphenoid sinus only
4. Through the nose and wall of the orbit

The relevance is related to size of perforation and the direction of perforation. How did ancient Egyptians guide their tools/instruments? In modern surgery, when undertaking a procedure 'blind' it is common practice to follow a sight line related to existing observable anatomy. In the case of the trans-nasal route the 'site line' may have been the anterior surface of the nose. If followed this would produce a more vertical alignment. If the instrument were angled more horizontally this would result in perforation of more posterior structures. This general rule of 'the more horizontal the sight line, the more posterior the structures breached ' is followed in the subsequent discussion of one of the more esoteric routes used for excerebration. Reference to section 4.1.1 will reveal the use of each of these routes in the trans-nasal approach. Each site of perforation will be considered to determine whether there is any relationship between the route and era or location. In relation to excerebration a final technique needs to be included – that is a total lack of excerebration.

First the ethmoid only perforation group will be considered. These mummies are shown grouped initially by era and, subsequently by location in Tables 9.1 and 9.2. It can be seen that this particular approach was used during a wide range of historical dates from Dynasty 20 to the Roman Period and in a wide range of locations from the Fayum and Hawara in the north to Thebes in the south of the Nile valley.

NUMBER	ERA	LOCATION
III	Dyn. 20-21	Thebes
XXVIII	Dyn. 21	Akhmim
XXIX	Dyn. 22	Thebes
XXXIII	Dyn. 22	Thebes
XXV	Dyn. 22-25	Thebes
LIII	Dyn. 25	Thebes
XXX	Dyn. 25	Thebes
XXXI	Dyn. 25	Thebes
XVII	3 IP	Thebes
XL	3 IP	Unknown
LIV	3 IP	Unknown
VI	Dyn. 26	Thebes
XI	Dyn. 26	Thebes
XXXVIII	Dyn. 26	Thebes
L	Dyn. 26	Akhmim/Thebes
XXIII	Ptolemaic	Akhmim
XXXVI	Ptolemaic	Akhmim
XXXVII	Ptolemaic	Akhmim
XLIII	Ptolemaic	Fayum
LI	Dyn. 19 / Ptolemaic	Unknown
I	Roman	Unknown
XVIII	Roman	Thebes
XIX	Roman	Unknown
XXVII	Roman	Hawara
XLI	Roman	Unknown
XLV	Roman	Hawara
LVI	Roman	Hawara
LVII	Roman	Hawara
LX	Roman	Thebes
XXVI	Unknown	Unknown

TABLE 9.1 MUMMIES WITH ETHMOID SINUS PERFORATION ONLY GROUPED BY ERA

NUMBER	ERA	LOCATION
XLIII	Ptolemaic	Fayum
XXVII	Roman	Hawara
XLV	Roman	Hawara
LVI	Roman	Hawara
LVII	Roman	Hawara
XXIII	Ptolemaic	Akhmim
XXVIII	Dyn. 21	Akhmim
XXXVI	Ptolemaic	Akhmim
XXXVII	Ptolemaic	Akhmim
L	Dyn. 26	Akhmim/Thebes
III	Dyn. 20-21	Thebes

NUMBER	ERA	LOCATION
VI	Dyn. 26	Thebes
XI	Dyn. 26	Thebes
XVII	3 IP	Thebes
XVIII	Roman	Thebes
XXV	Dyn. 22-25	Thebes
XXIX	Dyn. 22	Thebes
XXX	Dyn. 25	Thebes
XXXI	Dyn. 25	Thebes
XXXIII	Dyn. 22	Thebes
XXXVIII	Dyn. 26	Thebes
LIII	Dyn. 25	Thebes
LX	Roman	Thebes
I	Roman	Unknown
XIX	Roman	Unknown
XXVI	Unknown	Unknown
XL	3 IP	Unknown
XLI	Roman	Unknown
LI	Dyn. 19 / Ptolemaic	Unknown
LIV	3 IP	Unknown

TABLE 9.2 MUMMIES WITH ETHMOID SINUS PERFORATION ONLY GROUPED BY LOCATION

When considering the slightly more horizontal approach resulting in perforation of both ethmoid and sphenoid sinuses the cohort is shown in the Tables 9.3 and 9.4 grouped by era and then location. It can be seen that the technique was used in a wide time frame and in several locations.

NUMBER	ERA	LOCATION
VIII	Dyn. 22	Thebes
XXXIV	Dyn. 22	Thebes
XXXV	Dyn. 22	Thebes/Fayum
V	Dyn. 25	Thebes
XL	3 IP	Unknown
X	Ptolemaic	Akhmim
XLII	Ptolemaic	Fayum
XLIV	Ptolemaic	Unknown
XVI	Roman	Thebes
XXII	Unknown	Unknown

TABLE 9.3 MUMMIES WITH ETHMOID AND SPHENOID SINUS PERFORATION BY ERA

NUMBER	ERA	LOCATION
XLII	Ptolemaic	Fayum
X	Ptolemaic	Akhmim
V	Dyn. 25	Thebes
VIII	Dyn. 22	Thebes
XVI	Roman	Thebes
XXXIV	Dyn. 22	Thebes
XXXV	Dyn. 22	Thebes/Fayum
XXII	Unknown	Unknown
XL	3 IP	Unknown
XLIV	Ptolemaic	Unknown

TABLE 9.4 MUMMIES WITH ETHMOID AND SPHENOID SINUS PERFORATION BY LOCATION

Sphenoid sinus perforation in isolation is represented in Table 9.5. Again there is no particular influence from either era or location, although it has to be admitted that the cohort size is very small.

NUMBER	ERA	LOCATION
XLIX	D 22	Thebes
XLVI	D 26	Thebes
LIX	Roman	Hawara

TABLE 9.5 MUMMIES WITH EXCLUSIVELY SPHENOID PERFORATION.

The final section in variations of trans-nasal excerebration is the trans-nasal orbital route. There are only two examples here and these may represent an accidental 'wandering' from the normal route rather than a deliberate attempt to vary the route used for excerebration. These are shown in Table 9.6 and do not adhere to any particular era or location.

NUMBER	ERA	LOCATION
IX	D 25	Thebes
XLVII	Roman	Hawara

TABLE 9.6 MUMMIES WITH A TRANS-NASAL ORBITAL ROUTE FOR EXCEREBRATION

Before considering the final method of approach to the brain (namely no excerebration – leaving the brain in situ), the efficacy of the various routes should be assessed. The question is, 'how effective are the various routes at achieving full excerebration?'. Three levels of result will be considered – full excerebration (FE), a small amount of cerebral material remaining (Sm.) and significant remnants of the brain left in the cranial cavity. In fact there are no cases where there is a significant amount of cerebral material remaining.

NUMBER	Ethmoid	Eth. + Sph.	Sphenoid	T/N Orb.
I	Sm.			
III	FE			
VI	Sm.			
XI	Sm.			
XVII	FE			
XVIII	FE			
XIX	FE			
XXIII	FE			
XXV	FE			
XXVI	FE			
XXVII	FE			
XXVIII	FE			
XXIX	FE			
XXX	Sm.			
XXXI	Sm.			
XXXIII	FE			
XXXVI	FE			
XXXVII	FE			
XXXVIII	FE			
XLI	FE			

DISCUSSION OF SPECIFIC MUMMIFICATION TECHNIQUES

NUMBER	Ethmoid	Eth. + Sph.	Sphenoid	T/N Orb.
XLIII	FE			
XLV	FE			
L	FE			
LI	FE			
LIII	FE			
LIV	Sm.			
LVI	FE			
LVII	Sm.			
LX	FE			
V		FE		
VIII		FE		
X		FE		
XVI		FE		
XXII		FE		
XXXIV		FE		
XXXV		FE		
XL		FE		
XLII		FE		
XLIV		FE		
XLIX			Sm.	
XLVI			Sm.	
LIX			FE	
IX				FE
XLVII				FE

FE=FULL EXCEREBRATION SM.= A SMALL AMOUNT OF BRAIN REMAINING

TABLE 9.7 EFFECT OF EXCEREBRATION ROUTE ON EFFICIENCY OF EXCEREBRATION

Table 9.7 shows the numbers involved. In the case of the exclusively ethmoid route, complete removal of the brain occurs in 75%. Where the combined Ethmoid and sphenoid sinus route has been used, complete excerebration has been achieved in 100%. The sphenoid sinus route (more horizontal) has achieved only 33% of full excerebration, whilst the rather unusual trans-nasal orbital route has achieved 100%. However, the caveat is that the cohort numbers are unbalanced and small.

9.3 No excerebration

In six of the mummies in this series no excerebration has been attempted. These are shown in Table 9.8.

This table illustrates the fact that, in the mummies studied for this resaerch, the practice of not excerebrating a mummy appeared in Dynasty 26, was seen in a mummy from the Ptolemaic Period and was most prevalent in the Roman Period. In the Late Period (Dynasty 26) the lack of excerebration was not associated with a lack of evisceration. The eyes were incised and packed with linen and the mouth was also packed with linen.

There are four mummies from the Roman Period of which three had no evisceration, the fourth being eviscerated via the perineum. However, the eyes were removed from one of these mummies and the orbits packed with linen. Whilst there was resin in the mouth of one of these Roman Period mummies, it may have seeped into the oral cavity 'accidentally' from resin poured onto the face (*).

Whilst a lack of excerebration may have been an indication of 'cheap' mummification, this does not appear to be confirmed by these findings where proper attention to other parts of the head and body has been evident. Furthermore there is no relationship to age, location or era. The only consistent fact is the sex of the individuals subjected to this technique – namely they are all male.

9.4 More unusual routes used for excerebration

9.4.1 Trans-basal route

In the past the absence of brain tissue and the associated absence of damage to the ethmoid and sphenoid bones have been taken as evidence of presumed trans-foraminal excerebration (Wade, Nelson and Garvin, 2011: 250). Having reviewed the evidence for definite trans-foraminal excerebration, where disturbance of the atlanto-occipital area is obvious, it would be safer to cease making this assumption and look for other routes used for the process of excerebration. In this series there is one such case where perforation of the base of the skull can be identified. This is in the case of Mummy XXXII from the British Museum. The mummy is of a Dynasty 22 female and comes from Deir el Bahari. The age is somewhat contentious, as the skeletal and dental ages do not correspond. However, it is the mummy of someone not yet skeletally mature. The perforations in the base of the skull are clearly seen and the route used to achieve this would have been very horizontal and possibly through the mouth rather than the nose. If a line is drawn from the front teeth to the back of the bony palate, this projects very closely to the points of basal perforation (See Figs. 9.1 and 9.2, where parallel lines are shown). Noting that this mummy comes from a site unique to this series, the question to be posed is, 'does this phenomenon reflect a particular style of embalming

NUM.	ERA	LOC.	AGE	EYES	MOUTH	EVISC	SEX
II	Dyn. 26	Thebes	MA	L	LINEN	Abd.	M
LV	Ptol.	Unknown	C- 2-3	Des.	EMPTY	None	M
XII	Roman	Fayum	YA	Des.	RESIN *	None	M
XIII	Roman	Fayum	MA	Rem.	EMPTY	None	M
XXIV	Roman	El-Hibe	MA	Des.	EMPTY	P	M
LII	Roman	Hawara	C- 2	Des.	EMPTY	None	M

C=CHILD YA=YOUNG ADULT MA=MIDDLE AGED E=ELDERLY DES=DESICCATED REM=REMOVED L=LINEN P=PERINEAL

TABLE 9.8 MUMMIES WITH NO EXCEREBRATION

peculiar to Deir el Bahari or to a single embalming / mummification workshop?'. Until other mummies from Deir el Bahari (and from the same dynasty or era) are studied, the question will remain open.

Other techniques used in mummification in this particular case are retention and desiccation of the eyes, multiple substances used in the packing of the mouth (radio-dense granular material and linen) (See Fig. 9.3), retention of both leaves of the diaphragm and the mediastinum and the use of a left flank incision but no perineal disturbance. In the abdomen, evisceration has been performed with return of the viscera in both loose form and in canopic packages along with the introduction of foreign material (granular).

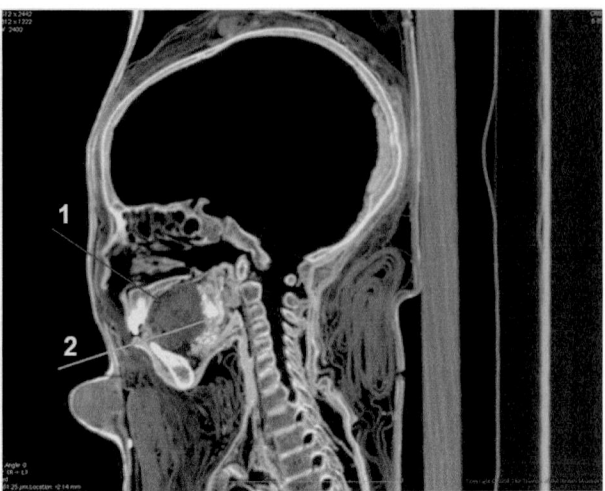

FIG. 9.3 SAGITTAL VIEW OF SKULL - MOUTH PACKING
COURTESY OF THE TRUSTEES OF THE BRITISH MUSEUM

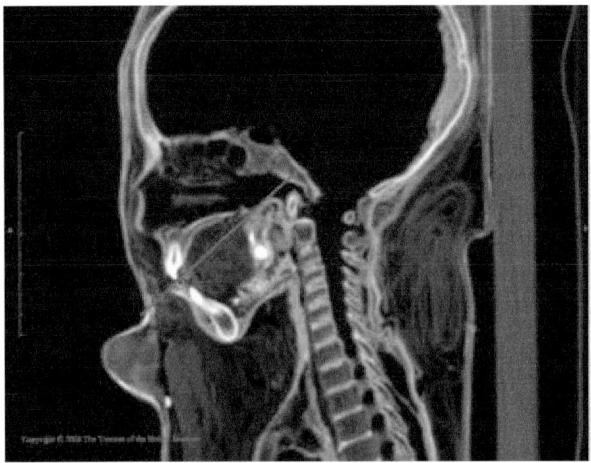

FIG. 9.1 SAGITTAL VIEW OF SKULL - LINE DRAWN IN THE MID LINE FROM UPPER FRONT TEETH TO POSTERIOR EDGE OF HARD PALATE
COURTESY OF THE TRUSTEES OF THE BRITISH MUSEUM

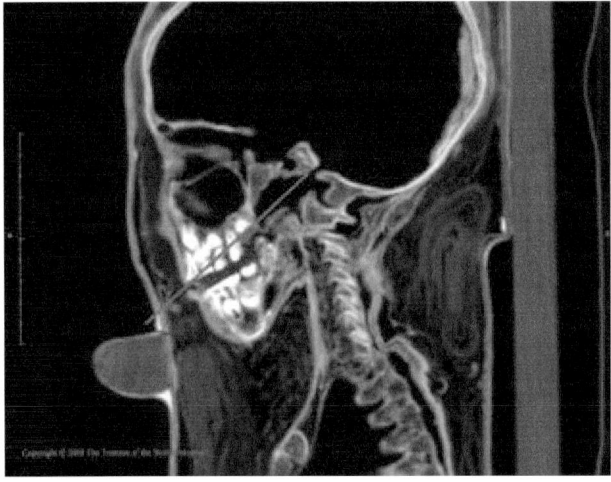

FIG. 9.2 SAGITTAL VIEW OF SKULL - PARALLEL LINE TO THAT IN FIG. 9.1, SHOWN ON CT 'SLICE' SHOWING TRANS-BASAL PERFORATION
COURTESY OF THE TRUSTEES OF THE BRITISH MUSEUM

9.4.2 Trans-orbital route

The second unusual route used for excerebration is the trans-orbital route. This is seen in Mummy XIV, Asru, from Manchester Museum. The mummy is female, probably elderly (judged by the dental condition and skeletal degenerative changes) and from Dynasty 26 Thebes. There is no perforation of the ethmoid or sphenoid sinuses, but excerebration has been performed. The eyes are an unusual shape with superior 'indentations' in the globes that lead directly to the superior orbital fissures that are slightly larger than normal (See Figs. 4.109 and 4.110). There is no fracturing of bone at the margins of the superior orbital fissures but the harder bone in this region would probably allow slight widening of the space without such obvious fracturing occurring.

A so-called 'trans-orbital' route has been described previously (Macke, Macke-Ribet and Connan J., 2002: 73), but with the route commencing in the orbit and proceeding superiorly through the roof of the orbit into the anterior cranial fossa. In the case of Mummy XIV the route is different and leads into the middle cranial fossa via a horizontal route. It is also noteworthy that Macke's description relates to a mummy from the Roman Period whilst Mummy XIV is from Dynasty 26 – the commencement of the Late Period.

Other features of the mummification of Mummy XIV are the presence of granular material in the mouth, retention of the leaves of the diaphragm and retention of the mediastinum. There is a left flank incision with evisceration but little in the way of returned viscera and no packing material in the abdominal cavity. The perineum is intact.

9.5 Treament of the eyes

As mentioned by Aufderheide (Aufderheide, 2010: 318) the obvious accessibility of the eyes does not appear to have resulted in any previous 'in depth' study. The results of eye treatment have been presented in chapter four (sections 4.2.1, 4.2.2, 4.2.3 and 4.2.4, and been grouped into removal, left in situ with only desiccation, packing the globe and the use of 'False Eyes' - Eye Plates). The crude numbers of mummies processed in each manner is shown in Table 9.9.

Des	Packing	Plates	Removal
33	12	5	4
DES = DESICCATION			

TABLE 9.9 DISTRIBUTION OF TREATMENT OF THE EYES (AS DISCUSSED IN CHAPTER 4 – 4.1)

The first group to be analysed is that in which no action has been taken – that is from the group of thirty-three mummies where the eyes were left in situ and therefore were subjected to desiccation, either without any further procedure or with the addition of plates or being opened and packed or opened and no further procedure undertaken. The mummies in this group, their origin, era, age at death and sex are shown in Table 9.10. Within this group some twenty-one had no procedure performed following desiccation. These are shown in Table 9.11, ordered by era.

NUMBER	ORIGIN	ERA	AGE	SEX
I	Unknown	Roman	YA	M
III	Thebes	D20-21	MA	M
IX	Thebes	D25	MA	M
X	Akhmim	Ptolemaic	MA	M
XII	Fayum	Roman	YA	M
XIV	Thebes	D26	MA	F
XV	Hawara	Roman	C - 5	M
XVIII	Thebes	Roman	YA	F
XIX	Unknown	Roman	C - 3-4	M
XXII	Unknown	Unknown	MA	?F
XXIV	El-Hibe	Roman	MA	M
XXVI	Unknown	Unknown	C - 6	M
XXVII	Hawara	Roman	YA	F
XXVIII	Akhmim	D21	YA	F
XXXI	Thebes	D25	MA	M
XXXII	Deir El Bahari	D22	C - 15-19	F
XXXIII	Thebes	D22	MA	F
XXXVI	Akhmim	Ptolemaic	YA	M
XXXVII	Akhmim	Ptolemaic	MA	?M
XL	Unknown	3IP	MA	F
XLI	Unknown	Roman	C - 3-6	?
XLIII	Fayum	Ptolemaic??	YA	F
XLIV	Unknown	Ptolemaic??	YA	M
XLV	Hawara	Roman	YA	F
XLVII	Hawara	Roman	C - 6	?F
LII	?Hawara	Roman	C - 2	M
LIII	Thebes	D25	MA	F
LIV	Unknown	3IP	YA	F
LV	Unknown	Ptolemaic	C - 2-3	M
LVI	Hawara	Roman	C - 2-3	M
LVII	Hawara	Roman	MA	M
LIX	Hawara	Roman	C - 2-3	M
LX	Thebes	Roman	MA	M

TABLE 9.10 ALL MUMMIES WITH DESICCATED EYES

NUMBER	ORIGIN	ERA	AGE	SEX
XXVIII	Akhmim	D21	YA	F
XXXII	Deir El Bahari	D22	C - 15-19	F
LIII	Thebes	D25	MA	F
XL	Unknown	3IP	MA	F
LIV	Unknown	3IP	YA	F
XXXVII	Akhmim	Ptolemaic	MA	?M
XLIV	Unknown	Ptolemaic??	YA	M
LV	Unknown	Ptolemaic	C - 2-3	M
I	Unknown	Roman	YA	M
XII	Fayum	Roman	YA	M
XVIII	Thebes	Roman	YA	F
XXIV	El-Hibe	Roman	MA	M
XXVII	Hawara	Roman	YA	F
XLI	Unknown	Roman	C - 3-6	?
XLVII	Hawara	Roman	C - 6	?F
LII	?Hawara	Roman	C - 2	M
LVI	Hawara	Roman	C - 2-3	M
LVII	Hawara	Roman	MA	M
LIX	Hawara	Roman	C - 2-3	M
XXII	Unknown	Unknown	MA	?F
XXVI	Unknown	Unknown	C - 6	M

TABLE 9.11 MUMMIES WITH EYE DESICCATION ALONE BY ERA

The conclusion is that the absence of any treatment of the eyes was not restricted to any particular era and spans time from Dynasty 21 to the Roman Period. It can also be seen that there was no specific site related to this technique (or lack of technique), nor any bias towards either sex.

There are twelve examples where the eye globe has been left in situ, opened and packed with material. These are shown in Table 9.12. In five cases the eyes were subsequently covered with 'false eyes' or eye plates.

NUMBER	ORIGIN	ERA	AGE	PLATES	SEX
VIII	Thebes	D22	YA		M
XXXIV	Thebes	D22	MA	YES	F
XLIX	Thebes	D22	E		F
XXV	Thebes	D22-25	E		F
XXX	Thebes	D25	MA	YES	M
V	Thebes	D25	?	YES	F
XVII	Thebes	3IP	MA	YES	F
II	Thebes	D26	MA		M
XI	Thebes	D26	E	YES	M
L	Akhmim/Thebes	D26	E		?F
LI	?Thebes	D19/Ptol.	MA		M
XVI	Thebes	Roman	YA		F

TABLE 9.12 MUMMIES WITH PACKED GLOBES – IN ORDER OF ERA

It is interesting to note that the use of eye plates with packing of the globe was only found in Thebes. There is a minor query about the veracity of location assigned to Mummies L and LI in that the origin is only 'possibly' Thebes. However, the overwhelming indication from Table 9.12 is that the mummies came from Thebes. The use of eye plates and packing seems to cover Dynasties 22 to 26 – in other words the Third Intermediate Period and into the Late Period. The sex distribution is more or less even. Although the numbers are small, the evidence is strong for the use of eye plates and packing being a Theban practice in the Third Intermediate Period, possibly fading out of use in the early Late Period. The foregoing discussion relates to the use of eye plates with globe packing, but it must not be forgotten that eye plates were used in two mummies where the eyes had been retained and desiccated but were not opened and packed. These are Mummies III and XXXIII from the Dynasties 20/21 and 22 respectively both from Thebes. Mummy III is male and Mummy XXXIII female. Although the use of 'false eyes' has been noted by some authors (Ikram, Dodson,1998:127; Aufderheide, 2010: 244) no association with a particular site has previously been noted.

The final type of eye 'treatment' is removal. This technique was used in four cases shown in Table 9.13. As can be seen, eye plates were used to cover the orbits that had been packed with linen after removal of the eyes. This case was from Dynasty 22 Thebes. No other association with either era or location appears evident.

NUMBER	ORIGIN	ERA	AGE	SEX	EYES
VII	Thebes	D25	YA	F	REMOVED
XIII	Fayum	Roman	MA	M	REMOVED REPLACED WITH LINEN
XXIII	Akhmim	Ptolemaic	E	M	REMOVED
XXIX	Thebes	D22	MA	M	REMOVED, REPLACED LINEN and PLATES

TABLE 9.13 MUMMIES IN WHICH THE EYES WERE REMOVED.

9.6 Use of the perineal route for evisceration

Although this evisceration route has been described extensively in the past there are not numerous examples of its use. Wade and Watson (Wade and Watson, 2013: 4202) reviewed fifty mummy CT scans and found only three cases of perineal evisceration. They postulated that the technique was restricted to 'elite females'. In this research project a total of fourteen cases were found (of these thirteen were definite cases of use of the perineal route – Mummy XXXVI had some evidence of use of the route, but was not a 'definite' case – only probable). They are shown in Table 9.14.

These represent 23% of the cases in this series. At one stage in the research it appeared that there might be an unrepresentatively large proportion of cases from Akhmim. However, with the addition of more cases this bias seems to have disappeared. It is noted that there is only a slight bias towards the use of this technique in females (8:6). Whilst there is only one case from each of the Dynasties 21, 22 and 23, there are five examples from each of the Ptolemaic and Roman eras. This would indicate that the technique became more popular after the invasion of the Macedonians and continued thereafter. Geographic location, with four cases from Akhmim and six from Thebes, seems to indicate a bias towards that area as opposed to the more northerly locations. In ten of the fourteen cases a left flank incision was used in conjunction with the perineal approach with all cases from Thebes having such a second approach. It is also notable that the Theban method included return of the viscera in all cases and that the three cases in which viscera were not returned to the body cavity came from Hawara, Assiut and Akhmim.

If a different approach is taken and two other cases from Akhmim are considered, these are Mummies XXVIII a Dynasty 21 mummy from Manchester Museum and Mummy L from Dynasty 26 from Perth Museum and Art Gallery. In the case of the latter, the location of origin is not firmly established, being either Akhmim or Thebes. The case for Akhmim as a provenance depends upon a name on the coffin containing the appellation Min. However this is the name of the occupant's mother.

Looking closely at the images of Mummy XXVIII, although there is insufficient evidence to be absolutely convinced of a perineal approach, the images do not show the perineal orifices clearly. There is a very straight appearance to the linen covering the perineum and resin from the abdominal cavity sits on the inner surface of this linen 'membrane' (see Figs. 9.4 and 9.5).

Mummy	Sex	Era	Location	Other inc.	Visc. Ret.
X	M	Ptol.	Akhmim	L.Flank	CP
XVI	F	Roman	Thebes	L.Flank	CP
XVIII	F	Roman	Thebes	L.Flank	CP
XXII	?F	Unknown	Unknown	L.Flank	CP
XXIII	M	Ptol.	Akhmim	L.Flank	CP
XXIV	?M	Roman	El-Hibe	None	?CP
XXXVI	M	Ptol.	Akhmim	L.Flank	CP
XXXVII	M	Ptol.	Akhmim	None	None
XXXVIII	F	D26	Thebes	L.Flank	CP
XXXIX	M	D21	Thebes	L.Flank	Loose
XLII	?F	Ptol.	Assiut	None	None
XLV	F	Roman	Hawara	None	None
LIII	F	D25	Thebes	L.Flank	CP
LX	F	Roman	Thebes	L.Flank	CP

TABLE 9.14 MUMMIES WITH USE OF THE PERINEAL ROUTE FOR EVISCERATION

Akhmim and the use of the perineal approach – possibly 100% association. Of the five mummies definitely from Akhmim, four were male and one female.

Examining the use of the perineal approach in Thebes reveals that this technique is found in 22% of cases. – a distinct difference from the rate of usage in Akhmim.

9.7 Techniques used in the Roman Period

9.7.1 Thoracic disruption

The striking feature of the Roman Period is the high proportion of mummies with distorted chest walls. Mummies from the Roman Period were found in the following locations (see Table 9.15).

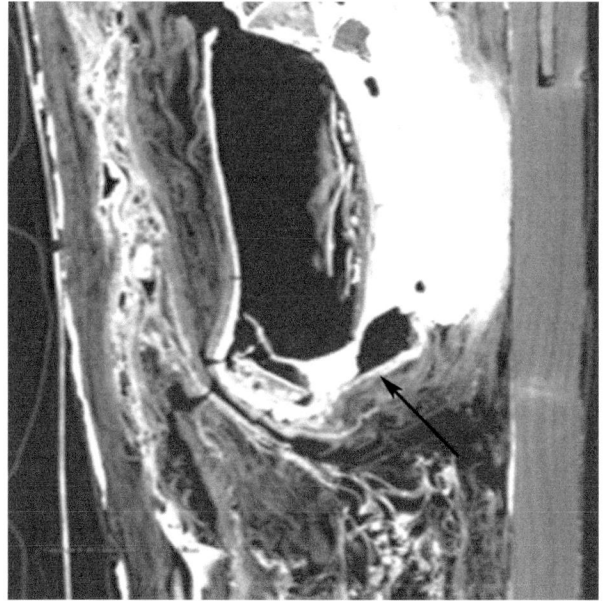

FIG. 9.4 SAGITTAL VIEW OF THE PERINEUM WITH ARROW SHOWING THE VERY STRAIGHT LINEN 'MEMBRANE'.

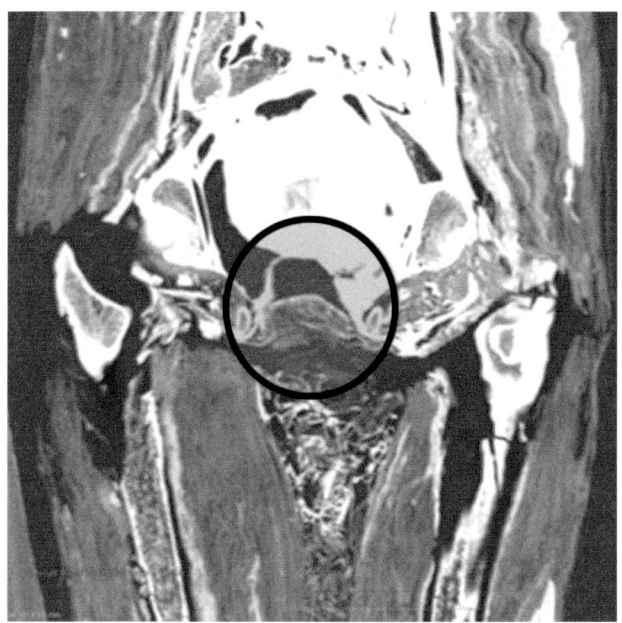

FIG. 9.5 CORONAL VIEW OF THE PERINEUM SHOWING THE LINEN WRAPPINGS.

NUMBER	ORIGIN	LOCATION
XII	Manchester - M1768	Fayum
XIII	Manchester - M1767	Fayum
XV	Liverpool - 13.10.11.25	Hawara
XXVII	Manchester - Demetria - 11630	Hawara
XLV	Manchester - M1766	Hawara
XLVII	Manchester - M1769	Hawara
LII	Manchester - M9319 - child	?Hawara
LVI	Manchester - MM2109	Hawara
LVII	Manchester - MM1775 - Artemidorus	Hawara
LIX	BM - EA 22108 Child	Hawara
XXIV	Zurich - Basel - BSAE.1030	El-Hibe
XVI	Liverpool - M13997a	Thebes
XVIII	Liverpool- M14048	Thebes
LX	BM - EA 6704	Thebes
I	Birmingham - Graeco-Roman	Unknown
XIX	Zurich - Altdorf Child	Unknown
XLI	Zurich - Lenzburg - K10351	Unknown

TABLE 9.15 MUMMIES FROM THE ROMAN PERIOD AND THEIR LOCATIONS

Table 9.15 is reconfigured to show the mummies in which chest distortion occurred, on which side (or symmetrically), whether it was accompanied by thoracic and/or abdominal compression, whether there was fracture and/or dislocation of the costo-vertebral joints and whether evisceration had been performed (See Table 9.16).

Although there is insufficient evidence to classify this as a definite perineal approach, there remains a distinct suspicion that this might be the case. A left flank incision is also used in this case. In the case of Mummy L the damage to the mummy excludes assessment of the perineum.

If Mummy XXVIII is accepted as probably having a perineal approach (as well as a left flank incision) then the origin of this mummy from Dynasty 21 may indicate that from this dynasty onwards such a method of evisceration was established in Akhmim as well as Thebes, although there is the possibility that the practice was discontinued and then re-introduced later. Furthermore it can be said that there is a very strong relationship between the site of

Of the seventeen mummies, one was disrupted in parts so making assessment of rib damage difficult. Of the seventeen, thirteen had evidence of chest wall compression. The four mummies without compression were of three children at or below the age of six years (See Table 9.17). The fourth was a mummy of a middle-aged person, probably male (but in the coffin of a female) from Thebes. The coffin is dated to Dynasty 19 or 20 but the wrapping of the mummy is similar to other mummies (in the National Museums, Liverpool) from the Roman Period – hence its assignment to this period.

Having analysed the thirteen mummies with chest compression it can be noted that eight had symmetrical antero-posterior compression and only five had

NUMBER	RIB FRACT.	C/V DIS.	ASYMM	COMP.	ABDO. COMP.	EVISC.
XII	DIS.	DIS.	N	Y	Y	N
XIII	N	R and L	N	Y	Y	?N
XV	N	N	N	Y	Y	N
XXVII	N	R and L	N	Y	Y	Y
XLV	N	R and L	Y	Y - R	Y	Y
XLVII	N	R and L	N	Y	Y	N
LII	N	N	N	N	N	N
LVI	N	R and L	N	Y	Y	N
LVII	Y - L	Y - R	Y	Y - L	N	N
LIX	N	R and L	N	Y	Y	N
XXIV	Y L and R	R and L	Sl.	Sl.	Y	Y
XVI	Y L and R	N	N	Sl.	Sl.	Y
XVIII	Y - L	R and L	Y	Y - L	Sl.	Y
LX	N	N	N	N	N	Y
I	N	R and L	Y	Y - L	Sl.	Y
XIX	N	N	N	N	N	Y
XLI	N	N	N	N	Sl.	Y

TABLE 9.16 ROMAN MUMMIES WITH DAMAGE TO THE CHEST WALL AND ITS DETAIL.

asymmetrical compression (that is of one side of the rib cage), three of these being of the left ribs. Twelve rib cages could be analysed in detail and of these four exhibited fractures – bilateral in two cases. In contrast, ten of the twelve had costo-vertebral dislocation, of which nine were bilateral and only one unilateral (the right ribs).

NUMBER	ABDO. COMP.	EVISC.	AGE	LOC.
LII	N	N	C - 2	Hawara
LX	N	Y	MA	Thebes
XIX	N	Y	C - 3-4	Unknown
XLI	Sl.	Y	C - 3-6	Unknown

TABLE 9.17 MUMMIES OF THE ROMAN PERIOD WITHOUT CHEST COMPRESSION

Disruption (dislocation or subluxation) of the costo-vertebral joints rarely occurs in the live human - the only recorded examples being in association with neurofibromatosis. As a traumatic event it is not seen in the human. The other notable factor is that the dislocations in these mummies have occurred without adjacent bony trauma. These facts reflect the point that the costo-vertebral joint is a very stable joint. It is, therefore, intrinsically strong. Figure 9.6 shows the two components of the costo-vertebral joint. These are articulations with the bodies of two adjacent vertebrae and with the transverse process of the same vertebra. The joint with the vertebral bodies is synovial but has a strong capsule. The joint with the transverse process is between the tubercle and neck of the rib and the transverse process and is largely ligamentous. It is very stable and strong. To achieve disruption of these joints whilst avoiding bony damage implies that the ligaments have been weakened in some way prior to applying compressive pressure to the chest wall. Weakening these ligaments could be achieved in one or both of two ways. The first is to surgically incise them and the second is to apply some chemical agent to soften/weaken the collagenous tissue.

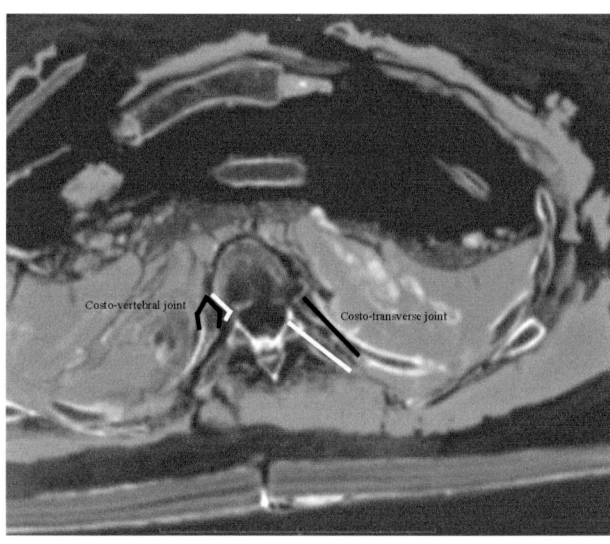

FIG. 9.6 THE COSTO-VERTEBRAL JOINTS SEEN ON A CT SCAN (AXIAL) OF THE MID-THORAX

If incision is used it could be performed either from without or within the thorax. If from without, the surgical route would be preserved and, therefore, visible. This is not the case. Surgical incision of the ligaments of both the component joints would have to be performed 'blind' if from within the thoracic cavity. Although theoretically possible, it would require a great deal of anatomical knowledge and considerable surgical dexterity and control to achieve.

The alternative explanation – that of chemical weakening of the ligaments - is more attractive. However, the obvious question is 'what chemical'? The most likely candidate is a substance that is normally used in mummification. This would be natron. Nevertheless, it is necessary to explain why a substance that had been used for millennia started to be employed this way only in the Roman Period. The possibilities include a subtle change in the composition of the natron – perhaps due to sourcing from a different location or exposing the body to its effects for a longer period. Analysis of the composition of natron from different eras and locations is required as well as experimental mummification using different exposure times. A further possibility is that the cost-vertebral joints were always weakened to an extent but that the difference in the Roman Period was the addition of a compressive force.

Following weakening of the costo-vertebral joints a compressive force would have had to be applied to 'flatten' or compress the chest. It is interesting to note that in only one case of the thirteen with chest compression was compression of the abdomen absent. This was in Mummy LVII from Hawara. In this case there was asymmetry of the rib-cage (shown in Fig. 5.279 on P 169) with fractures on the left and dislocations on the right. The fact that there was compression of both the abdomen and chest in over 90% of cases indicates the probability that the same technique was used to compress both areas of the body – possibly at the same time.

One further point of interest is the frequency of the combination of rib compression and distortion and accompanying abdominal compression in relationship to lack of evisceration. Evisceration via an abdominal or perineal route was absent in seven of the cases of abdominal compression and present in another seven, indicating that compression was not exclusively related to either technique.

Although these seventeen mummies represents just under 30% of the cohort in this study, it remains a relatively small sample and scrutiny of the CT scans of more Roman Period mummies would help to confirm the observations made here.

To complete the picture it is necessary to assess the frequency of rib-cage damage and distortion in mummies from other eras. There are four such mummies from the total cohort of non-Roman mummies of forty-three. These are shown in Table 9.18. As can be seen, although there is technically damage to the chest wall in these cases, it is minor and does not appear similar to the abnormalities seen in the Roman Period mummies.

MUMMY	ERA	LOC.	DAMAGE
VII	D25	Thebes	Thoracic asymmetry
X	Ptolemaic	Akhmim	Three undisplaced fractured left ribs + Fractured left wrist
XXIX	D22	Thebes	Fractured ribs (1 left and 3 right). No distortion of rib cage
XLVIII	D18	Gurob	3 fractured left ribs. No distortion of rib cage

TABLE 9.18 CHEST INJURY IN NON-ROMAN MUMMIES

9.7.2 Lack of an evisceration route

Where no route for evisceration exists the question of the use of enemas has to be discussed. The two methods of enema usage related by Herodotus are to clear the lower bowel (the 'cheapest' option) or to attempt to dissolve the bowel by the use of a lytic or corrosive substance (thought to be turpentine by some authors; Wade and Nelson 2013: 4204). However, Ikram reported that use of this chemical resulted in almost complete removal of the viscera rather than leaving evidence of their structure as seen in the CT scans in this project (Ikram 2005: 16-43). The implication is that, if an enema was used it was just a lower bowel cleansing exercise rather than dissolution of the viscera. This was found in seven cases as seen in Table 9.16.

9.7.3 Pelvic disruption

Consideration of the proposition that a compressive pressure was applied to the thorax and abdomen leads to the need to consider the possibility of this pressure having an effect on the bony pelvis. The twelve mummies with abdominal and thoracic compression are shown in Table 9.19 along with the recording of pelvic damage.

NUMBER	RIB FRACT.	C/V DIS.	COMP.	ABDO. COMP.	EVISC.	PELVIS
XII	DIS.	DIS.	Y	Y	N	S B
XIII	N	R and L	Y	Y	?N	N
XV	N	N	Y	Y	N	N
XXVII	N	R and L	Y	Y	Y	S B P
XLV	N	R and L	Y - R	Y	Y	S B P F
XLVII	N	R and L	Y	Y	N	S
LVI	N	R and L	Y	Y	N	N
LIX	N	R and L	Y	Y	N	S
XXIV	Y L and R	R and L	Sl.	Y	Y	S B F
XVI	Y L and R	N	Sl.	Sl.	Y	N
XVIII	Y - L	R and L	Y - L	Sl.	Y	S B P F
I	N	R and L	Y - L	Sl.	Y	S B P

S=SIJ DISRUPTION B=BILATERAL P=PUBIC SYMPHYSIS DISRUPTION F=FRACTURE OF THE PELVIS N=NO DISRUPTION OR FRACTURE

TABLE 9.19 PELVIC INJURY WITH COMPRESSION OF THE CHEST AND ABDOMEN

Eight of the twelve mummies involved showed evidence of pelvic disruption that could have been caused by the proposed compression. Analysis of the four mummies without pelvic damage reveals a mixed picture but with a bias towards children and young adulthood and towards the male sex. However the numbers are small and may not indicate a reliable pattern (see Table 9.20). Furthermore, the incidence of such 'protection' from disruption in the young because of their greater elasticity of tissues is not supported as these age groups are well represented in the group with disruption. The final factor to be considered is that of location. Again no particular location stands out as being associated with a lack of pelvic disruption. Although the analysis of a larger cohort may reveal a pattern, it is just as likely that the observed differences are a reflection of minor differences in the practices of different embalming workshops.

NUMBER	SEX	AGE	LOC.	PELVIS
XII	M	YA	FAYUM	S B
XIII	M	MA	FAYUM	N
XV	M	C - 5	HAWARA	N
XXVII	F	YA	HAWARA	S B P
XLV	F	YA	HAWARA	S B P F
XLVII	?F	C - 6	HAWARA	S
LVI	M	C – 2-3	HAWARA	N
LIX	M	C – 2-3	HAWARA	S
XXIV	M	MA	EL-HIBE	S B F
XVI	F	YA	THEBES	N
XVIII	F	YA	THEBES	S B P F
I	M	YA	UNKNOWN	S B P

S=SIJ DISRUPTION B=BILATERAL P=PUBIC SYMPHYSIS DISRUPTION
F=FRACTURE OF THE PELVIS N=NO DISRUPTION OR FRACTURE

TABLE 9.20 SEX, AGE AND LOCATION OF MUMMIES WITH CHEST AND ABDOMINAL COMPRESSION

9.8 Stiffeners within the wrappings and mummies.

Ten of the sixty mummies in this series have some form of 'stiffener' within the wrappings. There were two types of such a supporting item: those within the wrappings and those within the body. They are shown in Table 9.21.

NUMBER	STIFFENER	ORIGIN	ERA	AGE
XII	BOARD	Faiyum	Roman	YA
XV	BOARD	Hawara	Roman	C - 5
XXIV	BOARD	El-Hibe	Roman	MA
LVII	BOARD	Hawara	Roman	MA
XXXV	PALM FROND	Thebes/Faiyum	D22	YA
XLI	PALM FROND	Unknown	Roman	C - 3-6
LII	PALM FROND	?Hawara	Roman	C - 2
XIII	REEDS	Faiyum	Roman	MA
XXII	METAL ROD	Unknown	Unknown	MA
XXXI	CERVICAL STICK	Thebes	D25	MA

TABLE 9.21 STIFFENERS IN MUMMIES

9.8.1 Stiffeners within the wrappings

Reference to Table 9.21 reveals that there were four mummies with a wooden board lying posterior to the body. All these were from the Roman Period, but not from the same location nor was the technique associated with a particular age group. Reference to Fig. 9.7 demonstrates the use of a double board (from Mummy XII) as a posterior support for the body. The boards had been re-used, as demonstrated by the sawn off dowels at the outer sides and the intact dowels joining the two boards (see Fig. 9.8).

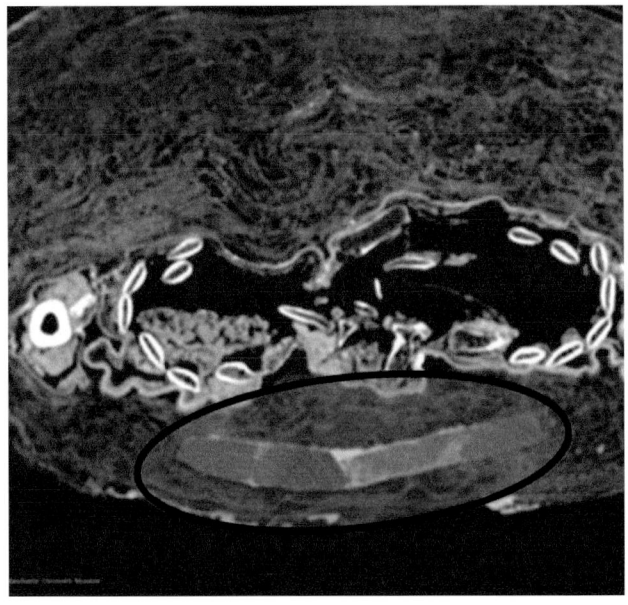

FIG. 9.7 AXIAL VIEW OF THORAX - DOUBLE BOARD USED FOR SUPPORT

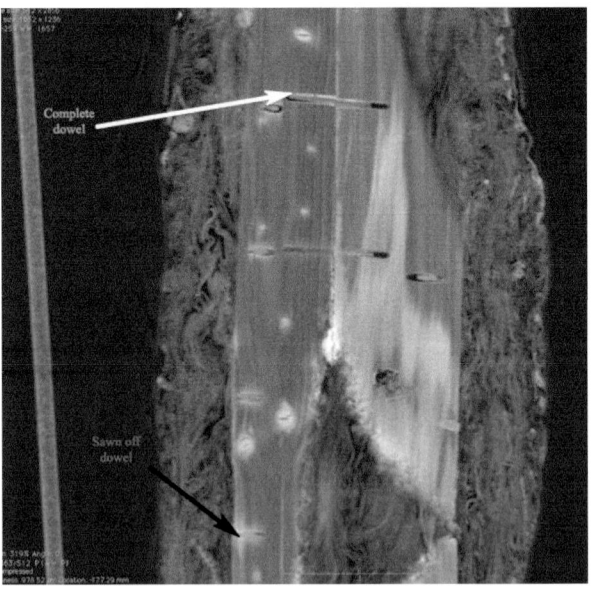

FIG. 9.8 CORONAL VIEW OF TRUNK - DOWELS IN RE-USED WOODEN PLANKS

Reference to Fig. 9.9 shows a single board used for support in Mummy XV.

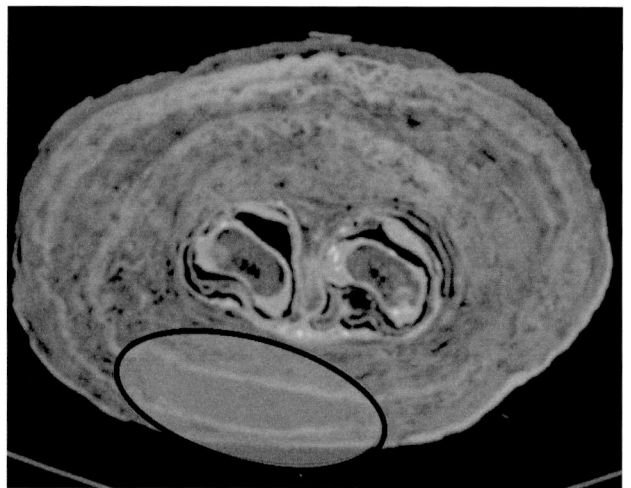

FIG. 9.9 AXIAL VIEW OF KNEES - SINGLE BOARD USED FOR SUPPORT

The boards used in Mummies XXIV and LVII were single boards. In all four cases the boards ran the entire length of the body from head to toe.

The second type of external support within the wrappings was a rod-like object used in multiples – sometimes in twos as in Mummy LII (See Fig. 9.10). Examination of the cross-sectional shape reveals that these are pericules or fronds from palm leaves (Dowson, 1982: 294). In the case of MummyXXXV the right pericule extends from the shoulder to the foot and on the left extends from hip to toe. In the case of Mummy XLI there are again two pericules running from shoulder to ankle. Whether these pericules add genuine strength or are symbolic is open to question and requires further investigation.

In the case of Mummy XIII there are four much thinner objects anterior to the body but within the wrappings. These objects are individually wrapped in linen and vary in length from nine to twenty-four centimetres. Whilst provisionally called 'reeds' their true identity remains a mystery. The ability of these objects to impart rigidity remains unknown until their identity is established. It is possible that they are no more than symbolic. They are shown in Figs. 9.11 and 9.12.

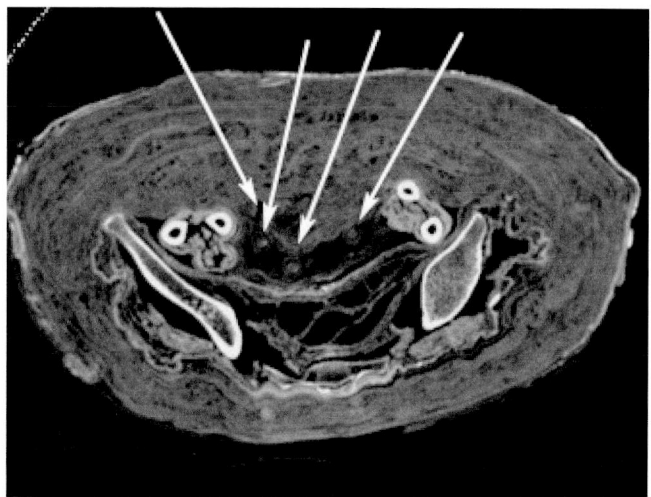

FIG. 9.11 AXIAL VIEW OF PELVIS - CROSS-SECTION OF 'REEDS' ANTERIOR TO THE ABDOMEN

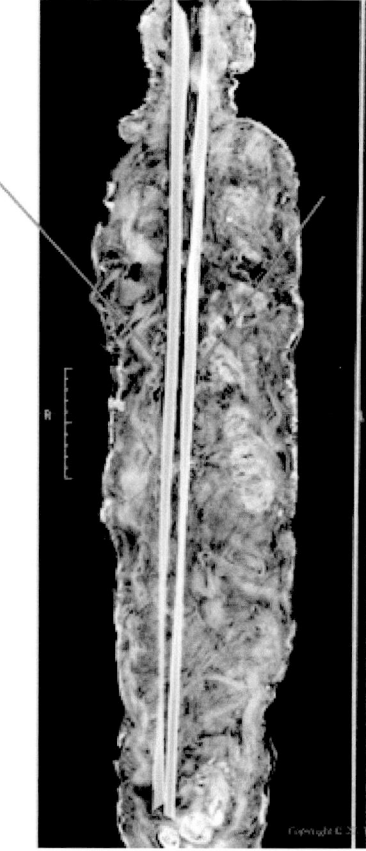

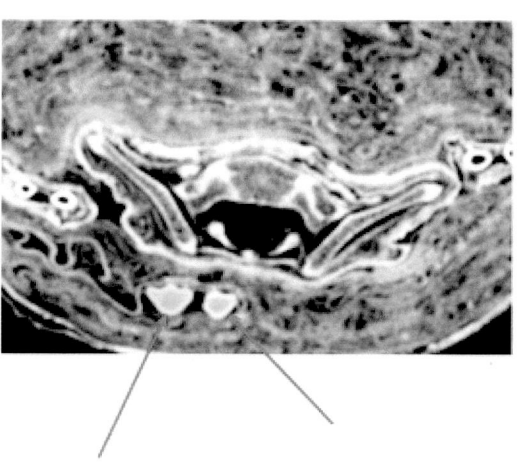

FIG. 9.10 CORONAL AND AXIAL VIEWS SHOWING TWO PERICULES USED IN MUMMY LII

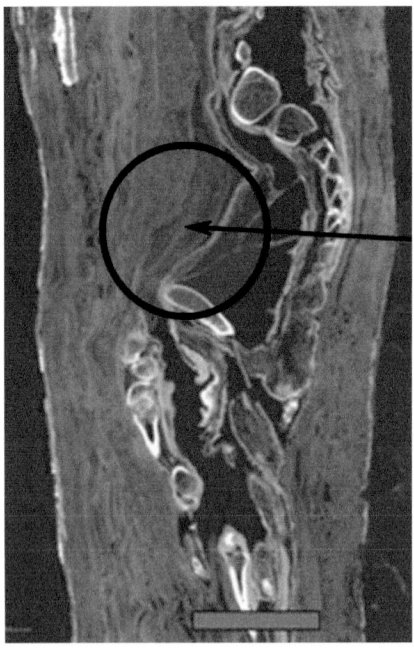

Fig. 9.12 Sagittal view of 'reeds' anterior to the abdomen

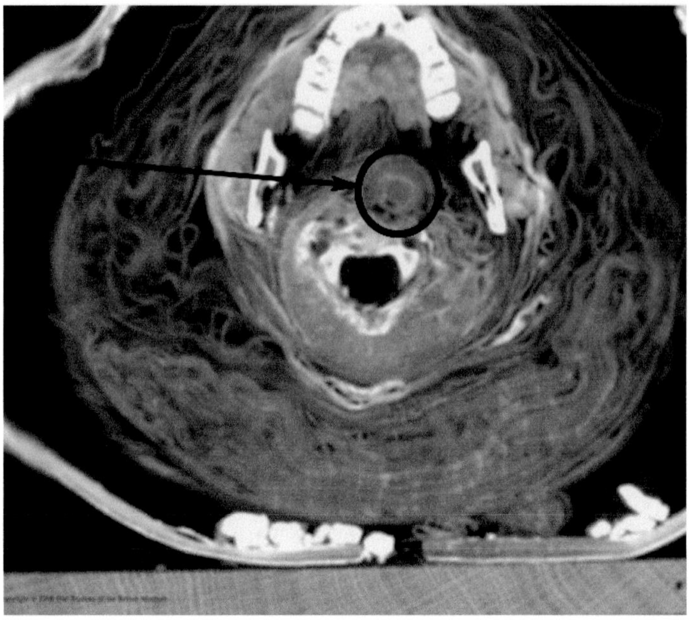

Fig. 9.14 Axial view of stick anterior to and supporting cervical spine
Courtesy of the Trustees of the British Museum

9.8.2 Stiffeners within the body

There are two examples of the use of a rod used within the body. On each occasion it is used to stabilize the neck. In Mummy XXXI it is in the form of a stick coverd in resin-soaked linen extending from the first cervical vertebra to the level of the seventh thoracic vertebra. It lies just anterior to the spine (See Figs. 9.13 and 9.14).

the fact that it has been inserted down the cervical spinal canal. As this structure is straight it implies that the neck was flexible at the time of insertion. Had this not been the case then the natural cervical lordosis would have become rigid after mummification and prevented insertion via the spinal canal (see Figs. 9.15, 9.16 and 9.17).

The use of internal supports during mummification is not unheard of but is infrequently seen. These examples seem specifically targeted.

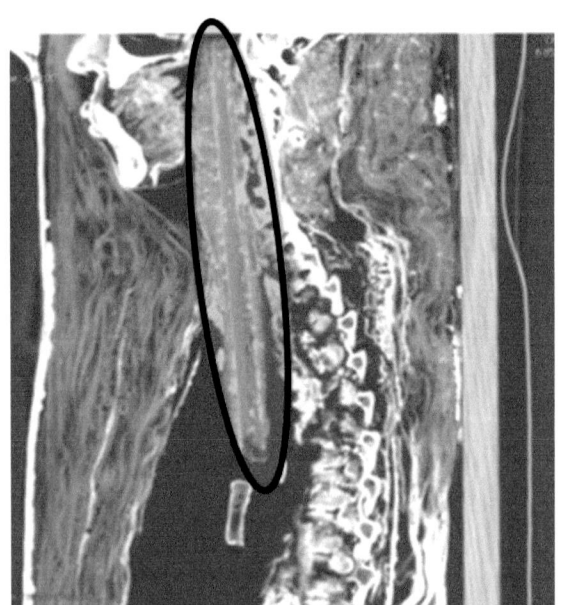

Fig. 9.13 Sagittal view of stick anterior to and supporting cervical spine
Courtesy of the Trustees of the British Museum

In Mummy XXII the rod is of metal and is used to connect the head to the trunk. It appears to have been inserted from the skull via a small trepanning hole in the occiput. The evidence for its insertion at the time of mummification is

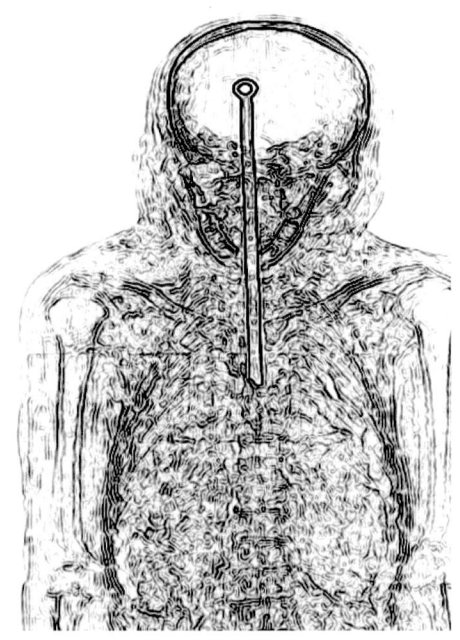

Fig. 9.15 Coronal view of metal rod through skull into thoracic spine (After IEM image)

Discussion of specific mummification techniques

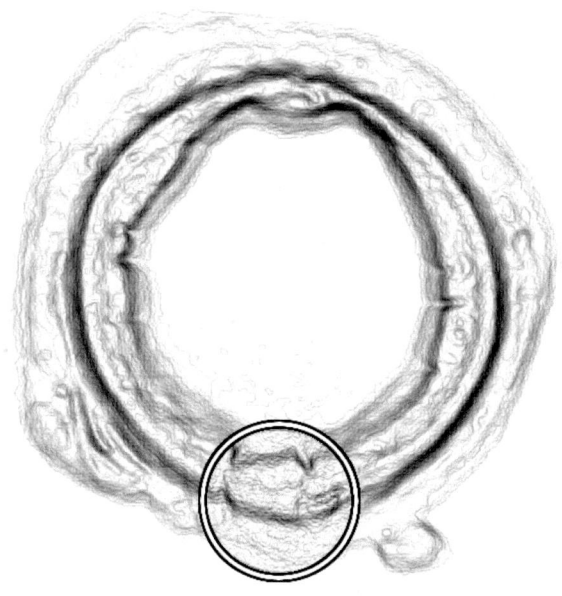

FIG. 9.16 AXIAL VIEW OF POINT OF TREPANATION IN SKULL, USED FOR ROD INSERTION (AFTER IEM IMAGE)

9.9 The effect of foreign rule in various eras

9.9.1 Introduction

This series of mummy CT scans includes one from the Middle Kingdom, three (possibly two) from the New Kingdom, twenty from the Third Intermediate Period, eight from the Late Period, nine from the Ptolemaic Period and seventeen from the Roman Period. Given the different cohort sizes and the wide variations seen in mummification practices within each era the comparison of techniques necessary to detect any influence from foreign invasion must be viewed with caution. Comparison between Middle and New Kingdom mummies excludes any influences that may have occurred in the Second Intermediate Period. For this reason it will not be undertaken.

Furthermore, the following statements indicate change that MAY have been the result of foreign influence, but there is no direct proof of this influence as opposed to the mere passage of time. However, the possibility of the influence of foreign intrusion cannot be ignored in this or any other culture.

9.9.2 New Kingdom to Third Intermediate Period

The comparison between the New Kingdom and the Third Intermediate Period uses the discussion on pages 197-203. There may be only two examples of New Kingdom mummies, these being Mummies III and XLVIII. The latter is of a young child with significant damage to the head, making analysis impossible. There is evidence of incomplete evisceration via a left flank incision. The other mummy is from Dynasty 20 or 21 exhibiting limited perforation of the ethmoid but thorough excerebration, retention of the eyes which were covered with eye plates, subcutaneous packing of the neck and evisceration via a left flank incision with retention of the mediastinum and return of the viscera after the introduction of resin.

Dynasty 22 commenced with the reign of Sheshonq I, a Libyan from the tribe of the Meshwesh (Shaw, 2000: 334). The Libyans then ruled Egypt until Dynasty 25, when the Nubians conquered the land.

The transition to the Third Intermediate Period saw the use of neck packing in many cases along with the use of a more horizontal approach to excerebration. Packing of the opened eye globe and of the mouth was also used in many cases. Although complete evisceration was the more common procedure, retention of the mediastinum was used on occasions. Return of the viscera, as either loose or as canopic packages was common. Foreign material – either resin or, more commonly, granular material (possibly earth, mud or saw-dust with resin) was used to pack the body cavity.

Although the numbers do not support the concept of 'proof' there is a strong argument to claim that these changes in mortuary practice were the effect of Libyan influence.

9.9.3 Dynasty 25

The conquest of Egypt by the Nubians of Dynasty 25 led to another change in funerary practice. The more vertical approach to trans-nasal excerebration was re-introduced but with a retention of the practice of cranial cavity

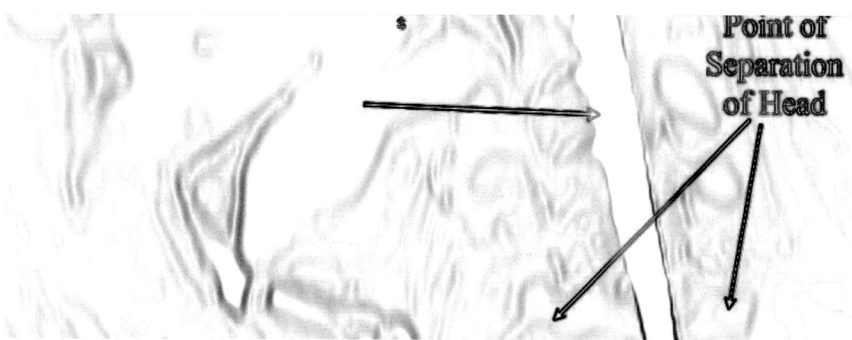

FIG. 9.17 SAGITTAL VIEW OF CERVICAL REGION - METAL ROD AND POINT OF SEPARATION OF THE HEAD FROM THE TORSO (AFTER IEM IMAGE)

packing. The eyes continued to be opened and packed. The mouth was packed but the neck packing used far less often. Complete evisceration was used more than the incomplete procedure and the viscera were returned either loose or as canopic packages. Packing material was used in the torso.

9.9.4 The Late Period

Dynasty 26 is the only representation of the Late Period in this series. This dynasty represents the rule of Egypt from Sais, in the Delta, by pharaohs at first controlled by the Assyrians although they later became totally independent. The eight mummies from this period show evidence of the continuing use of excerebration via a variety of routes from the traditional vertical trans-nasal route through the use of a more horizontal one via the sphenoid to the use of the trans-foraminal route. Cranial cavity packing was used less frequently but the eyes remained frequently packed, as was the mouth. Subcutaneous neck packing was no longer used. Evisceration continued to be performed via the left flank with (in this series) one example of an additional perineal route. The mediastinum was retained in all cases and the viscera returned to the body cavity. The only obvious change was mediastinal retention.

9.9.5 The Ptolemaic Period

This period followed conquest and subsequent rule by the Macedonians. Excerebration continued by the 'vertical' route of trans-nasal excerebration but with the much more frequent use of resin as a cranial filler. The eyes continued to be retained but were not opened and packed or covered with eye plates. Mouths were packed in just over half the cases. The left flank incision continued to be used but with the use of the perineal approach becoming more common. However, this latter fact needs to be seen in the context that most of these mummies came from Akhmim. Retention of the mediastinum continued but only in cases of the exclusive use of the perineal approach. Body cavity packing continued to be used in the majority of cases.

9.9.6 The Roman Period

Conquest by the Romans in 30 BC was followed by Roman rule until the fourth century AD. The seventeen mummies from the period provide a useful reflection on embalming practices with the introduction of a lack of excerebration coupled with a lack of evisceration. This and other changes are often interpreted as a 'decline' in mummification practices (Ikram and Dodson, 1998: 129). However, the fact that these mummies have survived to the present day does not accord well with this view. There certainly was a change in funerary practice but this does not necessarily mean a decline. The whole subject is discussed in section 9.7.

9.10 Practicalities from a surgeon's aspect

Many things have been written about the techniques used by the ancient Egyptians during mummification but certain practicalities have been ignored.

The first of these is the subject of trans-foraminal excerebration. Some authors have suggested that the absence of the brain combined with the presence of an intact cribriform plate should be taken as evidence of trans-foraminal excerebration.

Considering the incision needed to access the foramen magnum (along with the necessary displacement of the skull from the cervical spine) it can readily be seen that inevitably there will be considerable disturbance of the atlanto-occipital region, which would not go unnoticed. It is, therefore, not a concept that can be accepted in the future.

Turning now to the size of abdominal incision, it has to be accepted that to perform a proper evisceration, including that of the thoracic cavity as far superiorly as the suprapleural membrane, it would be necessary to introduce the operator's forearm almost as far as the elbow. To do this would entail the need to pass the proximal forearm through the incision. The measurement of the circumference of a 5ft 4ins female reveals this to be twenty-two centimetres. The likelihood of a male in ancient Egypt having such a slim arm is questionable. However, even with this measurement and allowing for a degree of skin and body wall elasticity, an incision of nine or ten centimetres would be required.

Consideration of the perineal approach to evisceration, if used alone, leads to the inevitable conclusion that access to any viscera beyond arm's length would be difficult if not impossible, unless instrumentation was used. It is therefore no surprise that evisceration through this route exclusively, often resulted in the retention of the mediastinum.

Excerebration or evisceration through the accepted routes means that most procedures were performed blind, with or without instruments which had themselves to be used blind. The implication is that the people who performed these tasks were extremely skillful and, probably, had a considerable knowledge of human anatomy.

Chapter Ten

Conclusions

10.1 Introduction

One of the objectives of this study was to obtain and analyse the CT scan images of ancient Egyptian human mummies thus permitting a search for patterns of the embalming techniques used. This objective has been achieved for fifty-nine of the sixty mummy images obtained.

It was a second intention to search for patterns of embalming methods associated with eras and locations. Although as previously noted there can be no certainty over the dating of some of the mummies, and sample size does not permit 'proof', strong indications of such patterns have been identified.

With the use of modern medical imaging techniques it has been possible to analyse the anatomical changes to the body in more detail than previously. As a result of this greater detail, the demonstrated minor differences in technique probably reflect the individual variations of each embalming workshop. This does not appear to have prevented the acceptance by those workshops of the general principles necessary to perform 'proper' mummification. However, the common themes previously assigned to each era have, in large measure, been confirmed.

The changes seen relating to different eras indicate that the overall theme of mummification practices did change with time. It is also noted that different locations seem to have had their own understanding of what constituted a 'proper' process. An example of this is the prevalence of perineal approach to evisceration seen in Akhmim. However, the caveat is that the numbers are small at present and a larger study needs to be performed to confirm or refute this observation.

Some previously described observations related to trans-foraminal excerebration (Wade et al., 2010 and 2011 and Wade and Nelson, 2013) have been challenged and a previously unreported technique associated with the Roman Period has been revealed, as has the indication of an emerging pattern of a specific technique associated with Akhmim.

A general and obvious statement to make is that in this study all the evidence supports the concept that pre- and post-desiccation procedures were performed with the body supine.

A précis of the findings related to head and torso (body) will now follow.

10.2 The head

The greater detailed analysis of excerebration routes has revealed that the more horizontal approach resulting in perforation of the sphenoid as well as, or as an alternative to, the ethmoid was used in a wide variety of eras and locations (see Tables 10.1 and 10.2). However, it is shown that this more horizontal route resulted in more effective removal of brain tissue only if the resulting perforation was larger and involved both structures. In contrast, complete lack of excerebration, although more common in the Roman Period is also seen in the Late and Ptolemaic Periods. It is a technique seen in 10% of the cases in this series but is not associated with any particular location or age group. If the ethmoid and sphenoid perforations are combined to reflect the 'horizontal' route the results are shown in Tables 10.3 and 10.4. To eliminate the effects of different cohort sizes these results are shown as percentages of each cohort in Table 10.5. This shows that although the horizontal route was indeed used over a wide range of eras, there was an increased usage in Dynasty 22 and a further increase in the Ptolemaic Period. Lack of excerebration is not associated with a lack of attention to mummification in other areas of the body.

ERA/DYN	Ethmoid	Eth.+Sph.	Sphenoid	None
MK	0	0	0	0
D18	0	0	0	0
D20	1	0	0	0
D21	1	0	0	0
3IP	3	1	0	0
D22	3	3	1	0
D25	3	1	0	0
D26	4	0	1	1
Ptolemaic	5	3	0	1
Roman	9	1	1	4

TABLE 10.1 STRUCTURE PERFORATED DURING TRANS-NASAL EXCEREBRATION

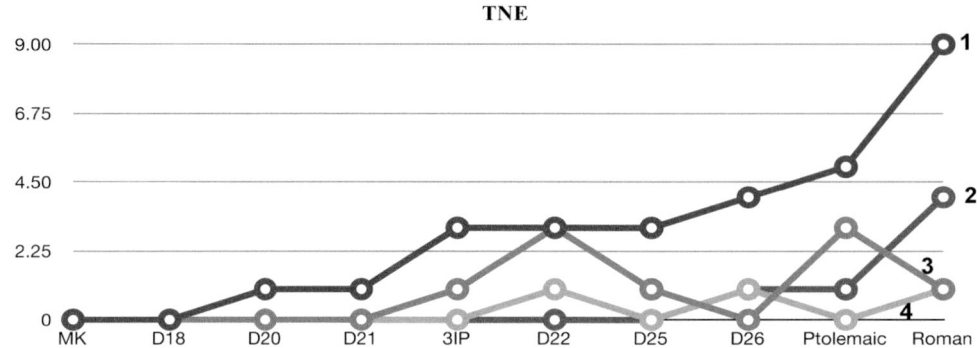

Table 10.2 Structure perforated during Trans-nasal Excerebration.
1 = Ethmoid perforation; 2 = No Excerebration; 3 = Ethmoid and Sphenoid; 4 = Sphenoid alone

ERA/DYN	Vertical	Horizontal	None
MK	0	0	0
D18	0	0	0
D20	1	0	0
D21	1	0	0
3IP	3	1	0
D22	3	4	0
D25	3	1	0
D26	4	1	1
Ptolemaic	5	3	1
Roman	9	2	4

Table 10.3 Vertical 'strike' c.f. Horizontal 'strike'

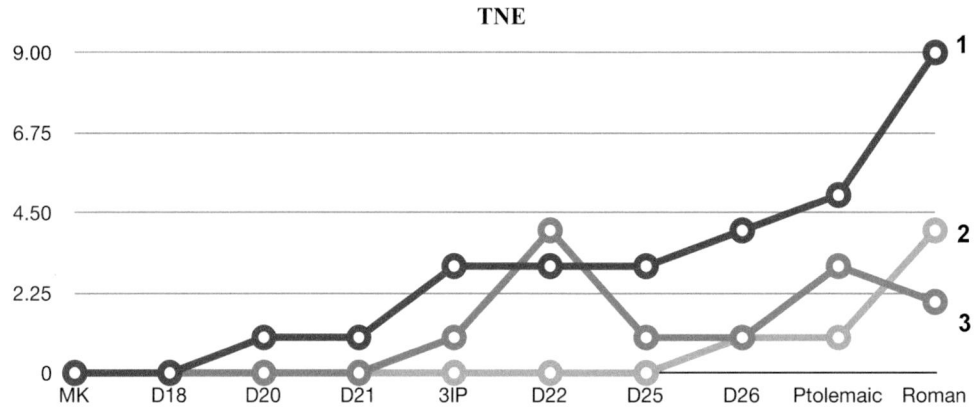

Table 10.4 Vertical 'strike' c.f. Horizontal 'strike'
1 = Vertical 'strike'; 2 = No excerebration; 3 = Horizontal 'strike'

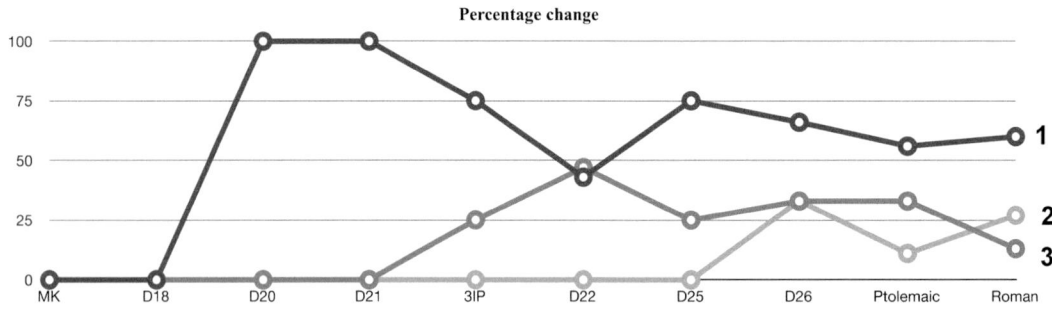

Table 10.5 Change in percentage of vertical c.f. horizontal 'strike'
key as in Table 10.4.

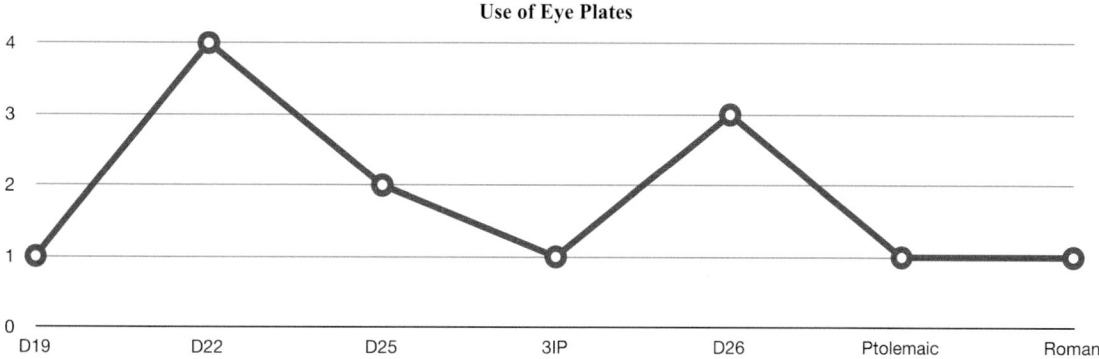

TABLE 10.6 FREQUENCY OF EYE PLATE USAGE

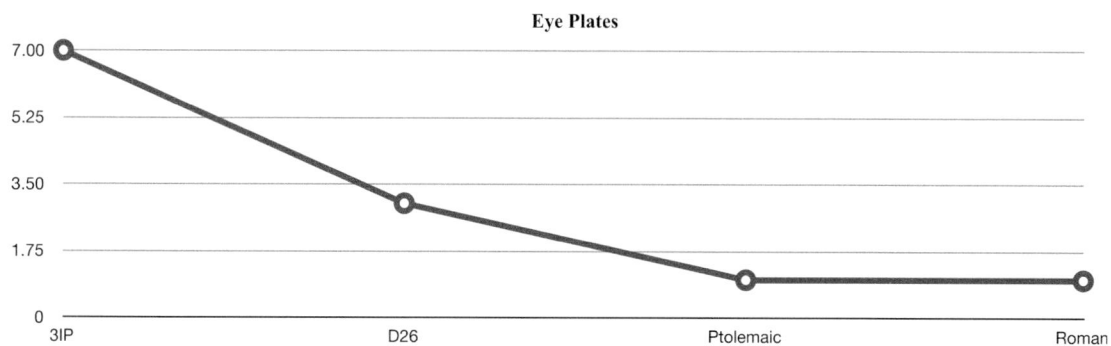

TABLE 10.7 REVISED FREQUENCY OF EYE PLATE USAGE

The more unusual routes used for excerebration are seen in mummies from Dynasty 22 Deir el Bahari (trans-basal) and Dynasty 26 Thebes (trans-orbital). Although the use of more esoteric routes is identified, the small number and distribution to possibly slightly different locations and points in history makes interpretation difficult. It is noted that the absence of brain tissue combined with the absence of a trans-nasal approach cannot be assumed to mean that a trans-foraminal approach has been used. However, the exposure of the perforated eyes (the route used for excerebration) in the case of Mummy XIV is unusual if it is accepted that one of the principles of mummification was to preserve the body 'intact' for the afterlife. It might reasonably be expected that the distorted eyes would at least have been covered by eye plates ('false eyes'). As the mummy has been unwrapped it is possible that eye plates were used but have been removed at a later date. The analysis of more mummies may reveal further examples of similar approaches to excerebration and help to explain the phenomenon.

The trans-foraminal route has been found in only four cases in this series and occurs in mummies from a wide range of eras and locations, with no particular pattern. The use of more 'esoteric' routes for excerebration appears to be more common in children. Where excerebration was performed it was complete in 80% of cases and in the remainder only a small amount of cerebral tissue persisted.

The method of treating the eyes has not been comprehensively addressed previously. The method of inaction (that is retention with desiccation alone) is found in a wide range of locations and eras in this series. The addition of a 'surgical procedure'; that is opening the globe of the eye and packing it with linen; is found most frequently in Theban mummies but covers the years from Dynasty 22 to the Roman Period. The only outlier in this series of twelve mummies is one where the origin of the mummy is designated as from either Thebes or Akhmim (see Table 9.12 – P 229).

The frequency of the use of packing in both the eyes and the mouth increases with the age of the individual in this series.

The use of 'false eyes' or eye plates is only found in mummies from Thebes but the timescale of the use of this method extended from Dynasty 20/21 to Dynasty 26 (spanning nearly four hundred years). See Table 10.6.

If Dynasties 22 and 25 are combined with the mummy from the Third Intermediate Period a different picture emerges. This is shown in Table 10.7.

Although the majority usage (five) of eye plates was in cases where the eyes had been opened and packed, there were two other mummies where the eyes were not opened (these mummies were from Dynasty 20/21 and Dynasty

22) and a further case; Mummy XXIX (from Dynasty 22 Thebes) where removal of the eyes was followed by packing of the orbits with linen and then covering the linen with eye plates. Again the cohort is small and further research may add more evidence to this topic.

The treatment of the mouth varied considerably with twenty-two of the fifty-five cases available for comment being empty (40%). The remaining 60% had some packing, linen being the commonest (24% of the total), the other cases having a combination of substances. There was no correlation between techniques of mouth packing and era or location.

The only examples of subcutaneous packing in this series were in the neck. All eight were from Thebes and the majority from the Third Intermediate Period.

10.3 The body

In general terms there are four different approaches seen to evisceration. These are an abdominal incision, a perineal approach, a combination of both routes and no attempt at evisceration via a 'surgical' route. The first three approaches have been described in the past and the perineal route has been associated with elite female burials by Wade and Watson (Wade and Watson vs.). That picture is not confirmed in this series. The perineal approach is seen in fourteen mummies (23% of the cohort) and is present in mummies from five different locations and from eras as diverse as Dynasty 21 and the Roman Period. The overall bias is towards increased use of this approach in the more southerly cities of Akhmim and Thebes and a more frequent use after the Ptolemaic Period (see Tables 10.8 and 10.9). When the influence of cohort size is minimized by using percentages, the result is shown in Table 10.10. If the mummies from Dynasties 22 and 25 are combined with those designated from the Third Intermediate Period, the result is as shown in Tables 10.11 and 10.12. The high rate of usage of the perineal approach in Akhmim compared to the rate in Thebes may have some association with the cult of Min, although this is, at present, far from proven. The analysis of more mummies from Akhmim would help to resolve this dilemma.

Regardless of the 'surgical' route used for evisceration there is wide variation in the subsequent diligence of evisceration with some mummies being completely eviscerated and others having evidence of some viscera being left in situ to be desiccated. There is no particular pattern to this practice other than a correlation between retention of mediastinal structures and a perineal approach and between retention of pelvic structures and an abdominal incision. The practical considerations of these findings are discussed in section 9.10.

Canopic packages were found in twenty-two of the thirty-eight mummies with an abdominal incision and of these twenty had convincing evidence of viscera within them.

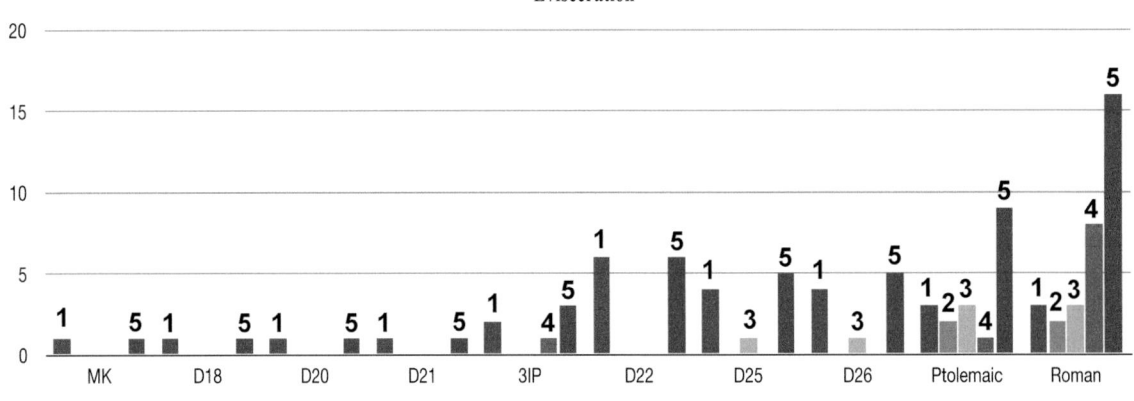

TABLE 10.8 EVISCERATION ROUTES.
1 = FLANK INCISION; 2 = PERINEAL; 3 = COMBINED; 4 = NO EVISCERATION; 5 = TOTAL IN EACH ERA.

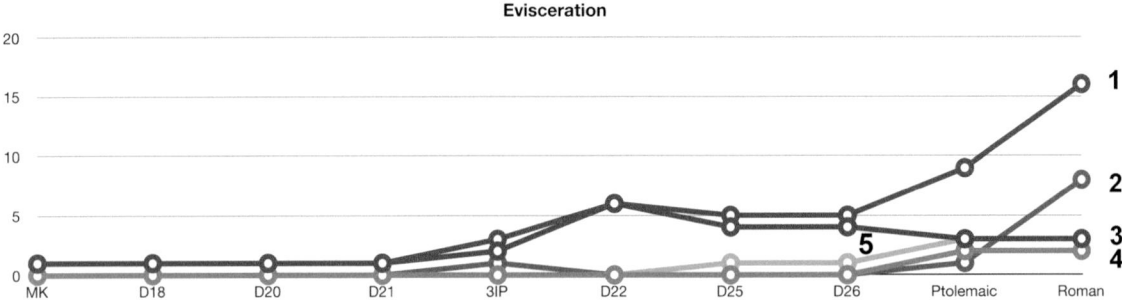

TABLE 10.9 EVISCERATION ROUTES.
1 = TOTAL IN EACH ERA; 2 = NO EVISCERATION; 3 = FLANK INCISION; 4 = PERINEAL; 5 = COMBINED.

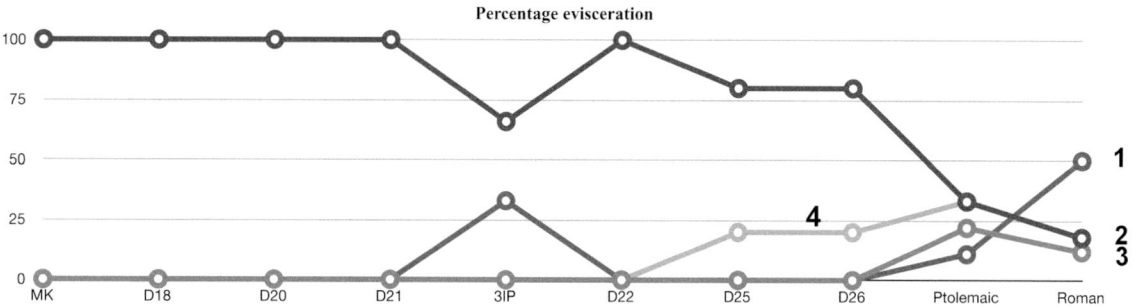

TABLE 10.10 EVISCERATION ROUTES AS PERCENTAGES OF EACH COHORT.
1 = NO EVISCERATION; 2 = FLANK INCISION; 3 = PERINEAL; 4 = COMBINED.

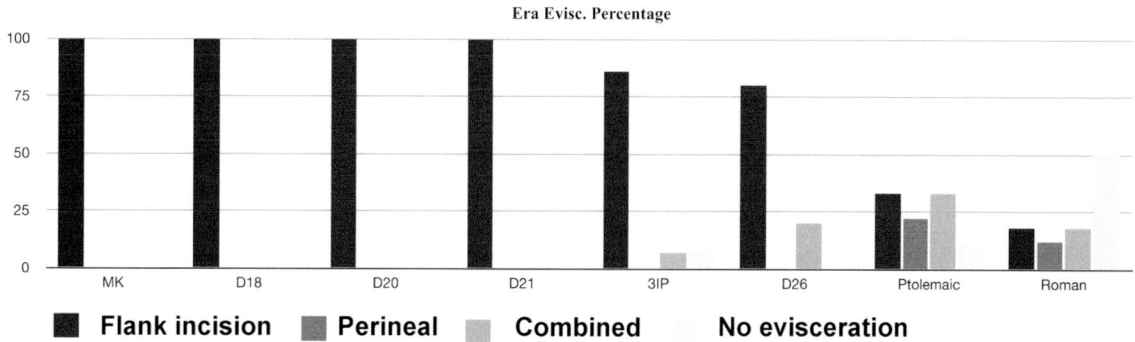

TABLE 10.11 EVISCERATION ROUTES AS PERCENTAGES OF EACH ERA.

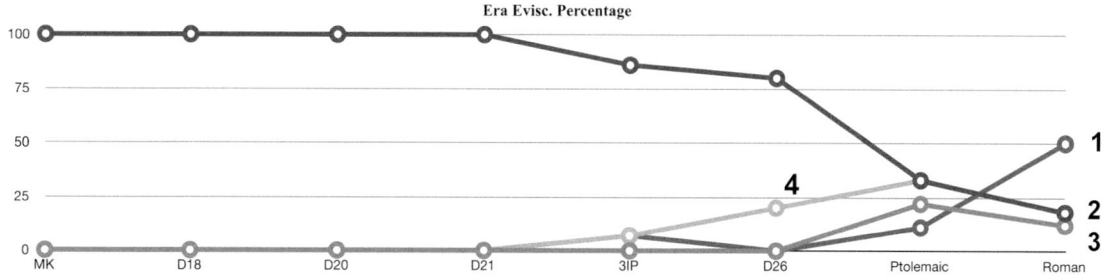

TABLE 10.12 EVISCERATION ROUTES AS PERCENTAGES OF EACH ERA.
1 = NO EVISCERATION; 2 = FLANK INCISION; 3 = PERINEAL; 4 = COMBINED.

One of the most striking findings in this series is the high rate of thoracic disruption and distortion in the Roman Period. There were seventeen mummies from this period. Thirteen of these exhibited compression of the chest wall. The strong association of this finding with an origin in Fayum or Hawara is noticeable as is the association with adult mummies (see Tables 10.13 and 10.14). Another feature of this technique is the high percentage of costo-vertebral dislocation (77%). In the absence of a local incision, the implication is that the collagen in the ligaments of these joints was weakened chemically. The fact that natron contains calcium carbonate, a strongly alkaline substance, and that the region of these joints would preferentially be exposed to natron and cadaveric fluids (in the supine position) may explain the process. However, unless the nature of natron was altered in the Roman Period or the exposure to it was altered, the addition of 'compressive forces' would need to be an innovative technique added in this era.

10.4 Caveats

Although a considerable effort was required to collect the sixty mummy image files in this series, the small cohort sizes found when the sample was broken down into eras and locations make firm conclusions difficult. There are strong indications of definitive findings, but these must be viewed with a degree of caution. The smaller the cohort size the less representative it may be.

Assigning a firm date (Kingdom, Period or Dynasty) to a mummy from the mummification techniques used is fraught with danger because of the varying techniques used and the influence of individual workshop practices on those techniques. However, there appears to be confirmation of

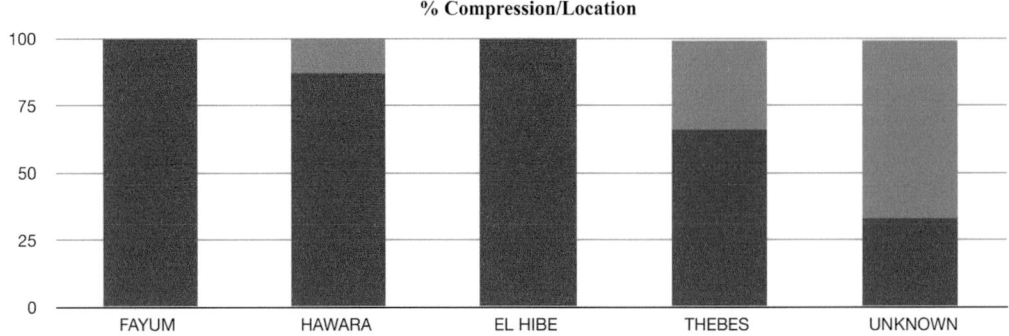

TABLE 10.13 INCIDENCE OF CHEST COMPRESSION.
DARK GREY = COMPRESSED; LIGHT GREY = NO COMPRESSION.

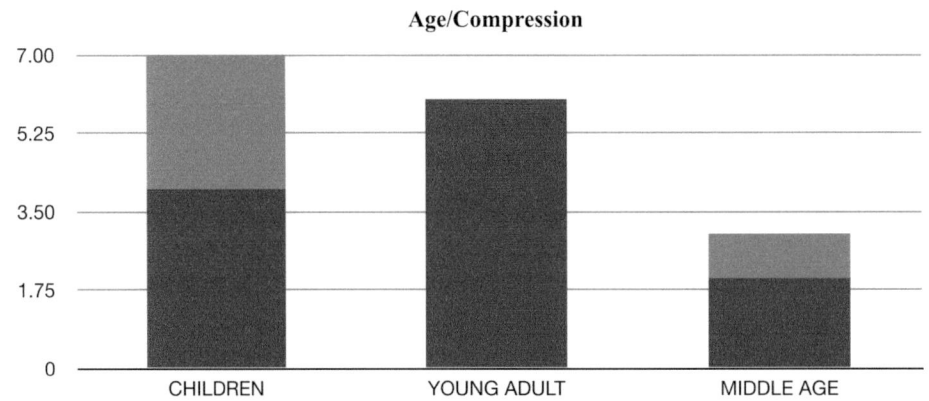

TABLE 10.14 INCIDENCE OF CHEST COMPRESSION.
DARK GREY = COMPRESSED; LIGHT GREY = NO COMPRESSION.

the well-established themes of mummification technique previously assigned to various eras, although there are significant variations on those 'themes' imposed by the workshops. Furthermore, there is support for the fact that foreign influence played a real part in the development of those 'themes'.

10.5 The Future

In view of the comments on cohort size it is intended to continue research in the subject of CT scan analysis of ancient Egyptian human mummies, with the objective of obtaining sufficient material to form more robust opinions regarding the mummification techniques employed. Clearly this will require the cooperation of institutions holding the mummies and of CT departments in hospitals. The feasibility of using mobile CT machines is also being explored. Publication of the new mummification techniques described in this document is also planned.

In general it may well become necessary to review the medical image material held relating to each mummy and decide on the need to perform more up to date investigations in the light of advances in medical imaging technology. It is arguable that this exercise should be performed on all image data relating to mummies. Both medical image acquisition techniques and the image manipulation software would be considered during such an exercise.

Bibliography

Adams C.V.A., 1990: Shepenmut – Priestess of Thebes. Her mummification and autopsy. *Discussion in Egyptology 16.* Oxford

Adam A, Dixon AK, eds. 2008: *Grainger and Allison's Diagnostic Radiology: A Textbook of Medical Imaging.* 5th ed. New York.

Aufderheide A.C., and Rodriguez-Martin C.1998: *The Cambridge Encyclopaedia of Human Paleopathology.* Cambridge

Aufderheide A.C., 2003: *The Scientific Study of Mummies,* Cambridge.

Bagnall R S., Frier B W., 1994: *The Demography of Roman Egypt.* Cambridge. (P100).

Bogen E. Pasternack D., 1954: Pleural adhesions, Their Incidence and Significance as Shown in Autopsies at the Los Angeles General Hospital, 1911-1952 *Chest.* 1954;25(2):166-171.

Bostock J, Roley H.T., 1855: *Pliny the Elder, The Natural History.* London.

Brier B., Wade R.S., 1997 : The Use of Natron in Human Mummification: A Modern Experiment. *ZAS* 124 (1997).

Brier B., Wade R.S., 1999 : Surgical Procedures during ancient Egyptian Mummification. *ZAS* 126 (1999).

Buckley S.A., Evershed R.P., 2001: Organic chemistry of embalming agents in Pharaonic and Graeco-Roman mummies. *Nature* 413.

Budge E A W., 1899: *Egyptian Magic.* London.

Capart J., Gardiner A H. and van de Walle B., 1936: New Light on the Ramesside Tomb-Robberies. *The Journal of Egyptian Archeology, Vol. 22 No. 2 (Dec. 1936).*

Cardiac Vascular and Thoracic Surgery Associates http://www.cvtsa.com Accessed on 1/12/13.

Cavka M., Petaros A., Boscic D., Kavur L., Janovic I., Despot R., Trajkovic J., Brkljacic B., 2012: CT-guided Endoscopic Recovery of a Foreign Object from the Cranial Cavity of an Ancient Egyptian Mummy. *Radiographics.* 32.

Chhem R.K., 2006: Paleoradiology: imaging disease in mummies and ancient skeletons. *Skeletal Radiology* 35.

Cicero. *Tusculanae Disputationes. Book 1. XLV.* The Loeb Classical Library Edition (Online. Accessed 23/7/14).

Clarysse W, Depauw M., 1973: *Zeitschrift für Papyrologie und Epigraphik.* Bonn.

Cobbold, R. S. C. (2007): *Foundations of Biomedical Ultrasound.* Oxford.

Cockburn,A.,CockburnE.,Reyman,T.A., 1998: *Mummies, Disease and Ancient Cultures.* Cambridge

Concise Oxford Dictionary , 1982, Oxford

Corcoran L.H. and Svoboda M., 2010: *Herakleides a Portrait Mummy from Roman Egypt.* Los Angeles.

Cull P., 1989: *The Source Book of Medical Illustration.* Carnforth.

David, A.R. (ed.), 1979: *Manchester Museum Mummy Project, multidisciplinary research on ancient Egyptian mummified remains.* Manchester.

David, A.R., 2002: *Religion and Magic in Ancient Egypt.* London.

Diodorus Siculus., *The Library of History.* Book 1, 69.

Dirnhofer R., Jackowski C., Vock P., Potter K.,Thali M.J., 2006: VIRTOPSY: Minimally Invasive, Imaging-guided Virtual Autopsy. *Radiographics.*

Dodson A., 2014: http://www.bris.ac.uk/archanth/research/dodson/ecpuk_files/exeter. Accessed 28/6/14.

Donchin Y, Rivkind AI, Bar-Ziv J, Hiss J, Almog J, Drescher M., 1994: Utility of postmortem computed tomography in trauma victims. *Journal of Trauma. 1994 Oct;37(4).*

Donoghue H D., Lee O Y-C., Minnikin D E., Besra G S., Taylor J H and Spigelman M., 2010: Tuberculosis in Dr Granville's mummy: a molecular re-examination of the earliest known Egyptian mummy to be scientifically examined and given a medical diagnosis. *Proceedings of the Royal Society B. vol.277 no. 1678.*

Dowson V.H.W., 1982: Date production and protection with special reference to North Africa and the Near East. *FAO Technical Bulletin No. 35.*

Dunand F.and Lichtenberg R, 1998: *Mummies and Death in Egypt.* New York

Eaton-Krauss M., 2008: Embalming Caches. *The Journal of Egyptian Archeology. Vol.94.*

Firkin. B.G., Whitworth, J.A. : *Dictionary of Medical Eponyms*, 1989, Carnforth,.

Gostner P., Bonelli M., Pertner P., Graefen A. and Zink A., 2013: New radiological approach for analysis and identification of foreign objects in ancient and historic mummies. *Journal of Archaeological Science. 40 (2013).*

Greulich W.W. and Pyle S., 1959: *Radiographic Atlas of Skeletal Development of the Hand and Wrist, 2nd edition.* Stanford

Gray P.H.K, 1971: Artificial eyes in Mummies. *The Journal of Egyptian Archaeology. Vol.57. Aug. 1971.*

Gray P.H.K., 1972: Notes concerning the position of arms and hands of mummies with a view to possible dating of the specimen. *The Journal of Egyptian Archaeology. Vol.58. Aug. 1972.*

Gupta R., Markowitz Y., Berman L., Chapman P., 2008: High-Resolution Imaging of an Ancient Egyptian Mummified Head: New Insights into the Mummification Process. *American Journal of Neurology.* 29

Herodotus, *The Histories* 2: 86. Translation by de Selincourt (1954: 115)

Hounsfield.G.N., 1973: Computerized transverse axial scanning (tomography): Part 1. Description of the system. *British Journal of Radiology (1973) 46.*

Hounsfield G. N., 1980: Computed Medical Imaging Nobel Lecture, 8th. December 1979. *Journal of Radiology. 1980 Jun-Jul;61(6-7).*

Ikram S., 2005: *Divine Creatures: Animal Mummies in ancient Egypt.* New York.

Ikram S., Dodson A., 1998: *The Mummy in Ancient Egypt.* London.

Isherwood, I., Jarvis.H. and Fawcitt.R.A. Radiology of the Manchester Mummies. In David A.R,(ed.), 1979: *The Manchester Museum Mummy Project.* Manchester

Janak J., Landgrafova R., 2011: New evidence on the Mummification Process in the Late Period. Hieratic Texts from the Embalmers' Cache in the Shaft Tomb of Menekhibnekau at Abusir. In Barta M., Coppens F., Krejci J. (ed) *Abusir and Saqqara in the year 2010/1.* Prague.

Johnston T.B., Davies D.V. and Davies F., 1958: *Gray's Anatomy. Descriptive and Applied.* London.

Jones H.L., 1917: *Strabo The Geography.* Harvard.

Karlik S. J., Bartha R., Kennedy K., and Chhem R., 2007. MRI and Multinuclear MR Spectroscopy of 3,200-Year-Old Egyptian Mummy Brain, 2007, *American Journal of Roentgenology,* Aug, 189: W105 - W110.

Kuffer A., Siegmann R., 2007: *Unter Dem Schutz Der Himmels-Gotten. Agyptische Sarge Mumien und Masken in der Schweiz.* Zurich.

Last R.J., 1966: *Anatomy Regional and Applied,* London

Leek F.F., 1969 : The Problem of Brain Removal During Embalming by the Ancient Egyptians. *JEA* 55 (1969).

Loynes R D., Ruhli F, David R, Chamberlain A, 2013: *Novel Medical and Egyptological findings in a Swiss CT scan data collection of Ancient Egyptian mummies.* Podium presentation. 8th World Congress on Mummy Studies. Rio. August 2013.

Macke A., Macke-Ribet C. and Connan J., 2002: *Ta Set Neferou, Une Necropole de Thebes-Ouest et son Histoire,* V. Momification, Chimie des Baumes, Anthropologie, Paleopathologie (Cairo 2002).

Magellan Geographic, 2014: www.maps.com. Accessed on 6/1/14.

Marx M. and Haney D'Auria S. : 1986, CT Examination of Eleven Egyptian Mummies. *RadioGraphics* Volume 6, Number 2 March: 321- 330

Maspero G., 1875: *Memoire sur quelques Papyrus du Louvre.* Paris.

Ohrstrom L., Bitzer A., Walter M., Ruhli F.J., 2010: Terahertz Imaging of ancient mummies and bone, *American Journal of Physical Anthropology* Vol. 142, Issue 3.

ONS, Office for National Statistics: ons.gov.uk. [Accessed December 2013].

Ouellette N. and Bourbeau R., 2011: Changes in the age-at-death distribution in four low mortality countries: A nonparametric approach. *Demographic Research.* Vol.25. 595-628.

PACS 2011. Available at <URL:http://www.connectingforhealth.nhs.uk/systemsandservices/pacs [Accessed 10 June 2011]

Pahor, A.L. and Cole.J., 1995. The Birmingham Mummy: the first torticollis in history. *The Journal of Laryngology and Otology.* April, Vol 109, 273-276

Panzer S., Borumandi F., Wanek J., Shved N., Colacicco G and Ruhli F., 2013: 'Modeling ancient Egyptian embalming': radiological assessment of experimentally mummified human tissue by CT and MRI. *Skeletal Radiology. Nov. 2013. Vol.42. Issue 11.*

Peedikayil F C., 2011: Delayed Tooth Eruption. *E-Journal of Dentistry.* Oct.-Dec. 2011 Vol 1 Issue 4> www.ejournalofdentistry.com

Peet T E., 1915a: The Great Tomb Robberies of the Ramesside Age. *The Journal of Egyptian Archaeology, Vol. 2 No. 3 (Jun 1915).*

Peet T E., 1915b: The Great Tomb Robberies of the Ramesside Age. *The Journal of Egyptian Archaeology, Vol. 2 No. 4 (Oct 1915).*

Peet T E., 1925a: Fresh Light on the Tomb Robberies of the Twentieth Dynasty at Thebes: Some New Papyri in London and Turin. *The Journal of Egyptian Archeology, Vol. 11 No. 1-2 (Apr. 1925).*

Peet T E., 1925b: Fresh Light on the Tomb Robberies of the Twentieth Dynasty at Thebes: An Additional Note. *The Journal of Egyptian Archeology, Vol. 11 No. 3-4 (Oct. 1925).*

Perthes. G., 1910: Uber Arthritis deformans juvenilis. *Deutsche Zeitschr. f. Chirurgie.* Vol. 107: 111

Pettigrew T.J., 1834 : *History of Egyptian Mummies.* London

Plutarch, 1928: *Septum Sapientium Convivium.* As published in Volume 2 of the Loeb Classical Library Edition (Online. Accessed 23/7/14).

Raven. M.J. and Taconis.W.K., 2005: Egyptian Mummies. *Radiological Atlas of the Collections in the National Museum of Antiquities in Leiden.* Turnhout, Belgium

Roaf R., 1966: *Scoliosis.* Edinburgh and London

Ruhli.F.J., Chhem.R.K. and Böni.T., 2004. Diagnostic paleoradiology of mummified tissue: interpretation and pitfalls. *Journal of the American College of Radiology,* 55(4), 218-227

Shaw. I. (ed.), 2000: *The Oxford History of Ancient Egypt.*

Scheuer L. and Black S., 2000: *Developmental Juvenile Osteology.* London.

Snape S, 2011: *Ancient Egyptian Tombs: The Culture of Life and Death.* Chichester.

Sutton, D., 1969: *A Textbook of Radiology.* London

Taylor, J.H., 2001: *Death and the afterlife in Ancient Egypt.* London

Taylor, J.H., 2004 : *Mummy: the inside story.* London

Taylor J.H., 2010: *Journey Through the Afterlife. Ancient Egyptian Book of the Dead.* London.

Taylor, R.E. 1985: 'The beginnings of radiocarbon dating in American Antiquity: a historical perspective'. *American Antiquity: Journal of the Society for American Archaeology* 50 (2): 309–325

Taylor T., 1823: *Porphyry, On abstinence from animal food.* Library of ancient Texts Online. Accessed 23/7/14.

thefullwiki.org

The British Museum http://www.britishmuseum.org : accessed 29/9/13

Tyldesley, J., 2010: *Myths and Legends of Ancient Egypt*, London.

Vallebona A., Una modalità di tecnica per la dissociazione radiografica delle ombre applicata allo studio del cranio. 1930: *Communication to the ninth Italian Congress of Radiology, Torino, May*

Wade AD., Nelson AJ. and Garvin GJ., 2010: Another Hole in the Head? Brain Treatment in Ancient Egyptian Mummies. *Anthropology Presentations.* Paper 5.

Wade,A.D., Nelson,A.J., Garvin,G.J., 2011: A synthetic radiological study of brain treatment in ancient Egyptian mummies. *Journal of Comparative Human Biology,* 62.

Wade A.D., Nelson A.J., 2013: Radiological evaluation of the evisceration tradition in ancient Egyptian mummies. *Journal of Comparative Human Biology,* 64. Issue1.

Wanek J, Speller R, Rühli F., 2013: Direct action of radiation on mummified cells: modeling of computed tomography by Monte Carlo algorithms *Radiat Enviro Biophys, 2013 Apr 25.*

Watson E.J. and Myers M. The Mummy of Baket-en-her-nakht in the Hancock Museum, 1993: A Radiological Update *The Journal of Egyptian Archaeology*, Vol. 79, 179-187

Appendix I

Museums and other institutions contacted

Aberdeen, Aberdeen Art Gallery and Museum - www.aagm.co.uk

Adelaide, South Australian Museum - www.samuseum.sa.gov.au

Amsterdam, Amsterdam Museum - www.amsterdammuseum.nl/en

Atlanta, Emery University - www.emory.edu

Barnsley, Barnsley Museums - www.barnsley-museums.com

Belfast, National Museums Northern Ireland - www.nmni.com/um

Blackpool, Blackpool Museum and Art Gallery - www.world-guides.com/.../blackpool/blackpool_museums.html

Berlin, Egyptian Museum - egyptian-museum-berlin.com

Blackburn, Blackburn Museum and Art Gallery - museum@blackburn.gov.uk

Bonn, Kunstmuseum- kunstmuseum-bonn.de

Bradford, Bradford Museum and Art Gallery - www.bradfordmuseums.org

Brighton, Brighton Museum and Art Gallery - www.brighton-hove rpml.org.uk/Museums

Bristol, Bristol Museum and Art Gallery - www.bristol.gov.uk/museums

Burnley, Burnley Art Gallery and Museum, Towneley Hall - www.burnley.gov.uk/residents/towneley

Bury, Bury Art Museum - www.bury.gov.uk/index.aspx?articleid=2537

Cambridge, The Fitzwilliam Museum -www.cam.ac.uk/museums

Cardiff, National Museum - www.museumwales.ac.uk/en/cardiff

Canterbury, Canterbury Museums - www.canterbury.co.uk/museums

Carlisle, Tullie house Museum and Art Galery - www.tulliehouse.co.uk

Cheltenham, The Wilson - www.cheltenhammuseum.org.uk

Chester, Grosvenor Museum - www.cheshirewestmuseums.org

Chesterfield, Chesterfield Museum - www.chesterfield.gov.uk/Chesterfield-Museum

Chicago, The Field Museum - Fieldmuseum.org

Copenhagen, Ny Carlsberg Glyptotek - www.glyptoteket.dk

Coventry, Herbert Art Gallery and Museum - www.theherbert.org

Denver, Denver Museums - www.denver.com/museums

Derby, Derby Museum and Art Gallery - www.derbymuseums.org

Dover, Dover Museum - www.dovermuseum.co.uk

Dudley, Dudley Museum and Art Gallery - www.dudley.gov.uk/see-and-do/museums

Dundee, The McManus - www.mcmanus.co.uk

Edinburgh, City Art Centre - www.edinburghmuseums.org.uk

Exeter, Royal Albert Memorial Museum and Art Gallery - www.rammuseum.org.uk

Glasgow, Kelvingrove Art Gallery and museum - www.glasgowlife.org.uk/museums

Gloucester, Gloucester City Museum and Art Gallery - www.thecityofgloucester.co.uk/.../museums-and-exhibitions

Grantham, Grantham Museum - www.granthammuseum.org.uk

Harrogate, Mercer Art Gallery - www.harrogate.gov.uk/musm

Hastings, Hastings museum and Art Gallery - www.hmag.org.uk

Hildersheim, Roemer und Pelizaeus Museum - www.rpmuseum.de

Hull, Hull an east riding Museum - www.hullcc.gov.uk/museums

Ipswich, Colchester and Ipswich Museums - www.cimuseums.org.uk

Lancaster, Lancaster City Museum - www.lancaster.gov.uk/sports-and-leisure/museums

Leeds, Leeds City Museum - www.leeds.gov.uk/museumsandgalleries

Leicester, Leicester Museums and Art Galleries - www.leicester.gov.uk/museums

Liverpool, National Museums - www.liverpoolmuseums.org.uk

London, British museum - www.britishmuseum.org

Manchester, Manchester Museum - www.museum.manchester.ac.uk

Melbourne, Melbourne Museum - museumvictoria.com.au/melbournemuseum

Middlesborough, Dorman museum - www.dormanmuseum.co.uk

Minnesota, Minnesota Association of Museums - www.minnesotamuseums.org/museums

Munich, New Egyptian museum - http://www.aegyptisches-museum-muenchen.de.

Newcastle, Great North Museum Hancock - www.newcastle.gov.uk/.../museums-and-galleries

Newport, Newport Museum and art Gallery- museum@newport.gov.uk

New York, Metropolital Museum of Art - www.metmuseum.org

Northampton, Northampton Museum and art Gallery - www.northampton.gov.uk/museums

Norwich, Norwich Castle museum and art Gallery - www.museums.norfolk.gov.uk

Nottingham, Nottingham Castle museum and Art Gallery - www.nottinghammuseums.org.uk

Oldham, Gallery Oldham - www.galleryoldham.org.uk

Oxford, Asmolean Museum - www.ashmolean.org

Pitt Rivers Museum - l prm@prm.ox.ac.uk

Perth (Australia), Western Australian Museum - museum.wa.gov.au

Perth, Scotland Perth Museum and Art Gsallery - www.museumsgalleriesscotland.org.uk/member/perth-museum

Peterborough, Peterborough Muaeum - museum@vivacity-peterborough.com

Philadelphia, Philadelphia Museum of Art - www.philamuseum.org

Plymouth, Plymouth Museum and Art Gallery - www.plymouth.gov.uk/museums

Portsmouth, Portsmouth Museums - www.portsmouthcitymuseums.co.uk

Preston, Museum of Lancashire - www.lancashire.gov.uk/museums

Reading, Reading Museum - www.readingmuseum.org.uk

Rochdale, (see Bury)

Salisbury, Salisbury and South Wiltshire Museum - www.salisburymuseum.org.uk

Scarborough, Scarborough Museums Trust - www.scarboroughmuseumstrust.org.uk

Sheffield, Museums Sheffield - www.museums-sheffield.org.uk

Southampton, Southanpton Museums - www.hampshireattractions.co.uk/.../southampton-museums

St. Albans, Museum of St. Albans - www.stalbansmuseums.org.uk

Stirling, Sterling Smith Museum and Art Gallery - www.stirlingdirectory.info/category/museums.html

Sunderland, Sunderland museum - www.twmuseums.org.uk/sunderland

Swansea, Swansea Museum - www.swanseamuseum.co.uk

Museum of Egyptian Antiquities - egyptcentre@swansea.ac.uk

Sydney, Nicholson Museum - sydney.edu.au/museums/collections/nicholson.shtml

Truro, Royal Cornwall Museum - www.royalcornwallmuseum.org.uk

Turin, Museo Egizio - www.museoegizio.it/pages/hp_en.jsp

Vancouver, Museum of Vancouver - www.museumofvancouver.ca

Vienna, Wien Museum - www.wienmuseum.at

Walsall, Walsall Museum - cms.walsall.gov.uk/museums

Washington, Washington DC Museums - www.world-guides.com/.../washington/washington_museums.html

Warrington, Warrington Museum and Art Gallery - www.warringtonmuseum.co.uk

Winchester, City Museum - www.winchester.gov.uk/museums

York - York Castle museum - www.yorkcastlemuseum.org.uk

Zurich – IEM, University of Zurich - www.anatom.uzh.ch/research/researchgrouppruhli